PANCREATITIS RESEARCH ADVANCES

PANCREATITIS RESEARCH ADVANCES

WILLIAM C. LANGLEY
EDITOR

Nova Biomedical Books
New York

Library of Congress Cataloging-in-Publication Data

Pancreatitis research advances / William C. Langley, editor.
p.; cm
Includes bibliographic references and index.
ISBN-13: 978-1-60021-883-5 (hardcover)
ISBN-10: 1-60021-883-0 (hardcover)
1. Pancreatitis. I. Langley, William C.
[DNLM: 1. Pancreatitis. 2. Pancreatic Neoplasms--diagnosis. 3. Pancreatitis--giagnosis. WI 805 P1926 2007]
RC858.P35 P363
616.3'7--dc22 2007027553

Published by Nova Science Publishers, Inc. ✣ New York

Contents

Preface

Pancreatitis is an inflammation of the pancreas. The pancreas is a large gland behind the stomach and close to the duodenum. The duodenum is the upper part of the small intestine. The pancreas secretes digestive enzymes into the small intestine through a tube called the pancreatic duct. These enzymes help digest fats, proteins, and carbohydrates in food. The pancreas also releases the hormones insulin and glucagon into the bloodstream. These hormones help the body use the glucose it takes from food for energy.

Normally, digestive enzymes do not become active until they reach the small intestine, where they begin digesting food. But if these enzymes become active inside the pancreas, they start "digesting" the pancreas itself. Acute pancreatitis occurs suddenly and lasts for a short period of time and usually resolves. Chronic pancreatitis does not resolve itself and results in a slow destruction of the pancreas. Either form can cause serious complications. In severe cases, bleeding, tissue damage, and infection may occur. Pseudocysts, accumulations of fluid and tissue debris, may also develop. And enzymes and toxins may enter the bloodstream, injuring the heart, lungs, and kidneys, or other organs.

This new book presents the latest research from around the world in this field.

Short Communication: Autoimmune pancreatitis (AIP) is a peculiar type of pancreatitis of presumed autoimmune etiology. As AIP dramatically responds to steroid therapy, accurate diagnosis of AIP is necessary to avoid unnecessary operation. Characteristic dense lymphoplasmacytic infiltration and fibrosis in the pancreas may prove to be the gold standard for diagnosis of AIP. However, since it is difficult to obtain sufficient pancreatic tissue, AIP should be diagnosed currently on the basis of combination of characteristic radiological findings (irregular narrowing of the main pancreatic duct and enlargement of the pancreas), serological findings (elevation of serum γglobulin, IgG, and IgG4, and presence of autoantibodies), clinical findings (elderly male preponderance, fluctuating obstructive jaundice without pain, occasional extrapancreatic lesions, and favorable response to steroid therapy), and histopathological findings (dense infiltration of IgG4-positive plasma cells and T lymphocytes with fibrosis and obliterative phlebitis in various organs).

In AIP patients, serum IgG4 concentration is rather specifically and significantly elevated, and various extrapancreatic lesions such as sclerosing cholangitis, sclerosing sialadenitis or retroperitoneal fibrosis are frequently associated. These extrapancreatic lesions showed similar histological features to those of the pancreas. Furthermore, it has been apparent that abundant infiltration of IgG4-positive plasma cell is observed specifically in various organs and extrapancreatic lesions of AIP patients. The author proposes the existence of a novel clinicopathological entity "IgG4-related sclerosing disease" and suggest that AIP is not simply a pancreatitis but a pancreatic lesion reflecting this systemic disease.

Short Communication: *Introduction:* Up to 30% of patients with acute pancreatitis are diagnosed of idiopathic acute pancreatitis (IAP) after an initial evaluation including a complete clinical history, physical examination, laboratory testing and abdominal imaging. Endosonography (EUS) has shown a high accuracy (60-80%) to diagnose biliary and pancreatic diseases in these patients.

Aims And Methods: Our aim was to evaluate the role of EUS in patients with IAP. The authors also wanted to find predictive factors of a positive finding on EUS in these patients. The authors defined IAP as those clinical pictures of acute pancreatitis where after a complete clinical history, physical examination, history of abdominal trauma or surgery, history of ethanol intake, laboratory analysis including calcium and triglycerides and at least two normal transabdominal ultrasound explorations the cause of the pancreatitis is not found. The authors prospectively performed an EUS to these patients with IAP from January 2005 until December 2006. All EUS procedures were performed by the same endoscopist. In order to analyze the possible influence of different factors on the findings of EUS, the authors recorded epidemiological data, number and severity of the previous bouts of pancreatitis and if patients had been previously cholecistectomized. Chi Square and Fisher tests were used to compare the influence of different factors on the EUS results. Quantitative variables are reported with mean value and standard deviation. P values over 0.05 were considered not significant.

Results: During the mentioned period we performed 552 EUS procedures in our unit, 37 of them were performed to patients with IAP who were included in the study. Sex distribution was 27 men and 10 women. Mean age was 60.54±16 yo (range: 23-83). All patients underwent at least 2 transabdominal ultrasound explorations before EUS, 35 a CT exploration and 12 a magnetic resonance cholangiopancreatography. None of those explorations found the etiology of the pancreatitis. EUS was performed after the first bout of pancreatitis in 19 patients while 18 patients had a recurrent disease (mean number of episodes: 3.67±3.05). Eight patients suffered a severe episode of pancreatitis before EUS. Twelve patients had a previous cholecystectomy. EUS was normal in 7 patients (19%), in the remaining 30 patients (81%) we found cholelithiasis (3 patients), microlithiasis (14 patients), chronic pancreatitis (14 patients), pancreas divisum (2 patients), pancreatic cancer (1 patient), apudoma (1 patient), intraductal papillary mucinous tumour (1 patient), cystic tumour of the pancreas (1 patient) and choledocholithiasis (2 patients). Microlithiasis was the only finding in 8 patients (21%) and chronic pancreatitis in 5 (13%). Positive findings in EUS were not influenced by age (older or younger than 65 yo: 62% vs 82%; p=0.25), sex (men vs women: 70% vs 90%; p=0.39), previous cholecystectomy (cholecystectomy vs non cholecystectomy: 60% vs 81%; p=0.21), previous severe pancreatitis (severe vs moderate: 75% vs 76%; p=1.00) or recurrent disease (recurrent vs first episode: 72% vs 79%; p=0.71).

Conclusions: EUS identifies the cause of IAP in 81% of patients. Epidemiological data, previous cholecystectomy, severe pancreatitis nor recurrent pancreatitis are predictors of positive findings in EUS.

Chapter I - Diagnostic endoscopic retrograde cholangiopancreatography (ERCP) has been replaced in many fields by magnetic resonance cholangiopancreatography (MRCP), a less invasive technique, and it is now limited to indications such as sphincter of Oddi dysfunction. Therapeutic ERCP has become an accepted interventional method for both biliary and pancreatic diseases despite complications. Post-ERCP pancreatitis, a complication associated to the technique and the endoscopist's skills, remains a burning issue since it has been reported to occur in 2-9% in unselected prospective series, and up to 30% in some series due to diverse definitions of post-ERCP pancreatitis and different methods of data collection. The severity of post-ERCP pancreatitis can range from a minor inconvenience, to a devastating illness (0.3% to 0.6% in prospective series) with pancreatic necrosis, multiorgan failure, permanent disability, and even death. Patient-related risk factors, such as patient selection, young age, sphincter of Oddi dysfunction, female sex, previous pancreatitis, potentially pancreatotoxic drugs, anatomic variations and endoscopy-related factors, such as precut sphincterotomy, injection of contrast media into the pancreatic duct and difficulty of cannulation, have been reported to increase the risk of developing post-ERCP pancreatitis. Numerous mechanisms (obstruction to outflow of pancreatic juice, hydrostatic injury, chemical or allergic injury to contrast medium, enzymatic injury, thermal injury, infection) have been postulated for the induction of post-ERCP pancreatitis. Regardless of the mechanism that initiates post-ERCP pancreatitis, the pathways of inflammation are similar to those for other forms of pancreatitis, including premature intracellular activation of proteolytic enzymes, autodigestion, impaired acinar secretion, and the inflammatory cascade, including chemokines and proinflammatory cytokines. Pharmacological agents, such as nifedipine, glucagon, calcitonin, n-acetylcysteine, allopurinol, corticosteroids, low-molecular weight heparin, gabexate, somatostatin and its analogues, have been proposed with the indication of avoiding post-ERCP pancreatitis. Novelties in cannulation techniques and improved equipment, along with specific endoscopic interventions, as prophylactic pancreatic stent placement, have been also proposed to effectively reduce the risk. This review provides an evidence- based assessment of published data on post-ERCP pancreatitis and current suggestions for its avoidance.

Chapter II - *Purpose*: To compare patients with chronic pancreatitis and patients without pancreatic disease in evaluating morphologic change of the main pancreatic duct (MPD) and pancreatic exocrine function estimated by measurement of duodenal fluid in dynamic MRCP after secretin stimulation (s-MRCP).

Materials and Methods: s-MRCP was performed in 14 patients with chronic pancreatitis (group 1) and 19 patients without pancreatic disease (group 2). Diameter of MPD and volume of duodenal fluid which reflect pancreatic exocrine function were measured quantitatively using area intensity measurement (AIM) method, which is a recently proposed hydrometry.

*Results: D*iameter of MPD was significantly larger and dilatation of MPD after secretin stimulation tended to be smaller in group 1 than those in group 2. Duodenal fluid after secretin stimulation in group 1 is significantly less than that in group 2.

Conclusions: s-MRCP can demonstrate noninvasively, even in general hospitals as well as in highly specialized laboratories, the stiffness of MPD and reduced exocrine function of the pancreas in patients with chronic pancreatitis. s-MRCP is considered to be useful for diagnosing chronic pancreatitis.

Chapter III - The insidious nature of disease taken into account, the majority of patients with chronic or malignant pancreatic disease present late in their course and even with early diagnosis, mortality rates of pancreatic cancer are high.

In anticipation of a better understanding of the molecular biology and the epigenesis in the origin and progression of disease, benign and malignant as well, the most challenging items in the diagnosis and management reside at present in endoscopic and radiological pancreatic imaging.

In these the diagnosis of early chronic pancreatitis, of early pancreatic cancer, the differentiation of a pancreatic mass in the setting of chronic pancreatitis and the accurate staging of potentially resectable pancreatic cancer with respect to the dorsal extension are of utmost importance. Focus in this chapter is on the diagnostic and imaging challenges of chronic pancreatitis and the differentiation with pancreatic cancer in an early stage.

Chapter IV - Acute pancreatitis is an emerging disease with great variability in severity. Whereas it runs a mild, self-limiting course in most patients, in others it can take a severe form characterized by extensive necrosis and in-hospital mortality rate in excess of 25%. It has been shown that many individuals facing severe pancreatitis develop multiple organ dysfunction syndrome (MODS), and much effort has been spent to improve understanding of the mechanism of disease progression from acinar cell injury to an overwhelming, life-threatening condition. Although the pathophysiology of acute pancreatitis has not been clearly established, emerging evidence suggests that dysregulation in immune response and interactions between leukocytes, soluble mediators (such as cytokines) and vascular endothelium contribute to the generalization of the inflammatory response.

The pleiotropic cytokine tumor necrosis factor (TNF)-α is considered one of the major mediators associated to the local and systemic tissue damage, being a key regulator of pro-inflammatory genes and a priming activator of immune and endothelial cells. Thus, investigators have regarded blocking its production or action as an attractive treatment option for pancreatitis, and various non-specific and specific anti-TNF-α agents have been tested in animal models with promising results. The authors group contributed to the present research line in the light of recent findings which evidenced an early up-regulation of the cytokine both in acinar and immune cells in the course of the disease. In addition, significantly elevated plasma levels have been demonstrated in patients with worse prognosis and outcome. Accordingly, the authors assessed in two studies the effects of thalidomide (an immunomodulatory agent which suppresses TNF-α biosynthesis and angiogenesis) and of Etanercept (a soluble TNF-α receptor construct which neutralizes the circulating cytokine) on the development of cerulein-induced acute pancreatitis in mice. The authors also evaluated, in the same model, the effects of genetic deletion of TNF-receptor I. In all our studies we observed a substantial amelioration of histological and biochemical features of pancreatitis, a decrease in the expression of pro-inflammatory cytokines, VEGF and adhesion molecules, a diminished neutrophil infiltration and pancreas apoptosis. Although a full extrapolation of experimental data has to be made with caution, acute pancreatitis may represent a suitable disease for TNF-α antagonism: timing of intervention and a careful selection of inclusion and exclusion criteria may aid in better defining the population most likely to benefit in future clinical trials.

Chapter V - In severe acute pancreatitis (SAP), multiple organ dysfunction syndrome (MODS) in the early phase and infectious complications in the late phase are contributors to high mortality. MODS is a consequence of the systemic inflammatory response syndrome, and infectious complication is thought to be a result of bacterial translocation from the gastrointestinal tract. The authors are researching these two major complications. Here the authors introduce their results.

Chapter VI - Characteristic imaging features of AIP are diffuse narrowing of the main pancreatic duct with an irregular wall, enlargement of the pancreas. However, with the increasing number of AIP cases, various imaging findings atypical to the classical definition of AIP are being encountered. First, the authors examined the imaging findings of 37 AIP cases and also examined misdiagnosed cases to determine their reasons for misdiagnosis. Only 7 cases showed typical AIP findings. Six cases were misdiagnosed with pancreatic cancer and two with bile duct cancer. Seven cases were surgically treated. Five cases were misdiagnosed due to non-existence of or unfamiliarity with the concept of AIP and of sclerosing cholangitis with AIP. Another three cases were diagnosed with pancreatic cancer because of segmental stenosis of the main pancreatic duct and no or focal enlargement of the pancreas. The authors also review characteristic imaging findings of AIP.

Second, AIP is often associated with systemic extrapancreatic lesions. Sclerosing cholangitis associated with AIP are different clinical entities from primary sclerosing cholangitis. Cholangiographic findings, clinical courses, effectiveness of steroid therapy, pathological findings are different. Similarly, sialadenitis associated with AIP are different clinical entities from Sjögren Syndrome. Pathological studies of AIP patients disclosed that plasma cells stained for anti-IgG4 antibody were seen mainly in the pancreas, biliary tract, salivary gland, and large intestine, and antibodies to the pancreas, biliary tract, salivary gland exist in the serum of patients with AIP. In addition, Inflammatory pseudotumors of liver, lung show similar pathologic findings to those of AIP. Inflammatory pseudotumors and AIP are closely related clinical entities in the category of IgG4-related autoimmune diseases.

From these results, the authors prepare new diagnostic criteria by modifying the Japanese version and propose the concept of "autoimmune sclerosing cholangiopancreatitis."

Chapter VII - The link between chronic inflammation and the development of cancer has been known for a number of years. Both, hereditary and sporadic forms of chronic pancreatitis represent inflammatory disorders associated with an increased risk of developing pancreatic cancer.

Pancreatic inflammation is associated with production of reactive oxygen species (ROS), cytokine release, and upregulation of pro-inflammatory transcription factors. Mediators of the inflammatory pathways (e.g., NF-κB and COX-2) have been shown to induce genetic damage, cell proliferation and inhibition of apoptosis in pancreas.

The oncogenesis of pancreatic ductal adenocarcinoma is a multistep process characterized by the progression from normal ductal epithelium through the spectrum of PanIN (pancreatic intraepithelial neoplasia) lesions to invasive ductal adenocarcinoma. PanIN lesions harbour a number of well-defined genetic alterations. The progression from normal ductal epithelium through mild to severe dysplasia is characterized by the sequence of genetic changes including activating K-*ras* point mutations, the overexpression of *HER-2/neu*, and the inactivation of *p16, p53, Smad4/DPC4,* and *BRCA2* tumor suppressor genes.

PanIN lesions are more frequently present in patients with chronic pancreatitis than in the general population. It has been suggested that PanINs represent a possible link between chronic pancreatitis and pancreatic cancer. p16 alterations were demonstrated in a significant number of PanIN lesions in chronic pancreatitis not associated with pancreatic cancer, and were suggested to indicate high risk precursors in chronic pancreatitis that might progress to pancreatic cancer.

Pancreatic inflammation seems to represent an early step in the development of malignancy with genetic alterations occuring as a manifestation of the prolonged inflammatory process. Suppression of inflammation and oxidative damage using a large spectrum of treatment strategies (e.g. anti-cytokine vaccines, inhibitors of pro-inflammatory COX-2 and NF-κB pathways, and anti-oxidants) was suggested as potentially useful for prevention or treatment of pancreatic neoplasia.

Chapter VIII - Chronic pancreatitis is a condition characterized by histopathological features of chronic changes including irregular pancreatic fibrosis, infiltration by inflammatory cells, parenchymal degeneration and shedding, and granulation tissue, along with impaired exocrine and endocrine functions. The most common causes of chronic pancreatitis are alcohol, idiopathic diseases, and gallstones. Pancreatic stones can develop within the pancreatic duct in patients with chronic pancreatitis, and may act as an outlet barrier to the pancreatic juice. Stenosis or obstruction of the pancreatic duct leads to raised pressure within the pancreatic duct, painful episodes, and progressive destruction of the pancreatic parenchyma. Similarly, the combination of protein plugs within the pancreatic duct and viscous pancreatic juice is thought to cause painful episodes and progressive destruction of the pancreatic parenchyma. Amelioration of stenosis or obstruction of the pancreatic duct relieves pain and halts progression of pancreatitis.

Although abstinence is usually considered a prerequisite for the successful treatment of alcoholic chronic pancreatitis, we often encounter patients with recurrent attacks from the compensatory period to the transitional period. In alcoholic chronic pancreatitis, continued alcohol consumption causes changes in the digestive hormones and vagal nerve function that induce the pancreatic acinar cells to oversecrete protein, increasing the protein concentration and viscosity of the pancreatic juice, allowing protein sedimentation from the pancreatic juice with consequent formation of protein plugs within the pancreatic duct. Recently, the main constituent proteins in these protein plugs have been identified, and accordingly several therapies have been tried, such as administration of secretin formulations and endoscopic removal.

Bromhexine hydrochloride, a bronchial mucolytic, has an affinity for the pancreatic acinar cells, inducing them to secrete pancreatic juice of low viscosity. In this chapter, the authors outline new medical treatments for alcoholic chronic pancreatitis, and in particular, the authors discuss the efficacy of bromhexine hydrochloride in the treatment of conditions where protein plug formation and increased viscosity of the pancreatic juice cause bouts of pancreatitis.

Chapter IX - Chronic pancreatitis is associated with intense desmoplastic reaction, replacing normal acinar and islet cells with fibrous tissue, thus leading to exocrine and endocrine pancreatic insufficiency. The risk of developing pancreatic cancer in patients with chronic pancreatitis is well established. Clinical differentiation between the two remains difficult and establishing the diagnosis of chronic pancreatitis, in the absence of calcifications, diabetes, malabsorbtion, with equivocal imaging tests remains a challenge.

Several large-scale expression profiling technologies have recently been employed in chronic pancreatitis research, both at RNA and protein level.

Microarray technologies using high-density oligonucleotide arrays fabricated by Affymetrix Inc. (Santa Clara, CA) have implicated various genes in the pathobiology of chronic pancreatitis, including genes encoding for extracellular matrix formation, cell structural components, immune and inflammatory factors, signal transduction and regulatory molecules.

Proteomic techniques, such as immunoblotting analysis (PowerBlot, BD Biosciences, NJ), revealed 30 proteins to be deregulated in comparison between chronic pancreatitis and normal pancreas, whereas a substantial proportion of proteins were similarly dysregulated in both chronic pancreatitis and pancreatic ductal adenocarcinoma. Two dimensional gel electrophoresis (2D gels) and isotope coded affinity tagged labeling (ICAT) with mass spectrometry (MS) have also been employed, revealing additional set of proteins deregulated in chronic pancreatitis, namely several antioxidants, calcium binding proteins, proteases and catalytic enzymes.

The data obtained from such large-scale profiling approaches will lay the foundation and provide further understanding of the underlying pathophysiological processes, thus providing novel targets for diagnosis and treatment of chronic pancreatitis.

Chapter X - The morphologic pattern of cell death,whether through an apoptotic or necrotic process, plays an important role in the degree of severity of an acute pancreatitis episode. In cases of biliary acute pancreatitis,which clinically is the most frequent (70%), a complex interrelationship of factors determine its main characteristics and probable outcome. Marked by the patient's genetic background and the *immuno-neuro-endocrine* peculiarities,closely similar types of injury may induce either a mild (edematous) or a very serious (necrotizing) episode of *pancreatic inflammation*.

This review was prompted by the authors conviction that in biliary acute pancreatitis duodeno-pancreatic autonomic-arc-reflexes induce,through several mechanisms (ischemia-reperfusion,free-oxygen-radicals) the expression and release of different types of cytokines, that either favour or abrogate the inflammatory response. This modulation is dependant of *adrenal glucocorticoids*, the last link of the *hypothalamic-pituitary-adrenal (HPA) axis*. This *immune-neuro-endocrine interaction* is set in motion by the cytokines themselves that prompt the fore-mentioned feedback loop between the *pancreatic immune system and the neuro-endocrine-system*.

Undoubtedly, genetically determined features of both the immunocytes,primarily the neutrophils granulocytes,and the neuro-endocrine apparatus, must play a pivotal influence in delineating the degree of reactivity of the pancreatic inflammatory response. It is probable that a blunted *HPA axis* response contributes to an episode of acute necrotizing pancreatitis. The same might occur in cases with genetically determined over-reactive immunocytes. In both clinical settings, the administration of glucocorticoids might have a sound justification.

Chapter XI - Acute pancreatitis (AP) has been drawing attention of many medical practitioners and researchers for more than a century. Much attention has been paid to its exact pathophysiological mechanism which is still not completely understood. Nevertheless, the authors understanding of the mechanistic processes that mediate the pathobiologic responses of pancreatitis is rapidly evolving in recent years. In addition, the authors now have initial evidence for potential treatment strategies for this disorder. Testing treatment strategies will lead to improved therapies and outcomes for patients with AP. Novel imaging techniques have been developed and appliced in diagnosis and severity grading of AP. Proinflammatory and anti-inflammatory cytokines have certain values in predicting the outcome of AP, and have shown promising in combination immunotherapy to decrease sepsis mortality in animal studies. For a given case, a multidisciplinary decision as treatment strategy is necessary to be made to benefit the sufferer by an early standard management.

Chapter XII - Acute severe hyperlipidemic pancreatitis although a rare condition (accounts for a small percentage 1.3-3.8% of the cases of acute pancreatitis) is a severe condition with considerable morbidity. It seems that this condition becomes more and more often. Severe acute hyperlipidemic pancreatitis has a clinical course which is characterized by an early toxic phase with organ dysfunction, acute pain due to triglycerides in circulation and may usually need the hospitalization in Intensive Care Unit. Plasmapheresis is an important procedure that should be done in these patients, resulting in acute regression of pain and improvement of their clinical course. Plasmapheresis is better to be applied the first 24 hours to provide maximal benefits and to be repeated as needed till triglyceride levels fall to normal levels. Afterwards these patients should be classified according to their lipidemic profile and treated with appropriate free fat diet and subsequent statin therapy. It seems important to these patients when triglyceride levels remain high during follow up although treatment, that plasmapheresis should be done prior to the attack of acute pancreatitis in order to prevent it. Acute pancreatitis involves a complex cascade of events. It is discussed that plasmapheresis should be done in order to decrease the effect of this cascade through the elimination of activated proteases, cytokines that are released by neutrophils and other inflammatory mediators.

Chapter XIII - Acute pancreatitis is a common clinical condition. The exact mechanisms by which diverse etiological factors induce an attack are still unclear but once the disease process is initiated common inflammatory and repair pathways are invoked. Acute pancreatitis is an inflammatory disorder, and inflammation not only affects the pathogenesis but also the course of the disease. Acinar cell injury early in acute pancreatitis leads to a local inflammatory reaction; if marked this leads to a systemic inflammatory response syndrome (SIRS). An excessive SIRS in acute pancreatitis leads to distant organ damage and multiple organ dysfunction syndrome (MODS), which is the primary cause of morbidity and mortality in this condition. Recent studies by us and other investigators have established the critical role played by inflammatory mediators such as TNF-α, IL-1β, IL-6, IL-8, CINC/GRO-α, MCP-1, PAF, IL-10, CD40L, C5a, ICAM-1, MIP1-α, RANTES, substance P, and hydrogen sulfide in acute pancreatitis and the resultant MODS. This chapter intends to present an overview of the role of inflammatory mediators in the pathogenesis of acute pancreatitis and associated MODS.

In: Pancreatitis Research Advances
Editor: William C. Langley, pp. 1-5
ISBN: 978-1-60021-883-5

Expert Commentary A

Bioethics Applied to the Study of Pancreatitis Using Animal Models

Marcelo Gustavo Binker and Laura Iris Cosen-Binker*
RHC-LICB Biomedical Research Institute, Buenos Aires, Argentina
"Programa de Estudios Pancreáticos", Hospital de Clínicas,
Universidad de Buenos Aires, Argentina
Cátedra de Gastroenterología y Enzimología Clínica,
Departamento de Bioquímica Clínica,
Facultad de Farmacia y Bioquímica,
Universidad de Buenos Aires, Argentina

The ultimate goal in biomedical research is to improve the diagnosis and treatment of diseases and/or find preventive procedures providing an understanding of the mechanisms involved in the development and evolution of the pathology [1]. This applies for research employing animals, their tissues, cells or sub-cellular fractions.

It is important to differentiate the clinical research from the pre-clinical one. Pre-clinical research has a clinical aim but it is not performed in humans; an example of this is the evaluation in animal models (rat, mouse, opposum, etc.) of physiopathological mechanisms and therapeutic strategies. In both circumstances when research procedures can be completed in animals before moving forward to their implementation in human beings the use of an appropriate *Experimental Animal Model* is essential. Let us emphasize that any experiment and/or procedure that can be performed in animals should not be done in humans [2-3].

An *Experimental Animal Model* is defined as a living organism with a pathologic process or disease that can be inherited, naturally acquired or induced reproducing as far as possible the same event as that observed in man [4]. The use of a reliable *Experimental Animal Model* implies an adequate breeding and care of the animals that are being used thus establishing what is known as the Laboratory Animal.

* Correspondence: Laura Iris Cosen-Binker, Biochemical Dr, PhD. laura.cosen.binker@utoronto.ca; labcosen@hotmail.com

The Laboratory Animal is a valuable living being that must be fully respected as such. Hence, it is mandatory to treat them with responsibility and employ them only when it is fully justified.

W. M. Russell and R. L. Burch in 1959 wrote their "Principals in Humanitarian Experimentation Techniques" establishing the "motto of the 3 Rs" in the use of animals in research:

1. *Reduction:* Use of the minimum number of animals that is required to obtain results that are statistically valid to correctly evaluate the hypothesis in study.
2. *Refinement:* Keep good control over the conditions in which the animals are before, during and after doing the experiments. Respect the international regulations that define the animals regarding genetic and microbiologic conditions.
3. *Replacement:* Try to find alternative methods that do not involve the use of animals in the experimental procedure.

If Laboratory Animals are employed the following issues have to be addressed [5]:

1. Provide adequate nourishment and housing allowing the animals to carry-on their usual routines/activities as naturally as possible.
2. Ensure good hygiene and optimum air renovation avoiding high concentration of ammonium.
3. Keep in mind that experimental results have to be reliable and reproducible. The role of a well-trained professional and technical team is required.
4. Evaluate the microbiologic condition of the animals considering the existence of:
   *Specific Pathogen Free (SPF) Animals.
   * Germ Free (GF) Animals.
5. Avoid and/or reduce to the minimum every type of procedure that is associated to pain and/or suffering. Use good practices in surgery, analgesia, anesthesia, and euthanasia.

The International Organization of Medical Sciences Council of the World Health Organizations (OMS) established in 1985 that:

1. The progress in the knowledge of biological processes, the improvement in health protection and the welfare of both men and animals obliges to perform experiments in animals of very different species.
2. Every-time that is possible, scientists should employ methods based on mathematical models, computer simulations and in vitro biological systems.
3. Experiments with animals will be done only when the results to be obtained will render an important benefit to human or animal health and the progress of biological knowledge.
4. The animals selected for a research project have to belong to the adequate species, gender, age and condition. The minimum number of animals that are required to obtain valid statistical and scientific results should not to be exceeded.

5. The animals should be well taken care of avoiding or minimizing any type of pain.
6. Keep in mind that any procedure that induces pain in humans may also do so in other type of vertebrate species.
7. Any procedure carried on in animals that may cause pain has to be done under proper sedation, analgesia and/or anesthesia according to veterinary guidelines. No painful maneuvers, be this surgical or of another nature, should be performed on animals that were paralyzed with chemical agents.
8. If article VII has to be over-run an external organism should view the decision. Article VII should not be put aside for teaching or demonstration reasons.
9. At the end of the experiment, animals should be painlessly sacrificed if left alive will mean that they will experience severe or chronic pain and/or irreversible inabilities.
10. Animals that will be employed for biomedical research have to be in the best possible conditions. Veterinaries with experience in Laboratory Animals should be in charge of the Animal Facility.
11. The Principal Investigator in charge of the laboratory should verify that those who will be performing research in animals are properly trained to work with them.

It is also important to provide appropriate information to the general public and the community stating that animals are used only when the research project justifies it reducing to the minimum the number of animals involved. It is also mandatory that well defined benefits for the community should arise from the project. Let us emphasize that animals are also used in other human activities such as: nourishment, dress, cosmetics, transport, sports, hunting, drug detection, entertainment, zoo, etc. [6-7].

In synthesis, the quality of the experimental studies is directly connected to the level of care received by the animals. In order to do so it is important to respect the "motto of the 3 Rs": reduction, refinement, and replacement. This will allow establishing an optimized study approach designing an experimental plan that will consider the exact dimension of the estimated sample considering the employment of alternative strategies to reduce the number of animals to be sacrificed.

To obtain reliable and reproducible results that justify the research project, the sanitary conditions of the animals should be excellent (nourishment, environmental conditions, pre-intra and post experimental treatment, analgesia and anesthesia) as these have a direct impact on the results. An example is the progress that represents the use of SPF and GF animals. It is fundamental to work with homogenous samples having established the corresponding genetic and biological conditions: species, gender, age, weight, and nourishment.

Requeriment of an "*Experimental Animal Model*" for the Study of "Acute Pancreatitis"

The efficiency and safety of new therapeutical procedures in human beings have to be properly tested and evaluated according to the legal dispositions regulating the corresponding pre-clinical studies. Every biomedical research project involving human beings has to be preceded by a detailed analysis of risk factors that may be involved in relation to probable benefits [8].

To acquire a better understanding of the events involved in the triggering, evolution and outcome of Acute Pancreatitis as an Analytical Aim it is important to properly select, determine and standardize the Maneuver to be employed in the Experimental Method together with the assessment and recording of the Basal Conditions of the Entity form to then compare the biomedical parameters obtained before and after the stimuli.

The Longitudinal Nature of the Experimental Model should provide the means to unravel the triggering factor of Acute Pancreatitis and the efficiency of the possible therapeutic treatments [9].

It is very difficult to establish with exactitude the precise moment when Acute Pancreatitis is unchained in human beings. So far this instant is generally referred to as the moment when abdominal pain begins.

The anatomical location of the pancreas in the retro-peritoneum makes it relatively inaccessible, this is even more relevant if one considers how difficult it is to directly reach the pancreas during the first hours after the initial episode of Acute Pancreatitis. These factors explain the need of Experimental Animal Models, which, due their diversity have provided the means to study different degrees of severity in Acute Pancreatitis favoring the comprehension of the early and late events that characterize this disease [10].

The use of an Experimental Animal Model enables to achieve the appropriate standardization of the Method in use thus providing a scientific validation of the results. The experiments can be performed on an adequate "n" number of individuals so that the results obtained will be subsequently analyzed by the corresponding statistical tests. Animals have to be the same age – sex – species (preferably inbred) developing the pathology with equal degree of severity and time of evolution upon registration of the onset of the disease. The experiment can also be concluded at a given time defined in relationship to the induction of the "noxa/stimuli" and/or therapeutic treatment. Therefore pre-existing factors that have no direct connection with Acute Pancreatitis but can influence on its evolution (respiratory infections, renal pathologies, anemia, diabetes, arterial hypertension) are thus eliminated [11].

An ideal Experimental Animal Model of Acute Pancreatitis *should present* [12]:

1-Severe, necrotizing Acute Pancreatitis:
  a) Intra and extra parenchymal necrosis.
  b) Signs and symptoms of Systemic Inflammation and Multi Organic Dysfunction Syndrome (MODS).
  c) Reproducible percentage of mortality.

2-Sequential Evolution of the Pathology:
  a) Initial Systemic Inflammatory Respiratory Syndrome (SIRS) with pancreatic lesions and early MODS.
  b) Secondary inflammatory reactions and/or exacerbation of the pathology corresponding to late pluriparenchymatose failure associated to shock and/or sepsis.

3-Evaluation of the employed therapy:

a)Improvement in the early symptoms of the pluriparenchymatose failure.

b)Decrease in the number and magnitude of the complications and mortality, lower morbid-mortality.

4-Monitoring biomedical parameters:

a)The severity of Acute Pancreatitis Models have to be standardized, reproducible and verifiable.

References

[1] Cosen, J. Investigación en Humanos: Proyecto de Normalización. Revista de la *Sociedad de Ética en Medicina*, 2000; 5:19-21. (1005-I).

[2] Cosen, J. *De la Investigación y Experimentación en humanos.* 73-80. En: Hurtado Hoyos, E.; Dolcini, H.; Yansenson J. Código de Ética para el Equipo de Salud. *Asociación Medica Argentina – Sociedad de Ética en Medicina*, Bs. As., Argentina, 2001.

[3] Cosen J.; Cosen, R. H. *Deontología e Investigación Clínica – Bases para un Código Deontológico Aplicado a Investigación Medica.* http://www.intramed.net.ar.

[4] Scwartz, A. Animal models for human diseases. *J. Biol. Med.*, 1978; 51: 191-197.

[5] Barassi, N.; Benavidez, F.; Ceccarelli A. Ética en el uso de animales de experimentación. *Medicina*, 1996; 56: 531-532.

[6] Schunemann de Aluja, A. Consideraciones finales. Gac. *Med. Mex.*, 1995; 131(1): 62-63.

[7] Hernández González, R. Educación en la ciencia de los animales de laboratorio. *Gac. Med. Mex.*, 1995; 131(1): 56-62.

[8] *Declaración de Helsinki.* Asociación Medica Mundial, 1964 – Helsinki, Finlandia; 1975 – Tokio, Japón; 1983 – Venecia, Italia; Apéndice 2, Articulo 5.

[9] Wikinski, J. Comentarios sobre la taxonomia del trabajo de Investigación Clínica. *Revista de la Facultad de Medicina*, 1981; 4(2): 31-32.

[10] Lerch, M.; Adler, G. experimental animal models of acute pancreatitis. *Int. J. Pancreatol.*, 1994; 15: 159-170.

[11] Rattner, D. *Experimental models of acute pancreatitis an their relevance to human disease.* Scand. J. Gastroenterol., 1996; 31(suppl. 219): 6-9.

[12] Foitzik, T.; Hotz, H.; Eibl, G.; Buhr, H. Experimental models of acute pancreatitis: are they suitable for evaluating therapy? *Int. J. Colorectal. Dis.*, 2000; 15: 127-135.

In: Pancreatitis Research Advances
Editor: William C. Langley, pp. 7-10

ISBN: 978-1-60021-883-5

Expert Commentary B

Challenging Research Items in Diagnosis and Imaging of Chronic Pancreatitis: Differentiating Early Chronic Pancreatitis from (Early) Pancreatic Cancer

Kenneth Coenegrachts[1]*, Vincent De Wilde[2], Vincent Denolin[3] and Hans Rigauts[1]

[1]Department of Radiology, AZ St.-Jan AV, Bruges, Belgium
[2]Department of Gastroenterology and Hepatology, AZ St.-Jan AV, Bruges, Belgium
[3]Philips Medical Systems, Best, the Netherlands

To differentiate between a focal inflammatory and neoplastic pancreatic mass may be extremely difficult, even in view of the different clinical histories and features. Microscopically, desmoplastic change leads to hypovascularity of pancreatic ductal adenocarcinomas. Another reason for hypovascularity of ductal adenocarcinomas is vascular encasement, causing arterial stenosis or obstruction [1]. On the contrary, an inflammatory pancreatic mass, which is a focal swelling of the pancreas, consists of inflammatory changes such as interlobular fibrosis and chronic inflammatory infiltrate around lobules and ducts [2]. Those inflammatory changes usually require blood flow and result in hypervascularity. Therefore most inflammatory masses show more vascularity than pancreatic adenocarcinomas. However, severe fibrosis can replace pancreatic acinar cells and inhibit vascular development in an inflammatory lesion which is probably the reason why a focal inflammatory pancreatic mass can be hypovascular [3]. Johnson and Outwater [4] found that masses of pancreatic adenocarcinoma and those due to Chronic Pancreatitis (CP) showed

* Corresponding author: Kenneth Coenegrachts, M.D. Department of Radiology, AZ St.-Jan AV, Ruddershove 10, B-8000 Bruges, Belgium, Phone: ++32-50 452103; Fax: ++32-50 452146. E-mail: kenneth.coenegrachts@azbrugge.be (kcoenegrachts74@yahoo.com)

more gradual progressive enhancement on dynamic Magnetic Resonance Imaging (MRI) than did normal pancreatic parenchyma, and they histologically found abundant fibrosis in both pathologic conditions, which was thought to account for the similar imaging appearances of the two kinds of masses. Especially when differentiating early focal CP and early pancreatic cancer, this causes differential diagnostic problems.

In this commentary focus is on future developments using perfusion-based contrast-enhanced (CE) MRI and developments in co-registration and post-processing tools.

Perfusion-Based Contrast-Enhanced MRI of the Pancreas

Perfusion-based CE MRI of the pancreas has been used for the study of the pancreatic parenchyma [5] but has never been used in the differentiation between focal pancreatitis and a solid pancreatic tumor.

Keyhole imaging was introduced independently in 1993 by van Vaals et al. [6] and Jones et al. [7] as a simple method to increase the temporal resolution of dynamic imaging studies while maintaining a high spatial resolution. It was later pointed out that the dynamic information of a keyhole imaging study has only low spatial resolution and that for an examination of dynamic changes, low-resolution studies might be sufficient [8]. However, the authors of this commentary want to stress the importance of high spatial resolution when evaluating perfusion-based imaging sets allowing better qualitative and quantitative analysis of the perfusion data. Keyhole imaging has now been introduced into a wide variety of different applications. These include CE perfusion studies [6, 9-11].

A newly developed and so-called 4D THRIVE Centra Keyhole sequence (specialized sequence further developed based on 3D T1w gradient echo acquisition using centra and keyhole imaging; Philips Medical Systems, Best, The Netherlands) during and following IV injection of a gadolinium-based contrast agent combines the advantages of keyhole imaging with minimal compromise in spatial resolution when compared with "state-of-the-art" 3D T1w gradient echo sequences. Specifically designed co-registration software and post-processing software allowing optimized data analysis by pixel mapping rather than Region-Of-Interest (ROI) placement has additionally been developed for optimized analysis (pixel mapping) of these 4D THRIVE Centra Keyhole imaging sets. Pixel mapping allows a rapid and robust evaluation of the whole pancreatic parenchyma for use in a clinical (and research) setting. In the author's department, further developments concerning the above mentioned 4D THRIVE Centra Keyhole sequence and co-registration and post-processing software are ongoing.

Analysis and presentation of perfusion-based imaging data needs to take into account the heterogeneity of vascular characteristics within the investigated area of (focal) pathology. User-defined whole focal CP or tumor ROI (lesion ROI) yield graphical outputs with good signal-to-noise ratio, but lack spatial resolution and are prone to partial volume averaging errors and thus are unable to evaluate tumor heterogeneity. As a result, whole lesion ROIs may not reflect small areas of rapid change and so may be insensitive to specific alterations in areas of focal CP or early pancreatic cancer. Whole lesion ROI assessment may be inappropriate particularly for the evaluation of malignant lesions where heterogeneous areas of enhancement are diagnostically important [12-14]. Pixel mapping has a number of advantages including the appreciation of heterogeneity of enhancement and removal for the need to selectively placed user-defined ROIs. The risk of missing important diagnostic information and of creating ROIs that contain more than one tissue type is reduced. An important advantage of pixel mapping is being able to spatially match lesional vascular characteristics such as blood volume, blood flow, permeability and leakage space. Such displays provide unique insights into lesional structures, function and therapeutic response.

Comparing perfusion-based 4D THRIVE Centra Keyhole CE MRI examinations of patients suffering from focal CP or early focal pancreatic cancer, it is hoped by the authors that differences in perfusion (heterogeneity of perfusion, differences in enhancement and wash-out, differences in vessel distribution within the area of focal CP or within focal early pancreatic cancer) can be found.

Contrast-Enhanced Endoscopic Ultrasound of the Pancreas

Contrast-Enhanced Endoscopic ultrasound (CE-EUS) has been used for the differential diagnosis of pancreatic tumor masses for a better assessment of perfusion in the pancreatic tissue and inside the mass [15,16]. Pancreatic adenocarcinoma was shown to be relatively hypovascular compared with surrounding pancreatic tissue, whereas markedly hypervascular lesions were inflammatory masses. Recent advances in technology have supported the development of new echo-endoscopic systems making it possible to use real-time, low mechanical index, contrast-enhanced imaging techniques with endoscopic ultrasound [17].

In conclusion, perfusion-based CE MRI and CE-EUS studies (separate studies or combined) might be valuable for diagnostic work-up of patients suffering from focal pancreatic pathology (focal CP vs focal pancreatic cancer). To the authors of this commentary perfusion-based studies using CE MRI and/or CE-EUS seem useful for future research projects. Hopefully, the near future will allow optimized diagnosis of (focal) pancreatic disease in an early stage, thus avoiding unnecessary operation or delayed adequate treatment in patients suffering from (focal) pancreatic disease.

References

[1] Hosoki T. Dynamic CT of pancreatic tumors. *AJR*, 1983; 140: 959-965.

[2] Robbins S, Cotran R. The pancreas. In: Robbins SL, Cotran RS, eds. *Pathologic basis of disease*, 2nd ed. Philadelphia: Saunders; 1979: 1101-1102.

[3] Koito K, Namieno T, Nagakawa T, Morita K. Inflammatory Pancreatic Masses: Differentiation from Ductal Carcinomas with Contrast-Enhanced Sonography Using Carbon Dioxide Microbubbles. *AJR*, 1997; 169:1263-1267.

[4] Johnson P, Outwater E. Pancreatic carcinoma versus chronic pancreatitis: dynamic MR imaging. *Radiology,* 1999; 212: 213-218.

[5] Coenegrachts K, Van Steenbergen W, De Keyzer F, Vanbeckevoort D, Bielen D, Chen F, Dockx S, Maes F, Bosmans H. Dynamic contrast-enhanced MRI of the pancreas: initial results in healthy volunteers and patients with chronic pancreatitis. *JMRI,* 2004; 20: 990-997.

[6] Van Vaals J, Brummer M, Dixon W, Tuithof H, Engels H, Nelson R, Gerety B, Chezmar J, den Boer J. Keyhole method for accelerating imaging of contrast agent uptake. *JMRI,* 1993; 3: 671-675.

[7] Jones R, Haraldseth O, Muller T, Rinck P, Oksendahl A. K-space substitution: a novel dynamic imaging technique. *MRM,* 1993; 29: 830-834.

[8] Hu X. On the keyhole technique. *JMRI,* 1994; 4: 231.

[9] Strouse P, Prince M, Chenevert T. Effect of the rate of gadopentetate dimeglumine administration on abdominal vascular and soft-tissue MR imaging enhancement patterns. *Radiology,* 1996; 201: 809-816.

[10] Miyati T, Banno T, Mase M, Kasai H, Shundo H, Imazawa M, Ohba S. Dual dynamic contrast-enhanced MR imaging. *JMRI,* 1997; 7: 230-235.

[11] Medic J, Tomazic S, Sersa I, Demsar F. Improved keyhole approach with motion-correction technique in contrast-enhanced dynamic MRI. *Proc ISMRM,* 1998; 2064.

[12] Aronen H, Gazit I, Louis D, Pardo F, Weisskoff R, Harsh G, Cosgrove G, Halpern E, Hochberg F, et al. Cerebral blood volume maps of gliomas: comparison with tumor grade and histologic findings. *Radiology,* 1994; 191: 41-51.

[13] Parker G, Suckling J, Tanner S, Padhani A, Revell P, Husband J, Leach M. Probing tumor microvascularity by measurement, analysis and display of contrast agent uptake kinetics. *JMRI,* 1997; 7: 564-574.

[14] Gribbestad I, Nilsen G, Fjosne H, Kvinnsland S, Haugen O, Rinck P. Comparative signal intensity measurements in dynamic gadolinium-enhanced MR mammography. *JMRI,* 1994; 4: 477-480.

[15] Bhutani M, Hoffman B, van Velse A, Hawes R. Contrast-enhanced endoscopic ultrasonography with galactose microparticles: SHU508A (Levovist). *Endoscopy,* 1997; 29: 635-639.

[16] Becker D, Strobel D, Bernatik T, Hahn E. Echo-enhanced and power Doppler EUS for the discrimination between focal pancreatitis and pancreatic carcinoma. *Gastrointest Endosc,* 2001; 53: 784-789.

[17] Dietrich C, Ignee A, Frey H. Contrast-enhanced endoscopic ultrasound with low mechanical index: a new technique. *Z Gastroenterol,* 2005; 43: 1219-1223.

In: Pancreatitis Research Advances
Editor: William C. Langley, pp. 11-13

ISBN: 978-1-60021-883-5

Expert Commentary C

The Pancreas: A Hidden Organ with Many Unknowns

Michael G. Wayne*
Cabrini Medical Center
New York, NY 10003

The pancreas is a wonderful organ, serving many functions for the body including endocrine and exocrine. It is relatively hidden in its retroperitoneal location and not thought about often unless a problem arises with it. Unfortunately these problems are usually significant.

Medicine has made great advances over the years; unfortunately the same cannot be said about treating the pancreas. There are many diseases that affect the pancreas, which are not diagnosed until late. Worse, when they are diagnosed there are not many successful treatments for them. Our aim going forward should continue to be finding earlier diagnostic tools and better treatment strategies.

A new focus of interest is autoimmune pancreatitis, which is being diagnosed more frequently now. We are seeing an increase in this diagnosis because of awareness. In the past this entity was often called idiopathic pancreatitis. Unfortunately this diagnosis is usually made on surgical specimens. Going forward we need to find serum markers, which will support the diagnosis of autoimmune pancreatitis in the appropriate clinical setting. This may preclude the need for surgery and allow the patients to obtain relief from steroids or other immunosuppressive medications.

There is still much to learn about the pathogenesis of chronic pancreatitis, which is still not clearly understood. Theories range from 1. Bile reflux into the pancreatic duct, 2. Secretory changes within the duct, 3. Early acinar cell injury leading to necrosis and fibrosis. The pathogenesis of early acinar cell injury is speculative but may be a consequence of unopposed free radical injury, activity of pancreatic stellate cells, or as a result of cholinergic hyperstimulation. Cigarette smoking, nutritional and racial factors influence the

* 227 East 19th St., Room D231; Phone: (212) 995-6611; E-mail: waynedocny@hotmail.com

predisposition to pancreatitis. The role of genes and immunomodulators are currently under evaluation. Another area of focus should center on the relationship of chronic pancreatitis and pancreatic cancer. I recently operated on three cases of patients with long standing pancreatitis who were found to have pancreatic cancer. These results will be published soon. We need to find a way to monitor the progression of chronic pancreatitis and be aware that it can degenerate into a malignancy.

In the past surgery was a mainstay for the treatment for pancreatic psuedocysts and fluid collections. Today, radiological imaging and intervention play important roles. CT evaluation of the severity of pancreatitis and assessment of its course are now routine. Percutaneous drainage of pancreatic psuedocysts and abscesses are commonly performed as an adjunct to surgical treatment and is frequently definitive therapy. Endoscopy and endoscopic ultrasound has also emerged as valuable options for diagnosing and treating pancreatic psuedocysts and fluid collections.

Surgery for chronic pancreatitis should only be considered for complications of this disease. Surgeons beware that unbridled enthusiasm is best replaced by tempered judgement. The complications requiring treatment include pain, obstruction, psuedocyst, and bleeding. Treatment requires a careful evaluation including knowledge of pancreatic anatomy, the presence of chemical dependency, and the psychosocial setting of the patient. Small duct disease requires resection, whereas large duct disease is managed by ductal drainage. Denervation procedures are used only very selectively. In well-selected patients, results can be satisfactory.

Because of the increased sensitivity of radiologic screening, there has been an increase in the number of patients with cystic lesions of the pancreas. What to do with them is still in the process of evolution. Size is an important factor for determining surgical intervention, but at what size. The differentiation of serous cystic lesions from the mucinous neoplasms is crucial because of the radically different biologic characteristics of these two neoplasms. We know that mucinous cystic lesions are premalignant and should be removed. Serous cystic lesions can be safely observed unless the patient is symptomatic from it. Clinical presentation and state-of-the-art imaging permit the differentiation of most cystic pancreatic neoplasms, not only from other cystic pancreatic disorders but also from one another.

Islet cell carcinomas are rare neuroendocrine tumors that arise from the Islets of Langerhans in the pancreas. Up to half of these tumors secrete one or more biologically active peptides. These tumors cause morbidity and mortality by tumor progression and excess hormone production. Surgical resection offers the only chance at cure and may alter the natural history of the disease by preventing the development of hjepatic metastasis. Palliative surgical intervention and hepatic arterial embolization have a limited role in the setting of refractory hormone symptoms of pain, rapid tumor expansion, and life-threatening complications. Current chemotherpies have only modest efficacy, and therfore patients should be encouraged to enroll in clinical trials testing newer antineoplastic agents to and treatment modalities.

There is a survival diference among periampullary cancers. Overall survival after pancreaticoduodenectomy is greatest for patients with ampullary and duodenal cancers, intermediate for patients with bile duct cancer, and least for patients with pancreatic cancer. Moreover, survival for each tumor stage is greater for nonpancreatic periampullary cancers than for pancreatic cancers. Invasion of the pancreas by nonpancreatic periampullary cancers is a major factor adversely affecting survival. Recent data suggest that the inherent differences in tumor biology rather than embryonic, anatomic, or histologic factors probably account for these differences in survival. Although pancreaticoduodenectomy remains the procedure of choice for resectable periampullary cancers, further increases in survival will likely evolve through more effective neoadjuvant therapies rather than modifications in the surgical approach.

Pancreatic cancer, for the most part, remains a lethal disease. Diagnostic and surgical advances have increased diagnostic accuracy and therapeutic safety, but have not improved survival. Multimodality approaches, including chemoradiation and novel biologic therapy, preceding or following surgery, are important components of therapy. Finding the most efficacious agents is our goal.

In: Pancreatitis Research Advances
Editor: William C. Langley, pp. 15-17
ISBN: 978-1-60021-883-5

Expert Commentary D

Inflammatory Mediators in Acute Pancreatitis: The Story So Far and Future Directions

Madhav Bhatia*
Department of Pharmacology, National University of Singapore, Singapore

The pathogenesis of acute pancreatitis involves the interplay of local and systemic immune responses that are often difficult to characterize. It is an intricate balance between localized tissue damage with the systemic production of pro-inflammatory and anti-inflammatory mediators. In recent years, significant contributions have been made to enhance our understanding of the role of inflammatory mediators as potential therapeutic targets for acute pancreatitis and associated multiple organ dysfunction syndrome (MODS). We and other investigators have focused on the role of these mediators in the pathogenesis of acute pancreatitis and associated lung injury.

Recent data have shown the importance of inflammatory mediators such as substance P, chemokines, and the recently identified mediator hydrogen sulfide in the pathogenesis of acute pancreatitis and associated MODS. Amongst these mediators, H_2S is a special case, as although it can act as a pro-inflammatory mediator on its own, a slow H_2S releasing non-steroidal anti-inflammatory drug (NSAID), diclofenac, shows a potentiation of its anti-inflammatory action [1]. Diclofenac is an NSAID and has been shown to have anti-inflammatory, analgesic, and antipyretic activity. ACS15 is an H_2S-releasing derivative of diclofenac. In that report [1], we described the effect of diclofenac and its H_2S-releasing derivative on acute pancreatitis and associated lung injury in the mouse. Acute pancreatitis was induced in mice by hourly intraperitoneal injections of caerulein. Diclofenac and ACS15 were administered either one hour before or one hour after starting caerulein injections and the severity of acute pancreatitis and associated lung injury were assessed. ACS15, given

* Madhav Bhatia, Ph.D. Department of Pharmacology, National University of Singapore, Yong Loo Lin School of Medicine, Centre for life Sciences, 28 Medical Drive. Singapore 117456 Tel. (65)-6516-8256. Fax. (65)-6775-7674. email. mbhatia@nus.edu.sg

prophylactically as well as therapeutically, significantly reduced lung inflammation without having any significant effect on pancreatic injury [1]. The anti-inflammatory effect may be caused by slow release of H_2S from ACS15. ACS15 causes significantly less gastric toxicity than diclofenac. ACS15 is likely to have less GI toxicity compared to the parent compound diclofenac in view of the recently discovered GI-protective properties of H_2S. These results suggested the usefulness of H_2S-releasing NSAIDs as potential treatments for pancreatitis-associated lung injury. These results also pointed to a dual – pro- and anti-inflammatory action of H_2S.

More recent work shows the inter-relationship of these mediators. For example, H2S acts as an inflammatory mediator by stimulating the synthesis of substance P [2]. Substance P, on the other hand, stimulates chemokine production by pancreatic acinar cells [3], and treatment with an antagonist of the receptor for substance P (neurokinin-1 receptor) attenuates chemokine production in experimental acute pancreatitis [4].

In a more recent study, we have further investigated the interaction between hydrogen sulphide and substance P in acute pancreatitis, using isolated pancreatic acini as the experimental system [5]. In that study, we investigated the presence of H_2S and the expression of H_2S synthesizing enzymes, CSE and CBS, in isolated mouse pancreatic acini. Pancreatic acinar cells from mice were incubated with or without a supramaximal dose of caerulein. Caerulein increased the levels of H_2S and CSE mRNA expression while CBS mRNA expression was decreased. In addition, cells pretreated with DL-propargylglycine, a CSE inhibitor, reduced the formation of H_2S in caerulein treated cells, suggesting that CSE may be the main enzyme involved in H_2S formation in mouse acinar cells. These results also showed acinar cell origin of H_2S in the pancreas. Furthermore, substance P (SP) concentration in the acini and expression of SP gene (preprotachykinin-A, PPT-A) and neurokinin-1 receptor (NK-1R), the primary receptor for SP, are increased in secretagogue caerulein-induced acinar cells. Inhibition of endogenous production of H_2S by PAG significantly suppressed SP concentration, PPT-A expression and NK1-R expression in the acini. To determine whether H_2S itself provoked inflammation in acinar cells, the cells were treated with H_2S donor drug, sodium hydrosulfide (NaHS), that resulted in a significant increase in SP concentration and expression of PPT-A and NK1-R in acinar cells [5]. These results suggest that the pro-inflammatory effect of H_2S may be mediated by SP-NK-1R related pathway in mouse pancreatic acinar cells.

It is, therefore, important to see different mediators of inflammation not in isolation, but as a part of a cascade, with some redundancy/overlap of function, as well as to try and understand the inter-relationship of these different inflammatory mediators.

In light of the critical role played by inflammatory mediators in the pathogenesis of acute pancreatitis and associated lung injury, and early clinical data emerging that show the clinical relevance of these findings, it is reasonable to speculate that elucidation of the key mediators in acute pancreatitis and associated MODS coupled with the discovery of specific inhibitors will make it possible to develop clinically effective anti-inflammatory therapy. Recent findings by us and other investigators have further substantiated the importance of these mediators as potential therapeutic targets. It is, therefore, important to investigate the clinical relevance of these mediators as therapeutic targets, in order to take therapy along these lines to the clinic.

Acknowledgement

The author would like to acknowledge grant support from National Medical Research Council, Biomedical Research Council, and Academic Research Fund.

References

[1] Bhatia M, Sidhapuriwala J, Sparatore A, and Moore PK. Treatment with H_2S-releasing diclofenac protects mice against acute pancreatitis-associated lung injury. *Shock.* 2007 (in press)

[2] Bhatia, M., et al. Role of substance P in hydrogen sulfide-induced pulmonary inflammation in mice. *Am. J. Physiol. Lung Cell Mol. Physiol.* 2006; 291: L896-L904.

[3] Ramnath, R.D., and Bhatia, M. Substance P treatment stimulates chemokine synthesis in pancreatic acinar cells via the activation of NF-κB. *Am. J. Physiol. Gastrointest Liver Physiol.* 2006; 291:G1113-1119.

[4] Sun, J., and Bhatia M. Blockade of neurokinin 1 receptor attenuates CC and CXC chemokine production in experimental acute pancreatitis and associated lung injury. *Am. J. Physiol. Gastrointest Liver Physiol.* 2007; 292: G143-G153.

[5] Ramasamy T, Moore PK, and Bhatia M. The mechanism by which hydrogen sulfide acts as a mediator of inflammation in acute pancreatitis: in vitro studies using isolated mouse pancreatic acinar cells. *J. Cell Mol. Med.* 2007; 11: 315-326.

In: Pancreatitis Research Advances
Editor: William C. Langley, pp. 19-30

ISBN: 978-1-60021-883-5

Short Communication A

Autoimmune Pancreatitis

Terumi Kamisawa*
Department of Internal Medicine,
Tokyo Metropolitan Komagome Hospital,
Tokyo, Japan

Abstract

Autoimmune pancreatitis (AIP) is a peculiar type of pancreatitis of presumed autoimmune etiology. As AIP dramatically responds to steroid therapy, accurate diagnosis of AIP is necessary to avoid unnecessary operation. Characteristic dense lymphoplasmacytic infiltration and fibrosis in the pancreas may prove to be the gold standard for diagnosis of AIP. However, since it is difficult to obtain sufficient pancreatic tissue, AIP should be diagnosed currently on the basis of combination of characteristic radiological findings (irregular narrowing of the main pancreatic duct and enlargement of the pancreas), serological findings (elevation of serum γglobulin, IgG, and IgG4, and presence of autoantibodies), clinical findings (elderly male preponderance, fluctuating obstructive jaundice without pain, occasional extrapancreatic lesions, and favorable response to steroid therapy), and histopathological findings (dense infiltration of IgG4-positive plasma cells and T lymphocytes with fibrosis and obliterative phlebitis in various organs).

In AIP patients, serum IgG4 concentration is rather specifically and significantly elevated, and various extrapancreatic lesions such as sclerosing cholangitis, sclerosing sialadenitis or retroperitoneal fibrosis are frequently associated. These extrapancreatic lesions showed similar histological features to those of the pancreas. Furthermore, it has been apparent that abundant infiltration of IgG4-positive plasma cell is observed specifically in various organs and extrapancreatic lesions of AIP patients. I propose the existence of a novel clinicopathological entity "IgG4-related sclerosing disease" and suggest that AIP is not simply a pancreatitis but a pancreatic lesion reflecting this systemic disease.

* 3-18-22 Honkomagome, Bunkyo-ku, Tokyo 113-8677, Japan. Tel: 81-3-3823-2101. Fax: 81-3-3824-1552. E-mail: kamisawa@cick.jp

Keywords: *autoimmune pancreatitis, IgG4, chronic pancreatitis, sclerosing cholangitis, retroperitoneal fibrosis.*

Introduction

In 1961, Sarles et al. [1]. first reported pancreatitis associated with hypergammaglobulinemia and suggested autoimmunity as a pathogenetic mechanism. Afterwards, the possible role of autoimmunity in causing chronic pancreatitis has drawn the attention of several investigators. Since Yoshida et al. [2]. proposed the concept of autoimmune pancreatitis (AIP) in 1995, many cases of AIP have been reported in the Western countries as well as in Japan. In this chapter, I review about the clinical, laboratory, imaging, and histopathological features of AIP based on my experience of 32 AIP cases.

Cocept and Pathogenesis

AIP is a unique form of pancreatitis in which autoimmune mechanisms are suspected to be involved in the pathogenesis. AIP has many clinical, radiological, serological and histopathological characteristics as follows: (1) elderly male preponderance; (2) frequent initial symptom of obstructive jaundice without pain; (3) occasional association with impaired pancreatic endocrine or exocrine function, and various extrapancreatic lesions (4) favorable response to steroid therapy; (5) radiological findings of irregular narrowing of the main pancreatic duct and enlargement of the pancreas; (6) serological findings of elevation of serum γglobulin, IgG, or IgG4 levels, along with the presence of some autoandibodies; (7) histopathological findings of dense lymphoplasmacytic infiltration with fibrosis and obliterative phlebitis in the pancreas [3, 4]. AIP is a rare disorder, but its exact incidence is unknown. In nationwide survey [5] conducted in Japan, 900 patients with AIP were collected and prevalence rate of AIP among patients with chronic pancreatitis was 1.95%.

Serum IgG4, a subtype of IgG, levels are frequently elevated and are particularly high in AIP [6, 7]. Dense infiltration of IgG4-positive plasma cells is seen in various organs of AIP patients [8-12]. These results suggest that IgG4 plays a major role in the pathogenesis of AIP, although the trigger for the IgG4 elevation or its pathogenetic role in AIP has not been clearly disclosed.

Clinical Manifestations

AIP occurs predominantly in elderly males [13]. In my series, the mean age of the patients is 68.3 years (range, 29-83 years) and the male-to-female ratio is 4:1. Patients rarely show typical features of pancreatitis, and the major presenting complaint is painless obstructive jaundice due to associated sclerosing cholangitis (65% [4]-86% [14]). The jaundice sometimes fluctuates. Diabetes mellitus, usually type 2, is often (41% [15]-76% [4]) observed. In many cases, the diagnoses of diabetes mellitus and AIP are made simultaneously; some cases show exacerbation of preexisting diabetes mellitus with the onset of AIP [16]. Pancreatic exocrine function is frequently impaired, but marked pancreatic insufficiency is uncommon [17].

Laboratory Findings

Few patients show marked elevation of serum pancreatic enzymes. The patients with biliary lesions show elevation of serum bilirubin and hepatobiliary enzymes. Hypergammaglobulinemia (>2.0 g/dL) and elevated serum IgG levels (>1800 mg/dl) are detected in 59%-76% [18-20] and 53%[4]-71% [18] of AIP patients, respectively. A diagnostic autoantibody for AIP has not been detected. Autoantibodies including antinuclear antibody (ANA) and rheumatoid factor (RF) are present in 43%-75% [15, 19, 20] and 13%-30% [15, 19, 20] of them, respectively. Since Hamano et al. [6]. reported that serum IgG4 levels are significantly and specifically high in AIP patients and are closely associated with disease activity in 2001, serum IgG4 level has become useful diagnostic marker for AIP. However, the sensitivity of elevated serum IgG4 levels is 63%-68% in other reports [3, 4, 21].

Radiological Findings

Typical AIP cases show diffuse enlargement of the pancreas, the so-called "sausage-like" appearance, on computed tomography (CT), ultrasonography (US), and magnetic resonance image (MRI). On dynamic CT and MRI, there is delayed enhancement of the swollen pancreatic parenchyma (Figure 1) [20, 22, 23]. Affected pancreatic lesion shows decreased intensity on T1-weighted image and increased intensity on T2-weighted image compared with the signal intensity in the liver [22-24]. Since inflammatory and fibrous changes involve the peripancreatic adipose tissue, a capsule-like rim surrounding the pancreas, which appears as a low density on CT and, as a hypointense area on T2-weighted MRI, is detected in some cases [20, 22-24]. US shows an enlarged hypoechoic pancreas with hyperechoic spots [20, 22, 23] Pancreatic calcification or pseudocyst is uncommon. Some cases show a focal enlargement of the pancreas, similar to that seen with pancreatic cancer [20, 25]. On endoscopic retrograde cholangiopancreatography (ERCP), irregular, narrow (<3 mm in diameter) main pancreatic duct is seen diffusely throughout the pancreas in typical cases (Figure 2). Degree of narrowing of the main pancreatic duct is partly different in the same patient. In some cases, there is segmental narrowing of the main pancreatic duct, but upstream dilatation of the distal pancreatic duct is less noted compared with pancreatic cancer [20, 25]. Stenosis of the extrahepatic or intrahepatic bile duct is frequently observed (Figure 2). Marked wall thickening of the extrahepatic bile duct or gallbladder is sometimes detected on US or endoscopic ultrasonography (EUS) [23, 26]. Magnetic resonance cholangiopancreatography (MRCP) does not adequately show the narrow portion of the main pancreatic duct [24], but it can adequately demonstrate stenosis of the bile duct with dilatation of the upper biliary tract [23].

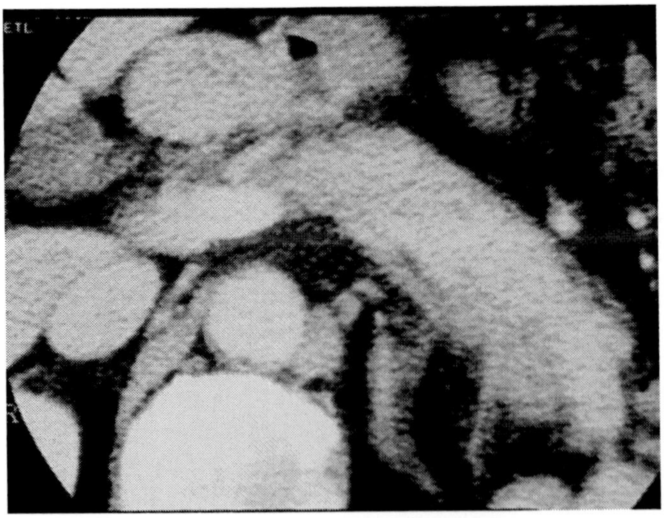

Figure 1. Diffuse enlargement of the pancreas showing delayed enhancement on CT scan.

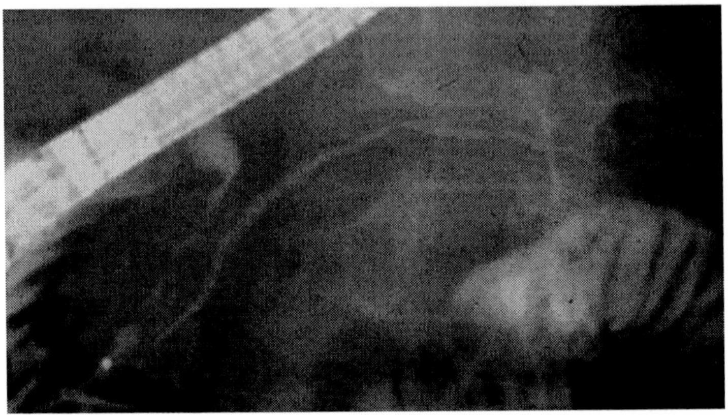

Figure 2. Diffuse irregular narrowing of the main pancreatic duct and stenosis of the lower bile duct on ERCP.

Histopathological and Immunohistochemical Findings

Gross appearance of the pancreas of AIP shows firm and mass-like enlargement with thick capsule. The hallmark of the histological findings in the pancreas of AIP is dense inflammatory cell infiltration and fibrosis in a periductal and interlobular distribution (Figure 3). The inflammatory infiltrate consists of mainly lymphocytes and plasma cells with occasional formation of lymphoid follicles. Pancreatic duct is narrowed by periductal fibrosis and lymphoplasmacytic infiltration. Another highly characteristic histological finding is obliterative phlebitis of the variably sized pancreatic veins and involvement of the portal vein with lymphoplasmacytic infiltrate and proliferation of fibroblasts in and around the wall of the vein.

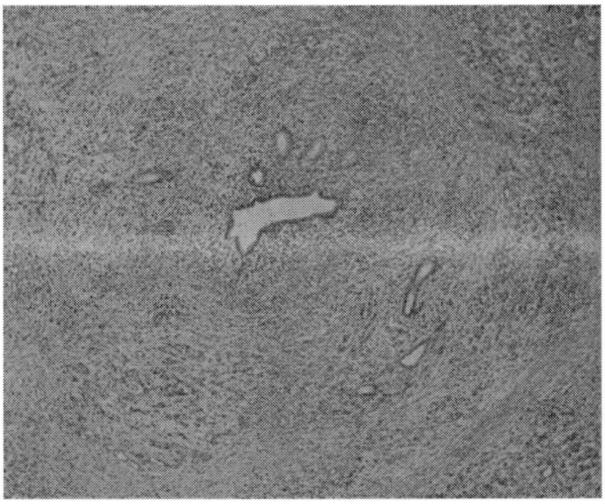

Figure 3. Prominent periductal and interlobular fibrosis with a dense lymphoplasmacytic infiltration and acinar destruction in the pancreas (Hematoxylin-eosin).

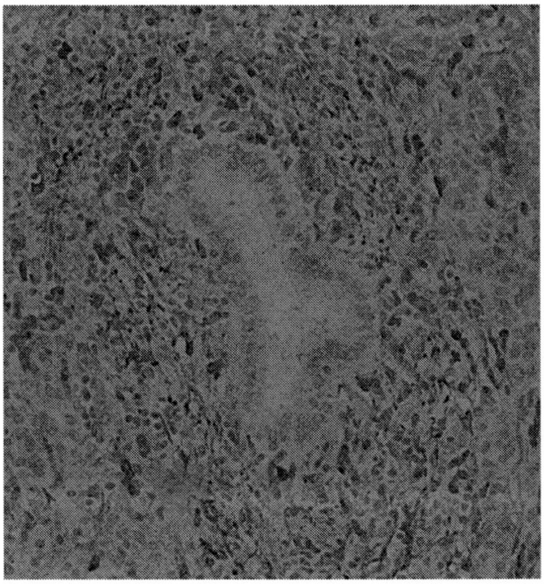

Figure 4. Dense infiltration of IgG4-positive plasma cells was detected in the pancreas (IgG4-immunostaining).

Such an inflammatory process widely and intensely involves the contiguous soft tissue and peripancreatic retroperitoneal tissue [10, 27]. The wall of the bile duct and gallbladder is thickening, histologically showing the same inflammatory process as that of the pancreas. Regional lymph nodes are swollen up to 2.0 cm in diameter, and show histologically marked follicular hyperplasia and dense plasmacytic infiltration in paracortical and medullary regions [10, 27].

Immunohistochemically, infiltrating inflammatory cells in the pancreas consist of CD4- or CD8-positive T lymphocytes and IgG4-positive plasma cells (Figure 4). Dense infiltration (>30/high power field (hpf)) of IgG4-positive plasma cells in the pancreas is not observed in chronic alcoholic pancreatitis or pancreatic cancer. Infiltration of abundant IgG4-positive plasma cells is also detected in various organs such as peripancreatic retroperitoneal tissue, major duodenal papilla, biliary tract, intrahepatic periportal area, salivary glands, gastric mucosa, colonic mucosa, lymph nodes and bone marrow of AIP patients [8-12].

Diagnostic Criteria and Differential Diagnosis

As it is usually difficult to take specimens from the pancreas, AIP should be diagnosed currently on the basis of combination with clinical, laboratory, and imaging studies. The Japan Pancreas Society proposed "Diagnostic Criteria for Autoimmune Pancreatitis" in 2002 [28], that was revised in 2006 [29]. It contained three items: (1) radiological imaging showing diffuse enlargement of the pancreas and diffuse irregular narrowing of the main pancreatic duct; (2) laboratory data demonstrating abnormally elevated levels of serum gammaglobulin and/or IgG and/or IgG4, or presence of autoantibodies; (3) histological examination of the pancreas showing lymphoplasmacytic infiltration and fibrosis. For the diagnosis of AIP, all of the criteria are present or criterion 1 together with either criterion 2 or criterion 3. The presence of the imaging criterion is essential for diagnosing AIP. The criteria are based on the minimum consensus of AIP to avoid misdiagnosing pancreatic cancer as far as possible.

The most important disease that should be differentiated from AIP is pancreatic cancer. Clinically, patients with pancreatic cancer and AIP share many features, such as being elderly, having painless jaundice, developing new-onset diabetes mellitus, and having elevated tumor markers [20]. Radiologically, focal swelling of the pancreas, the "double-duct sign" representing strictures in both the biliary and pancreatic ducts, as well as angiographic abnormalities, can sometimes be seen in both pancreatic cancer and AIP. As AIP responds dramatically to steroid therapy, accurate diagnosis of AIP can avoid unnecessary laparotomy or pancreatic resection. Imaging findings, such as a mass showing delayed enhancement and a capsule-like rim on dynamic CT or MRI, and segmental narrowing of the main pancreatic duct associated with less dilated upstream pancreatic duct, are all useful in differentiating pancreatic cancer from AIP. Measurement of serum IgG4 levels is a useful tool to differentiate between the two diseases. We preliminarily reported that IgG4-immunostaining of biopsy specimens taken from the major duodenal papilla of AIP patients may support the diagnosis of AIP [30]. Although improvement in clinical findings with steroid therapy may be useful in the differential diagnosis of AIP from pancreatic cancer, empiric administration of steroid should be avoided not to misdiagnose pancreatic cancer as AIP.

It is of uppermost important to consider the presence of AIP in elderly patients presenting obstructive jaundice and pancreatic mass.

Extrapancreatic Lesions

AIP patients frequently have various extrapancreatic lesions. Since they show similar histopathological findings to those in the pancreas, these extrapancreatic lesions are possibly induced by the same IgG4-related fibroinflammatory mechanisms as AIP.

Sclerosing Cholangitis

Sclerosing cholangitis is frequently associated with AIP. In many cases, the stenosis is located in the lower part of the common bile duct, but EUS or intraductal ultrasonography shows wall thickening of the common bile duct even in the segment in which abnormalities are not clearly observed with cholangiography [26]. When stenosis is found in the intrahepatic or the hilar hepatic bile duct, the cholangiographic appearance is very similar to that of primary sclerosing cholangitis (PSC) [31]. Sclerosing cholangitis associated with AIP dramatically respond well to steroid therapy [31, 32]. The histological findings of sclerosing cholangitis associated with AIP include transmural fibrosis and dense lymphoplasmacytic infiltration of the bile duct wall along with lymphoplasmacytic infiltration and fibrosis in the periportal area of the liver. Dense infiltration of IgG4-positive plasma cells was detected in the bile duct wall and the periportal area of patients with AIP, but it was not detected in those of patients with PSC [8, 9]. Furthermore, elevation of serum IgG4 levels was not detected in our 3 patients with PSC. Given the age at onset, associated diseases, pancreatographic findings, response to steroid therapy, prognosis, and IgG4-related serological and immunohistochemical data, sclerosing cholangitis associated with AIP should be differentiated from PSC [31].

Sclerosing Sialadenitis

In my series, swelling of the salivary glands was detected in 7 of 30 (23%) patients with AIP, and it was associated with cervical or mediastinal lymphadenopathy. Histology of these salivary glands was sclerosing sialadenitis with dense infiltration of IgG4-positive plasma cells and fibrosis. However, only a few (<3/hpf) IgG4-positive plasma cells were seen to infiltrate the salivary glands of 50 patients with Sjogren's syndrome, and serum IgG4 levels were not elevated in 10 patients with Sjogren's syndrome [9]. Salivary gland lesion associated with AIP is different from Sjogren's syndrome.

Retroperitoneal Fibrosis

A total of 10 cases (10 males; average age, 63.5 years) including my 4 cases have been reported to have retroperitoneal fibrosis associated with AIP [19, 33-36]. In 3 cases, retroperitoneal fibrosis occurred 10 to 18 months before the onset of AIP. Dense infiltration of IgG4-positive plasma cells and obliterative phlebitis were found in both the pancreas and retroperitoneal fibrous mass. These retroperitoneal fibrotic lesions associated with AIP seem to be the retroperitoneal lesions of IgG4-related systemic disease.

Lymphadenopathy

In a study using gallium-67 scintigraphy, pulmonary hilar gallium-67 uptake was found in 16 of 24 patients with AIP [37]. In our series, abdominal lymphadenopathy of up to 2 cm in diameter was observed in 5 of 8 patients at laparotomy, and cervical or mediastinal lymphadenopathy of up to 1.5 cm in diameter was observed in 7 of 28 patients on CT [9]. In all these cases, the lymphadenopathy disappeared after steroid therapy. Dense infiltration of IgG4-positive plasma cells was detected in abdominal or cervical lymph nodes of AIP patients, but only a few IgG4-positive plasma cells were seen to infiltrate abdominal lymph nodes of patients with chronic alcoholic pancreatitis and pancreatic cancer, and cervical lymph nodes of patients with Sjogren's syndrome [9].

Other reported major lesions associated with AIP were sclerosing cholecystitis [38], interstitial pneumonia [39], tubulointerstitial nephritis [40], and hepatic inflammatory pseudotumor [41].

Treatment and Prognosis

Steroid therapy is clinically, morphologically and serologically effective in AIP patients. The preferred initial dose of predonisolone is 30-40 mg/day, and it is tapered by 5 mg every 1-2 weeks. Serological and imaging tests are followed periodically after commencement of steroid therapy. Usually, pancreatic size is normalized within a few weeks, and biliary drainage becomes unnecessary during 1-2 months. Patients in whom complete radiological improvement is documented can stop their medication, but most other patients require continued maintenance therapy with predonisolone 5 mg/day [32]. In half of steroid-treated patients, impaired exocrine or endocrine function improved [16, 17]. Some AIP patients relapse during maintenance therapy or after stop of steroid medication, and should be retreated with high-dose steroid therapy.

The long-term prognosis of AIP is not well known. In my follow-up study of AIP patients, the prognosis is almost always good [42]. It is reported that recurrent attacks of AIP resulted in pancreatic stone formation in some cases [14].

IgG4-Related Sclerosing Disease

Dense infiltration of IgG4-positive plasma cells as well as CD4- or CD8-positive T lymphocytes and fibrosis have been observed in the peripancreatic retroperitoneal tissue, bile duct wall, gallbladder wall, periportal area of the liver, salivary glands, as well as the pancreas of AIP patients [8-10]. All extrapancreatic lesions associated with AIP such as sclerosing cholangitis, sclerosing sialadenitis or retroperitoneal fibrosis show infiltration of abundant IgG4-positive plasma cells, but the infiltration is not detected in those of PSC, Sjogren's syndrome, sialolithiasis, chronic alcoholic pancreatitis, or pancreatic cancer. Both pancreatic and extrapancreatic lesions of AIP respond well to steroid therapy, being different from PSC.

Table 1. Clinicopathological Findings of IgG4-related Sclerosing Disease

- Systemic disease characterized histopathologically by extensive IgG4-positive plasma cell infiltration of various organs together with T lymphocytes
- Major clinical manifestations are apparent in the organs in which tissues fibrosis with obstructive phlebitis is pathologically induced.

Pancreas	autoimmune pancreatitis
Bile duct	sclerosing cholangitis
Gallbladder	sclerosing cholecystitis
Salivary gland	sclerosing sialadenitis
Retroperitoneum	retroperitoneal fibrosis

- Some pseudotumors may be involved in this disease.
- Possibility of close relationship to multifocal fibrosclerosis
- Occasional association with lymphadenopathy
- Elderly male preponderance
- Frequent elevation of serum IgG4 levels
- Favorite response to steroid therapy
- Differentiation from malignant tumor is important.
- Precise pathogenesis and pathophysiology remain unclear

I would therefore propose the existence of a novel clinicopathological entity, an IgG4-related sclerosing disease incorporating sclerosing pancreatitis, cholangitis, sialadenitis, and retroperitoneal fibrosis with lymphadenopathy. It is histopathologically characterized by extensive IgG4-positive plasma cell and T lymphocyte infiltration of various organs. Major clinical manifestations are apparent in the pancreas, bile duct, salivary glands, and retroperitoneum, in which tissues fibrosis with obliterative phlebitis is pathologically induced. AIP is not simply a pancreatitis but that, in fact, it is a pancreatic lesion reflecting an IgG4-related systemic disease. Sclerosing cholangitis, sclerosing sialadenitis and retroperitoneal fibrosis associated with AIP are different from PSC, Sjogren's syndrome and so-called idiopathic retroperitoneal fibrosis. In some cases, only 1 or 2 organs are clinically involved, while in others 3 or 4 organs are affected. The disease occurs predominantly in elderly males, is frequently associated with lymphadenopathy, and responds well to steroid therapy. Serum IgG4 levels and immunostaining with anti-IgG4 antibody are useful in making the diagnosis [9]. Precise pathogenesis and pathophysiology of IgG4-related sclerosing disease remain unclear (Table 1).

Conclusion

AIP has many clinical, serological, morphological, and histopathological characteristic features. AIP should be diagnosed based on combination of these findings. In an elderly male presenting obstructive jaundice and pancreatic mass, AIP should be considered as one of differential diagnoses to avoid unnecessary surgery.

I proposed a new clinicopathological entity of IgG4-related sclerosing disease. It is characterized by extensive IgG4-positive plasma cell and T lymphocyte infiltration of various organs, and major clinical manifestations are apparent in the pancreas, bile duct, retroperitoneum, and salivary glands, in which tissues fibrosis with obliterative phlebitis is pathologically induced.

References

[1] Sarles H, Sarles JC, Muratoren R, et al. Chronic inflammatory sclerosing of the pancreas-An autonomous pancreatic disease? *Am. J. Dig. Dis.* 1961;6:688-98.

[2] Yoshida K, Toki F, Takeuchi T, Watanabe S, Shiratori K, Hayashi N. Chronic pancreatitis caused by an autoimmune abnormality. Proposal of the concept of autoimmune pancreatitis. *Dig. Dis. Sci.* 1995;40:1561-8.

[3] Okazaki K, Uchida K, Chiba T. Recent concept of autoimmune-related pancreatitis. *J. Gastroenterol* 2001;36:293-302.

[4] Kim KP, Kim MH, Song MH, Lee SS, Seo DW, Lee SK. Autoimmune chronic pancreatitis. *Am. J. Gastroenterol.* 2004;99:1605-16.

[5] Nishimori I, Tamaoki A, Kawa S, Tanaka S, Takeuchi K, Kamisawa T, et al. Influence of steroid therapy on the course of diabetes mellitus in patients with autoimmune pancreatitis: findings from a nationwide survey in Japan. *Pancreas* 2006;32:244-8.

[6] Hamano H, Kawa S, Horiuchi A, Unno H, Furuya N, Akamatsu T, et al. High serum IgG4 concentrations in patients with sclerosing pancreatitis. *N. Engl. J. Med.* 2001;344:732-8.

[7] Hirano K, Komatsu Y, Yamamoto N, Nakai Y, Sasahira N, Toda N, et al. Pancreatic mass lesions associated with raised concentration of IgG4. *Am. J. Gastroenterol.* 2004;99:2038-40.

[8] Kamisawa T, Funata N, Hayashi Y, Eishi Y, Koike M, Tsuruta K, et al. A new clinicopathological entity of IgG4-related autoimmune disease. *J. Gastroenterol.* 2003;38:982-4.

[9] Kamisawa T, Nakajima H, Egawa N, Funata N, Tsuruta K, Okamoto A. IgG4-related sclerosing disease incorporating sclerosing pancreatitis, cholangitis, sialadenitis and retroperitoneal fibrosis with lymphadenopathy. *Pancreatology* 2006;6:132-7.

[10] Kamisawa T, Funata N, Hayashi Y, Tsuruta K, Okamoto A, Amemiya K, et al. Close relationship between autoimmune pancreatitis and multifocal fibrosclerosis. *Gut* 2003;52:683-7.

[11] Kamisawa T, Egawa N, Nakajima H, Tsuruta K, Okamoto A, Hayashi Y, et al. Gastrointestinal findings in patients with autoimmune pancreatitis. *Endoscopy* 2005;37:1127-30.

[12] Kamisawa T, Nakajima H, Egawa N, Hayashi Y, Funata N. Autoimmune pancreatitis can be confirmed with gastroscopy. *Dig. Dis. Sci.* 2004;49:155-6.

[13] Kamisawa T, Yoshiike M, Egawa N, Nakajima H, Tsuruta K, Okamoto A, et al. Chronic pancreatitis in the elderly in Japan. *Pancreatology* 2004;4:223-7.

[14] Takayama M, Hamano H, Ochi Y, Saegusa H, Komatsu K, Muraki T, et al. Recurrent attacks of autoimmune pancreatitis result in pancreatic stone formation. *Am. J. Gastroenterol.* 2004;99:932-937.

[15] Horiuchi A, Kawa S, Hamano H, Hayama M, Kiyosawa K. ERCP features in 27 patients with autoimmune pancreatitis. *Gastrointest. Endosc.* 2002;55:494-9.

[16] Kamisawa T, Egawa N, Inokuma S, Tsuruta K, Okamoto A, Kamata N, et al. Pancreatic endocrine and exocrine function and salivary gland function in autoimmune pancreatitis before and after steroid therapy. *Pancreas* 2003;27:235-8.

[17] Kamisawa T, Nakamura T, Egawa N, Nakajima H, Tsuruta K, Okamoto A. Digestion and absorption of patients with autoimmune pancreatitis. *Hepatogastroenterology* 2006;53:138-40.

[18] Kawa S, Hamano H. Autoimmune pancreatitis and bile duct lesions. *J. Gastroenterol.* 2003;38:1201-3.

[19] Uchida K, Okazaki K, Asada M, Yazumi S, Ohana M, Chiba T. Case of chronic pancreatitis involving an autoimmune mechanism that extended to retroperitoneal fibrosis. *Pancreas* 2003;26: 92-4.

[20] Kamisawa T, Egawa N, Nakajima H, Tsuruta K, Okamoto A, Kamata N. Clinical difficulties in the differentiation of autoimmune pancreatitis and pancreatic carcinoma. *Am. J. Gastroenterol.* 2003;98:2694-9.

[21] Kamisawa T, Okamoto A, Funata N. Clinicopathological features of autoimmune pancreatitis in relation to elevation of serum IgG4. *Pancreas* 2005;31:28-31.

[22] Irie H, Honda H, Baba S, Kuroiwa T, Yoshimitsu K, Tajima T, et al. Autoimmune pancreatitis: CT and MR characteristics. AJR *Am. J. Roentogenol.* 1998;170:1323-7.

[23] Sahani DV, Kalva SP, Farrell J, Maker MM, Saini S, Mueller PR, et al. Autoimmune pancreatitis: image features. *Radiology* 2004;233:345-52.

[24] Kamisawa T, Chen PY, Tu Y, Nakajima H, Egawa N, Tsuruta K, et al. MRI and MRCP findings in autoimmune pancreatitis. *World J. Gastroenterol.* 2006;12:2919-22.

[25] Kamisawa T, Okamoto A, Funata N. Autoimmune pancreatitis. *Gastrointest Endosc.* 2004;59:865-6.

[26] Hyodo N, Hyodo T. Ultrasonographic evaluation in patients with autoimmune-related pancreatitis. *J. Gastroenterol.* 2003;38:1155-61.

[27] Kawaguchi K, Koike M, Tsuruta K, Okamoto A, Tabata I, Fujita N. Lymphoplasmacytic sclerosing pancreatitis with cholangitis: a variant of primary sclerosing cholangitis extensively involving pancreas. *Hum. Pathol.* 1991:22:387-395.

[28] Pearson RK, Longnecker DS, Chari ST, Smyrk TC, Okazaki K, Frulloni L, et al. Controversies in clinical pancreatology. Autoimmune pancreatitis: does it exist? *Pancreas* 2003;27:1-13.

[29] Okazaki K, Kawa S, Kamisawa T, Naruse S, Tanaka S, Nishimori I, et al. Clinical diagnostic criteria of autoimmune pancreatitis: revised proposal. *J. Gastroenterol.* 2006;41:626-31.

[30] Kamisawa T, Yu Y, Nakajima H, Egawa N, Tsuruta K, Okamoto A. Usefulness of biopsying the major duodenal papilla to diagnose autoimmune pancreatitis: a prospective study using IgG4-immunostaining. *World J. Gastroenterol.* 2006;12:2031-3.

[31] Kamisawa T, Egawa N, Tsuruta K, Okamoto A, Funata N. Primary sclerosing cholangitis may be overestimated in Japan. *J. Gastroenterol.* 2005;40:318-9.

[32] Kamisawa T, Egawa N, Nakajima H, Tsuruta K, Okamoto A. Morphological changes after steroid therapy in autoimmune pancreatitis. *Scand. J. Gastroenterol.* 2004;39:1154-8.

[33] Hamano H, Kawa S, Ochi Y, Unno H, Shiba N, Wajiki M, et al. Hydronephrosis associated with retroperitoneal fibrosis and sclerosing pancreatitis. *Lancet* 2002;359:1403-1404.

[34] Fukukura Y, Fujiyoshi F, Nakamura F, Hamada H, Nakajo M. Autoimmune pancreatitis associated with idiopathic retroperitoneal fibrosis. AJR 2003;181:993-995.

[35] Kamisawa T, Matsukawa M, Ohkawa M. Autoimmune pancreatitis associated with retroperitoneal fibrosis. *JOP* 2005;10:260-263.

[36] Kamisawa T, Chen PY, Tu Y, Nakajima H, Egawa N. Autoimmune pancreatitis metachronously associated with retroperitoneal fibrosis with IgG4-positive plasma cell infiltration. *World J. Gastroenterol.* 2006;12:2955-7.

[37] Saegusa H, Momose M, Kawa S, Hamano H, Ochi Y, Takayama M, et al. Hilar and pancreatic gallium-67 accumulation is characteristic feature of autoimmune pancreatitis. Pancreas 2003;27:20-25.

[38] Kamisawa T, Tu Y, Nakajima H, Egawa N, Tsuruta K, Okamoto A, et al. Sclerosing cholecystitis associated with autoimmune pancreatitis. *World J. Gastroenterol.*, 2006;12:3736-9.

[39] Taniguchi T, Ko M, Seko S, Nishida O, Inoue F, Kobayashi H, et al. Interstitial pneumonia associated with autoimmune pancreatitis. *Gut* 2004;53:770.

[40] Uchiyama-Tanaka Y, Mori Y, Kimura T, Sonomura K, Umemura S, Kishimoto N, et al. Acute tubulointerstitial nephritis associated with autoimmune-related pancreatitis. *Am. J. Kid Dis.* 2004;43:e18-e25.

[41] Sasahira N, Kawabe T, Nakamura A, Shimura K, Shimura H, Itobayashi E, et al. Inflammatory pseudotumor of the liver and peripheral eosinophilia in autoimmune pancreatitis. *World J. Gastroenterol.* 2005;11:922-925.

[42] Kamisawa T, Yoshiike M, Egawa N, Nakajima H, Tsuruta K, Okamoto A. Treating patients with autoimmune pancreatitis: results from a long-term follow-up study. *Pancreatology* 2005;5:234-40.

In: Pancreatitis Research Advances
Editor: William C. Langley, pp. 31-38

ISBN: 978-1-60021-883-5

Short Communication B

Influence of Endosonography in the Evaluation of Idiopathic Acute Pancreatitis

Juan J. Vila**, *Fernando Borda, F. Javier Jiménez, Erika Borobio, Inmaculada Elizalde and Antonio Arín
Gastroenterology Department, Hospital de Navarra,
Pamplona, Spain

Abstract

Introduction: Up to 30% of patients with acute pancreatitis are diagnosed of idiopathic acute pancreatitis (IAP) after an initial evaluation including a complete clinical history, physical examination, laboratory testing and abdominal imaging. Endosonography (EUS) has shown a high accuracy (60-80%) to diagnose biliary and pancreatic diseases in these patients.

Aims And Methods: Our aim was to evaluate the role of EUS in patients with IAP. We also wanted to find predictive factors of a positive finding on EUS in these patients. We defined IAP as those clinical pictures of acute pancreatitis where after a complete clinical history, physical examination, history of abdominal trauma or surgery, history of ethanol intake, laboratory analysis including calcium and triglycerides and at least two normal transabdominal ultrasound explorations the cause of the pancreatitis is not found. We prospectively performed an EUS to these patients with IAP from January 2005 until December 2006. All EUS procedures were performed by the same endoscopist. In order to analyze the possible influence of different factors on the findings of EUS, we recorded epidemiological data, number and severity of the previous bouts of pancreatitis and if patients had been previously cholecistectomized. Chi Square and Fisher tests were used to compare the influence of different factors on the EUS results. Quantitative variables

* Gastroenterology Dpt. Hospital de Navarra. Pamplona, Spain. Telephone: +34 848 422114. Fax: +34 848 422303. e-mail: xoanxose@hotmail.com

are reported with mean value and standard deviation. P values over 0.05 were considered not significant.

Results: During the mentioned period we performed 552 EUS procedures in our unit, 37 of them were performed to patients with IAP who were included in the study. Sex distribution was 27 men and 10 women. Mean age was 60.54±16 yo (range: 23-83). All patients underwent at least 2 transabdominal ultrasound explorations before EUS, 35 a CT exploration and 12 a magnetic resonance cholangiopancreatography. None of those explorations found the etiology of the pancreatitis. EUS was performed after the first bout of pancreatitis in 19 patients while 18 patients had a recurrent disease (mean number of episodes: 3.67±3.05). Eight patients suffered a severe episode of pancreatitis before EUS. Twelve patients had a previous cholecystectomy. EUS was normal in 7 patients (19%), in the remaining 30 patients (81%) we found cholelithiasis (3 patients), microlithiasis (14 patients), chronic pancreatitis (14 patients), pancreas divisum (2 patients), pancreatic cancer (1 patient), apudoma (1 patient), intraductal papillary mucinous tumour (1 patient), cystic tumour of the pancreas (1 patient) and choledocholithiasis (2 patients). Microlithiasis was the only finding in 8 patients (21%) and chronic pancreatitis in 5 (13%). Positive findings in EUS were not influenced by age (older or younger than 65 yo: 62% vs 82%; p=0.25), sex (men vs women: 70% vs 90%; p=0.39), previous cholecystectomy (cholecystectomy vs non cholecystectomy: 60% vs 81%; p=0.21), previous severe pancreatitis (severe vs moderate: 75% vs 76%; p=1.00) or recurrent disease (recurrent vs first episode: 72% vs 79%; p=0.71).

Conclusions: EUS identifies the cause of IAP in 81% of patients. Epidemiological data, previous cholecystectomy, severe pancreatitis nor recurrent pancreatitis are predictors of positive findings in EUS.

Introduction

In 10-30% of cases of acute pancreatitis, etiologic factors are not initially found, and patients are diagnosed of idiopathic acute pancreatitis (IAP).

Until recent years, ERCP was the first choice diagnostic procedure in these patients, with a diagnostic accuracy of 70-80% but with a rate of potentially severe complications of 10-15% [1]. Due to the risk of complications, some authors recommended ERCP performance only after the second episode of IAP or after the first if pancreatitis had been severe [2,3]. Other reports supported the indication of ERCP systematically after the first episode of IAP [4].

During the last few years, endoscopic ultrasonography (EUS) has proved to have similar diagnostic accuracy to ERCP with a lower complication rate, comparable with that of upper gastrointestinal endoscopy [5,6]. However, EUS does not allow any therapeutic manoeuvre.

Considering this background, we decided to perform a prospective study analysing the results of EUS in patients with IAP. The aim of the study was to evaluate in our own series of patients the diagnostic accuracy of EUS and to analyse the influence of different factors on EUS results in order to identify predictive variables of EUS positive findings.

Material and Methods

We designed a prospective study performing EUS to all patients diagnosed of IAP in our department from January 2005 until December 2006.

Patients were diagnosed of IAP when no cause was found after performing a basic etiologic study including complete clinical records (personal and family history of pancreatic disorders, personal history of recent infectious diseases, traumatisms or surgery and systemic autoimmune disease, and alcohol and drugs intake), physical examination, laboratory tests including calcium and triglycerides and whether two transabdominal ultrasonographies or an ultrasonography plus a CT scan with no pancreatic lesions or biliary lithiasis. Alcohol intake was considered important when higher than 40 g daily.

Recognized causes of acute pancreatitis were investigated with EUS. Therefore, we diagnosed biliary stones when echogenic elements that cast acoustic shadow were present in the gallbladder or bile duct. Biliary sludge was identifed as echogenic, layering nonshadowing material settled in the gallbladder or bile duct. Microlithiasis was diagnosed when mobile nonshadowing echogenic images were seen inside the gallbladder or bile duct.

Pancreas divisum was diagnosed when a patent dorsal duct was followed until the duodenal wall and communication between ventral and dorsal duct was not seen. Chronic pancreatitis was diagnosed when at least five ultrasonographic criteria were present or when pancreatic calcifications were found.

All procedures were performed by the same endoscopist (JJV). An Olympus UMQ 130 endoscope with frequencies of 7,5 and 20 MHz was used from January 2005 to August 2006, and a Pentax 3630 endoscope with frequencies ranging from 5 MHz until 12 MHz was used during the last months of the study. Every patient was informed about the procedure before signing an informed consent document, at least 24 hours before endoscopic examination. EUS was performed at least four weeks after hospital discharge to assure complete resolution of pancreatitis episode.

Besides EUS findings, other data were registered to analyze their possible influence on EUS results and to identify any predictive factor of EUS positive findings. These data included age, sex, number of pancreatitis episodes, severity of former pancreatitis bouts and previous cholecystectomy. According to age patients were divided in younger or older than 65 years. Fisher and Chi Square tests were used for statistical analysis. Variables were estimated as mean ± standard deviation, and p values lower than 0.05 were considered significant.

Results

During the study period 552 endosonographic procedures were performed in our unit, 37 of them in patients with IAP. These 37 patients (27 male, 10 female; mean age: 60.54±16 years, range: 23-83 years) were included in the study. Before EUS performance, transabdominal ultrasonography had been performed to all patients, a CT scan to 35 patients and Magnetic Resonance Cholangio-Pancreatography (MRCP) to 12 patients. No etiologic factors were found in any of these explorations.

In 19 patients EUS was indicated after the first episode of pancreatitis and in the remaining 18 cases after several episodes of pancreatitis (mean= 3.67±3.05). Eight patients had suffered at least one episode of severe pancreatitis. Cholecystectomy had been previously performed in 12 patients.

EUS showed no findings in 7 patients (19%). In 30 patients (81%) possible causes of pancreatitis were found: cholelithiasis (3 cases), microlithiasis (14 cases), pancreas divisum (2 cases), chronic pancreatitis (14 cases), pancreatic carcinoma (1 case), apudoma (1 case), intraductal papillary mucinous pancreatic tumour (1 case), cystic pancreatic tumour (1 case) and choledocolithiasis (2 patients with stones smaller than 4 mm). Results are summarized in Table I.

Microlithiasis was the only finding in 8 patients. It was associated with chronic pancreatitis in 5 patients and with pancreas divisum in another case. Chronic pancreatitis was the only finding in 5 patients and it was associated with microlithiasis in 5 patients, with pancreas divisum in 1 patient, choledocolithiasis in 1 patient, cystic pancreatic tumour in 1 patient and pancreatic apudoma in another patient. We did not find any association between positive EUS findings and age, sex, previous cholecystectomy, pancreatitis severity and number of previous episodes of pancreatitis. These results are shown in Table II.

Table I. EUS findings in patients with IAP

- Normal: 7 patients (19%).
- Cholelithiasis: 3 patients (8%).
- Microlithiasis: 14 patients (38%).
- Choledocholithiasis: 2 patients (5%).
- Chronic pancreatitis: 14 patients (38%).
- Pancreas divisum: 2 patients (5%).
- Pancreatic cancer: 1 patient (2,5%).
- Apudoma: 1 patient (2,5%).
- Intraductal papillary mucinous tumor: 1 patient (2,5%).
- Cystic tumour of the pancreas: 1 patient (2,5%).

Table II. Influence of analyzed factors on EUS findings

Factor	Categories	n	Patients with positive findings on EUS	p
Age	>65 yo	18	12 (66,7%)	0,269
	<65 yo	19	16 (84,2%)	
Sex	Women	10	9 (90%)	0,393
	Men	27	19 (70,4%)	
Number of IAP	First Episode	19	15 (78,9%)	0,710
	Recurrent IAP	18	13 (72,2%)	
Cholecystectomy	Cholecystectomy	10	6 (60%)	0,176
	Gallbladder in situ	27	22 (81,5%)	
Severity of IAP	Non severe	29	22 (75,9%)	1,00
	Severe	8	6 (75%)	

Discussion

Diagnostic yield of EUS in our series of patients was 81%, which is consistent with other published data [7,8, 9, 10, 11, 12, 13]. Biliary lithiasis was the most frequent finding, present in 19 cases (51%) with two cases of choledocolithiasis in two patients who had undergone previous cholecystectomy. This prevalence is similar to that reported in some papers [9, 14], although this rate is lower in other articles [10, 12] probably due to geographic variability.

This high detection rate of biliary lithiasis is probably the main support for performing EUS in IAP.

Dahan et al [15] compared the diagnostic accuracy of EUS and microscopic bile examination in detecting microlithiasis in patients with IAP or abdominal pain mimicking a biliary colic with transabdominal ultrasonography within normal limits. Results were significantly better with EUS than with microscopic bile examination, even the latter is considered the gold standard for the diagnosis of microlithiasis. However, up to our knowledge these results have not been confirmed by other groups.

Taking our and other authors results into account, it seems clear that EUS should be indicated as the first diagnostic procedure in patients with IAP and gallbladder "in situ". This indication can be rather controversial in patients with previous cholecystectomy.

Concerning chronic pancreatitis, EUS is presently considered one of the most sensitive techniques for diagnosis, even in early stages [16, 17], with good correlation with ERCP findings and acceptable interobserver variability and therefore acceptable reproducibility [18, 19, 20]. Ductal and parenchymal criteria are used for diagnosis, accepting that chronic pancreatitis can be diagnosed by the presence of 3 of these criteria. However, several authors including our group, consider that the presence of 5 criteria is needed to reach the diagnosis of chronic pancreatitis, thus increasing specificity and positive predictive value (>85%) and somehow avoiding overdiagnose [12, 21].

Sphincter of Oddi dysfunction diagnosis usually depends on ERCP performance with or without sphincter manometry. One article has been published presenting the utility of EUS in combination with Warshaw test performance in sphincter of Oddi dysfunction diagnosis [22]. However these results have not been reported by other groups.

Pancreas divisum diagnosis by means of EUS is technically difficult and requires expertise. Several signs have been described as suggestive of pancreas divisum. The stack sign is present in 33% of patients with pancreas divisum and in 83% of patients without this entity ($p=0.04$) [23]. According to our experience and in agreement with other authors [10, 12] we prefer to use other diagnostic criteria, as the finding of a persistent dorsal duct to the duodenal wall and the absence of a pancreatic duct crossing from ventral to dorsal pancreas. When this crossing duct is found negative predictive value is close to 100% for pancreas divisum diagnosis [12].

Taking into account that chronic pancreatitis, sphincter of Oddi dysfunction and pancreas divisum are the most frequent findings in patients with IAP without gallbladder, MRCP could be considered the first choice diagnostic technique in these patients. MRCP is a non invasive procedure which has shown good diagnostic accuracy for these entities [24, 25, 26, 27]. However EUS has proved to be superior in detecting choledocolithiasis smaller than 5 mm [28, 29]. If choledocolithiasis is strongly suspected, a negative MRCP should be followed by an EUS, as it happened in two of our patients in whom we finally found 4 mm stones in the bile duct which had been missed in MRCP. Considering EUS low complications rate, we routinely perform EUS in all patients with IAP with or without previous cholecystectomy.

Another factor, which has been a matter of debate in the literature, is pancreatitis course. Some authors have questioned the efficacy of EUS in cases of relapsing pancreatitis [21]. In our series, this fact has not played any influence on EUS findings, as we found no significant differences concerning diagnostic accuracy of EUS when comparing patients with single pancreatitis episode and patients with relapsing pancreatitis. These results are supported by previously published papers [12] and encourage us to perform EUS in every patient independently of the number of pancreatitis episodes.

We also believe that EUS could be considered as the first procedure to perform in patients with IAP. EUS diagnostic accuracy is similar to that of ERCP but with a lower complication rate. Perhaps, EUS main drawback is the impossibility of any therapeutic attitude, which is performed in 75% of patients initially studied by ERCP in other series [11, 30].

Another advantage of EUS is its high sensitivity for diagnosing pancreatic neoplasms, superior to CT scan, which is of great interest in patients with IAP older than 40 years of age [31, 32, 33]. Reported prevalence of pancreatic tumours in patients with IAP ranges from 0.8% to 0.9%, depending on certain predominant factors as patient age [11, 12]. In our series of patients, only one case of pancreatic cancer was detected (2,7%).

Conclusion

In conclusion, EUS shows a high diagnostic accuracy in patients with IAP. It allows the diagnosis of the cause of pancreatitis in the majority of these patients with a low complication rate. We perform EUS in every patient with IAP not taking into account neither the number of pancreatitis episodes nor previous history of cholecystectomy. Further studies are needed to demonstrate that EUS findings concerning pancreatitis etiology do not modify with the following of these patients and, so, can be considered really consistent.

References

[1] Standards of practice committee. ASGE guideline: complications of ERCP. *Gastrointest. Endosc.* 2005;57:633-638.

[2] Gregor JC, Ponich TP, Detsky AS. Should ERCP be routine after an episode of "idiopathic" pancreatitis? A cost-utility analysis. *Gastrointest. Endosc.* 1996;44:118-123.

[3] Bank S, Indaram A. Causes of acute and recurrent pancreatitis. Clinical considerations and clues to diagnosis. *Gastroenterol. Clin. North Am.* 1999;28:571-589.

[4] Baillie J. What should be done with idiopathic recurrent pancreatitis that remains "idiopathic" after standard investigation? *JOP J. Pancreas* 2001;2:401-405.

[5] Bournet B, Migueres I, Delacroix M, Vigouroux D, Bornet JL, Escourrou J, Buscail L. Early morbidity of endoscopic ultrasound:13 years′ experience at a referral center. *Endoscopy* 2006;38:349-54.

[6] Standards of practice committee. ASGE guideline: complications of EUS. *Gastrointest Endosc.* 2005;61:8-12.

[7] Norton SA, Alderson D. Endoscopic ultrasonography in the evaluation of idiopathic acute pancreatitis. *Br. J. Surgery* 2000;87:1650-1655.

[8] Frossard JL, Sosa-Valencia L, Amouyal G, Marty O, Hadengue A, Amouyal P. Usefulness of endoscopic ultrasonography in patients with "idiopathic" acute pancreatitis. *Am. J. Med.* 2000;109:196-200.

[9] Liu CL, Lo CM, Chan JFK, Poon RTP, Fan ST. EUS for detection of occult cholelithiasis in patients with idiopathic pancreatitis. *Gastrointest. Endosc.* 2000;51:28-32.

[10] Tandon M, Topazian M. Endoscopic ultrasound in idiopathic acute pancreatitis. *Am. J. Gastroenterol.* 2001;96:705-709.

[11] Coyle WJ, Pineau BC, Tarnasky PR, Knapple WL, Aabakken L, Hoffman BJ, Cunningham JT, Hawes RH, Cotton PB. Evaluation of unexplained acute and acute recurrent pancreatitis using endoscopic retrograde cholangiopancreatography, sphincter of Oddi manometry and endoscopic ultrasound. *Endoscopy* 2002;34:617-623.

[12] Yusoff IF, Raymond G, Sahai AV. A prospective comparison of the yield of EUS in primary vs. recurrent idiopathic acute pancreatitis. *Gastrointest. Endosc.* 2004;60:673.

[13] Garg PK, Tandon RK, Madan K. Is Biliary microlithiasis a significant cause of idiopathic recurrent acute pancreatitis? A long-term follow-up study. *Clin. Gastroenterol. Hepatol.* 2007;5:75-79.

[14] Ros E, Navarro S, Bru C, García-Puges A, Valderrama R. Occult microlithiasis in idiopatic acute pancreatitis: prevention of relapses by cholecystectomy or ursodeoxycholic acid therapy. *Gastroenterology* 1991;101:1701-1709.

[15] Dahan P, Andant C, Levy P, Amouyal P, Amouyal G, Dumont M, Erlinger S, Sauvanet A, Belghiti J, Zins M, Vilgrain V, Bernades P. *Gut* 1996;38:277-281.

[16] Irisawa A, Katakura K, Ohira H, Sato A, Bhutani MS, Hernandez LV, Koizumi M. Usefulness of endoscopic ultrasound to diagnose the severity of chronic pancreatitis. *J. Gastroenterol.* 2007;42[Suppl XVII]:90-94.

[17] Catalano MF. Diagnosing early-stage chronic pancreatitis: is endoscopic ultrasound a reliable modality? *J. Gastroenterol.* 2007;42[Suppl XVII]:78-84.

[18] Sahai AV, Zimmerman M, Aabakken L, Tarnasky PR, Cunningham JT, van Velse A, Hawes RH, Hoffman BJ. Prospective assessment of the ability of endoscopic ultrasound to diagnose,exclude, or establish the severity of chronic pancreatitis found by endoscopic retrograde cholangiopancreatography. *Gastrointest. Endosc.* 1998;48:18-25.

[19] Wallace MB, Hawes RH, Durkalski V, Chak A, Mallery S, Catalano MF, Wiersema MJ, Bhutani MS, Ciaccia D, Kochman ML, Gress FG, Van Velse A, Hoffman BJ. The reliability of EUS for the diagnosis of chronic pancreatitis: interobserver agreement among experienced endosonographers. *Gastrointest. Endosc.* 2001;53:294-9.

[20] Raimondo M, Wallace MB. Diagnosis of early chronic pancreatitis by endoscopic ultrasound. Are we there yet? *JOP. J. pancreas* 2004;5:1-7.

[21] Chen RYM, Hawes RH. Idiopathic acute pancreatitis: is EUS worth doing? *Am. J. Gastroenterol.* 2002;97:1244-1246.

[22] Catalano MF, Lahoti S, Alcocer E, Geenen JE, Walter JH. Dynamic imaging of the pancreas using real-time endoscopic ultrasonography with secretin stimulation. *Gastrointest. Endosc.* 1998;48:580-7.

[23] Bhutani MS, Hoffman BJ, Hawes RH. Diagnosis of pancreas divisum by endoscopic ultrasonography. *Endoscopy* 1999;31:167-9.

[24] Khalid A, Peterson M, Slivka A. Secretin-stimulated magnetic resonance pancreaticogram to assess pancreatic duct outflow obstruction in evaluation of idiopathic acute recurrent pancreatitis: a pilot study. *Dig. Dis. Sci.* 2003;48:1475-81.

[25] Matos C, Winant C, Delhaye M, Deviere J. Functional MRCP in pancreatic and periampullary disease. *Int. J. Gastrointest Cancer* 2001;30:5-18.

[26] Sugiyama M, Haradome H, Atomi Y. Magnetic resonance imaging for diagnosing chronic pancreatitis. *J. Gastroenterol.* 2007;42[Suppl XVII]:108-112.

[27] Hellerhoff KJ, Helmberger H 3rd, Rosch T, Settles MR, Link TM, Rummeny EJ. Dynamic MR pancreatography after secretin administration: image quality and diagnostic accuracy. *AJR Am. J. Roentgenol.* 2002;179:121-9.

[28] Kondo S, Isayama H, Akahane M, Toda N, Sasahira N, Nakai Y, Yamamoto N, Hirano K, Komatsu Y, Tada M, Yoshida H, Kawabe T, Ohtomo K, Omata M. Detection of common bile duct stones: comparison between endoscopic ultrasonography, magnetic resonance cholangiography, and helical-computed-tomographic cholangiography. *Eur. J. Radiol.* 2005;54:271-5.

[29] Verma D, Kapadia A, Eisen GM, Adler DG. EUS vs MRCP for detection of choledocholithiasis. *Gastrointest Endosc.* 2006;64:248-54.

[30] Kaw M, Brodmerkel GJ. ERCP, biliary crystal analysis, and sphincter of Oddi manometry in idiopathic recurrent pancreatitis. *Gastrointest. Endosc.* 2002;55:157-162.

[31] DeWitt J, Devereaux B, Chriswell M, McGreevy K, Howard T, Imperiale TF, Ciaccia D, Lane KA, Maglinte D, Kopecky K, LeBlanc J, McHenry L, Madura J, Aisen A, Cramer H, Cummings O, Sherman S. Comparison of endoscopic ultrasonography and multidetector computed tomography for detecting and staging pancreatic cancer. *Ann. Intern. Med.* 2004;141:753-63.

[32] Ho S, Bonasera RJ, Pollack BJ, Grendell J, Feuerman M, Gress F. A single-center experience of endoscopic ultrasonography for enlarged pancreas on computed tomography. *Clin. Gastroenterol. Hepatol.* 2006;4:98-103.

[33] Draganov P, Forsmark E. Idiopathic pancreatitis. *Gastroenterology* 2005;128:756-763.

In: Pancreatitis Research Advances
Editor: William C. Langley, pp. 39-77

ISBN: 978-1-60021-883-5

Chapter I

Post ERCP Pancreatitis

Georgia Lazaraki, Dimitrios Paikos and Panagiotis Katsinelos*

Department of Endoscopy and Motility Unit,
Central Hospital, Thessaloniki, Greece

Abstract

Diagnostic endoscopic retrograde cholangiopancreatography (ERCP) has been replaced in many fields by magnetic resonance cholangiopancreatography (MRCP), a less invasive technique, and it is now limited to indications such as sphincter of Oddi dysfunction. Therapeutic ERCP has become an accepted interventional method for both biliary and pancreatic diseases despite complications. Post-ERCP pancreatitis, a complication associated to the technique and the endoscopist's skills, remains a burning issue since it has been reported to occur in 2-9% in unselected prospective series, and up to 30% in some series due to diverse definitions of post-ERCP pancreatitis and different methods of data collection. The severity of post-ERCP pancreatitis can range from a minor inconvenience, to a devastating illness (0.3% to 0.6% in prospective series) with pancreatic necrosis, multiorgan failure, permanent disability, and even death. Patient-related risk factors, such as patient selection, young age, sphincter of Oddi dysfunction, female sex, previous pancreatitis, potentially pancreatotoxic drugs, anatomic variations and endoscopy-related factors, such as precut sphincterotomy, injection of contrast media into the pancreatic duct and difficulty of cannulation, have been reported to increase the risk of developing post-ERCP pancreatitis. Numerous mechanisms (obstruction to outflow of pancreatic juice, hydrostatic injury, chemical or allergic injury to contrast medium, enzymatic injury, thermal injury, infection) have been postulated for the induction of post-ERCP pancreatitis. Regardless of the mechanism that initiates post-ERCP pancreatitis, the pathways of inflammation are similar to those for other forms of pancreatitis, including premature intracellular activation of proteolytic enzymes, autodigestion, impaired acinar secretion, and the inflammatory cascade, including chemokines and proinflammatory cytokines. Pharmacological agents, such as nifedipine,

* Corresponding Author: Dr Panagiotis Katsinelos, Ethnikis Aminis 41, 54635, Thessaloniki, Greece. Tel: +302310963341, FAX:+302310210401. e-mail: akis_katsinelos@yahoo.gr

glucagon, calcitonin, n-acetylcysteine, allopurinol, corticosteroids, low-molecular weight heparin, gabexate, somatostatin and its analogues, have been proposed with the indication of avoiding post-ERCP pancreatitis. Novelties in cannulation techniques and improved equipment, along with specific endoscopic interventions, as prophylactic pancreatic stent placement, have been also proposed to effectively reduce the risk. This review provides an evidence- based assessment of published data on post-ERCP pancreatitis and current suggestions for its avoidance.

Introduction

The role of diagnostic endoscopic retrograde cholangiopancreatography (ERCP) is now limited to a handful of indications such as sphincter of Oddi dysfunction - due to the high number of complications associated with the technique and the development of novel, often less invasive diagnostic techniques (magnetic resonance cholangiopancreatography and endoscopic ultrasonography). Therapeutic ERCP, on the other hand, has become an established interventional method for biliary and pancreatic disease (biliary drainage due to malignancies, pancreatic pesudocyst drainage, biliary duct stones, etc).

Acute pancreatitis remains one of the major and most fearful complications of ERCP. Prospective series of non-selected patients reported a frequency of post-ERCP pancreatitis (PEP) that ranged between 2.1 and 39%. This varying incidence has been considered a result of multiple factors such as thoroughness of follow-up, definition used, and parameters relating to patient susceptibility, case mix, types of manoeuvres performed, and the endoscopist. Recently, two large studies reported incidence of PEP 15.1% and 12.1% respectively. The first one was a prospective multicenter study where the elevated PEP incidence was attributed to a high percentage (33.9%) of suspicion of Oddi dysfunction as indication for the procedure [1]. The second one was a retrospective study reporting risk factors in a population of patients that had undergone pancreatic sphincterotomy, which is "per se" a well-known risk factor [2]. Nonetheless, the largest prospective studies typically report an incidence of post-ERCP pancreatitis ranging from 1-9 % in unselected patients [3-9]. Although most episodes of PEP are mild (about 90%), a small percentage of patients (about 10%) [10-12] may develop severe pancreatitis; these patients have a significant morbidity and mortality since systemic inflammatory response, pseudocysts development and multisystem organ failure may occur.

This review provides a comprehensive, evidence-based assessment of published data on post-ERCP pancreatitis, mechanisms, risk factors, proposed prevention methods and current suggestions to avoid this complication. We searched the MEDLINE database (January 2007-January 1990) by using the following medical subject headings (MESH): post ERCP pancreatitis, pancreatitis, ERCP, ERCP complications, ERCP and risk factors, post ERCP pancreatitis and risk factors. The references lists cited in all articles retrieved from Medline were searched for additional studies not found in the computerized database search.

Pathogenesis

The aetiology of acute pancreatitis can be very different, but the concurrent acute phase response is uniform and is dependent on the severity of the disease. The pathophysiology and mechanism of acute pancreatitis are complex and humoral and cellular interactions are involved in the network of the proteolytic induced pathomechanism.

Regardless of the mechanism that initiates post-ERCP pancreatitis, once activated, the pathways of inflammation are similar to those for other forms of pancreatitis and multiple studies have indicated the usefulness of ERCP as a model for studying the early inflammatory response in acute pancreatitis [13-15]. In normal conditions, intrapancreatic digestive enzyme activation occurs within the pancreatic ductal space or in the duodenum. In experimental models of acute pancreatitis, it has been suggested that digestive enzyme activation might occur within acinar cells and it has been shown that in the early stages of acute pancreatitis there is a co-localization of digestive enzymes and lysosomal hydrolases within large cytoplasm vacuoles [16-19]. As the lysosomal enzyme cathepsin B is known to be capable of activating trypsinogen [20] and trypsin can activate the remaining digestive enzyme zymogens, the co-localization phenomenon could result in intravacuolar digestive enzyme activation. This is very quickly followed by the release of reactive oxygen intermediates (ROI) (within minutes) [21] and oxidative stress responsible for the lesions of cells membranes and cytoskeleton, lipidic peroxidation, intra-cellular depletion of anti-oxidants such as reduced glutathione (GSH) and vitamins E, A, C and the translocation of the nuclear factor kappa B (NF-Kappa B) into the nucleus [22-25]. Within the nucleus, NF-Kappa B units will induce the transcription of several target genes. Within the first 30 minutes, intra-acinar transcription of chemokines [monocyte chemoattractant protein 1 (MCP-1), MOB-1, interleukin 8 (IL-8), interferon inducible protein 10 (IP-10), etc] [24, 26, 27] begins. Transcription of pro-inflammatory cytokines such as IL-1, tumor necrosis factor alpha (TNFa), IL-6 or those of adhesion molecules (i.e., intercellular adhesion molecule: ICAM-1) [28] occurs within the following hour. These expression and release of chemokines, adhesion molecules and pro-inflammatory cytokines is responsible for the pancreatic invasion by monomacrophages, T lymphocytes and polymorphonuclear neutrophils (PMN), but also for their activation and for their own release of pro-inflammatory mediators (including chemokines, cytokines, NO, elastase, etc). This amplifies the intra-pancreatic pro-inflammatory cascade of events and finally activates hepatic Kupffer cells. These hepatic monomacrophages are the major systemic source of pro-inflammatory cytokines inducing systemic inflammatory response syndrome (SIRS) and multiple organ failure [29]. Data from experimental models of acute pancreatitis have shown that hepatic Kupffer cell blockade reduces plasma levels of pro-inflammatory cytokines, the severity of acute respiratory distress syndrome (ARDS) lesions and related mortality [30, 31].

In the literature, there are limited data from human studies describing the effect of ERCP on circulating proinflammatory and anti-inflammatory cytokines, as well as the correlation between these cytokines and pancreatic enzymes [15, 32-34]. Elucidation of the timing of the different pathophysiologic factors involved in acute pancreatitis will advance our understanding of the importance of the individual factors. If intracellular activation of trypsinogen is an important event, the leakage of trypsinogen and the appearance of markers of trypsinogen activation should be found at the same time. Conversely, if extracellular activation of trypsinogen is of importance, the leakage of trypsinogen should precede the appearance of markers of trypsinogen activation. If active trypsin is what initiates inflammation in the pancreas, markers for this event should precede early markers of inflammation such as cytokines and activated neutrophils. If trypsinogen activation were secondary to the inflammatory process, the opposite would be expected. Peterson et al showed that urinary concentrations of anionic trypsinogen 6 hours after ERCP have been shown to correlate with the development development of pancreatitis. Typsinogen activation, measured as elevated urinary CAPAP levels, occurs even in mild PEP, delayed in comparison with the leakage of anionic trypsinogen, suggesting that this activation occurs in the extracellular space and perhaps not until the interstitial trypsinogen concentration has reached a certain level [34].

Chen et al [35] reported serum levels of tumor necrosis factor α, interleukin-1β, interleukin-6, interleukin-8, and interleukin-10 significantly increased at 8 and 24 hours but not at 1 and 4 hours after ERCP in patients with post-ERCP pancreatitis, in comparison with patients without pancreatitis. In this study, serum levels of interleukin-6 and interleukin-8 modestly increased from baseline values, 1 to 24 hours after uncomplicated ERCP. Although this study had the limitation of small statistic sample, their data confirmed that serum IL-6 reaches maximal concentrations at 24–48 hours after ERCP in patients with post-ERCP pancreatitis as reported from other works [13, 15, 32, 34]. It has been shown a close relation between the concentrations and the time courses of serum IL-6 and CRP, suggesting that during this inflammatory condition IL-6 is the main inducer of acute phase protein synthesis in humans [36]. Devière et al [37] also noted that IL-6 levels increased with severity among patients with post-ERCP pancreatitis. Serum IL-8 was shown to present a significant increase after onset of post-ERCP pancreatitis [32, 35]. The changes in serum TNFα and IL-1β at the early stage of ERCP-induced pancreatitis are controversial in the literature [15, 32, 37]. Two groups reported that that TNFα significantly increased compared to baseline within 24 hours after ERCP in patients with post-ERCP pancreatitis [35, 37]. Conversely, other investigators observed that TNFα and IL-1β [13, 15, 32] were not increased in patients with post-ERCP pancreatitis. The concentrations of plasma soluble TNF Receptor-I were not altered at any investigation time point in the study of Peterson et al [34]. The discrepancy in the literature may be related in part to the severity of post-ERCP pancreatitis in different studies and activation of antiinflammatory response [15, 32]. Serum IL-10 levels were found to be significantly correlated with the degree of ampullar irritation, duration of ERCP, and pain score after ERCP [13]. This was confirmed by Chen et al [35] who reported IL-10 significant increase at 8 and 24 hours after ERCP in patients with post-ERCP pancreatitis. IL-10 is mainly secreted by T-cells and in part by some other cell types. IL-10 inhibits cytokine synthesis and therefore plays a central role as a down-re gulator of immune responses [13]. Numerous mechanisms, mechanical, chemical, enzymatic and infectious have been postulated for the induction of post-ERCP pancreatitis. Nonetheless, currently, the exact cause of activation of this inflammatory cascade during post-ERCP pancreatitis has not been identified.

Mechanical reasons include elevation of intrapancreatic duct pressure due to obstruction of the pancreatic juice flow. Direct trauma from endoscopy rarely causes pancreatitis [38].

Cannulation trauma to the papilla is the most common cause of sphincter of Oddi spasm [39] and/or an edema of the papilla, thus creating an obstacle to the flow of pancreatic juice, and subsequently determines an acute pancreatic inflammation [40]. This mechanism is highlighted by a Japanese group study [41] where the authors showed that, although the frequency of Endoscopic Spicterotomy (ES)-induced pancreatitis is significantly higher than that of post-ERCP pancreatitis, the frequency of severe pancreatitis within 48 hours, and the worsening of pancreatitis after 48 hours are significantly lower within the group of patients who contracted ES-induced pancreatitis. Thus, the lowering of intraductal pressure after ES mitigates the severity of post-procedural pancreatitis. To further support this, Freeman et al have demonstrated that multiple pancreatic duct injections are an independent risk factor in the etiology of acute pancreatitis following ERCP [3]. Another study by Freeman et al confirmed these results, showing that despite pancreatic duct multiple injections and small acinar ducts depiction, the risk for post-ERCP pancreatitis disappeared when endoscopic sphincterotomy was performed [4]. Patients with a patent minor papilla and an accessory pancreatic duct are reported to have a lower incidence of pancreatitis after ERCP despite transient major papilla trauma/edema [42], perhaps due to pancreatic juice flow via the secondary route, thus protecting the ductal system from overinjection. On the basis of the concept that pancreatic outflow obstruction is a major risk factor for post-ERCP pancreatitis, temporary placement of a pancreatic stent may be beneficial, particularly in high-risk candidates [43]. Injection pressure, during contrast media or other fluid injection into the pancreatic duct contributes to ductal epithelial or acinar injury. This injury probably occurs from the disruption of cellular membranes or tight junctions between the cells and the backflow of the intraductal contents, especially into the interstitial space [44, 45]. Previous studies have demonstrated a ducto-interstitial-venous pathway, and if enough radiographic contrast is injected into the pancreatic duct, the collecting system of the kidney can be seen during ERCP [45]. In their experimental study, Vaquero et al [24] demonstrated that saline injection and secondary hyperpression within the rat pancreatic duct leads to nuclear translocation of NF-Kappa B and to the subsequent intra-acinar transcription of IL-6, MCP-1, KC, etc., but without any trypsinogen activation and this finding was consistant with data from other experimental studies [46]. Therefore, the primary trigger of intra-acinar activation of trypsinogen is still not identified in post-ERCP pancreatitis. Nevertheless, intra-pancreatic transcription of pro-inflammatory cytokines is probably multifactorial in this case: activation of trypsinogen, intraductal hyperpression, oxidative stress, ischemia, etc. [29].

Several studies have demonstrated a correlation between the elevation of serum pancreatic enzyme levels, the volume of the contrast medium injected [47] and the degree of duct opacification [48-50]. Acinarization occurs when the volume injected into the pancreatic duct exceeds the ductal capacity and has been found to be associated with an increased incidence of post-ERCP pancreatic enzyme level elevation and pancreatitis [51, 52]. A rapid rate and high-pressure injection contributes to the development of acinarization [50-53]. Acinarization and intra-ductal hyperpression may probably increase the ischemia of the pancreatic tissue that occurs during acute pancreatitis. During tissue hypoperfusion, cells become ischemic and their reperfusion leads to oxidative stress, release of ROI, lipids peroxidation, transcription of pro-inflammatory cytokines, and finally chemoattraction of monomacrophages and PMN which, in turn, increase the pro-inflammatory cascade and induce tissue necrosis [29]. Post ERCP pancreatitis is a unique model of acute pancreatitis that exists in human, during which, the cascade of inflammatory events occur as in every acute pancreatitis (whatever its etiology); therefore it represents ideal target for immunomodulation.

In this context, immune mechanisms and their modulation (general inhibition of cytokine transcription using drugs or cytokines which block or reduce nuclear translocation of NF-Kappa B, post-transcriptional specific inhibition by administration of IL-10, IL-11, specific inhibition of bioactivity using monoclonal antibodies and receptor antagonists) have become a major topic of interest in acute pancreatitis [23, 37, 54-74]. However, in clinical practice, there is only a narrow therapeutic window, before or shortly after the appearance of the disease, during which it is still possible to modulate the severity of acute pancreatitis by administrating these factors [29].

The contrast media used for pancreatography can provoke pancreatitis. The osmolarity and ionic nature of the contrast media are believed to be the major factors responsible for many of the adverse effects that occur after intravascular administration [75]; thus they have been held responsible for the occurrence of post-procedure pancreatitis. Contrast media, not used in clinical practice at present, may also activate the conversion of trypsinogen into trypsin in the pancreatic juice [76]. Data from previous studies comparing different contrast media, i.e. low-osmolarity agents, usually non-ionic, have been inconclusive. Of the several prospective randomized studies which have attempted to compare the frequency of pancreatic enzyme level elevation, clinical pancreatitis and the quality of pancreatograms with the low- and high-osmolarity agents, some [77, 78] have suggested that low-osmolarity media were safer, whereas others [52, 79, 80] have shown no difference between the media used.

According to the reflux pathogenesis of acute pancreatitis [81, 82], the amount of activated intestinal enzymes carried into the pancreatic ductal system by ERCP manoeuvres is unknown. On the other hand, this theory is contradictory to the fact that, although endoscopic sphincterotomy allows free duodenal content reflux in the pancreatic duct, seems to be prophylactic to post-ERCP pancreatitis as mentioned above [4, 41]. Furthermore, if enzyme activation at ERCP is a major cause of acute pancreatitis, enzyme inhibitors might have a therapeutic role. Previous studies using old protease inhibitors failed to demonstrate any beneficial effects in preventing acute pancreatitis [83, 84]. More recently, gabexate mesilate, a low molecular weight protease inhibitor, has been shown to have a prophylactic effect on ERCP-induced pancreatitis [5].

Introduction of activated intestinal enzymes and bacteria into the pancreatic ductal system by ERCP manoeuvres have been suggested as a possible pathogenetic mechanism. If enzyme activation and bacterial infection are causes of post-ERCP pancreatitis, enzyme inhibitors and antibiotic prophylaxis might have a therapeutic role [85]. Currently, antibiotic use during ERCP is recommended for prophylaxis in preventing cholanghitis, especially in those with jaundice. There is only one prospective randomized placebo controlled trial that identified the lack of antibiotic prophylaxis as independent risk factor for the development of post ERCP pancreatitis in a multivariate analysis suggesting bacteria could play a role in the pathogenesis of post-ERCP pancreatitis [86].

Definitions and Diagnosis

The definition of post-procedure pancreatitis still remains a controversial issue in the field of post-ERCP/sphincterotomy complications, due to the different parameters and criteria adopted. The varying incidence of pancreatitis [1-40% in unselected series of patients] reflects differences in patient populations, indications and endoscopic expertise and, on the other, different definitions of pancreatitis and methods of data collection [85, 87]. Duration of pancreatic-type pain and the amplitude and duration of serum amylase increase are both crucial points in the definition and grading of the pancreatic reaction. Controversy also exists regarding pancreatitis severity; thus definition criteria have been proposed. The Atlanta classification for pancreatitis severity, classifies this complication as mild or severe on the basis of the absence or presence of local (documented by CT scan) or systemic complications, independently of the duration of the hospital stay [88]. On the other hand, length of hospitalization and occurrence of local or systemic complications were used as criteria for establishing the severity of the disease; pancreatitis was defined mild or moderate when no complications occurred and when less than three days or between three and ten days of hospitalization were required, respectively; severe when either local or systemic complications occurred and more than ten days of hospitalization were required [89]. Early detection of those patients who will go on to develop moderate or severe pancreatitis can guide decisions regarding hospital admission and aggressive management. Additionally, early detection can help direct the use of targeted therapies that have the potential to prevent or mitigate pancreatic inflammation.

Early prediction of the occurrence of pancreatitis may be achieved by clinical assessment, laboratory tests or by a combined clinical and laboratory approach [76-78, 87-93]. Clinical assessment alone (i.e. pancreatic-type pain) is not useful since pain in the post-procedure period may occur for several non-pancreatitis-related reasons such as intolerance to air inflation during the procedure. As post-ERCP pancreatitis can take some hours to present clinically, the evaluation of pain alone in the first hours after the procedure is not useful in predicting the occurrence of the complication. Moreover, regarding pain duration, pain persisting for 24 hours, but disappearing within the next 12-24 hours and not requiring a prolonged hospital stay, cannot be considered reliable criteria for defining pancreatitis. It has been proposed that epigastric pain, as an indicator of pancreatitis in the postprocedure period, must persist for at least 24-48 hours [89], or should require a hospital stay of more than 48 hours. Severity of pain could also be a parameter in the classification of pancreatitis. However, in most reports, it has neither been graded nor standardized and its reliability remains uncertain since subjective evaluation makes it difficult to define the degree [85, 87].

Attempts have been made to investigate the role of laboratory tests as predictors of post-ERCP pancreatitis. Three categories of tests may be used: pancreatic enzymes as markers of pancreatic injury, markers of proteolytic activation, and markers of systemic inflammation. Hyperamylasemia cannot be considered a complication, unless the patient also has pain and other signs of pancreatitis. Although the early rise in serum enzyme levels in reaction to manipulations during ERCP may vary considerably in more than 70% of patients [10, 85, 87, 94] without clinical significance, the degree of elevation is much more marked in patients who develop pancreatitis. Serum amylasemia more than five times the upper normal limit lasting for 24 hours after the endoscopic procedure, although suggesting some pancreatic involvement, may occur without clinical symptoms in about one-third of patients, whereas only in about one-third of these cases there is also evidence of computed tomography (CT) scan-confirmed pancreatitis [93, 94]. In the absence of pancreatitis, serum amylase levels peak at 90 minutes to 4 hours after ERCP and return to normal levels within 24-48 hours. Thomas and Sengupta proposed an algorithm for patient management based on stratification by the 4-hour serum amylase level. A 4-hour post-ERCP amylase level less than 1.5 times the upper normal level has been reported predictive in ruling out the risk of developing pancreatitis (negative predictive value 100%) and the patient could be safely discharged home. An amylase level greater than 3 times or more the upper normal limit should be considered a predictor of ongoing pancreatitis [90]. If the value falls between 1.5 and 3.0 times the URL, then clinical assessment, concerns or risk factors should be taken under consideration for management. Two-hour and six-hour serum amylase levels greater than six times and five times the upper normal limit, respectively, have been reported highly predictive for post-ERCP pancreatitis [91, 93]. It has been proposed in a consensus statement based on more than 15,000 procedures [89] that a three-fold increase above the normal serum amylase levels associated with 24-hour persisting pancreatic-type pain is required to establish the presence of post ERCP pancreatitis. A small prospective study [95] suggested elastase-1 serum levels, a protease synthesized by the acinar cells, accurately predict post-ERCP pancreatitis 2 hours after the procedure. Since elastase-1 is not routinely measured in clinical practice while amylase levels associated to clinical settings accurately detect post ERCP pancreatitis, the method is not routinely used for PEP detection.

Trypsinogen, the well-known inactive precursor of trypsin, occurs as two major isoenzymes, trypsinogen 1 (cationic trypsinogen) and trypsinogen 2 (anionic trypsinogen). Trypsinogen Activation Peptide (TAP) is generated in the pancreas when trypsinogen is converted to its active form, trypsin. In healthy subjects, the serum concentration of trypsinogen 1 is higher than that of trypsinogen 2, whereas in acute pancreatitis the trypsinogen 2 levels are higher [96, 97]. Kempainnen et al showed that trypsinogen 2 and trypsin 2-AAT (bound trypsin 2-alpha-1-antitrypsin complex) reflect pancreatic injury after ERCP. In this study, in patients developing pancreatitis, raised trypsinogen 2 concentrations were already evident one hour after ERCP and peaked at six hours, whereas the trypsin 2-AAT complex did not show a clear rise until 24 hours, at which time the trend was still increasing. The sensitivity of a threefold rise in trypsinogen 2 at one hour was 74% and the specificity 87%. Although it did not reach statistical significance, the patients with severe pancreatitis had the highest concentrations of trypsinogen 2 and trypsin 2-AAT. A trypsinogen 2 concentration of over 3000 μg/l at six hours after ERCP was suggested to prompt the clinician to institute intensive monitoring, aggressive fluid transfusion, and antibiotic therapy [98].

Recently, Lempinen et al, using an immunofluorometric assay, studied the very early sequential changes of trypsinogen-1, trypsinogen-2, the trypsin-2-alpha1-antitrypsin complex (T2-AAT), and pancreatic secretory trypsin inhibitor (PSTI) in serum from patients that underwent ERCP with and without post ERCP pancreatitis [99]. Trypsinogen-1 and trypsinogen-2 showed an equally steep increase during the two first hours after ERCP in patients developing acute pancreatitis, but trypsinogen-1 decreased more rapidly than trypsinogen-2, which remained elevated during the 5-day study period. Serum PSTI also increased rapidly whereas T2-AAT increased more slowly peaking at 24 h. In patients developing post-ERCP pancreatitis the median concentration of trypsinogen-1 was markedly higher than in the controls already before the ERCP procedure [100]. The same group also investigated trypsinogen-2 levels in the urine as potential markers; the rapid urinary trypsinogen-2 test in the diagnosis of post-ERCP pancreatitis carried out 6 hours after the procedure, showed 81% sensitivity and 90% specificity. A negative urine dipstick test carried out 6 hours after the procedure seems therefore to be highly reliable for excluding pancreatitis [101]. Plasma and urine levels of TAP (trypsinogen activation peptide) have been found to be elevated and predictive of the development of acute pancreatitis [102]; however, in a study looking specifically at post-ERCP patients, urinary TAP 4 hours after the procedure was not found to be useful in predicting mild pancreatitis.

Since trypsinogen 2 and trypsin 2-AAT are not completely specific for acute pancreatitis but rather can be found elevated in other conditions such as pancreatic, biliary tract, hepatocellular, and colorectal cancers as well as in chronic pancreatitis, pancreatic pseudocysts, and purulent cholangitis, the diagnostic criterion to be used is not the absolute value but the increase in concentration that is induced by ERCP. Considering the fact that clinical and laboratory evaluation has also been found to adequately predict the risk of pancreatitis as soon as only 6 hours after the procedure, the lack of specificity indicates a major drawback for the wide use of trypsinogen 2 and trypsin 2-AAT.

C-reactive protein, an acute phase reactant synthesized by hepatocytes, has been shown to be elevated in patients with acute pancreatitis. In the study of Kiviniemi et al [103], where CRP levels were prospectively studied in patients undergoing ERCP, serum levels have been shown to be greatly elevated only at 48 hours post procedure. C-reactive protein accurately predicts disease severity, but it appears to be a late marker. In the study of Kaw and Singh [14], serum levels were measured before ERCP and at 12-24 hours and 36-48 hours after ERCP. In the 20 patients who developed pancreatitis, CRP serum levels correlated with severity of pancreatitis.

Serum Interleukin (IL-6, IL-10) levels seem to be indicative of the degree of pancreatic injury and inflammation [13, 15, 32, 36, 37], but these markers have been used only for investigational purposes up to now.

Risk Factors

Post-ERCP pancreatitis often has been viewed in the past as an unpredictable and unavoidable complication, with no realistic strategy for its avoidance. During the last 2 decades, many studies have addressed the issue of possible risk factors for PEP and thus, by identifying them, to prevent this complication. Multivariate analyses have delineated patient- and procedure-related factors associated with the risk of this complication, so that post-ERCP pancreatitis is now largely predictable [3, 4, 7-8, 104-106]

Patient Related Risk Factors

Multivariate analyses has revealed that the risk of post-ERCP pancreatitis is determined by patient characteristics as well as technique related factors [3, 4, 6-7, 104]. Therefore, the risk of pancreatitis can largely be estimated before ERCP allowing proper patient selection; ERCP should not be proposed when other less invasive or non-invasive techniques can achieve imaging of the pancreaticobiliary tree or in patients with a low pre-test probability of benefiting form the procedure. When ERCP is indicated, high-risk patients should be informed about the specific risk of postprocedure pancreatitis. Studies have implicated multiple patient related risk factors with female gender, young age, suspected Oddi sphincter dysfunction (SOD), history of prior PEP, recurrent acute pancreatitis and normal bilirubin levels being the most common.

Women have a higher risk of developing PEP. Female gender has been delineated as an independent risk factor by multivariate analysis in most large (>100 patients) retrospective [2, 107], prospective trials [3, 4, 7, 108, 109] and in a metanalysis (odds ratio [OR] 2.23: 95% confidence interval [CI][1.75, 2.84]) [7]. They are also more likely to develop a severe pancreatitis [3]. Almost exclusively, patients with syndrome of Oddi dysfunction are women and this may explain the increased susceptibility of the female gender to PEP development. Nevertheless, it is difficult to short out the contribution of sphincter of Oddi dysfunction to female gender susceptibility and patients with multiple risk factors have dramatically enhanced risk [110].

Sphincter of Oddi dysfunction (SOD) is syndrome of unknown origin, defined as recurrent abdominal pain caused by structural or function abnormalities of the sphincter in the absence of stone(s) or another overt biliary or pancreatic abnormality. A pancreatic variant of SOD can present with a dilated pancreatic duct and/or recurrent episodes of acute pancreatitis or pancreatic type of pain. Often there is no objective evidence of biliary or pancreatic disease, although some patients might have abnormalities in liver and/or pancreatic chemistry, or a dilated pancreatic or biliary duct [4]. Suspected sphincter of Oddi disease has been the dominant risk factor in studies from North America while it has been an infrequent problem in other European reports. Freeman et al demonstrated in a multicenter study of biliary sphincterotomy involving 2347 patients that PEP occurred in 19.1% (2.7% severe) of patients with suspected SOD vs. 3.6% (0.05% severe) of those with other indications for ERCP [4]. Most series report an increase of PEP rate up to 10-30% in patients with suspected SOD [1, 3, 4, 107, 111-113]. By meta-analysis, SOD was associated with post-ERCP pancreatitis of an OR 4.09: 95% CI[3.37, 4.96]) [7]. Patients with SOD comprise the majority of patients with severe post-procedure pancreatitis in most prospective studies - including 11 of the 15 severe cases among 4310 patients undergoing ERCP and/or biliary sphincterotomy in two studies [3, 4]. The heightened susceptibility of these patients for ERCP-related pancreatitis can be seen in patients with normal pancreatic sphincter of Oddi manometry, the frequency of post-ERCP pancreatitis being as high as 18% [113] to 26.3% [3]. It was believed originally that SOD manometry "per se" was a risk factor for PEP. More recently large prospective trials demonstrated that patients not undergoing manometry have a risk similar to that for patients with normal or abnormal manometry [4, 104, 107]. Continuous perfusion was used with early manometry catheters, which were not always directed selectively into the bile or pancreatic duct.

Table 1. Patient related risk factors for post ERCP pancreatitis

Young age	Independent risk factor*
Female gender	Independent risk factor*
Suspected SOD	Independent risk factor*
Prior post-ERCP pancreatitis	Independent risk factor*
Recurrent pancreatitis	Independent risk factor*
Absence of Chronic pancreatitis	Independent risk factor*
Normal serum bilirubin	Possible**
Absence of stone in common bile duct	Possible**
Normal common bile duct diameter	Inconclusive***
Periampullary diverticulum	Inconclusive***
Pancreas divisum	Inconclusive***

* Significant by multivariate analysis in most studies or by meta-analysis.

** Significant by multivariate analysis in some studies, not confirmed in a metanalysis.

***Univariate analysis and/or conflicting data between prospective studies.

These factors likely account for some cases of perfusion-related hydrostatic injury, particularly those occurring after placement of the catheter in the pancreatic duct [114]. With the widespread use of aspirating instead of conventional perfusion catheters, the risk of manometry has probably been reduced to that of cannulation with any other ERCP accessory [110, 112]. Furthermore, SOD manometry is performed in populations with suspected SOD, a high-risk population as it has been previously stated. Prior acute or recurrent pancreatitis appears to act synergistically with SOD for PEP induction (OR 2.46: 95% CI [1.93,3.12]) [7, 104].

Younger patients have been shown to have an increase risk for PEP. Unfortunately, the definition of younger age among studies varies considerably since cut-off values of 50, 60 and 70 years have been used [4, 6-8]. A history of post-ERCP pancreatitis was reported to be independent risk factor in three prospective studies (18%-26%) [1, 3, 104]. Variations in anatomy such as the presence of periampullary diverticulum, gastrectomy with Billroth II anastomosis, and pancreas divisum have all been implicated as possible variables for PEP induction but existing data are inconclusive [1, 3, 4, 105]. A non-dilated common bile duct in the pre-procedure setting has been implicated as an independent risk factor for the development of PEP by some studies by multivariate analysis [3, 8, 111] but other works have not confirmed this finding [7, 104, 106]. Conflicting data regarding patients with normal bile duct diameter may be due to the fact that these patients might not have a true biliary disease, thus a poor ERCP indication [115], or in earlier studies in which only univariate analysis small duct diameter may have been a surrogate marker for SOD [110].

Risk factors appear to be synergistic; in the study of Freeman et al female gender, suspected SOD, and a normal serum bilirubin were associated with a PEP developing risk of 16 times higher than that for male gender and jaundice, the increase being independent of any technique-related factors [3].

Procedure Related Risk Factors

Technical factors have long been recognized to be important in causing post-ERCP pancreatitis. Papillary trauma, difficult cannulation, precut sphincterotomy, biliary and pancreatic sphincterotomy, injection of contrast media into the pancreatic duct, balloon-dilation of the biliary sphincter have all been reported to lead to an increased risk of developing post-ERCP pancreatitis. However, in the metanalysis performed by an Italian group, several potential risk factors, such as the difficulty of cannulation, could not be analyzed due to the heterogeneity of the studies [7].

Table 2. Procedure related risk factors for post ERCP pancreatitis

Pancreatic duct injection	Independent risk factor*
Pancreatic sphincterotomy	Independent risk factor*
Balloon dilation of intact biliary sphincter	Independent risk factor*
Difficult or failed cannulation	Independent risk factor*
Pre-cut sphincterotomy	Independent risk factor*
Minor papilla sphincterotomy	Possible**
Pancreatic acinarization	Possible**
Pancreatic brush cytology	Possible**
Low endoscopist volume	Possible**
Prior failed ERCP	Inconclusive***
Intramural contrast injection	Inconclusive***
Therapeutic vs diagnostic	Inconclusive***
Biliary sphincterotomy	Inconclusive***
Sphincter of Oddi manometry	Inconclusive***

* Significant by multivariate analysis in most studies or by meta-analysis.
** Significant by multivariate analysis in some studies, not confirmed in a metanalysis.
***Univariate analysis and/or conflicting data between prospective studies.

Trauma of the Papilla

Papillary trauma induced by difficult cannulation has a negative effect that is independent of the number of pancreatic duct contrast injections [3, 4, 6, 104, 106, 109]. The term "difficult cannulation" refers to the need for numerous attempts at cannulation before deep biliary or pancreatic duct access can be obtained, or the use of additional techniques to facilitate access. Copious manipulations of the papilla may result to edema of the papilla and the pancreatic sphincter, thus leading to mechanical obstruction of the pancreatic juice outflow, elevation of the hydrostatic pressure in the pancreatic duct and initiation of the inflammatory cascade. The importance of this mechanism has been highlighted by a Japanese group [41]: in their study, the authors showed that, although the frequency of ES-induced pancreatitis is significantly higher than that of post-ERCP pancreatitis, the frequency of severe pancreatitis within 48 hours and the worsening of pancreatitis after 48 hours is significantly lower within the group of patients who contracted ES-induced pancreatitis. In the large prospective study of Freeman et al, pancreatitis occurred in 2.5% of ERCP in which there was no pancreatic duct contrast injection at all [3]. Two studies have shown that the incidence of post ERCP pancreatitis increases with the degree of difficulty in cannulation [4, 104]. Deep, blind cannulation increases the chances of submucosal papillary lesions or pancreatic duct perforation with associated submucosal or intraparenchymal contrast injection; submucosal injection renders further endoscopic manoeuvres difficult, while duct perforation more commonly causes acute pancreatic inflammation [111, 116].

Endoscopic papillary balloon-dilation is a procedure where the biliary sphincter is dilated to allow extraction of bile duct stones. This method has been introduced as an alternative to biliary sphincterotomy to avoid complications associated to the latter method (i.e. bacterial colonization, increased bile lithogenicity, contamination with cytotoxins) since the former technique preserves the integrity of the biliary sphincter [117]. Randomized trials from referral centres in Europe and Asia have shown complications to be equivalent to or less than for sphincterotomy [117-122]. On the other hand, balloon dilation has been associated with a markedly increased risk of pancreatitis (15,4%) in other U.S. studies compared with 0,8% for patients undergoing biliary sphincterotomy [3, 123]. Two deaths were also noted in one randomized controlled study [123]. In general, balloon dilation is not recommended for extraction of bile duct stones unless there is a relative contraindication to sphincterotomy such as coagulopathy or need for early anticoagulation. Balloon dilation should especially be avoided in higher-risk patients such as younger patients who are anicteric – the very patients in whom one might otherwise be most interested in sphincter preservation [110].

Thermal injury has been implicated in causing pancreatitis after biliary sphincterotomy. Two randomized studies showed that pure cutting current significantly reduced pancreatitis rates when compared with the more conventional blended current (3% vs 11% and 3,2 vs 12,9 respectively) [124, 125]. Bipolar cautery, which is seldom used, was shown in one study to result in significantly lower rates of pancreatitis than conventional monopolar cautery (0 vs 6 %) [126]. Automated current delivery systems that can be programmed to deliver a specific tissue effect, such as ERBE (Surgical Technology Group, Hampshire, England, UK) are now increasingly used, but their effect on pancreatitis is unclear [110]. Pancreatitis as a result of thermal injury from papillectomy has been reported in retrospective series from 6% to 17% [127-129].

Contrast Agent Injection

Opacification of the main pancreatic duct alone is associated with a 31% incidence of hyperamylasemia; this figure is similar to the 24% incidence of hyperamylasemia which occurs after cholangiography alone [48]. On the grounds that it is the toxicity of the injected material that triggers PEP, agents of high or low osmolarity (non-ionic vs ionic) have been evaluated as possible etiologic factors in multiple studies [52, 80, 130-132]; nonetheless no significant difference was demonstrated between groups of different contrast agents in a recent metanalysis of 13 randomized controlled trials and over 3300 patients included [133].

Multiple pancreatic duct injections significantly increase the risk of post-ERCP pancreatitis as shown by univariate analysis in most studies, multivariate analysis [1, 3, 4, 6, 7, 104, 106-108, 131, 134] and a metanalysis [7]. Injection pressure and volume of the contrast medium injected into the pancreatic duct both contribute to ductal epithelial or acinar injury. This injury probably occurs from the disruption of cellular membranes or tight junctions between the cells with a backflow of the intraductal content into the interstitial space as noted previously [44]. Elevation of the pancreatic enzyme level has been shown to correlate with the volume of the contrast medium injected [47] and the degree of pancreatic duct opacification [48, 49, 51, 53]. Acinarization of the pancreas, although undesirable, is probably less important than generally thought, because it has not been shown to be an independently significant risk factor in multivariate analyses [1, 3, 4, 7, 8, 106, 110]. In the study of Freeman et al [4], even if the acinarization of the pancreas was significantly more frequent in patients who developed pancreatitis at univariate analysis, this risk disappeared at multivariate analysis when ES was performed whereas in the large prospective multi-centre trial of Cheng et al acinarization was not associated with PEP either in univariate or multivariate analysis [1]. Other manipulations of the pancreatic duct (such as obtaining pancreatic cytology samples) have also been associated with increased risk of pancreatitis in univariate [108] and multivariate analysis [104].

Biliary, Pancreatic Sphincterotomy and Precut Technique

Overall, risk of pancreatitis is generally similar for diagnostic and therapeutic ERCP [3, 7, 91]. Most large prospective studies have not shown standard biliary sphincterotomy [BS] to add significant independent risk of pancreatitis to ERCP [1, 3, 7, 106, 108]. Nonetheless biliary sphincterotomy was widely considered as risk factor for PEP in the past [84] but this finding was confirmed by multivariate analysis only in two recent retrospective studies [107, 109]. This points not to the safety of sphincterotomy but instead to the risk associated with diagnostic ERCP [110]. Whether biliary sphincterotomy should be performed for placement of large-caliber biliary stents remains controversial; two studies, one retrospective and one randomized protective suggested no added risk of PEP and even a protective role with BS respectively [113, 135]. When sphincterotomy is not performed, the tip of the outer flange on a large-caliber biliary stent may push into the pancreatic duct orifice and may contribute to sphincter trauma and pancreatitis, especially if an inward traction effect on the stent is maintained by a tight biliary stricture [110].

Pancreatic sphincterotomy was found to be a significant risk factor for pancreatitis by multivariate analysis in the study of Freeman et al [3], although the risk of severe pancreatitis was very small (less than one percent), perhaps because nearly all of these patients had pancreatic drainage via a pancreatic stent. Cheng et al, in their large prospective multicenter study delineated pancreatic sphincterotomy of the major and the minor papilla to be PEP associated in the univariate analysis but multivariate analysis associated only minor papilla sphincterotomy with an increased risk of PEP [OR3.8, 95% CI(2.003–7.106)] [1]. This finding was further confirmed by multivariate analysis in a large retrospective study from a tertiary referral European center [2].

Precut papillotomy or needle-knife sphicterotomy is a technique to gain access to the common bile duct when, despite standard catheters and sphincterotomes use, selective deep biliary cathterization remains unsuccessfull. Cutting into the major papilla has the potential risk to lacerate and injure the pancreatic sphincter as well as to cause significant tissue injury, swelling, bleeding and perforation. Moreover, this often comes after prolonged attempts of cannulation [115]. Precut technique has been shown to be independent risk factor for PEP in multicenter studies [3, 4, 7, 8] and in a metanalysis (OR 2.71: 95% CI[2.02, 3.63]) [7], although it has been suggested that the added risk is rather due to multiple prolonged manoeuvres in the papilla while attempting to cannulate than to the technique itself [110, 136-138]. However, this elevated risk emerges even after adjusting for other variables such as difficulty of cannulation, number of pancreatic injections [4, 7]. In contrast, series from tertiary referral centers have found complication rates no different than for standard sphincterotomy [137, 139-143] suggesting that risk of precut sphincterotomy is highly operator-dependent. One explanation for the assumpted low risk of precut sphincterotomy could be case selection, such that pre-cutting is used only for patients at relatively low risk (e.g., older patients with obstructive jaundice) and with favorable anatomy, including a prominent papilla, whereas, standard traction sphincterotomy is performed in many other higher-risk circumstances, such as suspected SOD, only after free cannulation is achieved. Another explanation, also likely to be valid, is that the outcome of precut papillotomy is highly operator dependent [110] although this was not confirmed in a study reporting a single endocopist expert experience [144]. Use of pancreatic stents prior to needle-knife precut, different technique, or different case mix may account in part for lower rates of precut-induced pancreatitis by other advanced endoscopists [110]. Needle-knife papillotomy over a pancreatic stent placed during the early stages of the procedure was shown to be substantially safer than conventional pull-type sphincterotomy without a pancreatic stent in patients with SOD [112]. Complications of precut sphincterotomy probably vary with the indication for the procedure (most risky with sphincter of Oddi dysfunction in the absence of pancreatic stenting) and the interactive effect between anatomic factors such as small papillas and operator related factors [110].

Use of a sphincterotome for biliary cannulation has been prospectively compared to a standard catheter in two randomized trials [145, 146]. Although both showed significantly higher success with the sphincterotome, there was no difference in rates of pancreatitis or other complications. The use of a steerable catheter was prospectively evaluated vs standard catheter for initial cannulation in a randomized study, which did not show any increases risk of PEP [147]. A randomized trial found that placement of a guidewire in the pancreatic duct facilitated biliary cannulation compared with persistent attempts at cannulation by using conventional techniques, with no episodes of pancreatitis in either group [148].

Operator Related Risk Factors

Independently of the technique-related risk factors, operator experience also seems to be a potential risk-factor for post-ERCP/ES complications although most multicenter studies have failed to show a significant correlation between endoscopist ERCP case volumes and pancreatitis rates [3, 4, 149]. In one study, endoscopists averaging more than 100 ERCP per year did not have significantly lower pancreatitis rates, but did have substantially higher rates of success at bile duct access (96.5% versus 91.5% for lower volume endoscopists) [3]. It is possible that none of the participating endoscopists in those studies reached the threshold volume of ERCP above which pancreatitis rates would diminish (perhaps greater than 250-

500 cases per year) [110]. However, the reported rates of pancreatitis from the highest volume tertiary referral centers in the U.S. are often relatively higher than those in private practices [3, 4]. This finding is in consistence with data from a large Italian multicenter prospective studie [8] that showed significant differences in the outcome of ERCP between low- (less than 200 ERCPs/year) and large- (more than 200 ERCPs/year) volume centers. Large-volume centers had significantly less overall complications (2.0 % vs. 7.1 %, $P<0.001$) and less complication-related deaths (0.18 % vs. 0.75 %, $P<0.05$), while the risk of pancreatitis was significantly increased in low-volume centers in the univariate analysis (relative risk 2.8). Rabenstein et al [150] found that cumulative live-time volumes of the endoscopists ("ERCP-experience") had no influence on the occurrence of complications, while a low ERCP-frequency (ongoing volumes less than 40 procedures per year) was the only significant risk factor for complications (9.3 % vs. 5.6 %; $P<0.05$). The same group confirmed these data in a prospective study [151].

The interactive effect of multiple risk factors is reflected in the profile of patients developing severe post-ERCP pancreatitis. In two different studies, nearly all of the patients who developed severe or fatal pancreatitis were young to middle-aged women with recurrent abdominal pain, a normal serum bilirubin, and with no biliary obstructive pathology. Regarding the procedure, nearly half were purely diagnostic procedures whereas prophylactic pancreatic stent placement was not used [3, 134].

Factors That Can Reduce the Risk of Pancreatitis

Technique Related

1. Pancreatic Stents

Trans-sphincter placement of a pancreatic stent is a relatively new and increasingly popular approach to reducing the risk of PEP. Theoretically, stents mitigate instrumental papillary trauma and maintain the flow of pancreatic juice, and/or empty the gland of reactive enzyme substrate; therefore, the effects of hydrostatic overpressure to the pancreatic duct are minimized. According to the "plumbing" concept, drainage of manipulated pancreatic ducts should prevent pancreatitis, just as drainage of obstructed bile ducts prevents cholangitis. Five prospective randomized controlled trials (3 fully published, two in abstract form), at least 7 case-control studies, and one meta-analysis have compared rates of pancreatitis after ERCP with and without a pancreatic stent [112,113,150]. These studies have involved heterogeneous high-risk groups of patients (various combinations of pre-cut sphincterotomy, SOD, difficult cannulation, pancreatic sphincterotomy, biliary balloon dilation for stones, papillectomy, and attempted pancreatic stent insertion).

Eleven of the 12 studies, and all of those that enrolled more than 30 patients, found either a trend or a statistically significantly lower rate of PEP in patients who had a pancreatic stent placed (range 0%-20%) compared with patients in whom a pancreatic stent was not inserted (range 6%-67%); statistical significance was evident in 3 of the 5 randomized controlled trials [152, 153]. In a meta-analysis of 5 prospective studies involving 483 patients who were considered to be at high risk for developing PEP, the odds ratio of PEP without stent was 3-

fold higher than that with stent (15.5% vs. 5.8%; OR 3.2: 95% CI[1.6, 6.4]) [107]. In this metanalysis 11.4% of patients developed pancreatitis after ERCP. Statistical analysis disclosed that a pancreatic stent must be placed in 10 patients to prevent one episode of acute pancreatitis. In one study that was used in the metanalysis, the one with historical controls, it was found that in 436 patients treated for SOD with biliary sphincterotomy, with or without pancreatic sphincterotomy, the rate of pancreatitis rates was 28.2% (5.4% severe) in those who underwent simple pull-type biliary sphincterotomy without a pancreatic stent vs. 13.5% (0.4% severe) in those who had biliary sphincterotomy, with or without pancreatic sphincterotomy, plus placement of a pancreatic stent ($p < 0.05$); there was a tendency for the rate of pancreatitis to be lower if a pancreatic stent was placed before (10.7%) as opposed to after (19.2%) pancreaticobiliary sphincterotomy [112]. Moreover, it has been shown, that stenting seems to help minimize the severity of pancreatitis in those who develop it [113, 152,154-155]. In fact, data from the metanalysis show that among the patients who had pancreatic stent placement, all episodes of post-ERCP pancreatitis were mild in severity.

The type and size of pancreatic stents that have been made to reduce the risk of PEP remain nonstandardized [156]. Ideally, the pancreatic stent would be made of soft material, narrow, without flaps, thus allowing pancreatic duct drainage without causing any trauma during placement, while it would spontaneously migrate in the duodenum within a week. After stent insertion, sometimes only of brief duration, pancreatic ductal and parenchymal changes have been observed in approximately one third to two thirds of patients, especially those with previously normal pancreatic ducts. Stents made of newer materials that are softer than the traditional polyethylene and with smaller inner flanges will probably cause less duct injury, although this has not been established.

Ductal changes have been observed mostly with traditional flanged 5F or 7F stents, which may be of similar diameter to the pancreatic duct, are made of rigid polyethylene, and have large pointed inner flanges, all factors that may be injurious to the duct, including injury that occurs during stent removal [113]. Therefore, pancreatic stents used for this purpose are narrow [3-5 Fr in diameter] and short [5 cm in length, or less]. A recent study found that unflanged, longer 3F stents with a single duodenal pigtail were associated with a substantially lower frequency of ductal changes (24%) compared with 5F and 6F stents (80%) and were not observed to migrate proximally into the duct [157]. Insertion of a 3F stent was also associated with a slightly lower rate of PEP (7.5%) compared with a 5F (9.8% pancreatitis) or a 6F stent (14.6%).

Pancreatic injury may be related to the duration of time the stent remains in place; therefore, it is necessary either to document passage of a pancreatic stent with a plain abdominal radiograph or to remove it endoscopically, preferably within 2 weeks if placed as a prophylactic measure. The rate of spontaneous passage of a 3F, unflanged pancreatic stent has been shown to be substantially higher (86%) than that for traditional 4F to 6F stents (65%-73%) ($p < 0.001$) [157]. Placement of nasopancreatic drains has been proposed as an alternative to the pancreatic stent, because the former can be removed without an endoscopic procedure. Nasopancreatic catheters are of a relatively large diameter (4F or 5F), while some are flanged, thus a concern for possible ductal injury is raised when they are placed in the relatively narrower duct in the body or in the tail of the pancreas. Moreover, overnight hospitalization is required.

Ironically, attempts at pancreatic stent placement may cause pancreatic trauma. If attempts at pancreatic stent placement fail the risk of PEP is extremely high [158]. Moreover, it may be difficult to decide which patient and which procedure warrant pancreatic stent insertion. Brackbill et al [156] conducted a survey to assess the current practice patterns of expert biliary endoscopists regarding prophylactic pancreatic duct stents. Prophylactic pancreatic duct stents were used by 96% of respondents. Stent use was universal during ampullectomy and pancreatic sphincterotomy. Most also used stents for minor papillotomy (93%) and sphincter of Oddi dysfunction (SOD) confirmed by manometry (82%). Endoscopists disagreed on the following: precut sphincterotomy, prior post-ERCP pancreatitis, suspected SOD, and traumatic sphincterotomy. Endoscopists used straight stents, pigtail stents, or a combination. Internal flanges were always used by 14%, never used by 54%, and sometimes used by 32%. Recently, Das et al [159] published a cost effectiveness analysis to evaluate the most cost-effective strategy for preventing post-ERCP pancreatitis where they showed that pancreatic-stent placement for the prevention of post-ERCP pancreatitis in high-risk patients is a cost-effective strategy.

It is unclear whether pancreatic stent placement will achieve similar benefits outside major centers. Most non-tertiary center endoscopists and endoscopy units are unfamiliar with the techniques and equipment needed for placement of pancreatic stents, especially the small diameter guidewires (0.018-0.025 inch) used to place the smaller 3F and 4F stents that appear to be optimal for avoiding ductal injury and for preventing pancreatitis. The effectiveness and the safety of pancreatic stent placement by endoscopists in the community would be expected to be less than for advanced centers. Specific training in techniques for pancreatic stent placement is recommended [157]. Overall, pancreatic stent placement appears promising as a strategy for prevention of PEP, one that has dramatically altered outcomes for high-risk patients undergoing ERCP at centres where the technique is used.

2. Guidewire Cannulation

Guidewire cannulation has been proposed as a simple way to avoid PEP [160]. In this technique, the biliary or the pancreatic duct are not selectively catheterized after contrast injection but rather cannulated with a guidewire inserted through a catheter or a sphincterotome. Since selective catheterization is often achieved without previous duct opacification, guidewire cannulation possibly reduces the risk of PEP by minimizing the risk of hydrostatic injury to the pancreas. Michopoulos et al [160] reported a success rate of 95% in deep cannulation of the bile duct with the use of a hydrophilic guidewire. PEP was reported in 2.3% of patients. Lella et al [161] also reported a significant risk reduction for PEP by using a hydrophilic guidewire in selective catheterization of the bile duct with a reported success rate over 97%. This was a prospective randomized trial; with all procedures performed by the same endoscopist and in the study design a power analysis was conducted for detecting differences at the 5% level of significance. Although this study's results were encouraging, this technique was not studied in a high-risk group of population and more data are needed.

Pharmacologic Prevention

Pharmacotherapy has been widely studied in the prevention of PEP during the last three decades. Up to now, routine prophylaxis has been neither adopted in the majority of centers that conduct ERCP procedures nor recommended in guidelines. This means that most endoscopists in the ERCP field believe that expertise and technique, more than pharmacologic prophylaxis, play a major role in the prevention of postprocedure pancreatitis. Medications to prevent PEP can be classified into those that affect sphincter pressure or contractility and those that affect pancreatic secretion. Topical lidocaine spray on the papilla, IV nifedipine, glyceryl trinitrate, subcutaneous low molecular weight heparin, prednisone, allopurinol, N-acetylcysteine, IV recombinant human IL-10, diclofenac, somatostatin, octreotide, and gabexate have all been evaluated. Conclusions from these studies cannot be easily extracted since either a given drug has been tested with different dosages or modalities of administration with contradictory results, or results from small studies have not been confirmed.

Agents Affecting Sphincter Function

Several agents have been used in an effort to relax the sphincter of Oddi and to promote pancreatic drainage and, thereby, prevent pancreatitis. Nifedipine, a calcium channel antagonist, decreases the basal pressure at the sphincter of Oddi. It also lowers the amplitude, shortens the duration and decreases the frequency of sphincter contraction in healthy volunteers [162]. This agent was ineffective in two trials that randomized 321 patients to receive regular or long acting nifedipine or placebo [163, 164].

The results with nitroglycerine in two randomized trials were more encouraging. Nitroglycerine (glyceryl trinitrate, GTN) administered sublingually or transdermally reduces sphincter of Oddi basal pressure and motility in normal individuals and relaxes the sphincter [165]. In one study, 186 patients at average risk for pancreatitis were randomized to sublingual nitroglycerine or placebo before ERCP, and a significant reduction in the frequency of pancreatitis was observed in the nitroglycerine group (7.7% vs. 17.8%; $p < 0.05$); the drug was primarily effective in patients undergoing diagnostic ERCP and in those who had cholangiography alone, which generally is low risk [166]. In the other study, 144 patients at average risk were randomized to a nitroglycerine patch or a placebo [167,168]. There was a significant reduction in the frequency of pancreatitis in the nitroglycerine group (4% vs. 15%; p=0.03) and, by multivariate analysis; treatment with nitroglycerine was independently significant. The scepticism in both of these studies includes unusually high rates of pancreatitis in the control groups (low- to average-risk patient groups) and limited assessment of efficacy in higher-risk patients. Kaffes et al evaluated the effect of transdermal GTN in facilitating cannulation or PEP prevention in either average or high-risk patient groups [108]. No difference in cannulation times or difficulty was appreciated and there was no difference in the incidence of post-ERCP pancreatitis. This study also had the reservation of small statistical sample. Furthermore, it is not surprising that nitroglycerin had no apparent effect on facilitating cannulation. Mechanical factors such as the angle between the ducts and ampulla and papillary stiffness are probably more important determinants of successful cannulation than the size and patency of the papillary orifice [169].

A topical spray of lidocaine on the papilla has been proposed to have a relaxing effect based on the fact that this agent blocks intramural neural reflexes in the small intestine and the sphincter of Oddi. However, a randomized trial in average-risk patients with a low background rate of pancreatitis did not demonstrate efficacy [164].

Prophylactic Antibiotics

Administration of antibiotics was postulated by one group of investigators to prevent pancreatitis by limiting secondary infection. A randomized trial in 321 patients compared prophylactically administered ceftazidime to placebo: the frequency of pancreatitis was significantly lower in the antibiotic-treated group (2.6% vs. 9.4%; p=0.009), a finding sustained in a multivariate analysis with a limited number of potentially confounding variables [86]. In another randomized controlled trial of 100 patients no significant difference was found in the incidence of PEP between the group treated with intravenous cefotaxime and the group given placebo (4% versus 6%) [170]. These conflicting data need to be verified in larger studies.

Agents Interfering with the Inflammatory Cascade

Efforts to prevent PEP have focused on a variety of agents that interrupt the inflammatory cascade at various points. Corticosteroid in various forms (methylprednisolone, prednisone, and hydrocortisone) has been extensively investigated as possible means of reducing the incidence of PEP. One retrospective observational study (without adjustment for confounding variables or multivariate analysis) suggested that corticosteroids might be protective [171]. Subsequently, 5 randomized controlled trials, with over 2500 patients, demonstrated no benefit, or any trend toward a benefit, for various corticosteroid formulations [172-176]. Recently, a large multicenter prospective blinded controlled trial [177] enrolled 1115 patients in two groups to receive 40 mgr prednisone per os or placebo, evaluating whether prophylactic corticosteroids) will reduce the incidence of post-ERCP pancreatitis. There was no difference in the incidence of pancreatitis or the frequency of investigated potential pancreatitis risk factors between the corticosteroid and placebo groups.

In a similar approach, it was hoped that xanthine oxidase inhibitors, such as allopurinol, might prevent PEP by inhibiting generation of oxygen-derived free radicals. Allopurinol has been evaluated in two randomized controlled trials of approximately 1000 patients in total. Both trials found no difference in the frequency of PEP in patients given allopurinol compared with those given a placebo [172, 178]. In the prospective randomized controlled study of Katsinelos et al though, pre-treatment with high-dose, orally administered allopurinol decreased the frequency of PEP [179]. Of special interest is the fact that total rates of pancreatitis of all 3 studies in the allopurinol groups (62 of 579, 10.7%) and the placebo groups (71 of 565, 12.6%) are not statistically different [180]. Of note, the allopurinol dosage and the timing of administration differ among all 3 studies: 600 mg at 15 and 3 hours before ERCP in the Katsinelos study, 600 mg at 4 hours and 300 mg 1 hour before ERCP in the Mosler study, and 200 mg at 15 hours and 3 hours before ERCP in the Budzynska study. The negative findings in the Mosler study argue strongly against the theory that insufficient quantities of allopurinol explained the disparity in findings in the Katsinelos and Budzynska studies.

In a similar context, another free radical scavenger, N-acetylcysteine, was studied as a possible agent for PEP prevention. A prospective, double-blind, placebo-controlled trial was conducted in 256 patients randomized to receive intravenous N-acetylcysteine at a loading dose of 70 mg/kg 2 hours before and 35 mg/kg at 4-hour intervals for a total of 24 hours after the procedure, or to receive normal saline solution as placebo [181]. There were no statistical differences in the incidence of PEP, severity grades or the mean duration of hospitalization for pancreatitis between the groups.

There are studies of inhibitors of the platelet-activating factor for the experimental and clinical modulation of the severity of acute pancreatitis. Unfortunately, the preliminary results of a large, multicenter, prospective, randomized trial do not indicate any reduction in PEP when using these agents [182]. Recombinant interleukin 10 (IL-10) has been evaluated for prophylactic immunomodulation of the pro-inflammatory cascade, with encouraging results in experimental models [183, 184]. A randomized trial that included 144 higher-risk patients undergoing ERCP found lower rates of pancreatitis in each of two treatment groups (3% and 5%) vs. the control group (11%) ($p < 0.05$). Multivariate analysis showed the distribution of risk factors was somewhat imbalanced between the groups; however it disclosed Il-10 association with a decreased likehood of developing PEP [OR 0.46, 95% CI 0.22-0.96; p=0.39] [60]. In contrast, another study of average-risk patients in which a lower dose of IL-10 (8 mcg/kg) was administered failed to demonstrate any significant difference, or any trend toward a difference, in the frequency of pancreatitis in treated patients (11%) vs. those given a placebo (9%) [60]. A meta-analysis of published data suggested that IL-10 was effective in preventing PEP with a frequency of 7.1% in the treated group vs. 13.9% in the placebo group (p=0.003), thus, raising a hope that this drug is effective [185].

The newest but simplest agent for interrupting the inflammatory cascade, based partly on its ability to inhibit phospholipase A2, is diclofenac, an orally administered non-steroidal anti-inflammatory drug (NSAID). A single randomized trial in 220 patients suggested that diclofenac given as a rectal suppository immediately after ERCP was associated with a frequency of pancreatitis of 6.4% compared with 15.5% in a control group (p=0.049) [186]. NSAIDs can inhibit the early inflammatory cascade involving phospholipase-A2, prostaglandins, or endothelial neutrophil attachment during acute pancreatitis. A larger multicenter study is needed to confirm the protective role of NSAIDs since this was a single center study and diclofenac was not effective in the subgroup of patients with SOD, the very group of patients that are at greatest risk. And, there is the further concern for the potential adverse effects of a NSAID with respect to renal function and bleeding.

One of the most promising agents for prevention of PEP, one used in routine clinical practice in some parts of the world, especially in Asia, is the protease inhibitor gabexate [5, 187]. Prevention of intra-acinar trypsinogen activation to trypsin and the subsequent inflammatory cascade may be achieved by using antiprotease agents. In 1995, a study [188] on the first attempt at a using C1-inhibitor (C1-INH) plasma concentrate was published. The blockage of ongoing complement and contact system activation by high doses of C1-INH has been reported to improve the outcome of acute pancreatitis in experimental models [189]. Gabexate mesilate was shown to be effective in preventing post-ERCP pancreatitis in a prospective, multicenter, controlled trial involving 418 patients: the incidence of pancreatitis was reduced four-fold in the treatment group compared with the placebo group (2% vs. 8%)

[5, 190]. An initial meta-analysis of these two trials suggested that gabexate significantly reduced the risk of pancreatitis (OR 0.27: 95% CI [0.13, 0.57]); the number needed to treat to prevent one episode of pancreatitis was relatively high at 27 [190]. A subsequent large multicenter study of gabexate as a single dose before ERCP and continued for 2 hours thereafter found no significant difference in the frequency of pancreatitis in the treatment group (8.1%) vs. the placebo group (6.5%). A second meta-analysis from the same group including papers published up to 2003 on the prevention of post-ERCP pancreatitis with somatostatin and gabexate, in both standard and high-risk patients, suggested that when all studies were combined, gabexate was barely effective (OR 0.58: 95% CI [0.34, 0.99]), with the number needed to treat being 35; in addition, gabexate given as a short-term infusion (<4 hours) was found to be ineffective [106]. A disadvantage of the gabexate mesilate prophylaxis is the need for a 12-hour infusion; however, a recent multicenter study by the same group has demonstrated that a 6-hour infusion was as effective as a 12-hour infusion [187]. In the end of last year, Testoni et al reported the experience of their centre in over 2400 patients. Data from 1312 patients who underwent ERCP procedures without gabexate prophylaxis and from 1149 consecutive patients with 1g i.v. gabexate, were retrospectively evaluated during a 6-year period. Statistical analysis was also performed in groups of standard- and high-risk subjects and data for cost effectiveness were also assessed. The frequency of pancreatitis appeared significantly reduced in the gabexate period in comparison with before gabexate in overall cases (2.2% versus 3.9%; p=0.019); however, the reduction was significant only for high-risk patients (3.8% versus 7.3%; p=0.001). Furthermore, gabexate appeared unable to reduce the incidence of severe pancreatitis [191]. A double-blind multicenter prospective randomized controlled trial studied 1127 patients undergoing ERCP to receive intravenous administration of 750 mcg somatostatin, 500 mg gabexate mesylate, or placebo [192]. The drug infusion started 30 minutes before and continued for 6 hours after endoscopy. No significant differences in incidences of pancreatitis, hyperamylasemia, or abdominal pain were observed among the placebo (4.8%, 32.6%, and 5.3%, respectively), somatostatin (6.3%, 26.8%, and 5.1%, respectively), and gabexate mesylate groups (5.8%, 31.5%, and 6.3%, respectively). Recently a third metanalysis including 4 prospective randomized controlled trials; three from Italy and one from China were published [193]. The authors concluded that gabexate mesilate cannot prevent the pancreatic injury after ERCP. Overall, at present, routine prophylactic administration of gabexate mesilate in all patients undergoing ERCP cannot be suggested.

Heparin has been shown to have anti-inflammatory properties, to inhibit the activity of pancreatic proteases and improve pancreatic circulation. Salas et al [194] found that heparin reduces TNF-alpha-induced inflammation by inhibiting the interaction between leukocytes and endothelium. Rabenstein et al showed in a prospective analysis of risk factors for PEP after ERCP with endoscopic sphincterotomy that the administration of any type of heparin was associated with a reduction in the frequency of PEP from 7.9% (43/547) to 3.4% (9/268; p=0.005) [150]. There was no increase in the number of bleeding events in the heparin treated group compared with the placebo group. In a study that followed the preliminary report of this observation [195], heparin significantly improved the course in 3 different experimental animal models (rats) of mild to moderate pancreatitis [196]. Continuous intravenous treatment with unfractionated heparin was started before induction of pancreatitis, and it resulted in significantly reduced edema, inflammation, and peak serum amylase values compared with control animals. However, in a separate randomized controlled study by the same research group in 458 high-risk patients, there was no reduction in the incidence of PEP in the low-molecular-heparin group compared to placebo [197].

Agents Affecting Pancreatic Secretion

The antisecretory agent somatostatin and its long-acting analogue octreotide have been extensively evaluated for the prevention of PEP. Somatostain and octreotide affect the exocrine function of the pancreas directly by reducing the secretion of digestive enzymes and indirectly by inhibiting secretin and cholecystokinin production. Besides their antisecretory effects, somatostatin and octreotide modulate the cytokine cascade and may also have a protective effect on pancreatic cells [198, 199]. Furthermore, animal studies have shown that both substances have protective effects in experimental acute pancreatitis. Octreotide has the advantage of simple administration by subcutaneous injection, whereas somatostatin requires continuous parenteral infusion. On the other hand, octreotide stimulates and raises the pressure of the sphincter of Oddi.

Somatostatin has been administered for prophylactic purposes either by 2 to 26-hour prolonged i.v. infusion or by a single bolus administration immediately before the ERCP procedure. Over the last 15 years, over 15 randomized controlled trials and 2 metanalysis have been published. Somatostatin statistically significantly reduced the risk of PEP in only 3 [106,200,201] randomized controlled trials. In an initial meta-analysis, of 28 clinical trials with somatostatin (12 papers), octreotide (10 papers), and gabexate (6 papers), somatostatin was found to be effective (OR 0.38: 95% CI[0.22, 0.65]) [190]. None of these studies investigated the efficacy in high-risk patients. A subsequent large scale, multicenter, placebo-controlled trial in 382 patients found that a single dose of somatostatin at 750 μg and continued for 2 hours after infusion was ineffective in preventing pancreatitis; pancreatitis occurred in 11.5% of patients who received somatostatin vs. 6.5% of those given a placebo [106]. A second meta-analysis of somatostatin by the same investigators who performed the first, in which data from short- and long-term infusion studies were pooled, found somatostatin to be ineffective (OR 0.68: 95% CI[0.44 1.04]; p=0.075) [106,202]. After publication of the second meta-analysis, another study in 372 patients found that pancreatitis was significantly less frequent (1.7%) in patients treated with a bolus or a 12-hour infusion of somatostatin compared with those given a placebo (9.8%) [203]. In summary, somatostatin is possibly efficacious in the prevention of PEP.

Of 10 studies of octreotide, most show no significant reduction in the frequency of PEP compared with placebo [204,205]. Paradoxically, several studies have noted an increase in the frequency of pancreatitis in patients given octreotide, an observation that reached statistical significance in at least one study [205].

Table 3. Prospective controlled trials comparing pancreatic stent vs. no stent for the prevention of post-ERCP acute pancreatitis

Study, year	Sample size	High risk population	PEP Stent group	PEP No stent group	OR
Smithline, 1993	93	Yes	6/43	9/50	0.73 (0.25, 2.27)
Sherman, 1995	104	Yes	1/46	8/58	0.13 (0.017,1.15)
Tarnasky, 1998	80	Yes	3/41	10/39	0.07 (0.01, 0.59)
Aizawa, 2001	130	No	0/38	6/92	0.17 (0.009, 3.14)
Fazel, 2003	74	Yes	2/38	10/36	0.14 (0.02, 0.71)

Table 4. Proposed medications for PEP prevention

Drug	Suggested way of action	Effective in prospective RCT
Calcium channel blockers	Sphincter spasm	No
Nitroglycerine		Conflicting data
Topical lidocaine spray		No
Antibiotics	Infection	Conflicting data, need for more trials
Ocreotide	Pancreatic secretion	Conflicting data
Somatostatin		Conflicting data
Corticosteroids	Inflammation cascade	No
Allopurinol		Conflicting data
N-acetylcysteine		No
Platelet activating factor Inhibitors		No
Interleucin-10		Conflicting data
Heparin		Conflicting data
Gabexate		Conflicting data
Diclofenac (NSAIDs)		Yes in only one study, need for more trials

This may be explained by the fact that ocreotide also raises the pressure of the sphincter of Oddi, thus contributing to pancreatic outflow obstruction and, hence, pancreatitis [206]. A meta-analysis suggested that octreotide is ineffective in preventing pancreatitis after ERCP [190]. The drawback in this metanalysis data was that none of the studies included investigated the efficacy in high-risk patients. Lung et al [207] in a recent meta-analysis, included 11 randomized, controlled trials accepted as abstracts for Digestive Disease Week for the years 2000, 2001, and 2002, enrolling a total of 2770 patients. No beneficial effect of octreotide in the prevention of post-ERCP pancreatitis was found. Despite these disappointing results coming from 2 metanalysis, Thomopoulos et al, in a study in nonselected cases [208], published in the issue of November 2006 of Gastrointestinal Endoscopy, showed that it is possibly the way of administration and the dosage of the agent they should rather be changed in order to obtain favorable results, reporting postprocedure pancreatitis rates of 8.9% and 2% in the placebo and octreotide groups ($P < .03$), respectively. These investigators, keeping in mind some important aspects concerning the characteristics of the drug and that the pancreas should be depleted of the intracellular enzyme before the procedure to reduce local damage induced by enzyme activation, started an increased dosage of octreotide administration 24 hours before the ERCP, and not immediately before, as in previous studies; the 24-hour octreotide schedule seems to lower the pancreatic enzyme content [209,210]. To avoid potential effects of octreotide on the sphincter of Oddi motor function, the investigators administered the drug at least 1 hour before the procedure. There was no significant difference between the 2 groups with respect to the difficulty of cannulation, suggesting that giving octreotide at least 1 hour before the procedure does not cause any drug-related increase in cannulation problems. This has also been shown previously [211]. The major concern in this study is the fact that it has not included high-risk populations that would benefit the most from chemoprophylaxis. Furthermore, this study presents the same risk as previously considered promising agents, with no larger subsequent study to confirm these data.

References

[1] Cheng CL, Sherman S, Watkins JL, Barnett J, Freeman M, Geenen J, et al. Risk factors for post-ERCP pancreatitis: a prospective multicenter study. *Am. J. Gastroenterol.* 2006 ;101:139-147.

[2] Hookey LC, RioTinto R, Delhaye M, Baize M, Le Moine O, Deviere J. Risk factors for pancreatitis after pancreatic sphincterotomy: a review of 572 cases. *Endoscopy* 2006;38:670-676.

[3] Freeman ML, Di Sario JA, Nelson DB, Fennerty MB, Lee JG, Bjorkman DJ, et al. Risk factors for post-ERCP pancreatitis: a prospective, multicenter study. *Gastrointest Endosc.* 2001; 54:425-434.

[4] Freeman ML, Nelson DB, Sherman S, Haber GB, Herman ME, Dorsher PJ, et al. Complications of endoscopic biliary sphincterotomy. *N. Engl. J. Med.* 1996; 335:909-918.

[5] Cavallini G, Tittobello A, Frulloni L, Masci E, Mariani A, Di Francesco V. Gabexate for the prevention of pancreatic damage related to endoscopic retrograde cholangiopancreatography. Gabexate in digestive endoscopy--Italian Group. *N. Engl. J. Med.* 1996; 335:919-923

[6] Christoforidis E, Goulimaris I, Kanellos I, Tsalis K, Demetriades C, Betsis D. Post-ERCP pancreatitis and hyperamylasemia: patient-related and operative risk factors. *Endoscopy* 2002;34:286-292.

[7] Masci E, Mariani A, Curioni S, Testoni P. Risk Factors for Pancreatitis Following Endoscopic Retrograde Cholangiopancreatography: A Meta-Analysis. *Endoscopy* 2003; 35: 830-834.

[8] Loperfido S, Angelini G, Benedetti G, Chilovi F, Costan F, De Berardinis F, et al. Major early complications from diagnostic and therapeutic ERCP: a prospective multicenter study. *Gastrointest Endosc.* 1998; 48:1-10.

[9] Masci E, Toti G, Mariani A, Curioni S, Lomazzi A, Dinelli M, et al. Complications of diagnostic and therapeutic ERCP: a prospective multicenter study. *Am. J. Gastroenterol.* 2001; 96:417-23.

[10] Conn M, Goldenberger A, Concepcion L, Mandeli J. The effect of ERCP on circulating pancreatic enzymes and pancreatic protease inhibitors. *Am. J. Gastroenterol.* 1991; 86: 1011–1014.

[11] Sternlieb J, Aronchick C, Retig J, Dabezies M, Saunders F, Goosenberg E, et al. A multicenter, randomized, controlled trial to evaluate the effect of prophylactic octreotide on ERCP-induced pancreatitis. *Am. J. Gastroenterol.* 1992: 11: 1561–1566.

[12] Bhatia V, Garg PK, Tandon RK, Madan K. Endoscopic retrograde cholangiopancreatography-induced acute pancreatitis often has a benign outcome. *J. Clin. Gastroenterol.* 2006;40:726-731.

[13] Oezcueruemez-Porsch M, Kunz D, Hardt PD, Fadgyas T, Kress O, Schulz HU, et al. Diagnostic relevance of interleukin pattern, acute-phase proteins, and procalcitoninin early phase of post-ERCP pancreatitis. *Dig. Dis. Sci.* 1998; 43:1763-1769.

[14] Kaw M, Singh S. Serum lipase, C-reactive protein, and interleukin-6 levels in ERCP-induced pancreatitis. *Gastrointest. Endosc.* 2001; 54:435-440.

[15] Messman H, Vogt W, Holstege A, Lock G, Heinisch A, von Furstenberg A, et al. Post-ERCP pancreatitis as a model for cytokine induced acute phase response in acute pancreatitis. *Gut* 1997;40;80-85.

[16] Koike H, Steer ML, Meldolesi J. Pancreatic effects of ethionine: blockade of exocytosis and appearance of crinophagy and autophagy precede cellular necrosis. *Am. J. Physiol.* 1982; 242:G297-307.

[17] Watanabe O, Baccino FM, Steer ML, Meldolesi J. Supramaximal caerulein stimulation and ultrastructure of rat pancreatic acinar cell: early morphological changes during development of experimental pancreatitis. *Am. J. Physiol.* 1984; 246:G457-467.

[18] Saluja A, Hashimoto S, Saluja M, Powers RE, Meldolesi J, Steer ML. Subcellular redistribution of lysosomal enzymes during caerulein-induced pancreatitis. *Am. J. Physiol.* 1987; 253:G508-516.

[19] Saito I, Hashimoto S, Saluja A, Steer ML, and Meldolesi J. Intracellular transport of pancreatic zymogens during caerulein supramaximal stimulation. *Am. J. Physiol.* 1987; 253:G517-526.

[20] Greenbaum LA, Hirshkowitz A. Endogenous cathepsin activates trypsinogen in extracts of dog pancreas. *Proc. Soc. Exp. Biol. Med.* 1961; 107:74-76.

[21] Gough DB, Boyle B, Joyce WP, Delaney CP, McGeeney KF, Gorey TF, Fitzpatrick JM. Free radical inhibition and serial chemiluminescence in evolving experimental pancreatitis. *Br. J. Surg.* 1990; 77:1256-1259.

[22] Muller JM, Rupec RA, Baeuerle PA. Study of gene regulation by NF-kappa B and AP-1 in response to reactive oxygen intermediates. *Methods* 1997; 11:301-312.

[23] Gukovsky I, Gukovskaya AS, Blinman TA, Zaninovic V, Pandol SJ. Early NF-kappaB activation is associated with hormone-induced pancreatitis. *Am. J. Physiol.* 1998; 275:G1402-1414.

[24] Vaquero E, Gukovsky I, Zaninovic V, Gukovskaya AS, Pandol SJ. Localized pancreatic NF-kappaB activation and inflammatory response in taurocholate-induced pancreatitis. *Am. J. Physiol. Gastrointest Liver Physiol.* 2001; 280:G1197-1208.

[25] Dunn JA, Li C, Ha T, Kao RL, Browder W. Therapeutic modification of nuclear factor kappa B binding activity and tumor necrosis factor-alpha gene expression during acute biliary pancreatitis. *Am. Surg.* 1997; 63:1036-1043.

[26] Han B, Logsdon CD. Cholecystokinin induction of mob-1 chemokine expression in pancreatic acinar cells requires NF-kappaB activation. *Am. J. Physiol.* 1999; 277:C74-82.

[27] Demols A, Le Moine O, Desalle F, Quertinmont E, Van Laethem JL, Deviere J. CD4(+) T cells play an important role in acute experimental pancreatitis in mice. *Gastroenterology* 2000; 118:582-590.

[28] Zaninovic V, Gukovskaya AS, Gukovsky I, Mouria M, Pandol SJ. Cerulein upregulates ICAM-1 in pancreatic acinar cells, which mediates neutrophil adhesion to these cells. *Am. J. Physiol. Gastrointest Liver Physiol.* 2000; 279:G666-676.

[29] Demols A, Deviere J. New Frontiers in the Pharmacological Prevention of Post-ERCP *Pancreatitis: The Cytokines*. JOP 2003; 4:49-57.

[30] Gloor B, Todd KE, Lane JS, Lewis MP, Reber HA. Hepatic Kupffer cell blockade reduces mortality of acute hemorrhagic pancreatitis in mice. *J. Gastrointest. Surg.* 1998; 2:430-435.

[31] Gloor B, Blinman TA, Rigberg DA, Todd KE, Lane JS, Hines OJ, Reber HA. Kupffer cell blockade reduces hepatic and systemic cytokine levels and lung injury in hemorrhagic pancreatitis in rats. *Pancreas* 2000; 21:414-420.

[32] Messmann H, Vogt W, Falk W, Voql D, Zirnqibl H, Leser HG, et al. Interleukins and their antagonists but not TNF and its receptors are released in post-ERP pancreatitis. *Eur. J. Gastroenterol. Hepatol.* 1998; 10:611–617.

[33] Wozniak B, Wisniewska-Jarosinska M, Drzewoski J. Evaluation of selected parameters of the inflammatory response to endoscopic retrograde cholangiopancreatography. *Pancreas* 2001; 23:349–355.

[34] Petersson U, Borgström A, Ohlsson K, Fork FT, Toth E. Enzymes leakage, trypsinogen activation, and inflammatory response in endoscopic retrograde cholangiopancreatography- induced pancreatitis. *Pancreas* 2002; 24:321–328.

[35] Chen CC, Wang, SS, Lu RH, Lu CC, Chang FY, Lee SD. Early Changes of Serum Proinflammatory and Anti-inflammatory Cytokines after Endoscopic Retrograde Cholangiopancreatography. *Pancreas* 2003; 26:375-380.

[36] Leser H-G, Gross V, Scheibenbogen C, Heinisch A, Salm R,Lausen M, et al. Elevation of interleukin-6 concentration precedes acute-phase response and reflects severity in acute pancreatitis. *Gastroenterology* 1991; 101: 782-785.

[37] Deviere J, Le Moine O, van Laethem JL, Eisendrath P, Ghilain A, Severs N, Cohard M. Interleukin-10 reduces the incidence of pancreatitis after therapeutic endoscopic retrograde cholangiopancreatography. *Gastroenterology* 2001; 120:498-505.

[38] Deschamps JP, Allemand H, Janin Magnificat R, Camelot G, Gillet M, Carayon P. Acute pancreatitis following gastrointestinal endoscopy without ampullary cannulation. *Endoscopy* 1982; 14:105-106.

[39] Polack EP, Fainsinger MH, Bonnano SV. A death following complications of roentgenologic nonoperative manipulation of common bile duct calculi. *Radiology* 1977; 123:585-586.

[40] Saari A, Kivisaari L, Standertskjold-Nordenstam CG, Brackett K, Schroder T. Experimental pancreatography: a comparison of three contrast media. *Scand. J. Gastroenterol.* 1988; 23:53-8.

[41] Akashi R, Kiyozumi T, Tanaka T, Sakurai K, Oda Y, Sagara K. Mechanism of pancreatitis caused by ERCP. *Gastrointest. Endosc.* 2002; 55:50-54.

[42] Mairose UB, Wurbs D, Classen M. Santorini's duct--an insignificant variant from normal or an important overflow valve? *Endoscopy* 1978; 10:24-29.

[43] Singh P, Sivak MV, Agarwal D, Wong R, Isenberg G, Das A, et al. Prophylactic pancreatic stenting for prevention of post-ERCP acute pancreatitis: a meta-analysis of controlled trials [abstract]. *Gastrointest. Endosc.* 2003; 57: AB 89.

[44] Bockman DE, Schiller WR, Anderson MC. Route of retrograde flow in the exocrine pancreas during ductal hypertension. *Arch. Surg.* 1971; 103:321-329.

[45] Waldron RL, Luse SA, Wollowick HE, Seaman WB. Demonstration of a retrograde pancreatic pathway: correlation of roentgenographic and electron microscopic studies. *Am. J. Roentgenol.Radium. Ther Nucl. Med.* 1971; 111:695-699.

[46] Hietaranta AJ, Saluja AK, Bhagat L, Singh VP, Song AM, Steer ML. Relationship between NF-kappaB and trypsinogen activation in rat pancreas after supramaximal caerulein stimulation. *Biochem. Biophys. Res. Commun.* 2001; 280:388-395.

[47] Tulassay Z, Papp J, Koranyi L, Szathmari M, Tamas G Jr. Hormonal and biochemical changes following endoscopic retrograde cholangio-pancreatography. *Acta Gastroenterol. Belg.* 1981; 44:538-544.

[48] Skude G, Wehlin L, Maruyama T, Ariyama J. Hyperamylasaemia after duodenoscopy and retrograde cholangiopancreatography. *Gut* 1976; 17:127-132.

[49] Okuno M, Himeno S, Kurokawa M, Shinomura Y, Kuroshima T, Kanayama S, et al. Changes in serum levels of pancreatic isoamylase, lipase, trypsin, and elastase 1 after endoscopic retrograde pancreatography. *Hepatogastroenterology* 1985; 32:87-90.

[50] Kasugai T, Kuno N, Kizu M. Manometric endoscopic retrograde pancreatocholangiography. Technique, significance, and evaluation. *Am. J. Dig. Dis.* 1974; 19:485-502.

[51] Lavelle MI, Tait NP, Walsh T, Alderson D, Record CO. Demonstration of pancreatic parenchyma by digital subtraction techniques during endoscopic retrograde cholangiopancreatography. *Clin. Radiol.* 1985; 36:405-407.

[52] Johnson GK, Geenen JE, Bedford RA, Johanson J, Cass O, Sherman S, et al. A comparison of nonionic versus ionic contrast media: results of a prospective, multicenter study. Midwest Pancreaticobiliary Study Group. *Gastrointest. Endosc.* 1995; 42:312-316.

[53] Kivisaari L. Contrast absorption and pancreatic inflammation following experimental ERCP. *Invest. Radiol.* 1979; 14:493-497.

[54] Norman JG, Fink GW, Messina J, Carter G, Franz MG. Timing of tumor necrosis factor antagonism is critical in determining outcome in murine lethal acute pancreatitis. *Surgery* 1996; 120:515-521.

[55] Hughes CB, Gaber LW, Mohey el-Din AB, Grewal HP, Kotb M, Mann L, Gaber AO. Inhibition of TNF alpha improves survival in an experimental model of acute pancreatitis. *Am. Surg.* 1996; 62:8-13.

[56] Norman J, Franz M, Messina J, Riker A, Fabri PJ, Rosemurgy AS, Gower WR Jr. Interleukin-1 receptor antagonist decreases severity of experimental acute pancreatitis. *Surgery* 1995; 117:648-655.

[57] Tanaka N, Murata A, Uda K, Toda H, Kato T, Hayashida H, et al. Interleukin-1 receptor antagonist modifies the changes in vital organs induced by acute necrotizing pancreatitis in a rat experimental model. *Crit. Care Med.* 1995; 23:901-908.

[58] Fujimura K, Kubota Y, Ogura M, Yamaguchi T, Binnaka T, Tani K, et al. Role of endogenous platelet-activating factor in caerulein-induced acute pancreatitis in rats: protective effects of a PAF-antagonist. *J. Gastroenterol. Hepatol.* 1992; 7:199-202.

[59] Formela LJ, Wood LM, Whittaker M, Kingsnorth AN. Amelioration of experimental acute pancreatitis with a potent platelet-activating factor antagonist. *Br. J. Surg.* 1994; 81:1783-5.

[60] Dumot JA, Conwell DL, Zuccaro G Jr, Vargo JJ, Shay SS, Easley KA, Ponsky JL. A randomized, double blind study of interleukin 10 for the prevention of ERCP-induced pancreatitis. *Am. J. Gastroenterol.* 2001; 96:2098-2102.

[61] Van Deventer SJ, Elson CO, Fedorak RN. Multiple doses of intravenous interleukin 10 in steroid-refractory Crohn's disease. Crohn's Disease Study Group. *Gastroenterology* 1997; 113:383-389.

[62] Guice KS, Miller DE, Oldham KT, Townsend CM Jr, Thompson JC. Superoxide dismutase and catalase: a possible role in established pancreatitis. *Am. J. Surg.* 1986; 151:163-169.

[63] Wisner J, Green D, Ferrell L, Renner I. Evidence for a role of oxygen derived free radicals in the pathogenesis of caerulein induced acute pancreatitis in rats. *Gut* 1988; 29:1516-1523.

[64] Koichiro T, Manabe T, Tobe T. Effect of short-term-ischemia and reperfusion on the rat pancreas. *Nippon Geka Hokan* 1991; 60:335-341.

[65] Schoenberg MH, Buchler M, Schadlich H, Younes M, Bultmann B, Beger HG. Involvement of oxygen radicals and phospholipase A2 in acute pancreatitis of the rat. *Klin Wochenschr* 1989; 67:166-170.

[66] Schoenberg MH, Buchler M, Gaspar M, Stinner A, Younes M, Melzner I, et al. Oxygen free radicals in acute pancreatitis of the rat. *Gut* 1990; 31:1138-1143.

[67] Rutledge PL, Saluja AK, Powers RE, Steer ML. Role of oxygen-derived free radicals in diet-induced hemorrhagic pancreatitis in mice. *Gastroenterology* 1987; 93:41-47.

[68] Schoenberg MH, Buchler M, Younes M, Kirchmayr R, Bruckner UB, Beger HG. Effect of antioxidant treatment in rats with acute hemorrhagic pancreatitis. *Dig. Dis. Sci.* 1994; 39:1034-1040.

[69] Luthen R, Grendell JH, Haussinger D, Niederau C. Beneficial effects of L-2-oxothiazolidine-4-carboxylate on cerulein pancreatitis in mice. *Gastroenterology* 1997; 112:1681-1691.

[70] Neuschwander-Tetri BA, Barnidge M, Janney CG. Cerulein-induced pancreatic cysteine depletion: prevention does not diminish acute pancreatitis in the mouse. *Gastroenterology* 1994; 107:824-830.

[71] Wisner JR, Renner IG. Allopurinol attenuates caerulein induced acute pancreatitis in the rat. *Gut* 1988; 29:926-929.

[72] Niederau C, Niederau M, Borchard F, Ude K, Luthen R, Strohmeyer G, et al. Effects of antioxidants and free radical scavengers in three different models of acute pancreatitis. *Pancreas* 1992; 7:486-496.

[73] Lankisch PG, Pohl U, Otto J, Wereszczynska-Siemiatkowska U, Grone HJ. Xanthine oxidase inhibitor in acute experimental pancreatitis in rats and mice. *Pancreas* 1989; 4:436-440.

[74] Rau B, Bauer A, Wang A, Gansauge F, Weidenbach H, Nevalainen T, et al. Modulation of endogenous nitric oxide synthase in experimental acute pancreatitis: role of anti-ICAM-1 and oxygen free radical scavengers. *Ann. Surg.* 2001; 233:195-203.

[75] King BF, Hartman GW, Williamson B Jr, LeRoy AJ, Hattery RR. Low-osmolality contrast media: a current perspective. *Mayo Clin. Proc.* 1989; 64:976-985.

[76] Doubilet H, Pooppel MH, Mulholland JH. Pancreatography: techniques, principles, and observations. *Radiology* 1955; 64:325-339.

[77] Cunliffe WJ, Cobden I, Lavelle MI, Lendrum R, Tait NP, Venables CW. A randomised, prospective study comparing two contrast media in ERCP. *Endoscopy* 1987; 19:201-202.

[78] O'Connor HJ, Ellis WR, Manning AP, Lintott DJ, McMahon MJ, Axon AT. Iopamidol as contrast medium in endoscopic retrograde pancreatography: a prospective randomised comparison with diatrizoate. *Endoscopy* 1988; 20:244-247.

[79] Hamilton I, Lintott DJ, Rothwell J, Axon AT. Metrizamide as contrast medium in endoscopic retrograde cholangio-pancreatography. *Clin. Radiol.* 1982; 33:293-295.

[80] Hannigan BF, Keeling PW, Slavin B, Thompson RP. Hyperamylasemia after ERCP with ionic and non-ionic contrast media. *Gastrointest. Endosc.* 1985; 31:109-110.

[81] Seidel H. Bemerkungen zu meiner Methode der experimentellen Erzeugung der akuten hamorrhagischen Pankreatitis. *Zentralbl Chir.* 1910; 37:1601-1604.

[82] Pfeffer RB, Stasior O, Hinton JW. The clinical picture of the sequential development of acute hemorrhagic pancreatitis in the dog. *Surg .Forum* 1957; 8:248-251.

[83] Brust R, Thomson AB, Wensel RH, Sherbaniuk RW, Costopoulos L. Pancreatic injury following ERCP. Failure of prophylactic benefit of Trasylol. *Gastrointest. Endosc.* 1977; 24:77-79.

[84] Koch H, Belohlavek D, Schaffner O, Tympner F, Rosch W, Demling L. Prospective study for the prevention of pancreatitis following endoscopic retrograde cholangio-pancreatography (ERCP). *Endoscopy* 1975; 7:221-224.

[85] Testoni PA. Unresolved issues about post-ERCP pancreatitis: An overview. *JOP* 2002;3:156-161.

[86] Raty S, Sand J, Pulkkinen M, Matikainen M, Nordback I. Post-ERCP pancreatitis: reduction by routine antibiotics. *J. Gastrointest. Surg.* 2001;5:339-345.

[87] Testoni P, Bagnolo F, Natalie C, Primignani M. Incidence of post-endoscopic retrograde cholanghiopancreatography/sphincterotomy pancreatitis depends upon definition criteria. *Dig. Liver Dis*. 2000; 32:412-418.

[88] Bradley EL. A clinically-based classification system for acute pancreatitis. *Arch. Surg.* 1993; 128:586-590.

[89] Cotton PB, Lehman G, Vennes J, Geenen JE, Russell RCG, Meyers WC, et al. Endoscopic sphincterotomy complications and their management: an attempt at consensus. *Gastrointest Endosc*. 1991; 37:383-393.

[90] Thomas PR, Sengupta S. Prediction of pancreatitis following endoscopic retrograde cholangiopancreatography by the 4-h post procedure amylase level. *J. Gastroenterol. Hepatol.* 2001; 16:923-926.

[91] Gottlieb K, Sherman S, Pezzi J, Esber E, Lehman GA. Early recognition of post-ERCP pancreatitis by clinical assessment and serum pancreatic enzymes. *Am. J. Gastroenterol.* 1996; 91:1553-1557.

[92] Testoni PA, Bagnolo F. Pain at 24 hours associated with amylase levels greater than 5 times the upper normal limit as the most reliable indicator of post-ERCP pancreatitis. *Gastrointest. Endosc*. 2001; 53:33-39.

[93] Testoni PA, Caporuscio S, Bagnolo F, Lella F. Twenty-four-hour serum amylase predicting pancreatic reaction after endoscopic sphincterotomy. *Endoscopy* 1999; 3 1:131-136.

[94] Shahnaz S, Baillie J. What Are the Predictors of Post-ERCP Pancreatitis, and How Useful Are They? *JOP* 2002; 3:188-194.

[95] Katsanos K, Tzambouras N, Baltayannis G, Kondodimou K, Kolios G, Christodoulou D, et al. The true value of serum elastase-1 in endoscopic retrograde cholangiopancreatography. *Eur. J. Intern. Med.* 2002; 13:329-335.

[96] Itkonen O, Koivunen E, Hurme M, Alftan H, Schröder T, Stenman UH. Time-resolved immunofluorometric assay for trypsinogen-1 and 2 in serum reveal preferential elevation of trypsinogen-2 in pancreatitis. *J. Lab. Clin. Med.* 1990; 115: 712–718.

[97] Hedström J, Sainio V, Kemppainen E, Haapiainen R, Kivilaakso E, Schröder T, et al. Serum complex of trypsin-2 and alpha-1-antitrypsin as diagnostic and prognostic marker of acute pancreatitis: clinical study in consecutive patients. *BMJ* 1996; 313: 333–337.

[98] Kemppainen E, Hedstrom J, Puolakkainen P, Halttunen J, Sainio V, Haapiainen R, et al. Increased serum trypsinogen 2 and trypsin 2-alpha 1 antitrypsin complex values identify endoscopic retrograde cholangiopancreatography induced pancreatitis with high accuracy. *Gut* 1997; 41:690-695.

[99] Lempinen M, Stenman UH, Halttunen J, Puolakkainen P, Haapiainen R, Kemppainen E. Early sequential changes in serum markers of acute pancreatitis induced by endoscopic retrograde cholangiopancreatography. *Pancreatology* 2005;5:157-164.

[100] Kemppainen E, Hedstrom J, Puolakkainen P, Halttunen J, Sainio V, Haapiainen R, Stenman UH. Urinary trypsinogen-2 test strip in detecting ERCP-induced pancreatitis. *Endoscopy* 1997; 29:247-251.

[101] Tenner S, Fernandez-del Castillo C, Warshaw A, Steinberg W, Hermon-Taylor J, Valenzuela JE, et al. Urinary trypsinogen activation peptide (TAP) predicts severity in patients with acute pancreatitis. *Int. J. Pancreatol.* 1997; 21:105-110.

[102] Banks PA, Carr-Locke DL, Slivka A, Van Dam J, Lichtenstein DR, Hughes M. Urinary trypsinogen activation peptides (TAP) are not increased in mild ERCP-induced pancreatitis. *Pancreas* 1996; 12:294-297

[103] Kiviniemi H, Juvonen T, Makela J. Acute phase response in patients with uncomplicated and complicated endoscopic retrogradic cholangiopancreaticography. *HPB Surg.* 1994; 8:129-131.

[104] Vandervoort J, Soetikno RM, Tham TC, Wong RC, Ferrari AP Jr., Montes H, et al. Risk factors for complications after performance of ERCP. *Gastrointest. Endosc.* 2002; 56:652-656.

[105] Rabenstein T, Schneider HT, Bulling D, Nicklas M, Katalinic A, Hahn EG, et al. Analysis of the risk factors associated with endoscopic sphincterotomy techniques: preliminary results of a prospective study, with emphasis on the reduced risk of acute pancreatitis with low-dose anticoagulation treatment. *Endoscopy* 2000;32:10-19.

[106] Andriulli A, Clemente R, Solmi L, Terruzzi V, Suriani R, Sigillito A, et al. Gabexate or somatostatin administration before ERCP in patients at high risk for post-ERCP pancreatitis: a multicenter, placebo-controlled, randomized clinical trial. *Gastrointest Endosc.* 2002;56:488-495.

[107] Singh P, Das A, Isenberg G, Wong RC, Sivak MV Jr, Agrawal D, Chak A. Does prophylactic pancreatic stent placement reduce the risk of post-ERCP acute pancreatitis? A meta-analysis of controlled trials. *Gastrointest. Endosc.* 2004; 60:544-550.

[108] Kaffes AJ, Bourke MJ, Ding S, Alrubaie A, Kwan V, Williams SJ. A prospective, randomized, placebo-controlled trial of transdermal glyceryl trinitrate in ERCP: effects on technical success and post-ERCP pancreatitis. *Gastrointest. Endosc.* 2006;64:351-357.

[109] Perney P, Berthier E, Pageaux GP, Hillaire-Buys D, Roques V, Fabbro-Peray P, Melki M, et al. Are drugs a risk factor of post-ERCP pancreatitis? *Gastrointest. Endosc.* 2003; 58:696-700.

[110] Freeman ML, Guda NM. Prevention of post-ERCP pancreatitis: a comprehensive review. Gastrointest Endosc 2004;59:845-64.

[111] Sherman S, Ruffolo TA, Hawes RH, Lehman GA. Complications of endoscopic sphincterotomy. A prospective series with emphasis on the increased risk associated with sphincter of Oddi dysfunction and nondilated bile ducts. *Gastroenterology* 1991;101:1068-1075.

[112] Fogel EL, Eversman D, Jamidar P, Sherman S, Lehman GA. Sphincter of Oddi dysfunction: pancreaticobiliary sphincterotomy with pancreatic stent placement has a lower rate of pancreatitis than biliary sphincterotomy alone. *Endoscopy* 2002;34:280-285.

[113] Tarnasky PR, Palesch YY, Cunningham JT, Mauldin PD, Cotton PB, Hawes RH. Pancreatic stenting prevents pancreatitis after biliary sphincterotomy in patients with sphincter of Oddi dysfunction. *Gastroenterology* 1998;115:1518-1524.

[114] Rolny P, Anderberg B, Ihse I, Lindstrom E, Olaison G, Arvill A. Pancreatitis after sphincter of Oddi manometry. *Gut* 1990;31:821-824.

[115] Frank CD, Adler DG. Post- ERCP pancreatitis and its prevention. *Nat. Clin. Pract. Gastroenterol. Hepatol.* 2006; 3:680-688.

[116] Sherman S, Lehman GA. ERCP- and endoscopic sphincterotomy-induced pancreatitis. *Pancreas* 1991; 6:350-367.

[117] Komatsu Y, Kawabe T, Toda N, Ohashi M, Isayama M, Tateishi K, et al. Endoscopic papillary balloon dilation for the management of common bile duct stones: experience of 226 cases. *Endoscopy* 1998;30:12-17.

[118] Bergman JJ, Rauws EA, Fockens P, van Berkel AM, Bossuyt PM, Tijssen JG, et al. Randomised trial of endoscopic balloon dilation versus endoscopic sphincterotomy for removal of bileduct stones. *Lancet* 1997;349:1124-1129.

[119] Fujita N, Maguchi H, Komatsu Y, Yasuda I, Hasebe O, Igarashi Y, et al. Endoscopic sphincterotomy and endoscopic papillary balloon dilatation for bile duct stones: a prospective randomized controlled multicenter trial. *Gastrointest. Endosc.* 2003;57:151-155.

[120] Ochi Y, Mukawa K, Kiyosawa K, Akamatsu T. Comparing the treatment outcomes of endoscopic papillary dilation and endoscopic sphincterotomy for removal of bile duct stones. *J. Gastroenterol. Hepatol.* 1999;14:90-96.

[121] Ueno N, Ozawa Y. Pancreatitis induced by endoscopic balloon sphincter dilation and changes in serum amylase levels after the procedure. *Gastrointest. Endosc.* 1999;49:472-476.

[122] Vlavianos P, Chopra K, Mandalia S, Anderson M, Thompson J, Westaby D. Endoscopic balloon dilatation versus endoscopic sphincterotomy for the removal of bile duct stones: a prospective randomised trial. *Gut* 2003;52:1165-1169.

[123] Disario JA, Freeman ML, Bjorkman DJ, Macmathuna P, Petersen BT, Jaffe PE, et al. Endoscopic balloon dilation compared with sphincterotomy for extraction of bile duct stones. *Gastroenterology* 2004; 127: 1291-1299.

[124] Elta GH, Barnett JL, Wille RT, Brown KA, Chey WD, Scheiman JM. Pure cut electrocautery current for sphincterotomy causes less post-procedure pancreatitis than blended current. *Gastrointest. Endosc.* 1998;47:149-153.

[125] Stefanidis G, Karamanolis G, Viazis N, Sgouros S, Papadopoulou E, Ntatsakis K, et al. A comparative study of postendoscopic sphincterotomy complications with various types of electrosurgical current in patients with choledocholithiasis. *Gastrointest Endosc.* 2003;57:192-197.

[126] Siegel JH, Veerappan A, Tucker R. Bipolar versus monopolar sphincterotomy: a prospective trial. *Am. J. Gastroenterol.* 1994;89:1827-1830.

[127] Norton ID, Gostout CJ, Baron TH, Geller A, Petersen BT, Wiersema MJ. Safety and outcome of endoscopic snare excision of the major duodenal papilla. *Gastrointest. Endosc.* 2002;56:239-243.

[128] Desilets DJ, Dy RM, Ku PM, Hanson BL, Elton E, Mattia A, et al. Endoscopic management of tumors of the major duodenal papilla: refined techniques to improve outcome and avoid complications. *Gastrointest. Endosc.* 2001;54:202-208.

[129] Zadorova Z, Dvofak M, Hajer J. Endoscopic therapy of benign tumors of the papilla of Vater. *Endoscopy* 2001;33:345-347.

[130] Cunliffe WJ, Cobden I, Lavelle MI, Lendrum R, Tait NP, Venables CW. A randomised, prospective study comparing two contrast media in ERCP. *Endoscopy;* 1987, 19:201-202.

[131] Johnson GK, Geenen JE, Johanson JF, Sherman S, Hogan WJ, Cass O. Evaluation of post-ERCP pancreatitis: potential causes noted during controlled study of differing contrast media. Midwest Pancreaticobiliary Study Group. *Gastrointest. Endosc.* 1997;46:217-222.

[132] Sherman S, Hawes RH, Rathgaber SW, Uzer MF, Smith MT, Khusro QE, et al. Post-ERCP pancreatitis: randomized, prospective study comparing a low- and high-osmolality contrast agent. *Gastrointest. Endosc.* 1994; 40:422-427.

[133] Suku G, Arvind KA, Stevens G, Forsmark CE, Draganov P. Role of osmolality of contrast media in the development of post ERCP pancreatitis: a metanalysis. *Dig. Dis. Sci.* 2004; 49: 503-508.

[134] Trap R, Adamsen S, Hart-Hansen O, Henriksen M. Severe and fatal complications after diagnostic and therapeutic ERCP: a prospective series of claims to insurance covering public hospitals. *Endoscopy* 1999; 31:125-130.

[135] Margulies C, Siqueira ES, Silverman WB, Lin XS, Martin JA, Rabinovitz M, et al. The effect of endoscopic sphincterotomy on acute and chronic complications of biliary endoprostheses. *Gastrointest. Endosc.* 1999;49:7.

[136] Cotton PB. Precut papillotomy: a risky technique for experts only. *Gastrointest. Endosc.* 1989;35:578-579.

[137] Freeman ML. Precut (access) sphincterotomy. *Techniques in Gastrointestinal Endoscopy* 1999;1:40-48.

[138] Rabenstein T, Ruppert T, Schneider HT, Hahn EG, Ell C. Benefits and risks of needle-knife papillotomy. *Gastrointest. Endosc.* 1997;46:207-211.

[139] Desilets DJ, Howell DA. Precut sphincterotomy: another perspective on efficacy and complications. UpToDate [serial online] 2004 Feb [cited 24 February, 2004];11.3.

[140] Bruins SW, Schoeman MN, DiSario JA, Wolters F, Tytgat GN, Huibregtse K. Needle-knife sphincterotomy as a precut procedure: a retrospective evaluation of efficacy and complications. *Endoscopy* 1996;28:334-339.

[141] Foutch PG. A prospective assessment of results for needle-knife papillotomy and standard endoscopic sphincterotomy. *Gastrointest. Endosc.* 1995;41:25-32.

[142] Kasmin FE, Cohen D, Batra S, Cohen SA, Siegel JH. Needle-knife sphincterotomy in a tertiary referral center: efficacy and complications. *Gastrointest. Endosc.* 1996;44:48-53.

[143] Rollhauser C, Johnson M, Al Kawas FH. Needle-knife papillotomy: a helpful and safe adjunct to endoscopic retrograde cholangiopancreatography in a selected p Harewood GC, Baron TH. An assessment of the learning curve for precut biliary sphincterotomy. *Am. J. Gastroenterol.* 2002;97:1708-1712.

[144] Harewood GC, Baron TH. An assessment of the learning curve for precut biliary sphincterotomy. *Am. J. Gastroenterol.* 2002;97:1708-1712.

[145] Cortas GA, Mehta SN, Abraham NS, Barkun AN. Selective cannulation of the common bile duct: a prospective randomized trial comparing standard catheters with sphincterotomes. *Gastrointest. Endosc.* 1999;50:775-779.

[146] Schwacha H, Allgaier HP, Deibert P, Olschewski M, Allgaier U, Blum HE. A sphincterotome-based technique for selective transpapillary common bile duct cannulation. *Gastrointest. Endosc.* 2000;5:387-391.

[147] Laasch HU, Tringali A, Wilbraham L, Marriott A, England RE, Mutignani M, et al. Comparison of standard and steerable catheters for bile duct cannulation in ERCP. *Endoscopy* 2003;35:669-674.

[148] Maeda S, Hayashi H, Hosokawa O, Dohden K, Hattori M, Morita M, et al. Prospective randomized pilot trial of selective biliary cannulation using pancreatic guide-wire placement. *Endoscopy* 2003; 35:721-724.

[149] Classen M. Endoscopic papillotomy. In: Sivak MV, ed. *Gastroenterologic Endoscopy.* Philadelphia: WB Saunders, 1987:631-651.

[150] Rabenstein T, Schneider HT, Nicklas M, Ruppert T, Katalinic A, Hahn EG, Ell C. Impact of skill and experience of the endoscopist on the outcome of endoscopic sphincterotomy techniques. *Gastrointest. Endosc.* 1999; 50:628-636.

[151] Rabenstein T, Roggenbuck S, Framke B, Martus P, Fischer B, Nusko G, et al. Complications of endoscopic sphincterotomy: can heparin prevent acute pancreatitis after ERCP? *Gastrointest. Endosc.* 2002; 55:476-483.

[152] Fazel A, Quadri A, Catalano MF, Meyerson SM, Geenen JE. Does a pancreatic duct stent prevent post-ERCP pancreatitis? A prospective randomized study. *Gastrointest Endosc.* 2003; 57:291-294.

[153] Sherman S, Earle DT, Bucksot L, Baute P, Gottlieb K, Lehman G. Does leaving a main pancreatic duct stent in place reduce the incidence of precut biliary sphincterotomy (ES)-induced pancreatitis? A final analysis of a randomized prospective study. [abstract]. *Gastrointest. Endosc.* 1996; 43:A489.

[154] Smithline A, Silverman W, Rogers D, Nisi R, Wiersema M, Jamidar P, Hawes R, Lehman G. Effect of prophylactic main pancreatic duct stenting on the incidence of biliary endoscopic sphincterotomy-induced pancreatitis in high-risk patients. *Gastrointest. Endosc.* 1993;39:652-657.

[155] Sherman S et al. Does leaving a main pancreatic duct stent in place reduce the incidence of precut biliary sphincterotomy induced pancreatitis? *Am. J. Gastroenterol.* 1995;90: 1614.

[156] Brackbill S, Young S, Schoenfeld P, Elta G. A survey of physician practices on prophylactic pancreatic stents. *Gastrointest. Endosc.* 2006;64:45-52.

[157] Rashdan A, Fogel E, McHenry L, Sherman S, Schmidt S, Lazzell L, et al. Pancreatic ductal changes following small diameter long length unflanged pancreatic stent placement. *Gastrointest. Endosc.* 2003;57:AB213.

[158] Rashdan A, Fogel EL, McHenry L Jr, Sherman S, Temkit M, Lehman GA. Improved stent characteristics for prophylaxis of post-ERCP pancreatitis. *Clin. Gastroenterol. Hepatol.* 2004;2:322-329.

[159] Das A, Singh P, Sivak MV Jr, Chak A. Pancreatic-stent placement for prevention of post-ERCP pancreatitis: a cost-effectiveness analysis. *Gastrointest. Endosc*. 2007 Feb 27; [Epub ahead of print].

[160] Lella F, Bagnolo F, Colombo E, Bonassi U. A simple way of avoiding post-ERCP pancreatitis. *Gastrointest Endosc*. 2004;59:830-834.

[161] Michopoulos S, Natsios A, Manthos G, Katsakos N, Stamatis G, Stamoulis I, et al. First intention of the biliary tree cannulation by means of a sphincterotome and a hydrophilic guidewire is a low-risk high-success ERCP method. *Gastrointest Endosc*. 2003; 57: AB201.

[162] Guelrud M, Mendoza S, Rossiter G, Ramirez L, Barkin J. Effect of nifedipine on sphincter of Oddi motor activity: studies in healthy volunteers and patients with biliary dyskinesia. *Gastroenterology* 1988;95:1050-1055.

[163] Prat F, Amaris J, Ducot B, Bocquentin M, Fritsch J, Choury AD, et al. Nifedipine for prevention of post-ERCP pancreatitis: a prospective, double-blind randomized study. *Gastrointest Endosc*. 2002;56:202-208.

[164] Sand J, Nordback I. Prospective randomized trial of the effect of nifedipine on pancreatic irritation after endoscopic retrograde cholangiopancreatography. *Digestion* 1993;54:105-111.

[165] Wehrmann T, Schmitt T, Stergiou N, Caspary WF, Seifert H. Topical application of nitrates onto the papilla of Vater: manometric and clinical results. *Endoscopy* 2001;33:323–328.

[166] Schwartz JJ, Lew RJ, Ahmad NA, Shah JN, Ginsberg GG, Kochman ML, et al. The effect of lidocaine sprayed on the major duodenal papilla on the frequency of post-ERCP pancreatitis. *Gastrointest Endosc*. 2004;59:179-184.

[167] Sudhindran S, Bromwich E, Edwards PR. Prospective randomized double-blind placebo-controlled trial of glyceryl trinitrate in endoscopic retrograde cholangiopancreatography-induced pancreatitis. *Br. J. Surg*. 2001;88:1178-1182.

[168] Moreto M, Zaballa M, Casado I, Merino O, Rueda M, Ramirez K, et al. Transdermal glyceryl trinitrate for prevention of post-ERCP pancreatitis: a randomized double-blind trial. *Gastrointest Endosc*. 2003;57:1-7.

[169] Muralidharan V, Jamidar P. Pharmacologic prevention of post-ERCP pancreatitis: is nitroglycerin a sangreal? *Gastrointest Endosc*. 2006;64:358-360.

[170] Niederau C, Pohlmann U, Lubke H, Thomas L. Prophylactic antibiotic treatment in therapeutic or complicated diagnostic ERCP: results of a randomized controlled clinical study. *Gastrointest Endosc*. 1994;40:533-537.

[171] Weiner GR, Geenen JE, Hogan WJ, Catalano MF. Use of corticosteroids in the prevention of post-ERCP pancreatitis. *Gastrointest Endosc*. 1995;42:579-583.

[172] Budzynska A, Marek T, Nowak A, Kaczor R, Nowakowska-Dulawa E. A prospective, randomized, placebo-controlled trial of prednisone and allopurinol in the prevention of ERCP-induced pancreatitis. *Endoscopy* 2001;33:766-772.

[173] De Palma GD, Catanzano C. Use of corticosteriods in the prevention of post-ERCP pancreatitis: results of a controlled prospective study. *Am. J. Gastroenterol*. 1999;94:982-985.

[174] Dumot JA, Conwell DL, O'Connor JB, Ferguson DR, Vargo JJ, Barnes DS, et al. Pretreatment with methylprednisolone to prevent ERCP-induced pancreatitis: a randomized, multicenter, placebo-controlled clinical trial. *Am. J. Gastroenterol.* 1998;93:61-65.

[175] Sherman S, Blaut U, Watkins JL, Barnett J, Freeman M, Geenen J, et al. Does prophylactic steroid administration reduce the risk and severity of post-ERCP pancreatitis: a randomized prospective multicenter study. *Gastrointest Endosc.* 2003;58:23-29.

[176] Manolakopoulos S, Avgerinos A, Vlachogiannakos J, Armonis A, Viazis N, Papadimitriou N, et al. Octreotide versus hydrocortisone versus placebo in the prevention of post-ERCP pancreatitis: a multicenter randomized controlled trial. *Gastrointest Endosc.* 2002;55:470-475.

[177] Testoni PA, Mariani A, Masci E, Curioni S. Frequency of post-ERCP pancreatitis in a single tertiary referral centre without and with routine prophylaxis with gabexate: a 6-year survey and cost-effectiveness analysis. *Dig. Liver Dis.* 2006;38:588-595.

[178] Mosler P, Sherman S, Marks J, Watkins JL, Geenen JE, Jamidar P, et al. Oral allopurinol does not prevent the frequency or the severity of post-ERCP pancreatitis. *Gastrointest Endosc.* 2005;62:245-250.

[179] Katsinelos P, Kountouras J, Chatzis J, Christodoulou K, Paroutoglou G, Mimidis K, Beltsis A, Zavos C. High-dose allopurinol for prevention of PEP : a prospective randomized double-blind controlled trial. *Gastrointest Endosc.* 2005;61:407-415.

[180] Harewood GC, Topazian M. Post-ERCP pancreatitis: is allopurinol the Holy Grail? *Gastrointest Endosc.* 2005;62:251-252.

[181] Katsinelos P, Kountouras J, Paroutoglou G, Beltsis A, Mimidis K, Zavos C. Intravenous N-acetylcysteine does not prevent post-ERCP pancreatitis. *Gastrointest Endosc.* 2005;62:105-111.

[182] Sherman S, Lehman G, Geenen JE, Chuttani R, Kozarek RA, Pribble J, et al. Evaluation of recombinant human platelet activating factor acetylhydolase (RPAF-AH) for reducing the incidence and severity of post-ERCP acute pancreatitis. [abstract]. *Gastrointest Endosc.* 2000;51:AB67.

[183] Rongione AJ, Kusske AM, Kwan K, Ashley SW, Reber HA, McFadden DW. Interleukin 10 reduces the severity of acute pancreatitis in rats. *Gastroenterology* 1997;112:960-967.

[184] Van Laethem JL, Marchant A, Delvaux A, Goldman M, Robberecht P, Velu T, et al. Interleukin 10 prevents necrosis in murine experimental acute pancreatitis. *Gastroenterology* 1995;108:1917-1922.

[185] Singh P, Lee T, Davidoff S, Bank S. Efficacy of Interleukin 10 (IL10) in the prevention of post-ERCP pancreatitis: a meta-analysis. *Gastrointest Endosc.* 2002;55:AB150.

[186] Murray B, Carter R, Imrie C, Evans S, O'Suilleabhain C. Diclofenac reduces the incidence of acute pancreatitis after endoscopic retrograde cholangiopancreatography. *Gastroenterology* 2003;124:1786-1791.

[187] Masci E, Cavallini G, Mariani A, Frulloni L, Testoni PA, Curioni S, et al. Comparison of two dosing regimens of gabexate in the prophylaxis of post-ERCP pancreatitis. *Am. J. Gastroenterol.* 2003;98:2182-2186.

[188] Testoni PA, Cicardi M, Bergamaschini L, Guzzoni S, Cugno M, Buizza M, et al. Infusion of C1-inhibitor plasma concentrate prevents hyperamylasemia induced by endoscopic sphincterotomy. *Gastrointest Endosc.* 1995; 42:301-305.

[189] Ruud TE, Aasen AO, Pillgram-Larsen J, Stadaas JO. Effects on peritoneal proteolysis and haemodynamics of prophylactic infusion with C1 inhibitor in experimental acute pancreatitis. *Scand. J. Gastroenterol.* 1986; 21:1018-1024.

[190] Andriulli A, Leandro G, Niro G, Mangia A, Festa V, Gambassi G, et al. Pharmacologic treatment can prevent pancreatic injury after ERCP: a meta-analysis. *Gastrointest. Endosc.* 2000;51:1-7.

[191] Testoni PA, Mariani A, Masci E, Curioni S. Frequency of post-ERCP pancreatitis in a single tertiary referral centre without and with routine prophylaxis with gabexate: a 6-year survey and cost-effectiveness analysis. *Dig. Liver Dis.* 2006;38:588-595.

[192] Andriulli A, Solmi L, Loperfido S, Leo P, Festa V, Belmonte A, et al. Prophylaxis of ERCP-related pancreatitis: a randomized, controlled trial of somatostatin and gabexate mesylate. *Clin. Gastroenterol. Hepatol.* 2004;2:713-718.

[193] Zheng M, Chen Y, Yang X, Li J, Zhang Y, Zeng Q. Gabexate in the prophylaxis of post-ERCP pancreatitis: a meta-analysis of randomized controlled trials. *BMC Gastroenterol.* 2007 Feb 12;7:6.

[194] Salas A, Sans M, Soriano A, Reverter JC, Anderson DC, Pique JM, et al. Heparin attenuates TNF-alpha induced inflammatory response through a CD11b dependent mechanism. *Gut* 2000;47:88-96.

[195] Rabenstein T, Schneider HT, Bulling D, Nicklas M, Katalinic A, Hahn EG, et al. Analysis of risk factors of endoscopic sphincterotomy techniques: preliminary results of a prospective study with emphasis on the reduced risk of acute pancreatitis under low-dose anticoagulation. *Endoscopy* 2000;32:10-19.

[196] Hackert T, Werner J, Gebhard MM, Herfarth C, Klar E. Prevention of post-ERCP pancreatitis by heparin in rats. *Gastroenterology* 2000;118:A42.

[197] Rabenstein T, Fischer B, Wiessner V, Schmidt H, Radespiel-Troger M, Hochberger J, et al. Low-molecular-weight heparin does not prevent acute post-ERCP pancreatitis. *Gastrointest Endosc.* 2004;59:606-613.

[198] Karalis K, Mastorakos G, Chrousos GP, Tolis G. Somatostatin analogues suppress the inflammatory reaction in vivo. *J. Clin. Invest.* 1994; 93:2000-2006.

[199] Baxter JN, Jenkins SA, Day DW, Roberts NB, Cowell DC, Mackie CR, Shields R. Effects of somatostatin and a long-acting somatostatin analogue on the prevention and treatment of experimentally induced acute pancreatitis in the rat. *Br. J. Surg.* 1985; 72:382-385.

[200] Poon RT, Yeung C, Lo CM, Yuen WK, Liu CL, Fan ST. Prophylactic effect of somatostatin on post-ERCP pancreatitis: a randomized controlled trial. *Gastrointest Endosc.* 1999;49:593-598.

[201] Poon RT, Yeung C, Liu CL, Lam CM, Yuen WK, Lo CM, Tang A, Fan ST. Intravenous bolus somatostatin after diagnostic cholangiopancreatography reduces the incidence of pancreatitis associated with therapeutic endoscopic retrograde cholangiopancreatography procedures: a randomised controlled trial. *Gut.* 2003;52:1768-1773.

[202] Andriulli A, Caruso N, Quitadamo M, Forlano R, Leandro G, Spirito F, et al. Antisecretory vs. antiproteasic drugs in the prevention of post-ERCP pancreatitis: the evidence-based medicine derived from a meta-analysis study. *JOP* 2003;4:41-48.

[203] Arvanitidis D, Anagnostopoulos GK, Giannopoulos D, Pantes A, Agaritsi R, Margantinis G, et al. Can somatostatin prevent post-ERCP pancreatitis? Results of a randomized controlled trial. *J. Gastroenterol. Hepatol.* 2004;19:278-282.

[204] Arvanitidis D, Hatzipanayiotis J, Koutsounopoulos G, Frangou E. The effect of octreotide on the prevention of acute pancreatitis and hyperamylasemia after diagnostic and therapeutic ERCP. *Hepatogastroenterology* 1998;45:248-252.

[205] Sternlieb JM, Aronchick CA, Retig JN, Dabezies M, Saunders F, Goosenberg E, et al. A multicenter, randomized, controlled trial to evaluate the effect of prophylactic octreotide on ERCP-induced pancreatitis. *Am. J. Gastroenterol.* 1992;87:1561-1566.

[206] Binmoeller KF, Dumas R, Harris AG, Delmont JP. Effect of somatostatin analog octreotide on human sphincter of Oddi. *Dig. Dis. Sci.* 1992;37:773-777.

[207] Lung E. The use of somatostatin or octreotide to prevent post-ERCP pancreatitis: a meta-analysis of randomized, controlled trials. *Gastrointest Endosc.* 2004;59:AB107.

[208] Thomopoulos K, Pagoni N, Vagenas K, Margaritis V, Theocharis G, Nikopoulou V, et al. Twenty-four hour prophylaxis with increased dosage of octreotide reduces the incidence of post ERCP pancreatitis. *Gastrointest Endosc.* 2006;64:726-731.

[209] Gullo L, Pezzilli R, Ancona D. Effect of octreotide, a long-acting somatostatin analogue, on plasma amino acid uptake by the pancreas. *Pancreas* 1991;6:668-672.

[210] Malfertheiner P, Mayer D, Buechler M. Treatment of pain in chronic pancreatitis by inhibition of pancreatic secretion with octreotide. *Gut* 1995;36:450-454.

[211] Testoni PA, Bagnolo F, Andriulli A. Octreotide 24-h prophylaxis in patients at high risk for post-ERCP pancreatitis: results of a multicenter, randomized, controlled trial. *Aliment Pharmacol. Ther.* 2001;15:965-972.

In: Pancreatitis Research Advances
Editor: William C. Langley, pp. 79-90

ISBN: 978-1-60021-883-5

Chapter II

Morphological and Functional Evaluation with Dynamic MRCP after Secretin Stimulation for Patients with Chronic Pancreatitis

Ryo Tamura, [1)2)]***, Kiyoshi Ishii*** [2)]***, Masaru Koizumi*** [3)]***,***
Tadashi Ishibashi [4)] ***and Shoki Takahashi*** [1)]

[1)] Department of Diagnostic Radiology, Tohoku University Graduate School of Medicine, 1-1 Seiryo-machi Aoba-ku, Sendai, Miyagi, 980-8574, Japan

[2)] Department of Radiology, Sendai City Hospital, 3-1 Shimizukoji, Wakabayashi-ku, Sendai, Miyagi, 984-8501, JAPAN

[3)] Department of Gastroenterology, Tohoku University Graduate School of Medicine, 1-1 Seiryo-machi Aoba-ku, Sendai, Miyagi, 980-8574, Japan

[4)] Course of Health Sciences, Tohoku University School of Medicine, 1-1 Seiryo-machi Aoba-ku, Sendai, Miyagi, 980-8574, Japan

Abstract

Purpose: To compare patients with chronic pancreatitis and patients without pancreatic disease in evaluating morphologic change of the main pancreatic duct (MPD) and pancreatic exocrine function estimated by measurement of duodenal fluid in dynamic MRCP after secretin stimulation (s-MRCP).

Materials and Methods: s-MRCP was performed in 14 patients with chronic pancreatitis (group 1) and 19 patients without pancreatic disease (group 2). Diameter of MPD and volume of duodenal fluid which reflect pancreatic exocrine function were measured quantitatively using area intensity measurement (AIM) method, which is a recently proposed hydrometry.

Results: Diameter of MPD was significantly larger and dilatation of MPD after secretin stimulation tended to be smaller in group 1 than those in group 2. Duodenal fluid after secretin stimulation in group 1 is significantly less than that in group 2.

Conclusions: s-MRCP can demonstrate noninvasively, even in general hospitals as well as in highly specialized laboratories, the stiffness of MPD and reduced exocrine function of the pancreas in patients with chronic pancreatitis. s-MRCP is considered to be useful for diagnosing chronic pancreatitis.

Background

ERCP has been regarded as the accepted standard for the morphological evaluation of pancreatic ductal abnormalities. Its spacial resolution is higher and more precise ductal lesion can be depicted compared with MRCP. However, ERCP is expensive and invasive, with a reported complication rate of 5%. Furthermore, in up to 30% of the cases, inadequate opacification of the pancreatic duct results in an incomplete examination [1].

For functional evaluation, tube examinations such as the secretin-cerulein test have been regarded as the accepted standard. The secretin-cerulein test has higher accuracy in the diagnosis of chronic pancreatitis compared with ERCP. However, the procedure and its evaluation are time-consuming, expensive, and can be performed in only a few highly specialized laboratories [2].

MR cholangiopancreatography (MRCP) is a noninvasive modality with high diagnostic accuracy and has become important in the diagnosis of pancreas disease. The secretion of pancreatic fluid and bicarbonate are stimulated by exogenous administration of secretin. Recently, dynamic MRCP after secretin stimulation (s-MRCP) is reported as a useful modality for both functional and morphological evaluation of the pancreas [1, 3, 4, 5 6, 7, 8, 9, 10, 11, 12, 13]. In addition to improvement of the pancreatic duct delineation, s-MRCP can inspect the pancreatic exocrine function by assessing the duodenal fluid and the ductal change after secretin stimulation simultaneously.

In all previous studies except for those by Heverhagen et.al. [2] [14], pancreatic exocrine function has been evaluated semiquantitatively by using visual grading of duodenal fluid. Heverhagen et. al. assessed the exocrine function of the pancreas quantitatively by using MR hydrometry.

On the measurement of the MPD in previous studies, lumen diameters were measured with electronic calipers or were presented without mention of what measurement methods were used [1, 3, 6, 7, 11, 12, 13].

The quantitative evaluation of secretory pancreatic fluid was done in only a limited patient population (2, 14) and the quantitative evaluation of the pancreatic duct diameter in s-MRCP using an accurate measurement method has not been reported.

A new caliber or lumen diameter measurement method called area intensity measurement (AIM) has more recently been proposed [15, 16]. With this method, the lumen diameter is calculated on the basis of signal intensity on MRCP images, permitting a more accurate measurement of diameter than is possible by using full width at half maximum method

(FWHM). The AIM is based on the hydrometry as well as Heverhagen`s method, therefore can be applied to measurement of duodenal fluid.

The purposes of our study were to compare patients with chronic pancreatitis and patients without pancreatic disease in evaluating morphologic change of the main pancreatic duct (MPD) and pancreatic exocrine function estimated by measurement of duodenal fluid in s-MRCP.

Materials and Methods

Patient Population

From May 1997 to May 2000, 53 consecutive patients with suspected pancreatobiliary diseases except for acute inflammation in the liver and the pancreas underwent s-MRCP with informed consent for the procedures in Tohoku University hospital. We had Institutional Review Board approval and waiver of informed consent for this study. None of these patients experienced abdominal pain or discomfort after secretin stimulation. After twenty patients were excluded because of having pancreatic neoplasm, patients were retrospectively classified into one of two groups. These were diagnosed by means of clinical history, laboratory findings, ultrasonography (US), computed tomography (CT), and MR findings.

Group 1 included 14 patients with chronic pancreatitis (11 male and 3 female patients) aged 26-76 years (mean age ± standard deviation (SD), 53 years ± 13).

Group 2 included 19 patients without pancreatic disease (10 male and 9 female patients) aged 15-87 years (61years ± 17). Patients included choledocholithiasis (n=5), cholecystolithiasis (n=3), anomalous arrangement of pancreattobiliary ductal system (n=1), GB cancer (n=1), no abnormality (n=6), state after choledochojejunostomy (n=3; one hepatolithiasis, one CBD cancer, and one duodenal stenosis due to Crohn disease).

Imaging Techniques

Coronal dynamic MRCP images were acquired with single-shot fast spin-echo (repetition time/echo time/flip angle, ∞/1100/150°; echo train length, 240; slice thickness, 30-50mm; number of slices, 1; field of view, 250×250mm; matrix, 240×256; number of excitation, 1; acquisition time, 7sec) using a 1.5T unit (Magnetom Vision, Siemens, Erlangen) with a phased-array coil. Chemical fat suppression and oral negative contrast (FerriSeltz, Otsuka, Tokushima) were applied.

MRCP images were acquired before and at every 30 seconds for 10 minutes after an intravenous injection of secretin (Secrepan; Eisai, Tokyo, Japan) at a dose of 1 clinical unit per kilogram of body weight. Therefore, 21 images were obtained in each patient.

Image Analysis (Figure 1, 2)

Analyses were performed in retrospective fashion on a display monitor by one experienced diagnostic radiologist (R.T., 10 years of experience regarding MRCP imaging analysis) without knowledge of clinical data or other images.

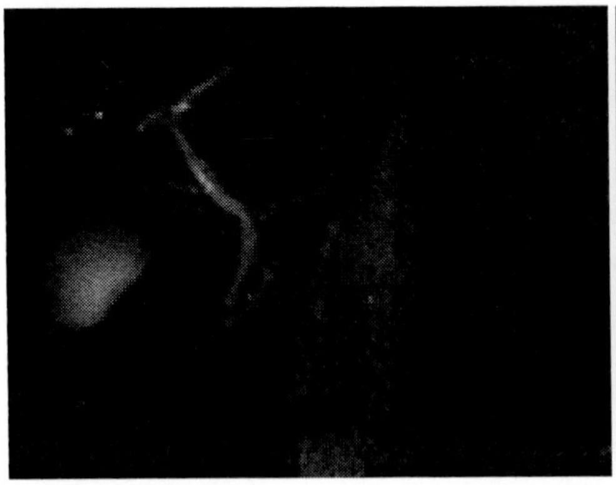

Figure 1a

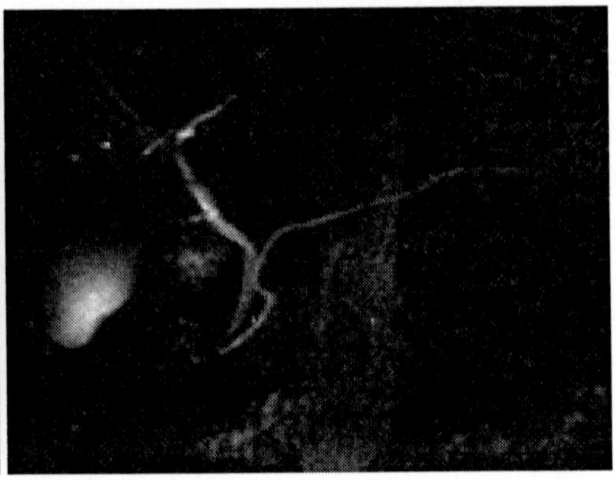

Figure 1b

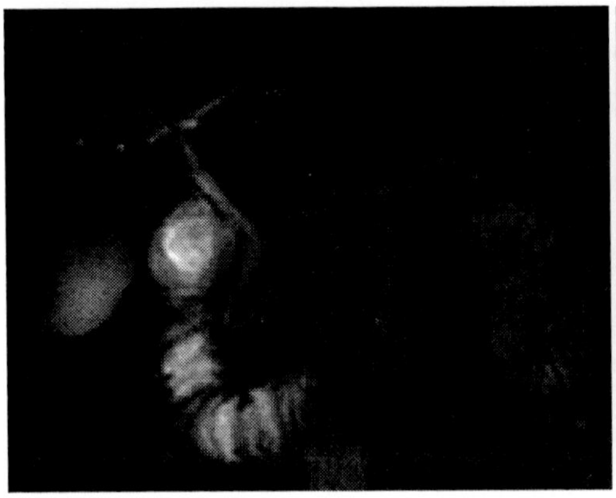

Figure 1c

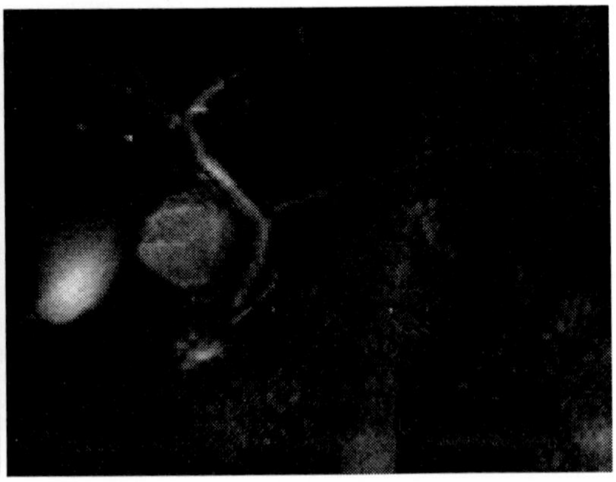

Figure 1d

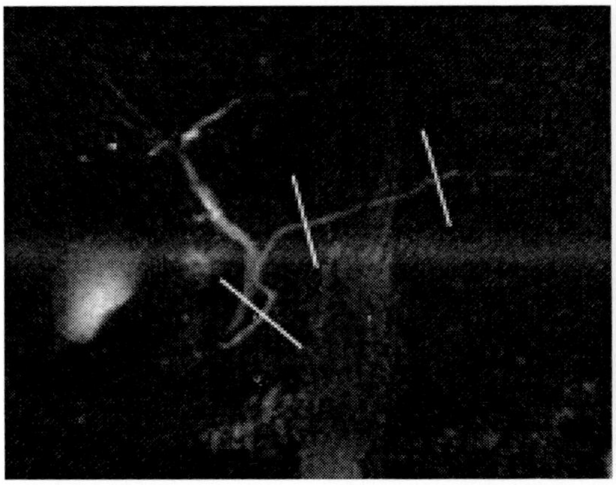

Figure 1e

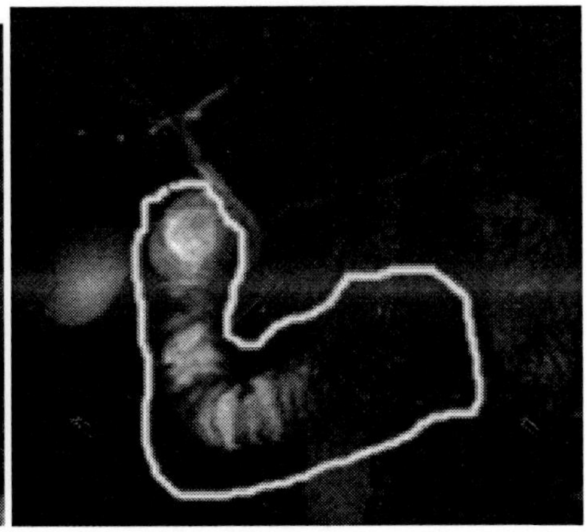

Figure 1f

Figure 1. Patient without pancreatic disease. Coronal MR cholangiopancreatograms (∞/1100) with fat-suppression obtained (a) before, (b) at maximal dilatation of the MPD, (c) at maximal secretory pancreatic fluid and (d) 10 minutes after secretin administration. The MPD is dilated and the duodenal fluid increases after secretin administration, and those diminished at 10 minutes after the administration. (e) Measurement of the MPD at head, body and tail portion in figure 1b. The measurement was performed at the same sites in 21 images of each patient. Lines indicate measurement sites. (f) Measurement of duodenal fluid in figure 1c. A region of interest was placed over the duodenal region, then, the duodenal fluid volume was calculated from the signal intensity of the region.

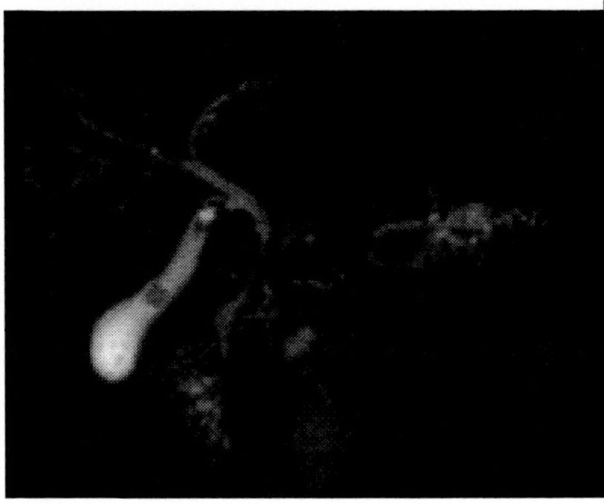

Figure 2a

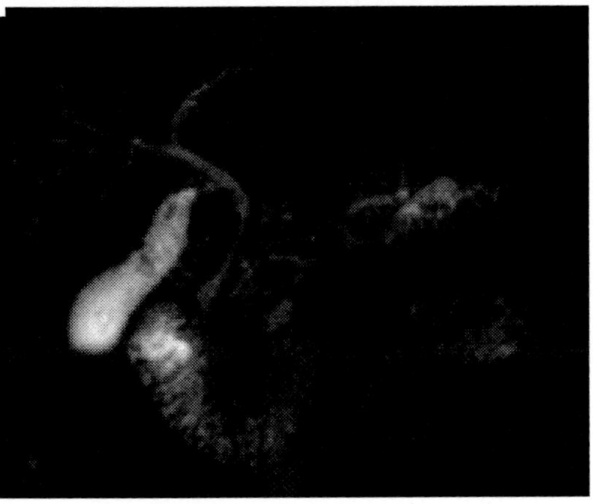

Figure 2b

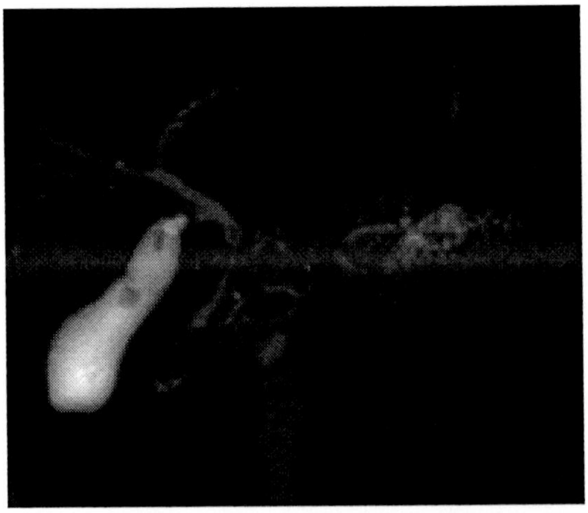

Figure 2c

Figure 2. Patient with chronic pancreatitis. Coronal MR cholangiopancreatograms (∞/1100) with fat-suppression obtained (a) before, (b) at maximal secretory pancreatic fluid and (c) 10 minutes after secretin administration. The degree of MPD dilatation and that of duodenal fluid increase are slighter in figure 2 than in figure 1. Those findings are considered to be indicative of the stiffness of the MPD and reduced exocrine function of the pancreas in patients with chronic pancreatitis.

1) Variations in the MPD Diameter

The diameter of the MPD was measured in each of the head, body and tail portions at the same sites in 21 images of each patient. The diameter of the MPD before secretin administration (Db), at maximal dilatation (Dm) and the time to achieve the Dm (Tmax), the diameter at 10 minutes after secretin administration (D10) in each of the three portions were recorded. The ratios among three values of diameters (Dm /Db, D10/Db, Dm/D10) were calculated.

The measurement was based on the AIM method, in which a caliber diameter is calculated on the basis of signal intensity. The procedure was performed as previously described [15, 16). Briefly, a phantom containing tubes with various lumen diameters that were filled with distilled water was initially imaged 30 times for calibration with the same MRCP sequences used to image the patients. Scanned images were transported in Digital Imaging and Communications in Medicine, or DICOM, format to a personal computer (Power Macintosh G3; Apple, Cupertino, Calif), and the signal intensity curves of the lumens were obtained along the cross sections perpendicular to the ducts by using an image analysis application (NIH Image, version 1.62; National Institutes of Health, Washington, DC). Net area under the curve (AUC) values were calculated by subtracting the signal intensity of the pancreatic parenchyma (used as a background signal intensity value) from the gross signal intensity curves. The following regression equation was then derived from the 30 images of the phantom and used to describe the relationship between the AUC value and the diameter of the duct: $\varphi = a \times \sqrt{AUC} + b$, where φ is the diameter of the duct as calculated in millimeters, the constant a is 0.22 ± 0.01 (SD), and the constant b is 0.20 ± 0.004.

Each patient's MRCP data were transformed into DICOM format and analyzed at the personal computer by using the same method used in the phantom study. Finally, the diameter of the MPD in the three portions of the pancreas was calculated for each patient by using the regression equation and inserting the values of the AUC into the equation.

2) Secretory Pancreatic Fluid Volume

Secretory pancreatic fluid was measured in all 21 images of each patient. The measurement was based on the method to which the AIM method applied.

Maximal secretory pancreatic fluid (V max) was determined as maximal fluid volume minus the volume before secretin administration. The maximal instantaneous secretory pancreatic fluid flow (ΔV max) (ml/min) was defined as the double value of the maximal increase volume in 30 seconds.

The time to achieve Vmax (T vmax) and ΔV max (T ΔV max) was also recorded.

In the same manner as the caliber measurement, the pancreatic fluid volume in the duodenum was calculated by inserting the values of the signal intensity of the pancreatic fluid into the equation.

The following regression equation was derived from the same phantom images as the caliber measurement and used to describe the relationship between the signal intensity and the volume of the fluid: $V = c \times I$ fluid $+d$, where V is the fluid volume in the duodenum as calculated in milliliters, I fluid is the signal intensity of the fluid, the constant c is 0.058 ± 0.009, and the constant d is 1.713 ± 0.109.

Each patient's MRCP data were transformed by using the same method used in the caliber measurement, then a region of interest was placed over the duodenal region and the signal intensity of the region was acquired. Finally, the pancreatic fluid volume was calculated for each patient by using the regression equation and inserting the values of the fluid signal intensity into the equation.

Secretin test, which is duodenal intubation test for exocrine pancreatic function, was performed in addition to s-MRCP for 6 patients of group 1. All 6 patients were with reduced exocrine pancreatic function, four patients were reduced in bicarbonate concentration only (1 factor-reduced group), two were both in bicarbonate concentration and in pancreatic exocrine fluid volume (2 factor-reduced group). The results were compared with those in s-MRCP.

Statistical Analysis

A two-tailed paired-t test and ANOVA were performed with a statistical analysis application (Stat View ver.5.0, 1998, Abacus Concepts, USA) in comparison between group 1 and 2 and among three segments of the main pancreatic duct, respectively. A *P* value of less than .05 was considered to indicate a statistically significant difference.

Results

Quantitative Analysis

1) Variations in the MPD diameter (table 1, 2) Db, Dm and D10 at all three segments of the MPD of group 1 were significantly larger than those of group 2. Concerning the ratios of Dm /Db, D10/Db and Dm/D10, Dm/D10 was significantly smaller in the head in group 1 compared to group 2, however, other ratios among three segments were not different significantly among two groups.

There was no significant difference in Tmax at all three segments between group 1 and 2. In both group, Tmax tended to be shorter in order of the tail, body and head portion. In group 1, Tmax in the body and tail was significantly shorter than that in the head. In group 2, the difference was not significant among three segments.

2) Secretory pancreatic fluid volume (table 3) Vmax and ΔV max were significantly lower than those in group 2. T vmax and T ΔV max were not significantly different between two groups.

In 6 patients of group 1 examined with secretin test, Vmax and ΔV max were lower in 1 factor-reduced group than in 2 factor-reduced group, however, without significance (Figure 3).

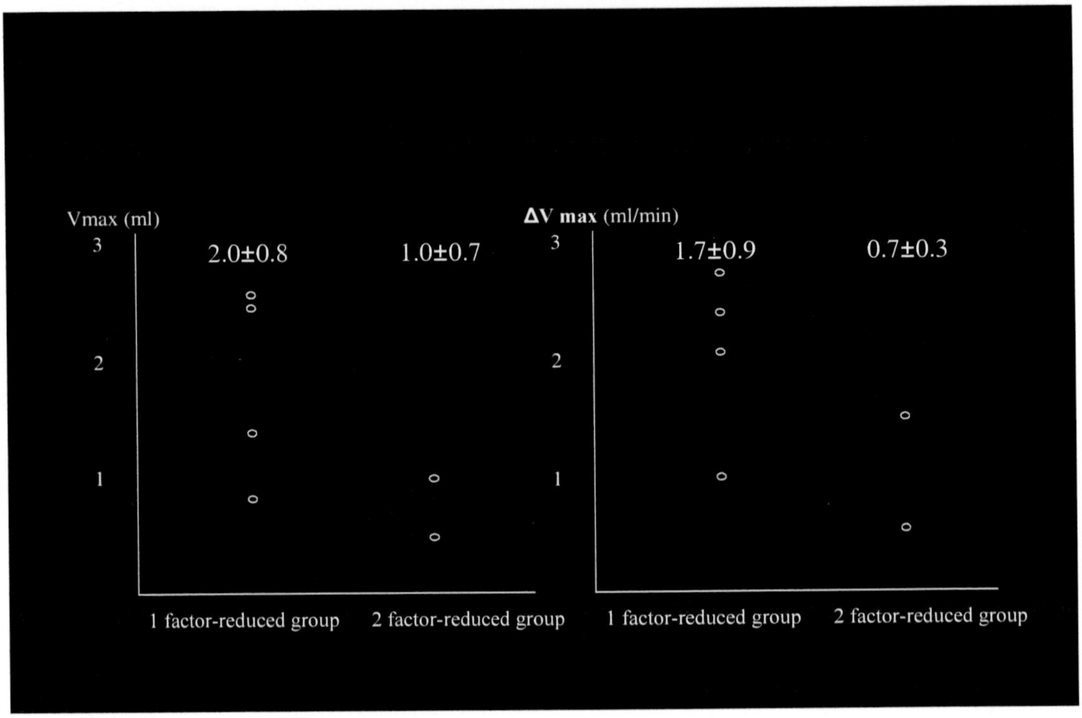

Figure 3. Comparison between s-MRCP and secretin test. Vmax and ΔV max in s-MRCP were lower in 1 factor-reduced group than in 2 factor-reduced group assessed in secretin test.

Discussion

In previous studies, the variations of the pancreatic duct diameter were analyzed in MRCP after secretin administration [1, 3, 6, 7, 11, 12, 13, 17]. However, in these studies, lumen diameters were measured with electronic calipers or were presented without mention of what measurement methods were used, and the values were reported by using units of less than 1 pixel in size. Because the minimum measurement unit in digital imaging is pixel size, any reported values that included units less than 1 pixel in size would have been inaccurate, even if electronic calipers had been used [16]. Since the normal upper limit of the diameter of the MPD are considered to be 2 mm in MRCP [18, 19] and the pixel sizes in the current versions of MRCP are about 1mm, measurements by counting pixels or using an electronic caliper are inappropriate because of their inadequate spatial resolution.

Matos et al. reported that mean MPD diameters in healthy volunteers before and 10 minutes after secretin administration and at maximal dilatation were 2.3mm, 2.2mm and 3.1mm, respectively (12). The measured values are larger than both of the normal upper limit of the MPD and values in our study. These findings suggest that measurement by using an electronic caliper couldn't have enough accuracy to evaluate MPD, thus, partial volume averaging effect might have caused overestimation of the caliber.

This is the first report that measured the diameter of the MPD in dynamic MRCP after secretin administration by not using electronic caliper, but by using the AIM method. This method is based on the supposition that a linear correlation exists between the volume and the signal intensity of fluid. The linear correlation and high reproducibility of this measurement have been confirmed in previous studies [2, 15, 16]. In the original in vitro study (15), mean measurement errors for 1-8 mm caliber ducts were significantly smaller with the AIM method (mean 6.8%) than with the FWHM (mean 30%). Caliber measurement by using electronic caliper might be a relatively less objective and less accurate method. Therefore, we believe the MPD diameter measured at MRCP by using the AIM method in this study should be more sensitive and accurate than those with electronic calipers.

The MPD diameter measured in group 1 was significantly larger than that in group 2. In contrast, Dm/Db as a parameter of dilatation tendency of the MPD after secretin stimulation tended to be smaller in group 1, however, without significant difference probably due to a small study population. Cappeliez et al. reported evaluation of pancreatic exocrine function in patients with chronic pancreatitis and in a normal control group with MR pancreatography after secretin stimulation [3]. In their study, all ductal diameters were significantly larger in patients with chronic pancreatitis and the maximal diameter variation after secretin stimulation was significantly higher in the control group. Bolondi et al. reported sonographic measurements of the MPD after secretin stimulation in chronic pancreatitis patients and normal control subjects [20]. In their study, the dilatation of the MPD in the control group showed a peak at the third minute and the MPD showed a flatter profile of the response curve with a slower increase in patients with chronic pancreatitis. The results in our study are compatible with those in those previous studies, and may be due to the fibrosis of pancreatic parenchyma and low elasticity of the pancreatic duct.

Tmax was significantly longer in the head region than in the body and tail region in group 1, however, it was not significantly different among the three regions in group 2. Cappeliez et al. reported that mean time until maximal diameter in patients with chronic pancreatitis and in the control group was 289 sec and 175 sec, respectively [3]. Fukukura et al. reported that the best visualization of the main pancreatic duct was achieved in 4.9 minutes and 4.7-4.8 minutes in patients with and without stenosis of the MPD, respectively [6]. The results in our study are similar to those of Fukukura et al. Besides; Dm/D10 was significantly smaller in the head in group 1, although the other ratios were not significantly different between the two groups. These results might suggest persistent dilatation of the MPD in the head region compared with those in other regions in patients with chronic pancreatitis due to lower compliance, and might be the early sign in s-MRCP. Results in this study agree with recent investigations that the head of the pancreas triggers the chronic inflammatory process [21]. In addition, the tendency may be emphasized by the fact that pancreatic fluid, which is secreted not only in the head but also in the body and the tail regions, pass the MPD in the head region.

In previous studies, the assessment of duodenal filling on dynamic MRCP after secretin stimulation was used to evaluate pancreatic secretion semiquantitatively by using visual evaluation [1, 3, 12, 13, 17]. Pancreatic secretion represents an indirect index of the pancreatic exocrine reserve, which is typically reduced in patients with chronic pancreatitis [22]. In this study, pancreatic secretion was evaluated quantitatively by using the method to which the AIM method applied, not semiquantitatively by visual evaluation as in previous reports. Similar quantitative measurement of pancreatic fluid has been done by Heverhagen et al. at an external workstation by using a specially designed histogram algorithm [2]. On the other hand, we used a general-purpose personal computer and free software in this study. The method of this study is less expensive, easily available and able to be widely used.

The result that ΔV max and V max in group 1 were significantly lower than in group 2 indicates reduced exocrine function in group 1. Not like tube examination, the AIM method can only measure duodenal fluid, and can not measure bicarbonate nor enzyme concentration in the pancreatic fluid which is thought to be the most reliable parameter in evaluating pancreatic exocrine function. However, s-MRCP can evaluate not only functional but also morphological aspects of the pancreas noninvasively and quickly. In measurement of pancreatic fluid volume, s-MRCP using AIM could substitute tube examination.

Another merit of the AIM method is the ability to measure ΔV max. Since the increment or decrement of duodenal fluid could be measured in a short period, measurement error caused by the inflow or outflow of duodenal fluid is expected to be smaller and the measurement might be more accurate and more sensitive to reduced pancreatic exocrine function than that on Vmax.

In 6 patients of group 1 examined with secretin test, Vmax and ΔV max were lower in the 1 factor-reduced group than in the 2 factor-reduced group. The difference was not statistically significant probably due to the small population, however, the results in tube examination agreed with that in s-MRCP.

Secretin is necessary not only at s-MRCP but also at tube examination. It was available in a form purified from porcine duodenum, however, it is now available in a synthetic form of human or porcine. In Japan, it is not commercially available in either form unfortunately.

Limitations

A limitation of our study is that we could establish a correlation with tube examination in only a small patient population. We desire further study in which tube examination and s-MRCP are compared in a large patient population.

Accurate quantitative measurement of pancreatic secretion on MRCP is difficult owing to inflow of gastric juice and outflow of pancreatic fluid. However, this difficulty is the same as for semiquantitative analysis. We think that application of oral negative contrast could reduce the inflow influence.

When the problem of inflow and outflow is eliminated, the measurement method in this study could evaluate pancreatic secretion as accurately as in caliber measurement by using AIM, and is thought to be more precise than semiquantitative analysis.

In summary, we evaluate variations in the MPD diameter and pancreatic fluid quantitatively in patients with chronic pancreatitis and patients without pancreatic disease by using the AIM method at s-MRCP. s-MRCP can demonstrate noninvasively, even in general hospitals as well as in highly specialized laboratories, the stiffness of MPD and reduced exocrine function of the pancreas in patients with chronic pancreatitis. s-MRCP is considered to be useful for diagnosing chronic pancreatitis.

References

[1] Manfredi R, Costamagna G, Brizi MG, Maresca G, Vecchioli A, Colagrande C, et al. Severe chronic pancreatitis versus suspected pancreatic disease: dynamic MR cholangiopancreatography after secretin stimulation. *Radiology* 2000;214(3):849-55.

[2] Heverhagen JT, Muller D, Battmann A, Ishaque N, Boehm D, Katschinski M, et al. MR hydrometry to assess exocrine function of the pancreas: initial results of noninvasive quantification of secretion. *Radiology* 2001;218(1):61-7.

[3] Cappeliez O, Delhaye M, Deviere J, Le Moine O, Metens T, Nicaise N, et al. Chronic pancreatitis: evaluation of pancreatic exocrine function with MR pancreatography after secretin stimulation. *Radiology* 2000;215(2):358-64.

[4] Matos C, Deviere J, Cremer M, Nicaise N, Struyven J, Metens T. Acinar filling during secretin-stimulated MR pancreatography. *AJR Am. J. Roentgenol.* 1998;171(1):165-9.

[5] Helmberger H, Hellerhoff K, Rull T, Brandt C, Gerhardt P. [Functional MR-pancreatography with secretin. A comparison of imaging quality and diagnostic value]. *Rofo* 2000;172(4):367-73.

[6] Fukukura Y, Fujiyoshi F, Sasaki M, Nakajo M. Pancreatic duct: morphologic evaluation with MR cholangiopancreatography after secretin stimulation. *Radiology* 2002;222(3):674-80.

[7] Hellerhoff KJ, Helmberger H, 3rd, Rosch T, Settles MR, Link TM, Rummeny EJ. Dynamic MR pancreatography after secretin administration: image quality and diagnostic accuracy. *AJR Am. J. Roentgenol.* 2002;179(1):121-9.

[8] Aube C, Lebigot J, Pessaux P, Tuech JJ, Kapel N, Burtin P, et al. Evaluation of the permeability of pancreaticogastric anastomoses (PGA) with dynamic magnetic resonance pancreatography after secretin stimulation (secretin MRCP). *Abdom Imaging* 2003;28(4):563-70.

[9] Petersein J, Reisinger W, Hamm B. [Diagnostic value of secretin injections in dynamic MR pancreatography]. *Rofo* 2002;174(4):437-43.

[10] Matos C, Nicaise N, Metens T, Cremer M, Deviere J. Secretin-enhanced MR pancreatography. *Semin Ultrasound* CT MR 1999;20(5):340-51.

[11] Manfredi R, Costamagna G, Brizi MG, Spina S, Maresca G, Vecchioli A, et al. Pancreas divisum and andquot;Santoriniceleandquot;: diagnosis with dynamic MR cholangiopancreatography with secretin stimulation. *Radiology* 2000;217(2):403-8.

[12] Matos C, Metens T, Deviere J, Nicaise N, Braude P, Van Yperen G, et al. Pancreatic duct: morphologic and functional evaluation with dynamic MR pancreatography after secretin stimulation. *Radiology* 1997;203(2):435-41.

[13] Manfredi R, Lucidi V, Gui B, Brizi MG, Vecchioli A, Maresca G, et al. Idiopathic chronic pancreatitis in children: MR cholangiopancreatography after secretin administration. *Radiology* 2002;224(3):675-82.

[14] Heverhagen JT, Wagner HJ, Ebel H, Levine AL, Klose KJ, Hellinger A. Pancreatic transplants: noninvasive evaluation with secretin-augmented mr pancreatography and MR perfusion measurements--preliminary results. *Radiology* 2004;233(1):273-80.

[15] Tamura R, Ishibashi T, Saito H, Majima K, Tsuda M, Takahashi S, et al. [New duct caliber measurement methods on magnetic resonance cholangiopancreatography][In Process Citation]. *Nippon Igaku Hoshasen Gakkai Zasshi* 2000;60(13):738-45.

[16] Tamura R, Ishibashi T, Takahashi S. Chronic pancreatitis: MRCP versus ERCP for quantitative caliber measurement and qualitative evaluation. *Radiology* 2006;238(3):920-8.

[17] Monill J, Pernas J, Clavero J, Farre A, Morales A, Gonzalez M, et al. Pancreatic duct after pancreatoduodenectomy: morphologic and functional evaluation with secretin-stimulated MR pancreatography. *AJR Am. J. Roentgenol.* 2004;183(5):1267-74.

[18] Soto JA, Barish MA, Yucel EK, Clarke P, Siegenberg D, Chuttani R, et al. Pancreatic duct: MR cholangiopancreatography with a three-dimensional fast spin-echo technique. *Radiology* 1995;196(2):459-64.

[19] Bret PM, Reinhold C, Taourel P, Guibaud L, Atri M, Barkun AN. Pancreas divisum: evaluation with MR cholangiopancreatography. *Radiology* 1996;199(1):99-103.

[20] Bolondi L, Li Bassi S, Gaiani S, Santi V, Gullo L, Barbara L. Impaired response of main pancreatic duct to secretin stimulation in early chronic pancreatitis. *Dig. Dis. Sci.* 1989;34(6):834-40.

[21] Koninger J, Friess H, Muller M, Buchler MW. Duodenum preserving pancreatic head resection in the treatment of chronic pancreatitis. *Rocz. Akad. Med. Bialymst.* 2004;49:53-60.

[22] Lankisch PG, Lohr-Happe A, Otto J, Creutzfeldt W. Natural course in chronic pancreatitis. Pain, exocrine and endocrine pancreatic insufficiency and prognosis of the disease. *Digestion* 1993;54(3):148-55.

In: Pancreatitis Research Advances
Editor: William C. Langley, pp. 91-148
ISBN: 978-1-60021-883-5

Chapter III

Challenging Items in Diagnosis and Imaging of Chronic Pancreatitis: Early Chronic Pancreatitis and Differentiation with (Early) Pancreatic Cancer

Kenneth Coenegrachts[1,*], Vincent De Wilde[2], Vincent Denolin[3] and Hans Rigauts[1]
[1]Department of Radiology, AZ St.-Jan AV,
Bruges, Belgium
[2]Department of Gastroenterology and Hepatology,
AZ St.-Jan AV, Bruges, Belgium
[3]Philips Medical Systems,
Best, the Netherlands

Abstract

The insidious nature of disease taken into account, the majority of patients with chronic or malignant pancreatic disease present late in their course and even with early diagnosis, mortality rates of pancreatic cancer are high.

In anticipation of a better understanding of the molecular biology and the epigenesis in the origin and progression of disease, benign and malignant as well, the most challenging items in the diagnosis and management reside at present in endoscopic and radiological pancreatic imaging.

In these the diagnosis of early chronic pancreatitis, of early pancreatic cancer, the differentiation of a pancreatic mass in the setting of chronic pancreatitis and the accurate staging of potentially resectable pancreatic cancer with respect to the dorsal extension are

* Corresponding author: Kenneth Coenegrachts, M.D. Department of Radiology, AZ St.-Jan AV. Ruddershove 10, B-8000 Bruges, Belgium. Phone: ++32-50 452103; Fax: ++32-50 452146. E-mail: kenneth.coenegrachts@azbrugge.be (kcoenegrachts74@yahoo.com)

of utmost importance. Focus in this chapter is on the diagnostic and imaging challenges of chronic pancreatitis and the differentiation with pancreatic cancer in an early stage.

1. Early Chronic Pancreatitis

Chronic pancreatitis (CP) is a disease of prolonged inflammation, induced by the fibrogenic pancreatic stellate cells and turning into irreversible morphologic and/or functional disturbances [1, 2, 3]. The triggers, thresholds, immunologic response and mechanisms of CP remain unclear and are still under investigation.[4] Despite marked progress in diagnostic tools and imaging methods there is no consensus in the grading of CP up till now. The various classification systems include the Marseilles (1963), Cambridge (1984), Marseilles (1984), Rome (1988), Chari (1994), Ammann (1997) and ABC system (2002).[5, 6, 7, 8, 9, 10, 11]. The diagnosis of CP at an early stage remains the biggest clinical challenge. Tissue biopsy, considered to be the gold standard [12, 13, 14], is generally not performed in view of the high complication rate [14] and may not be diagnostic in case of a patchy distribution of the histological lesions.[15] On the other hand currently available imaging modalities (Endoscopic Retrograde Pancreatography (ERP), Computed Tomography (CT), Endoscopic UltraSound (EUS), Magnetic Resonance Imaging (MRI)) have limited sensitivity and/or specificity for early CP and rely on quantitative criteria. As a consequence efforts are being made to search for biological and functional markers of early-stage CP [16, 17].

ERP has long been considered the gold standard imaging procedure for CP but gives no information with regard to parenchymal abnormalities [18, 19, 20].

The value of CT in identifying early ductal and parenchymal changes is negligible.[18, 21, 22, 23]. Endoscopic ultrasound is superior to the other imaging techniques with CP being likely once 5 of more criteria out of 9 to 11 have been reached.[24] The EUS criteria for CP are the presence of hyperechoic foci, hyperechoic strands, a lobular outer gland margin, lobularity, stones, calcifications, ductal dilation, side branch dilation, duct irregularity, hyperechoic duct margins, cysts, atrophy and a non-homogeneous echo pattern.[24] Not all criteria may be equally important and age-related changes as well may affect the diagnostic threshold.[25] In this respect the presence of intraductal calcifications on their own are highly suggestive of CP even in the absence of additional criteria and the widening of the pancreatic duct together with a hyperechogenic wall may be normal above the age of 70. As more criteria are reached, the specificity (positive predictive value) rises and the sensitivity (negative predictive value) lowers [24]. MRI of the pancreas in general uses a combination of T2-weighted (T2w) and T1-weighted (T1w) sequences. In most cases an MRI examination is started with T2w imaging in the axial plane. Additional coronal T2w imaging can be useful to depict the pancreatic and bile ducts more accurately. A T2w Half-Fourier Acquisition Single-Shot Turbo Spin Echo (HASTE) or Single-Shot-Fast Spin Echo (SS-FSE) sequence is a single-shot technique that acquires just over half of k-space in a single echo train, using k-space symmetry to reconstruct the image. The main advantage of the HASTE-sequence is its insensitivity to motion artifacts, even without breath-holding. The drawbacks of the HASTE-sequence include poorer Signal-to-Noise Ratio (SNR) when compared with multi-shot FSE-techniques, and blurring as a result of T2-decay during the long echo train. The resultant decreased sensitivity for detecting small, low-contrast lesions in the liver can be partially remedied by adding fat-suppression. These drawbacks, however, are not considered diagnostically significant when combined with the information obtained from the T1w unenhanced and dynamic contrast-enhanced sequences [26]. Nonetheless, non-fat-suppressed T2w imaging allows an improved evaluation of the fat stranding when compared with fat-suppressed imaging. For very ill patients who are unable to tolerate breath-holding, breathing-independent sequences using single-shot techniques such as T2w HASTE or SS-FSE are very useful.

In most cases T2w imaging is combined with so-called MRCP images. MRCP imaging uses heavily T2w imaging displaying only fluid. This allows depiction of the bile ducts and pancreatic ducts. Dynamic MRCP imaging furthermore allows evaluation of the repetitive contractions at the level of the sphincter of Oddi.

Concerning T1w imaging, two types of breath-hold sequences are mostly employed [26]:

1. In-and-out-of-phase gradient-echo (GE) imaging
Three-dimensional T1w GE imaging with fat-suppression

Fat-Suppression (FS) results in improvement in the (contrast-enhanced) dynamic range of non-fatty tissues, enhancing the contrast between different tissues and reducing motion artifacts from high signal intensity fat. The in-phase GE-sequence and T1w FS GE sequence are excellent for demonstrating areas of low signal intensity indicating pathologic changes within a normal spontaneously hyperintense pancreatic parenchyma. The decreased signal intensity on T1w FS images reflects the loss of soluble proteins in the acini of the pancreas. To our experience this finding is often more helpful when compared with the information obtained with contrast-enhanced T1w imaging.

Magnetic Resonance Imaging in the Diagnosis of Chronic Pancreatitis

The diagnosis of CP on MRI is based on signal intensity and enhancement changes as well as on morphologic abnormalities in the pancreatic parenchyma, pancreatic duct, and biliary tract. The imaging features of CP can be divided into early and late findings. Early findings include low-signal-intensity pancreas on T1w FS images, decreased and delayed enhancement after IV contrast administration, and dilated side branches. Late findings include parenchymal atrophy or enlargement, pseudocysts, and dilatation and beading of the pancreatic duct often with intraductal calcifications.

MRI allows early recognition of CP based on changes in pancreatic signal intensity; these changes are best visualized on unenhanced and gadolinium-enhanced T1w FS images. Chronic inflammation and fibrosis diminish the proteinaceous fluid content of the pancreas, resulting in the loss of the usual high signal intensity on T1w FS images. The normal pancreas enhances uniformly and intensely on late arterial phase contrast-enhanced T1w FS images and exhibits rapid washout of gadolinium on subsequent images. In contrast, a pancreas with chronic fibrosis and glandular atrophy exhibits decreased and heterogeneous enhancement on late arterial phase images and increased relative enhancement on delayed images [27].

Until recently, the role of MRCP in cases of CP was limited to diagnosis and follow-up of advanced cases.[28, 29] Owing to spatial resolution that is lower than that of ERP, ductal abnormalities in cases of mild CP cannot be assessed at MRCP. Side branches usually are depicted only when dilated. Moreover, the condition in which the pancreatic ductal system is demonstrated at MRCP differs from that in which it is depicted during ERP. Indeed, in ERP, retrograde injection of contrast medium creates enlargement of the ducts, whereas in MRCP, the physiologic or physiopathologic ductal liquid content is demonstrated.

ERP by many is the standard of reference for imaging the pancreaticobiliary system because of its high image resolution and the advantage of allowing therapeutic intervention. ERP is useful especially for depicting side branch changes of early CP. Today, diagnostic ERP is challenged by MRCP, which is a noninvasive diagnostic alternative to ERP for the morphologic evaluation of normal and diseased pancreatic ducts.[28, 29, 30, 31] The administration of secretin during MRCP may help detect subtle side branch abnormalities and allows noninvasive assessment of exocrine pancreatic function. Duct abnormalities such as dilatation, irregularity, and stones and complications of CP such as pseudocysts are best depicted by thin-section T2w and thick-slab T2w MRCP images. MRCP is accurate in depicting strictures of the pancreatic duct or biliary tract. The beaded main pancreatic duct with its dilated side branches may have a chain-of-lakes appearance when more extensive.

CT is more sensitive than MRI for the detection of calcifications associated with CP; however, MRI best depicts intraductal stones and duct obstruction. Unlike ERP, MRCP can show the dilated duct upstream from an obstructing stone. Nevertheless, visualizing intraductal stones not surrounded by fluid may be difficult on MRI [32].

Recent technical issues with regard to MRCP include monitoring of pancreatic flow dynamics and duodenal filling after pancreatic hormonal stimulation with secretin. This is made possible by the advent of single-shot heavily T2w MRI sequences. This technique improves depiction of the pancreatic ducts and may allow estimation of pancreatic exocrine reserve [33]. Cappeliez O. et al. [34] compared duodenal filling as measured on MRCP obtained 10 minutes after secretin injection with biochemical parameters in pure pancreatic juice (PPJ) collected during the intraductal secretin test.

Dynamic variations in main pancreatic ductal diameter after secretin stimulation can be monitored. Measurable dilatation of the main pancreatic duct is mostly observed within 2–6 minutes of secretin injection. [34] This is explained by a secretin-stimulated increase in fluid secretion by the ductal cells in the ductal system and by simultaneously increased tonus of the sphincter of Oddi during the first 5 minutes, which inhibits the release of fluid through the papilla of Vater. [35] After that time, the tonus of the sphincter decreases, and the caliber of the main pancreatic duct returns to the baseline value as the pancreatic juice flows out through the papilla and progressively fills the duodenum. All main pancreatic ductal diameters measured on the dynamic MRI studies were significantly higher in patients with CP in the study by Cappeliez et al. [34]. Furthermore, the time to reach peak ductal diameter was longer, and the percentage increase in diameter was lower in patients with CP than in control patients. This probably reflects the fibrotic process involving pancreatic parenchyma in patients with CP. Cappeliez et al. [34] provide additional data regarding the relevance of duodenal filling observed during MRCP after secretin stimulation. Until now, there has been only speculation that duodenal filling could be correlated with exocrine pancreatic function [33]. Currently, the most valuable pancreatic function tests are the duodenal and intraductal secretin tests with sampling of duodenal juice or PPJ. [36, 37, 38, 39] With these invasive techniques, the best evaluation of the pancreatic exocrine function is given by measuring bicarbonate output and concentration in PPJ collected after secretin stimulation [37, 40, 41].

Cappeliez O. et al. [34] indicate a strong association between reduced duodenal filling and impaired pancreatic exocrine function. Patients with reduced duodenal filling observed at MRCP are 17.6 times more likely to have deficient pancreatic function (ie, ≤50% of normal function) than are patients with normal duodenal filling. By considering duodenal filling alone in patients with reduced pancreatic function, reduced duodenal filling is specific (87%) but less sensitive (72%) for detection of impaired pancreatic exocrine function; therefore, normal duodenal filling seen at MRCP after secretin stimulation does not exclude reduced pancreatic exocrine function.

Although some investigators [42, 43, 44] have shown a correlation between secretin stimulation test and ERP results in patients with CP, others [34, 45] have shown that exocrine pancreatic function as assessed with PPJ analysis (and with findings of duodenal filling, in our study) may be normal in patients with abnormal ERP findings and vice versa, with discordant results in 12%–29% of cases [43, 44, 45].

Matos C. et al. [46] describe progressive hydrographic enhancement of the pancreatic parenchyma, termed acinar filling, during dynamic secretin MRCP studies probably being a specific, although insensitive, finding of early CP. The cause of this acinar filling remains unclear, with subtle or no ductal changes on ERCP and without calcifications. However, Matos C. et al. [46] state that acinar filling might illustrate the ductal and tissue hypertension that have been described in humans [47] and in animal models in the early stages of CP.[48, 49] Ductal and tissue hypertension are due to both outflow impairment and a lack of compliance of the diseased pancreas. Progressive acinar filling could represent fluid leakage caused by increased ductal and tissue pressure in a pancreas that has lost its elasticity [47, 50].

Perfusion-Based Contrast-Enhanced MRI of the Pancreas

In a prospective study by K.Coenegrachts et al. [51], the potential of a non-invasive technique, namely perfusion-based contrast-enhanced MRI, has been explored as a diagnostic tool for CP (Figure 1). The rationale for this study came from the observation of a decreased pancreatic tissue perfusion in animal studies [52, 53], as well as in humans with CP.[54, 55] This study was performed on a 1.5T MRI scanner (Intera, Philips, Best, The Netherlands), using the synergy body phased-array coil. The imaging protocol consisted of a scout acquisition, a reference scan for the use of Sensitivity Encoding (SENSE) reconstruction in subsequent acquisitions and coronal T2-weighted Half-Fourier Turbo Spin Echo (Haste) acquisitions. The Haste images were used to accurately localize the pancreatic parenchyma in all subjects and to position the 3D imaging volume on the pancreas. The perfusion study was performed with a series of 3D RF spoiled T1w gradient echo acquisitions.

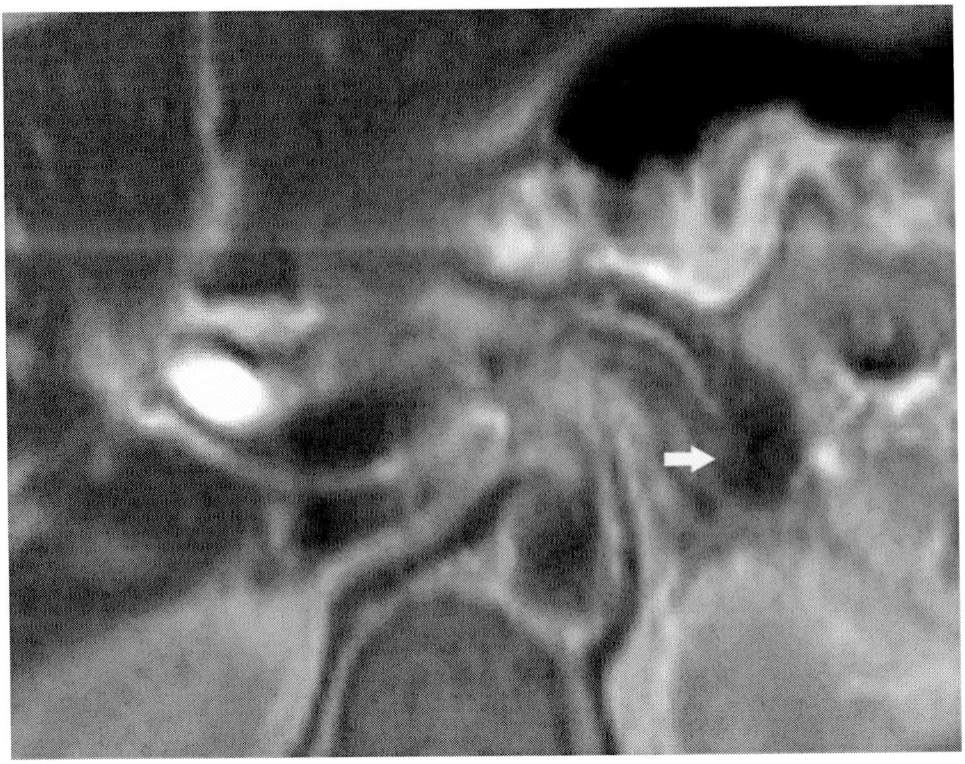

Figure 1a. T2w TSE (short TE) MRI-sequence displaying an area of pathologic signal intensity changes (white arrow) between normal and pathologic (proximal part of pancreatic tail) pancreatic parenchyma.

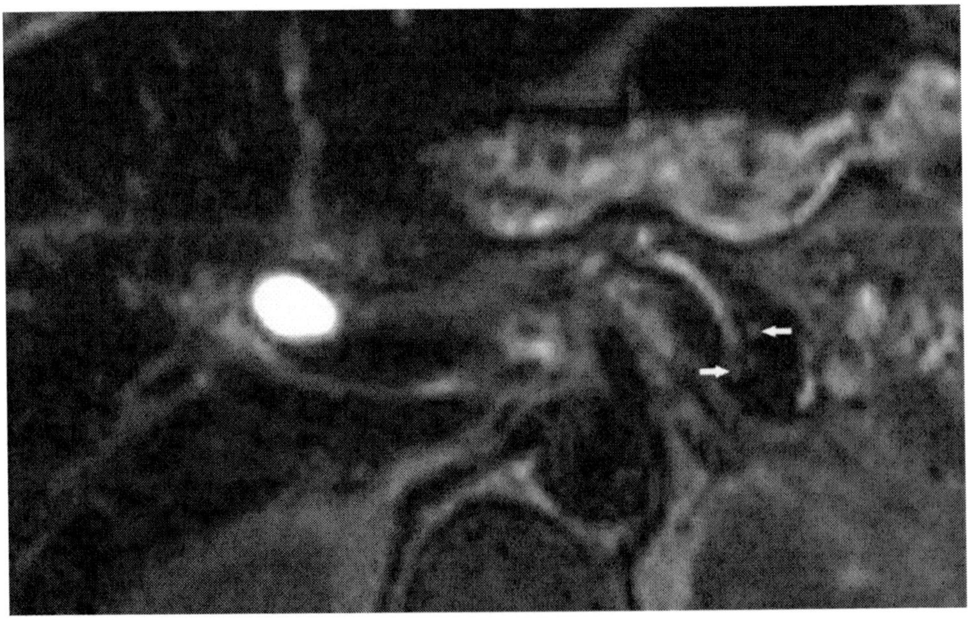

Figure 1b. T2w TSE (long TE) MRI-sequence displaying the above mentioned area of pathologic signal intensity changes. In this area some dilated side branches (white arrows) can be detected.

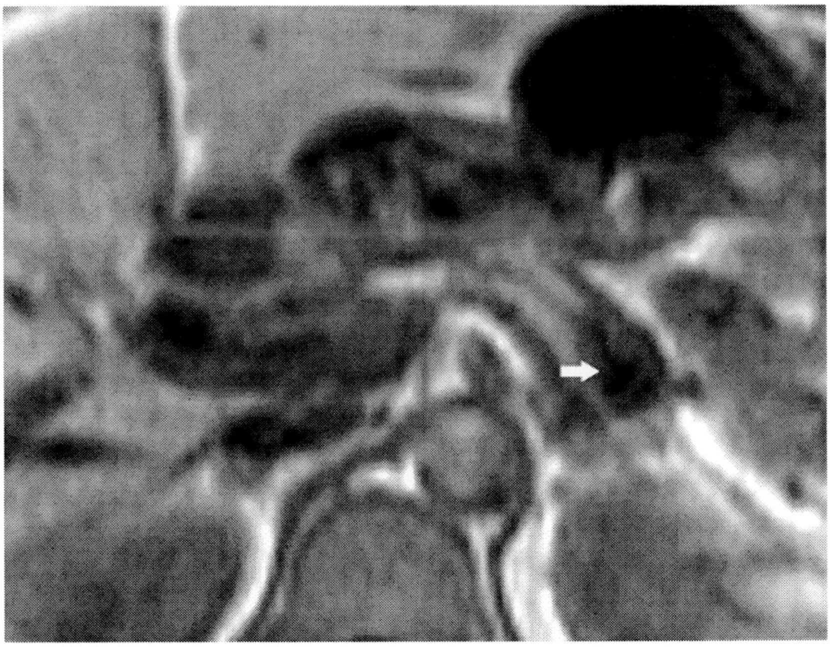

Figure 1c. T1w GE MRI-sequence before IV injection of contrast agent and without fat suppression also displays the above mentioned area of pathologic signal intensity changes (white arrow).

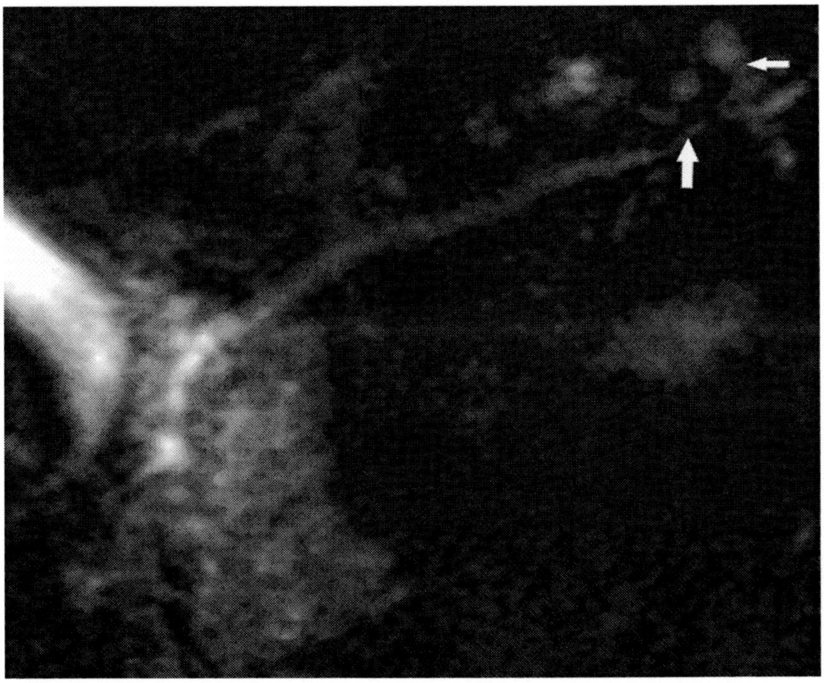

Figure 1d. MRCP-sequence displays a focal distinctive narrowing of the main pancreatic duct and accompanying dilated side branches (white arrows) at the level of the above mentioned signal intensity changes.

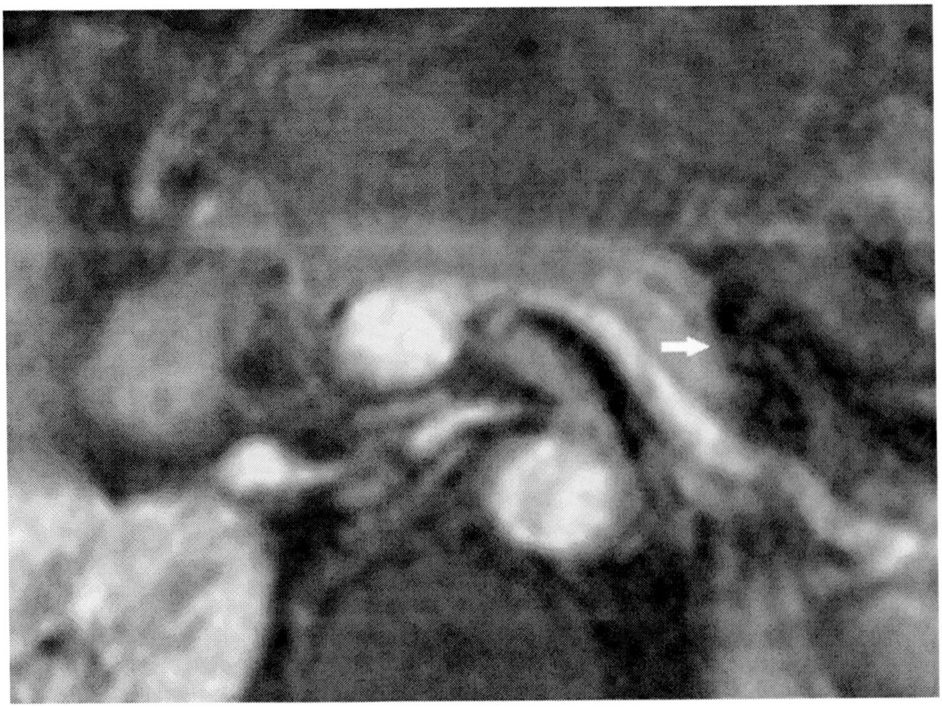

Figure 1e

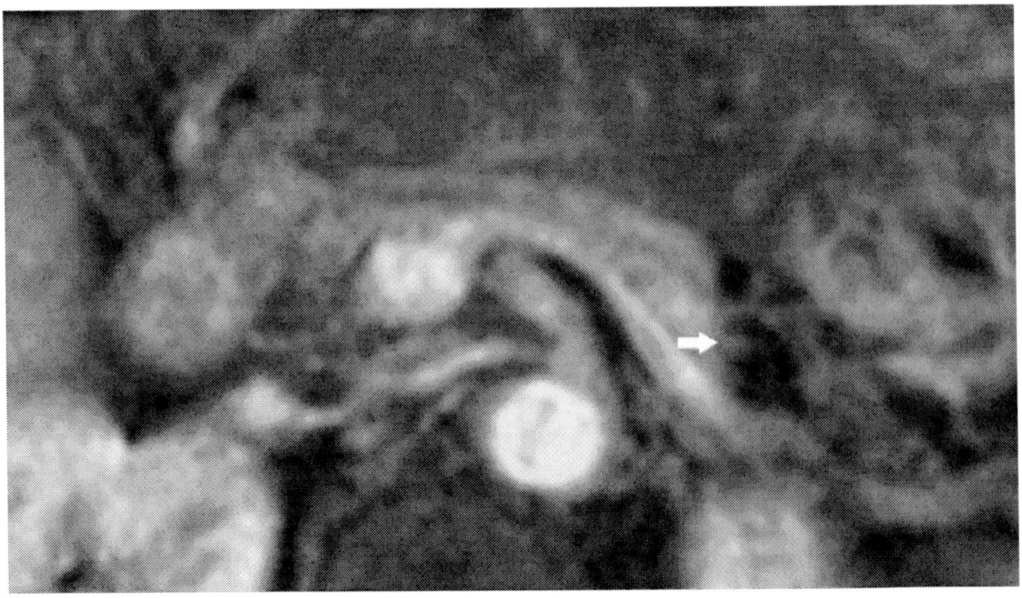

Figure 1f

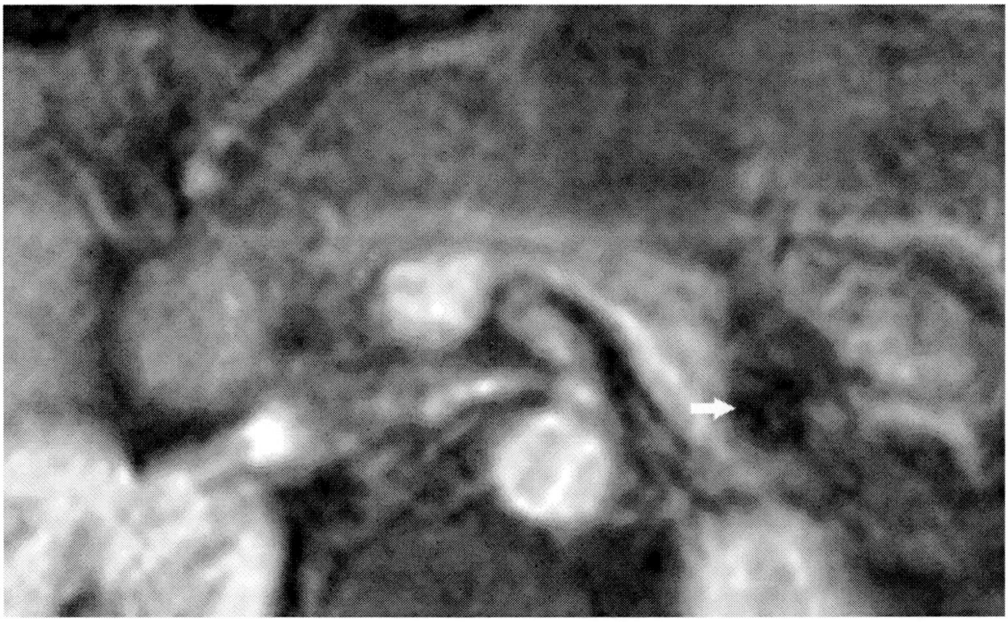

Figure 1g

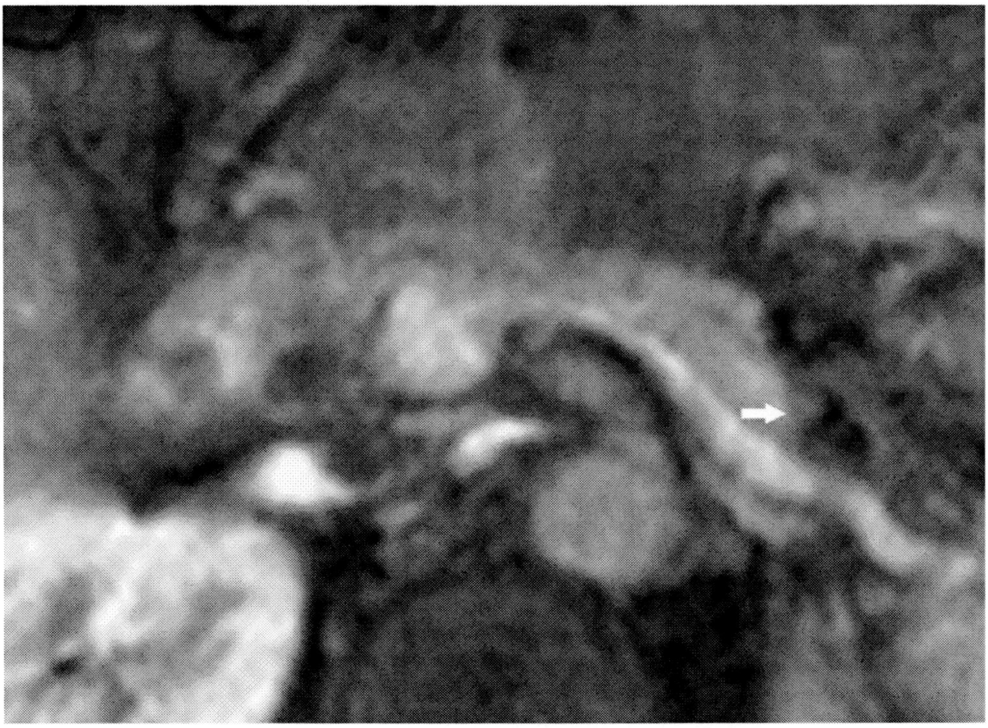

Figure 1h

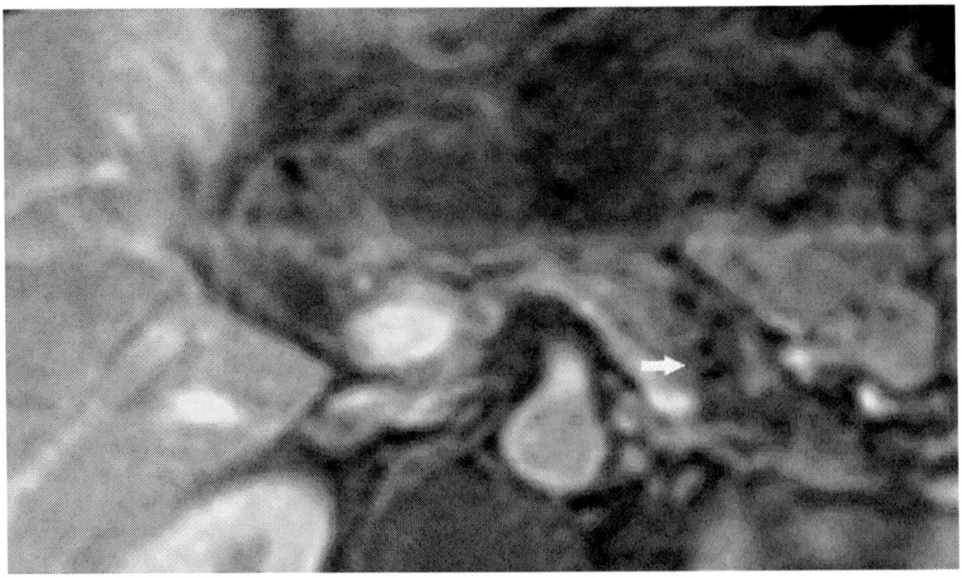

Figure 1i

Figure 1e-i. T1w GE MRI-sequence with fat suppression during IV injection of contrast agent. Dynamic "perfusion-based" MRI was performed obtaining images of the entire pancreatic parenchyma every 2 seconds (modified sequence from the one used in earlier study by Coenegrachts K. et al. reference [51]) displaying a gradually increasing contrast-enhancement at the level of the above mentioned signal intensity changes. Further study needs to be done to find a reliable threshold (reliable Time-Intensity-Curve) for the differentiation between focal chronic pancreatitis and a focal pancreatic cancer.

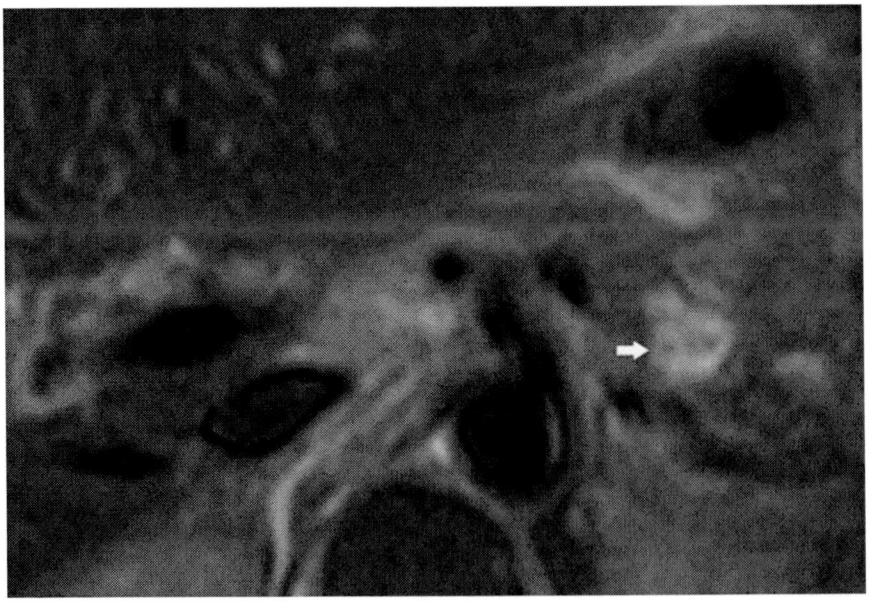

Figure 1j. Follow-up T2w TSE (short TE) MRI-sequence after two weeks displaying a strong hyperintense signal (white arrow) at the earlier detected level of pathologic signal intensity change. This finding suggests evolution toward development of a pseudocyst.

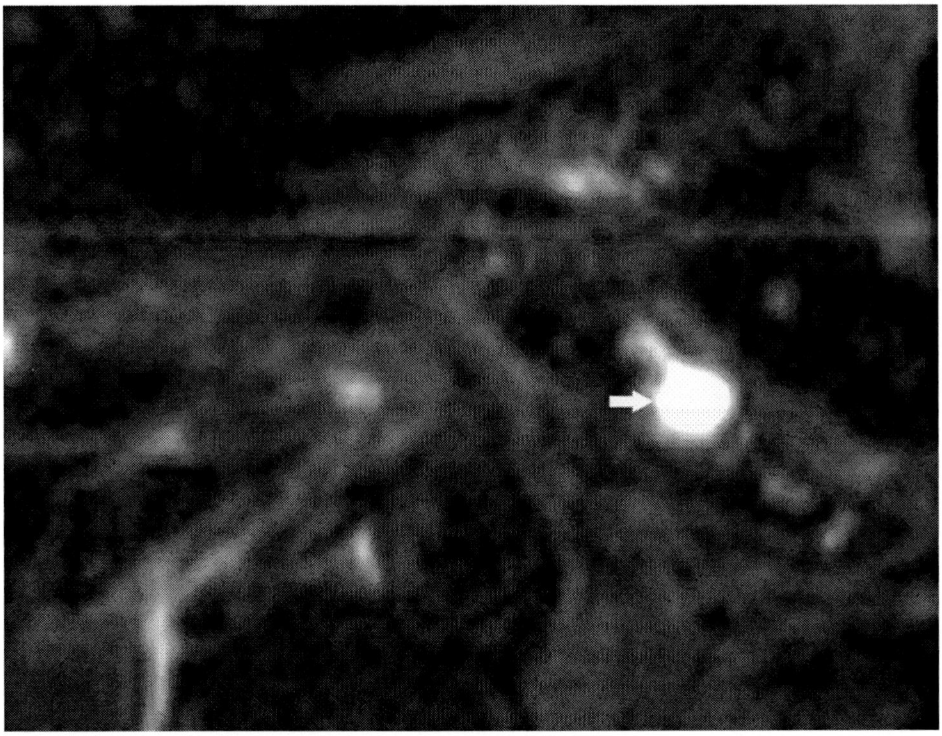

Figure 1k. Follow-up T2w TSE (long TE) MRI-sequence after two weeks again displaying a strong hyperintense signal compatible with fluid (pseudocyst).

A dose of 0.1mmol/kg Gd-DTPA (Omniscan®, Nycomed, Ireland) contrast agent was used followed by a bolus of 20 ml of physiologic saline (NaCl 0,9%). The patient inclusion criteria for moderate to severe CP were imaging findings considered diagnostic of moderate to severe CP (Cambridge classification type II or III) with or without a concommittant functional exocrine or endocrine insufficiency. Criteria for exocrine insufficiency were an abnormal mixed triglycerides breathing test and/or the presence of abnormal fecal fat measurements. Criteria for endocrine insufficiency were an abnormal oral glucose tolerance test. Patients with prior abdominal surgery were excluded.

Patients with thrombosis or obstruction in the portal vein and its branches were excluded from the study. The signal enhancement curve from data in the aorta was used to check for unknown cardiovascular pathologies with influence on the aortic flow. In all cases the complete first pass of the bolus was visualized. Three Regions-Of-Interest (ROIs) (at the level of pancreatic head, body and tail respectively) could be chosen in all subjects. In patients suffering from CP, some dilated side branches were inevitably included within the ROI. Regions of interest (ROIs) were selected in the pancreatic head, body and tail and enhancement curves (Time-Intensity-Curves (TICs)) were calculated. Typical TICs in the pancreas of both a volunteer and a patient with CP are shown in figure 2. In the volunteer, the enhancement curve shows the baseline signal prior to the arrival of the contrast agent in the pancreatic parenchyma and an earlier and steeper increase in signal intensity during the early phase of contrast bolus when compared with the patient suffering from CP. Semi-quantitative parameters were calculated from the TICs in the pancreas of both healthy volunteers and patients with moderate to severe CP. The purpose was to compare the perfusion-related data in both groups. This is considered a first step towards a possible protocol for perfusion-based contrast-enhanced MRI for the diagnosis of early CP.

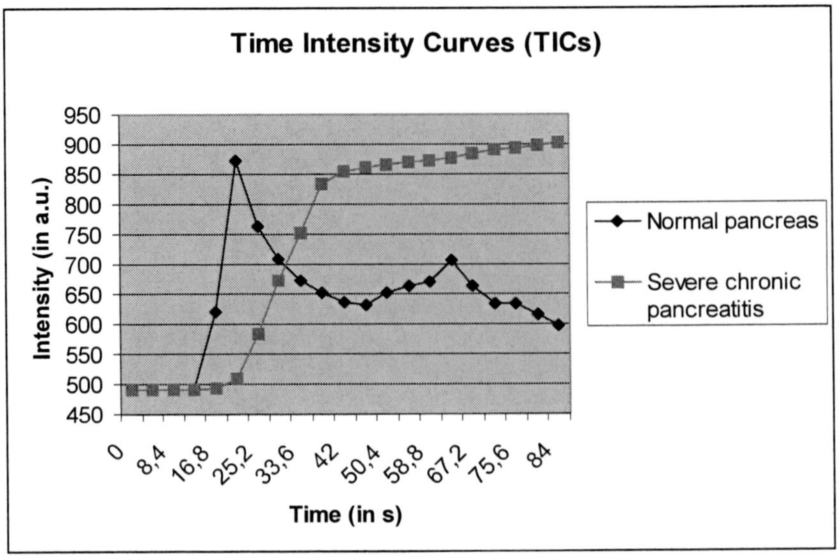

Figure 2. shows a typical Time Intensity Curve (TIC) in a healthy subject and in a patient with severe chronic pancreatitis. The first and second pass of contrast material can clearly be appreciated in the healthy subject.

A first reason to use the 3D T1w FS GE technique is the better spatial resolution when compared, e.g. to T2*w perfusion acquisitions. In addition, bowel loops within the imaging volume don not induce susceptibility artefacts. The 3D volume included the complete pancreatic parenchyma and different parts of the pancreas were readily distinguished. A good spatial resolution is crucial for adequate placement of the different ROIs at the level of the pancreatic parenchyma. Especially in patients with moderate to severe CP, there can be a pronounced atrophy of the pancreatic parenchyma. A good spatial resolution is therefore a determining factor for the practical applicability of the technique. The dynamic 3D acquisition allows a temporal resolution of 4.2 sec per 3D-stack. It remains to be studied whether a shorter acquisition time, when using as an example a 2D gradient echo measurement, would change the values of the perfusion parameters.

Two parameters were found promising in this regard: the Time-to-Inflow Deceleration (TID) and the wash-in rate (Figure 3). The TID in the pancreatic head, body and tail of patients with CP is significantly longer than in volunteers. The wash-in rate at the level of the pancreatic head and body is significantly slower in patients with CP. These findings might be explained by a combination of microcirculatory disturbances, changes in compliance/elasticity of the pancreatic parenchyma, by an increased tissue pancreatic interstitial pressure and possibly also by an important diffusion of the contrast agent into the pancreatic parenchyma. A laser Doppler flow study, performed in patients with alcoholic pancreatitis undergoing laparatomy for pancreatic head resection, showed a significantly decreased pancreatic blood flow and also alterations in the blood flow wave or pulsatile index as compared to normal controls [55].

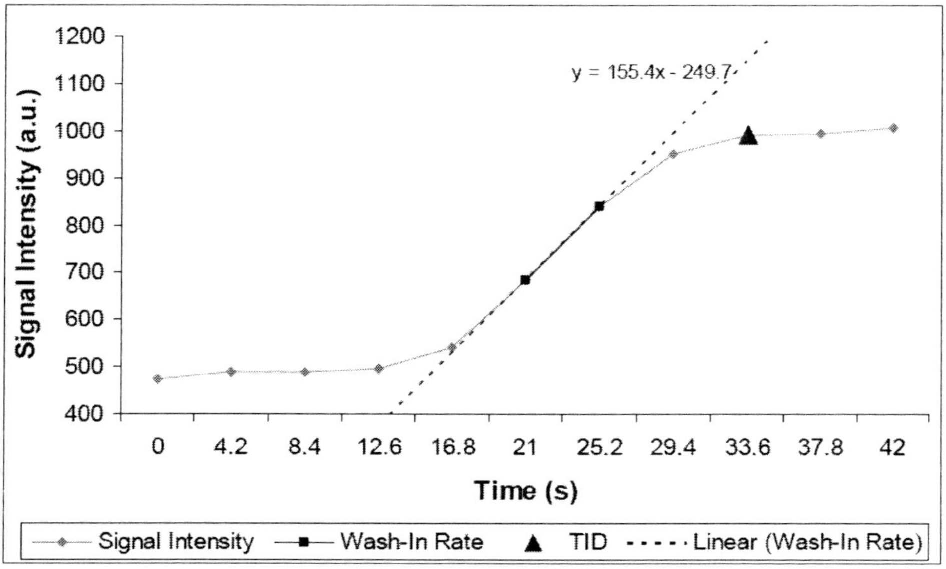

Figure 3. A TIC of a patient with chronic pancreatitis is shown, displaying how the Time-to-Inflow Deceleration (TID) parameter and wash-in are measured. The wash-in rate was defined as the maximal signal intensity gradient or slope that can be calculated between successive measured time points; the TID is the duration from the onset of the signal enhancement to the point where the wash-in rate decreases to less than 10% of its maximal value.

In a series of studies performed in both animals with experimentally induced CP as well as in patients with CP, Reber and coworkers demonstrated a decreased pancreatic perfusion but also an increased pancreatic interstitial pressure as compared to controls.[52] According to the latter authors, stimulation of the pancreas by the administration of secretin and cholecystokinin leads to an increase in blood flow in the normal pancreas but to a further reduction in blood flow and a further increase in interstitial pressure when dealing with CP. Duct decompression, especially by surgical pancreaticojejunostomy, improves pancreatic blood flow, decreases interstitial pressure, and prevents any further deterioration on pancreatic secretagogue stimulation [56].

When using the non-specific contrast agents, the enhancement slope always expresses tissue vascularisation given by the number and dimension of vessels and capillary permeability.[57, 58] During the first pass, approximately 50% of the contrast agent (or even more in pathologic tissues) enters the interstitial space through the capillary network. The complete enhancement curve (TIC) is therefore mainly determined by the capillary permeability and the composition of the interstitial space. [59] The use of blood pool agents, i.e. contrast agents that remain for a much longer time in the vessels, visualises the perfusion more selectively [60].

Differences in signal intensity on fat-suppressed, T1-weighted images and percent contrast enhancement on dynamic images have been previously observed between healthy persons and patients with CP.[27, 61, 62] Only in one recent study, two quantitative signs were described to characterize patients with an apparent "early or mild" CP by dynamic contrast-enhanced MRI.[63] In this retrospective study, 24 patients with suspected early or mild CP, classified by imaging criteria of equivocal CP (ultrasound, computed tomography (CT) or ERCP) grading, had dynamic MRI that included unenhanced, arterial, early venous, and late venous phases of contrast enhancement. Twenty patients without pancreatic diseases also had the dynamic sequence as a control group. The signal intensity was measured at the pancreatic head, body, and tail on all phases, and for each, the signal intensity ratio (SIR, the signal intensity in postcontrast divided by that in precontrast) was calculated. Two radiologists independently reviewed the images of the patients with suspected early or mild CP for pancreatic morphologic abnormalities without knowing the results of signal intensity measurements. Patients with CP had a relative signal enhancement of 1.65 ± 0.23 in the arterial phase. This was significantly lower than the corresponding value in normal controls, 1.89 ± 0.31, and that was also significantly lower than in the early venous phase: 1.75 ± 0.22. The presence of a signal intensity ratio < 1.73 in the arterial phase and/or a delayed peak enhancement after contrast had a sensitivity of 92% and a specificity of 75% for early CP. This is significantly higher than the 50% sensitivity for diagnosis based on morphological abnormalities alone.[64] The parameters were calculated from 3 successive 3D GE acquisitions (lasting 20s each) during the injection of a contrast agent. In this study we found two quantitative signs of suspected early or mild CP on dynamic contrast-enhanced MRI. The arterial phase SIR of the pancreatitis group was significantly lower than that of the control group ($P < 0.01$). Additionally, enhancement in the pancreatitis group was greatest in the early or late venous phase, rather than in the arterial phase, as in the control group ($P < 0.05$). The sensitivity of 92% for diagnosing suspected early or mild CP by measuring pancreatic signal intensity on dynamic contrast-enhanced images was significantly higher than the sensitivity of 50% depending on visible pancreatic morphologic changes ($P < 0.05$). Additionally, we found that pancreatic morphologic abnormalities did not correlate significantly with pancreatic enhancement measurements. This indicates that abnormal pancreatic enhancement may precede or be independent of pancreatic morphologic abnormalities. Our population with suspected early or mild CP had unenhanced pancreatic signal intensity that was not significantly different from that of our control group. Measuring pancreatic signal intensity on gadolinium chelate dynamic MRI is helpful for diagnosing early or mild CP, especially before apparent pancreatic morphologic or signal intensity changes are present. This method is different from present approach. Therefore the results cannot be correlated with the values obtained in this work. In addition, also the selection of patients was different.

Endoscopic Ultrasound

EUS has developed significantly over the last two decades and has had a considerable impact on the imaging and staging of mass lesions within or in close proximity to the gastrointestinal (GI) tract. In conjunction with conventional imaging such as helical CT and MRI, among others some indications for EUS include assessing suspected pancreatic lesions that are either equivocal or not seen on conventional imaging and staging malignant tumors of the pancreas prior to surgery or oncological treatment. The introduction of linear scanning instruments has also allowed tissue sampling of suspicious lesions under real time EUS control to become feasible (EUS-guided fine needle aspiration or FNA), and in many cases can be performed more safely than with conventional techniques [65].

Endoscopic Ultrasound in the Diagnosis of Chronic Pancreatitis

EUS has been proposed as a diagnostic test for early CP. A number of features of CP that might not be obvious on other imaging or functional tests can be demonstrated on EUS, including hyperechoic foci, hyperechoic strands, lobularity, cysts, calcification, stones, ductal dilatation, side branch dilatation, ductal irregularity, and hyperechoic duct margins.[24] Currently, it is generally accepted that the presence of five or more of the above criteria make the diagnosis of CP likely, but the significance of one to four criteria remains unclear and there is a need for a reliable gold standard for diagnosing CP. Studies comparing EUS criteria for CP with EUS-guided FNA cytology are ongoing. Two other factors must be taken into account when diagnosing CP based on EUS criteria. All criteria may not be equally important. For example, the presence of intraductal calcifications alone is highly suggestive of CP even in the absence of other criteria. In addition, there are age-related changes in the pancreas that may affect the diagnostic threshold.[25] The pancreatic duct becomes progressively wider with hyperechogenic wall as the individual ages. A 4 mm main pancreatic duct may be normal for a 70-year-old, but abnormal for a 30-year-old. Currently, there is no accepted scoring system that factors in these effects. One common practice is to require a higher threshold (e.g., 5 or more criteria for older individuals) and a lower threshold (e.g. 4 or more criteria for a younger individual). EUS criteria other than being solely quantified should also be correlated to the patient's clinical history along with the presence of risk factors (ethanol, smoking) [24].

Endoscopic Ultrasound in the Diagnosis of Early Chronic Pancreatitis

The diagnosis of CP is based on clinical features, morphologic changes and functional abnormalities. In the early stages of the disease, the diagnosis remains challenging and agreement between various methods is poor. [18, 19, 66, 67] Functional tests probably miss the diagnosis in the early stages because of exocrine pancreas functional reserve. Imaging studies, such as CT, have poor resolution, especially in the initial stages. ERP is still considered the most accurate method of assessing ductal anatomy [13, 18]. However, parenchymal abnormalities can be missed and post-procedure acute pancreatitis may occur in 5-10% of patients.[68, 69] Although these exams may be good indicators in the advanced stages, the same is not true in early-stage disease. Therefore, a method able to assess the early stages of both parenchymal and ductal irregularities with minimal risk would be of great value. EUS generates high-resolution images of parenchymal and ductal structures without the use of contrast without risk of post-procedure pancreatitis and minimal risk of sedation. EUS can also be used to obtain pancreatic tissue and juice samples. [13, 18, 20, 67, 70, 71]

EUS provides better resolution images than US, CT and ERP. Hence, both parenchymal and ductal morphology can be assessed without fluoroscopy or contrast injection. It is therefore possible to assume that EUS might be able to detect abnormalities not previously seen by other methods. Its complication rate is similar to diagnostic upper gastrointestinal endoscopy [66, 72]. EUS criteria for pancreatic disease are useful but have some limitations. Abnormalities may be similar in acute and chronic disease and slight changes of CP may be seen in the elderly population secondary to fibrotic changes related to age.[20, 70] Pancreatic abnormalities depicted by EUS can possibly be asymptomatic; on the other hand, patients highly suspected of having CP might present only mild EUS pancreatitis.[73, 74, 75] Yusoff and Sahai [76] prospectively studied the effect of ethanol and other variables on the endosonographic appearance of the pancreas and found that the number of criteria correlated most strongly with ethanol ingestion and smoking history. Wiersema et al. [20] prospectively evaluated 69 patients and 20 controls to assess pancreatic EUS features, demonstrating that sensitivity and specificity were optimal when 3 or more criteria were found. For all forms of CP, sensitivity was 80% and specificity was 86%. When considering initial pancreatic disease, sensitivity was 86%. In the study by Sahai et al. [66] 126 patients underwent EUS followed by ERP. The prevalence of CP in the population studied was 76% with 47% having moderate to severe disease. The authors found that this diagnosis can be made with an 85% certainty when more than 2 criteria are present and moderate to severe forms when more than 6 features are seen. Moderate to severe CP is unlikely (negative predictive value greater than 85%) when less than 3 criteria are found. Independent features predictive of CP were the sum of the criteria and alcohol abuse. Catalano et al. [19] evaluated 80 patients with non-alcoholic, acute, recurrent pancreatitis by EUS, ERP and pancreatic juice examination. The agreement between EUS and, both the secretin test and ERP was excellent for normal and severe pancreatitis, but poor for mild to moderate disease. When at least 3 EUS features were used to diagnose CP, the sensitivity was 86% and specificity 98%. This prospective study compared EUS appearance in patients with and without alcohol abuse excluding those with suspicious or confirmed diagnosis of CP. When comparing alcoholic and non-alcoholic groups, they found that the mean number of criteria was significantly higher in the alcoholic group. This suggests that although asymptomatic, alcoholic patients might have pancreatic abnormalities, which may be missed by other procedures, and EUS might be useful in screening patients with suspected initial stage CP. Still related to such findings, we can also argue that EUS is able to show early structural damage to the pancreas. The threshold of features needed to diagnose CP can vary according to whether or not we wish to maximize sensitivity and specificity. Once EUS detects structural changes not detected by other diagnostic methods, follow-up is necessary in order to rule out whether or not these patients who have been diagnosed with mild CP by EUS will develop signs of pancreatic disease.[77] Patients presenting more than 1 and 2 EUS features of the Catalano and Sahai score systems, respectively, are at great risk of having CP [77].

There is now some evidence in the literature suggesting that these early changes detected by EUS correlate with the histological changes of CP and may predict progression to more advanced disease. The EUS diagnosis of CP relies on quantitative (more than qualitative) parenchymal and ductal criteria found during evaluation of the pancreas. It is generally accepted that, in the absence of any criteria, CP is unlikely, whereas in the presence of 5 or more criteria (out of 9-11) CP is likely although ERP and pancreatic function tests may still be normal. The diagnostic significance of patients with fewer (1-4) criteria found on EUS is currently unclear, particularly when other diagnostic tests such as ERP and function testing are normal. In these cases, there is a potential for "over-diagnosis" of CP, since the EUS changes cannot be confirmed by other modalities.[24] One measure of early CP is whether a patient responds to pancreatic specific therapy. Walsh et al. [78] identified 43 patients who had characteristic symptoms of pancreatic disease but normal or equivocal US, CT or ERP. Those patients (16 patients), whose symptoms failed to respond to medical therapy (enzyme replacement, low fat diet, and at least 3 trials of bowel rest with total parenteral nutrition), underwent pancreatic resection. The histologic appearance in the pancreas of these patients showed subtle but distinct evidence of minimal-change CP. These changes were "focally" distributed throughout the gland and included lymphocytic cell infiltrates, intralobular and periductal fibrosis, and focal ductal dilation with inspissated protein plugs. Nine of the 16 patients had complete or significant improvement in pain after total pancreatectomy, whereas 5 did not respond and 1 died of unrelated causes. The histologic changes and response to pancreatectomy suggest that these patients had CP despite normal imaging and functional testing. However, a placebo response cannot be excluded. In the absence of a gold standard, diagnostic tests must meet other accepted criteria to be considered valuable. These include inter- and intra-observer reliability, correlation with other validated (albeit non-gold standard) tests of the disease, and prediction of response to therapy. EUS meets some, but not all of these criteria. A fundamental requirement for any test is reliability. When no gold standard is available, this is often measured as the degree to which practitioners agree on a diagnosis. Wiersema et al. [20] compared the degree of agreement among 3 experienced endosonographers reading individual criteria of CP. The agreement was 88% for hyperechoic foci, 94% for focal reduced echogenicity, 94% for lobularity, 83% for hyperechoic duct margins and 94% for duct irregularity. To further improve the reliability, an "International Working Group" has published a set of "Minimum Standard Terminology (MST)", including definitions, for many of the EUS criteria of CP.[79] Zimmerman et al. [80] and Dr. Brenda Hoffman (personal communication) reported the EUS criteria in comparison to the histologic features of CP in 34 patients who underwent EUS followed by pancreatectomy or open surgical biopsy (at the time of a lateral pancreatico-duodenostomy) (21 for CP, 13 for pancreatic adenocarcinoma). Overall, 68% of the patients met the histologic criteria for CP. The total number of EUS criteria present was predictive of histologic CP. The sensitivity and specificity were 87% and 64% using a threshold diagnosis for 3 or more criteria, 78% and 73% for 4 or more criteria, 60% and 83% for 5 or more criteria, and 43% and 91% for 6 or more criteria. From these results, it was concluded that a threshold of 4 or more criteria was the optimal threshold. Hollerbach et al. [81] reported their experience with EUS-FNA in CP. These authors evaluated 27 patients with CP and compared the results of EUS with 22-gauge needle FNA with the results of ERCP. EUS-FNA increased the negative predictive value to 100% and the specificity to 64%. EUS results were in agreement with regard to the severity of CP according to the Cambridge classification at ERP in 5 of 8 patients with grade I, 11 of 13 patients with grade II, and 10 of 10 patients with grade III disease. Complications in the form of mild acute pancreatitis occurred in 2 patients (7%). On the average, 2.3 needle passes were needed to obtain a sufficient amount of tissue for diagnosis. This study better supports the role of EUS-FNA "in ruling out" rather than " in ruling in" CP. However, it is already well known that a normal EUS examination virtually rules out CP in the appropriate clinical context. Larger needles, improvements in tissue processing, and molecular biology markers could, in the future, expand the application of EUS-FNA in patients with CP.

As with the comparison to ERP, it is unknown if EUS is more sensitive to mild changes of CP than functional testing or if it is overdiagnosing early CP.[24] The natural history may be the most definitive gold standard for early CP. A diagnosis of "mild" CP based on EUS, which then progresses to more severe CP as diagnosed by other tests (EUS positive, ERCP, positive functional test), is likely to be a correct diagnosis. Unfortunately, there are only limited data on the long-term natural history of "mild" CP diagnosed by EUS. Hastier et al. [82] reported the short-term (mean: 22 months) progression of pancreatic disease in 17 asymptomatic alcoholics with an abnormal EUS but a normal ERP. Follow-up EUS examinations for 12-38 months did not identify any progression to more overt (ERP positive) disease. It is likely, however, that patients who took more than 55 years (mean age of study patients was 55.5 years) to develop "mild" disease, require more than 2-3 years to progress from mild to more severe disease. A cross-sectional study of alcoholic patients with and without abdominal pain by Bhutani [74] showed that the EUS diagnosis of CP (4 or more criteria) was positive in 89% of alcoholics with abdominal pain but also in 58% of alcoholics without pain, and 0% of control patients (non-alcoholic, no abdominal pain). More recently, Kahl et al. [75] reported a subgroup of 38 patients with a history of chronic alcohol use and recurrent abdominal pain. At the time of enrollment in the study, 32 of 38 patients had an abnormal EUS but a normal ERP. After a median follow-up of 18 months (range: 6-25 months), 22 of 32 patients developed changes of CP at ERP (12 patients grade I and 10 patients grade II according to the Cambridge classification). Contrary to the study of Hastier et al. [82], Kahl et al. [77] observed ERP changes of CP in a short follow-up (18 months). The only significant differences between the 2 studies appeared to be the presence of alcoholic cirrhosis in Hastier's study and the presence of abdominal pain and recurrent pancreatitis in Kahl's study. Further long-term follow up data are needed.

Nonetheless, there are also several disadvantages of EUS. EUS still remains confined to very few centers, and it is not widely available. Parada et al. [83] retrospectively reviewed the indications for EUS at three major EUS centers. Based on these data, they calculated the hypothetical demand for EUS in the United States to be 79,572 per year for all indications. Second, the value of EUS is directly proportional to the training, skill, and experience of the endosonographer. Virtually all of the data and published information pertaining to EUS are the work of a relatively small group of experts. Third, the principal concern in using EUS for the diagnosis of CP is the possibility that it may overdiagnose the features of CP, causing patients to be falsely diagnosed with CP when they do not have pancreatic disease. Because experts cannot agree on a gold standard for the diagnosis of CP, it has been difficult to determine the extent to which overdiagnosis occurs. In patients with EUS evidence of changes of CP but a normal secretin test or a normal ERP, it is not clear whether the EUS is more sensitive for early changes or if it is truly overdiagnosing CP [84].

2. Pancreatic Cancer

Pancreatic cancer is the most deadly of all gastrointestinal malignancies, the fourth leading cause of cancer-related deaths in the United States and has a very poor prognosis; almost all pancreatic cancer patients will die from this disease. The 5-year survival rate is less than 5%.[85] Pancreatic cancer is a major health problem for several reasons: the aggressive behavior of the tumor and the relative frequency which appears to be increasing; approximately 30,000 new cases in 2002 and about 32,000 in 2004 were diagnosed in the United States.[85] As pancreatic mass lesions are aggressive neoplasms, patients would benefit from early detection, diagnosis, and surgical intervention [86, 87].

Unfortunately most patients present late in the course of their disease with advanced cancer either locally or with metastatic spread.[88, 89] Even though surgery represents the only chance for cure, at the time of diagnosis only 10 to 25% (in the more optimistic series) of pancreatic cancer patients will be eligible for potentially curative resection [89, 90, 91, 92] and the prognosis remains dismal even for patients with potentially curative resections. This is clearly demonstrated by a 5-year survival rate which does not surpass 20% even after surgical resection.[93, 94, 95] Furthermore, considering the high cost of major pancreatic surgery, not only in terms of money but also in terms of morbidity and mortality even in the most experienced surgical hands [96, 97], it is clear that all efforts must be oriented towards the need for an early diagnosis and towards reliably identifying patients who really can benefit from major surgical intervention. A recent study [98] indeed found that a complete resection with negative margins could be achieved in almost half of 53 patients with suspicion of locoregional pancreatic cancer when state-of-the-art preoperative imaging is used.

3. Differentiation of an Early Neoplastic and Inflammatory Mass in Chronic Pancreatitis

Patients with CP have an increased risk of pancreatic cancer, most probably due to increased cell turnover and defective DNA repair with loss of p16 expression and K-ras mutations [99, 100].

Allowing for the relationship between CP and pancreatic cancer to differentiate between a neoplastic and inflammatory pancreatic mass may be extremely difficult, even in view of the different clinical histories and features. A further confounding factor is that some pancreatic cancers are associated with a marked desmoplastic reaction in the pancreas, creating peritumour fibrosis [101].

Microscopically, desmoplastic change leads to hypovascularity of pancreatic ductal adenocarcinomas. Another reason for hypovascularity of ductal adenocarcinomas is vascular encasement, causing arterial stenosis or obstruction.[102] On the contrary, an inflammatory pancreatic mass which is a focal swelling of the pancreas, consists of inflammatory changes such as interlobular fibrosis and chronic inflammatory infiltrate around lobules and ducts.[103] Those inflammatory changes usually require blood flow and result in hypervascularity. Therefore most inflammatory masses show more vascularity than pancreatic adenocarcinomas. However, severe fibrosis can replace pancreatic acinar cells and inhibit vascular development in an inflammatory lesion which is probably the reason why a focal inflammatory pancreatic mass can be hypovascular [104].

Nonetheless, tissue diagnosis (cytologic or histologic examination) often is used in the differentiation of focal CP and pancreatic adenocarcinoma, with EUS-guided fine-needle aspiration (EUS-FNA) usually performed. EUS-FNA is becoming the standard for obtaining cytologic diagnosis, although the sensitivity of EUS-FNA for the differential diagnosis of a focal pancreatic mass is variable in the literature, being as low as 75% in some studies [105]. Moreover, the sensitivity was reported to be unacceptably lower (about 54%) in the context of focal CP, whereas surgical resection was still necessary to confirm the diagnosis [106].

Overall, imaging examinations (CT, MRI, PET, EUS) and EUS FNA have limited success in differentiating between focal CP and pancreatic adenocarcinoma [107].

General CT and MRI Features in the Diagnosis of Pancreatic Adenocarcinoma

Dilatation of the main pancreatic duct, parenchymal atrophy, pancreatic calcification, fluid collection, focal pancreatic enlargement (pancreatic mass due to CP), biliary ductal dilatation, and changes in attenuation in peripancreatic fat or fascia are frequent findings in patients with CP.[108] These findings are also often seen as secondary changes in patients with pancreatic adenocarcinoma.[109] These overlaps of imaging findings make it difficult to distinguish a focal pancreatic mass due to CP from a pancreatic adenocarcinoma or other tumors.

Helical CT and dynamic MRI have been reported useful for detecting and characterizing pancreatic cancers.[110, 111, 112, 113] Pancreatic duct adenocarcinoma is usually hypovascular and appears as a hypoenhanced lesion relative to surrounding pancreatic parenchyma on pancreatic phase images of helical CT and on dynamic MRI.[111, 112] However, these studies didn't focus on early pancreatic cancer. Johnson and Outwater [110] found that masses of pancreatic adenocarcinoma and those due to CP showed more gradual progressive enhancement on dynamic MRI than did normal pancreatic parenchyma, and they histologically found abundant fibrosis in both pathologic conditions, which was thought to account for the similar imaging appearances of the two kinds of masses. Especially when differentiating early focal CP and early pancreatic cancer, this causes differential diagnostic problems.

Computed Tomography in the Differentiation of Focal Chronic Pancreatitis and Pancreatic Adenocarcinoma

A CT examination is limited in identifying (early) ductal adenocarcinoma which begins during CP because of the reduced difference in density between the cancerous lesion, which is typically hypovascularized, and the pancreatic parenchyma, which is also hypovascularized due to the fibrosis. Furthermore, the main pancreatic duct, obstructed upstream by the lesion, already appears dilated due to the pre-existing chronic inflammatory processes. In rare cases, the onset of an adenocarcinoma in CP can sometimes be detected due to the displacement of ductal calcifications (Figure 4) with respect to previous CT examinations, indicating the presence of an expansive lesion.[114] Further, the presence of foci of calcification within the mass is believed to be a crucial radiologic criterion almost never seen in pancreatic duct adenocarcinoma.[115] This criterion only rarely is useful to aid in the differentiation between early CP and early pancreatic adenocarcinoma.

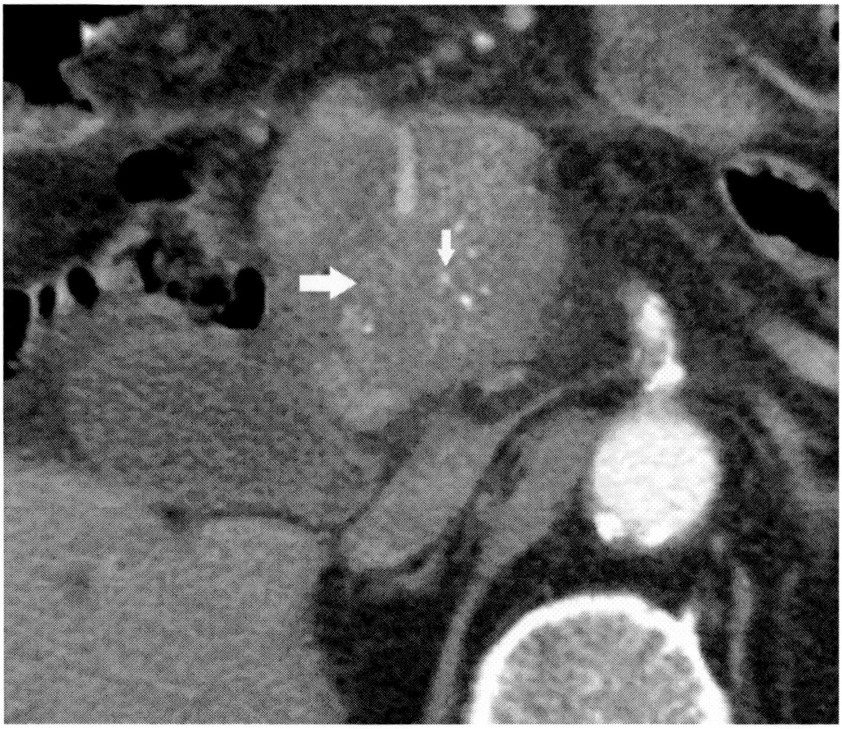

Figure 4a. CT-scan in the dynamic late arterial phase after IV injection of contrast agent displays an area of hypodensity (large white arrow) displacing some intrapancreatic calcifications. An underlying pancreatic cancer is likely in this case.

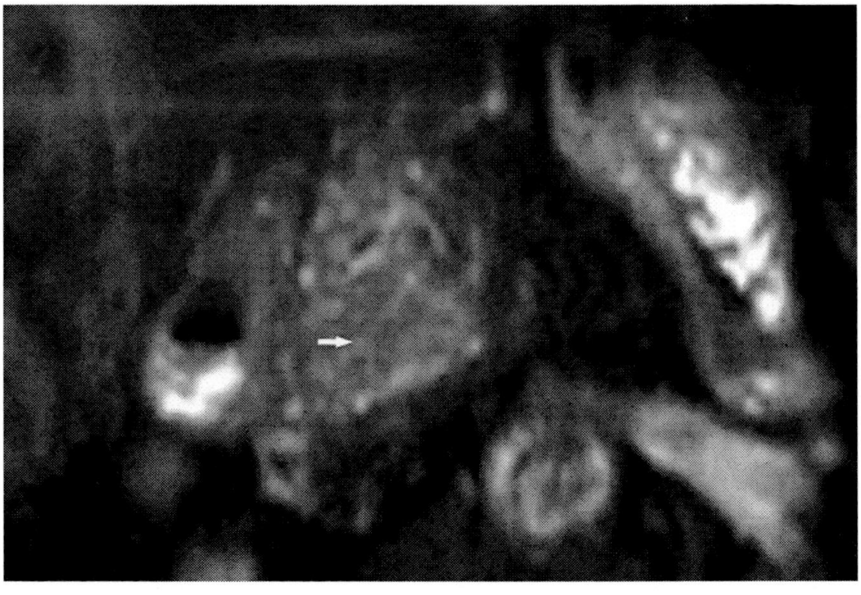

Figure 4b

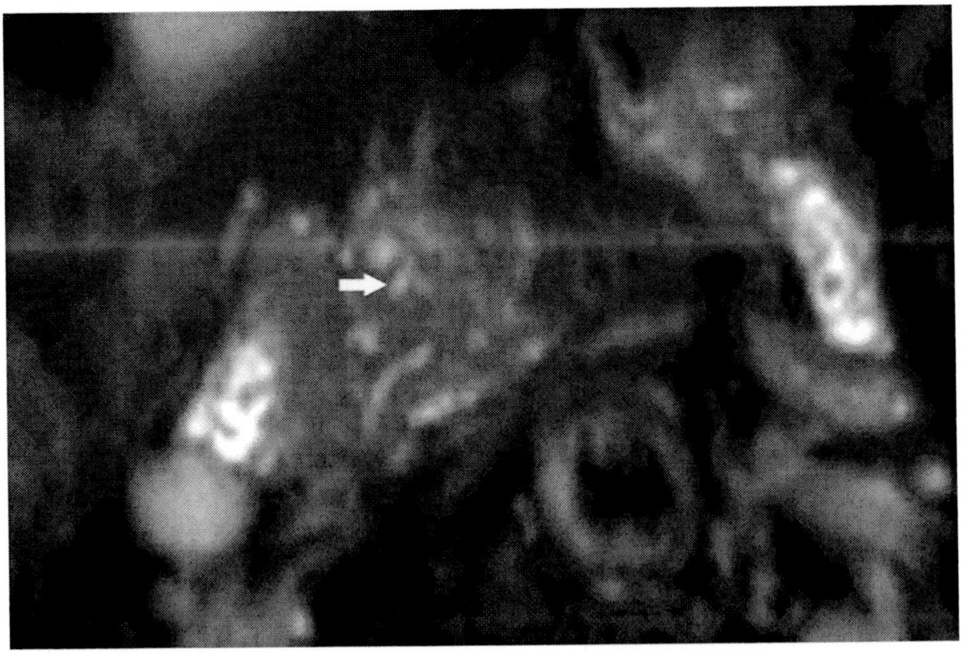

Figure 4c

Figure 4b, 4c. T2w TSE (short TE) MRI-sequence in the transverse plane displays some dilated side branches ("duct-penetrating sign) in the pathologic area (white arrow).

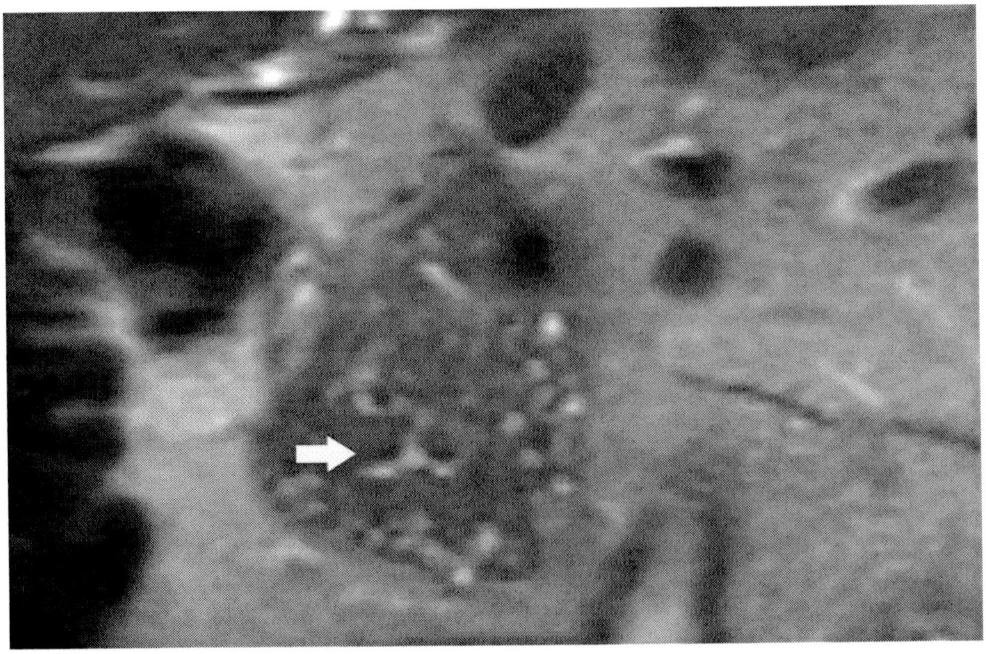

Figure 4d

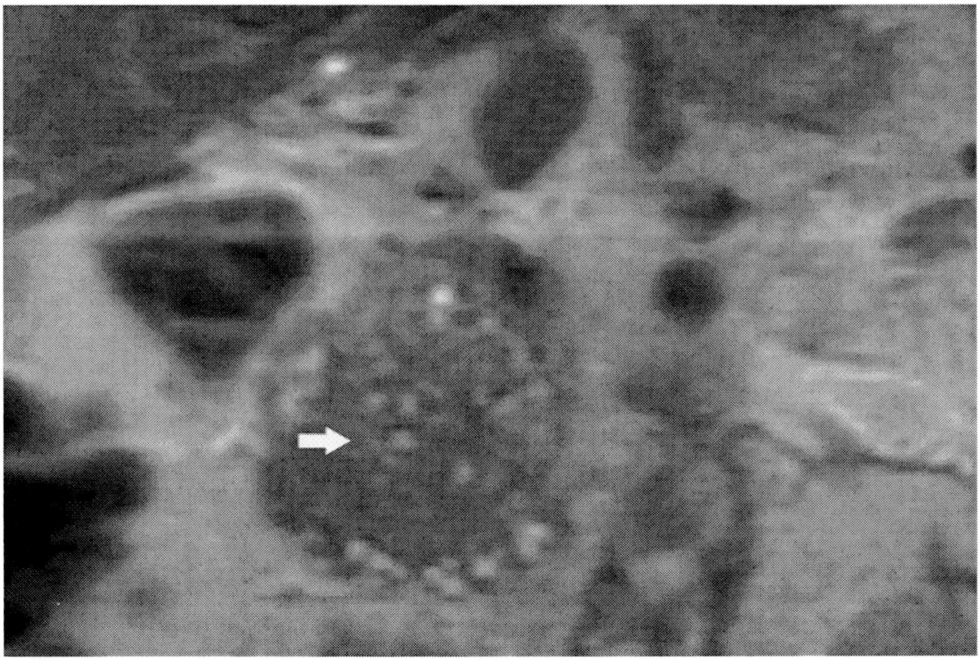

Figure 4e
Figure 4d, 4e. T2w TSE (short TE) MRI-sequence in the coronal plane displays some dilated side branches ("duct-penetrating sign) in the pathologic area (white arrow).

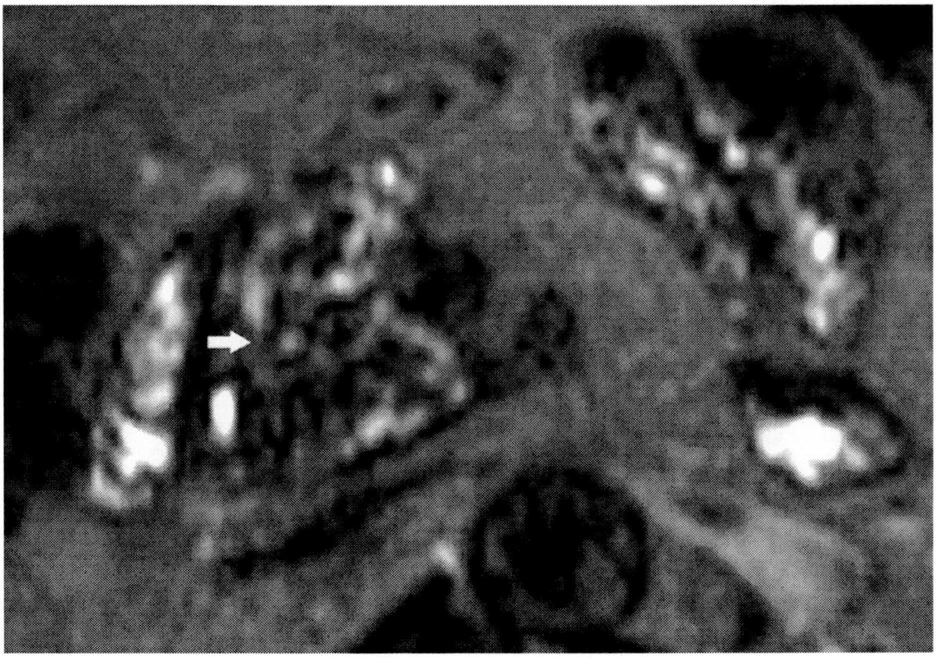

Figure 4f

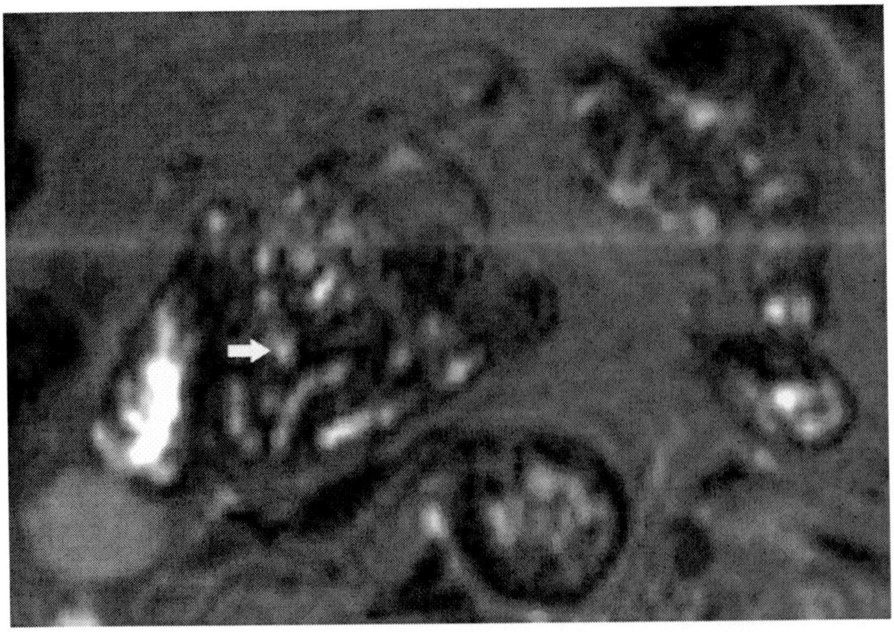

Figure 4g

Figure 4f, 4g. T2w TSE (long TE) MRI-sequence in the transverse plane nicely displays some dilated side branches in the pathologic area (white arrow) indicative of the so-called "duct-penetrating" sign.

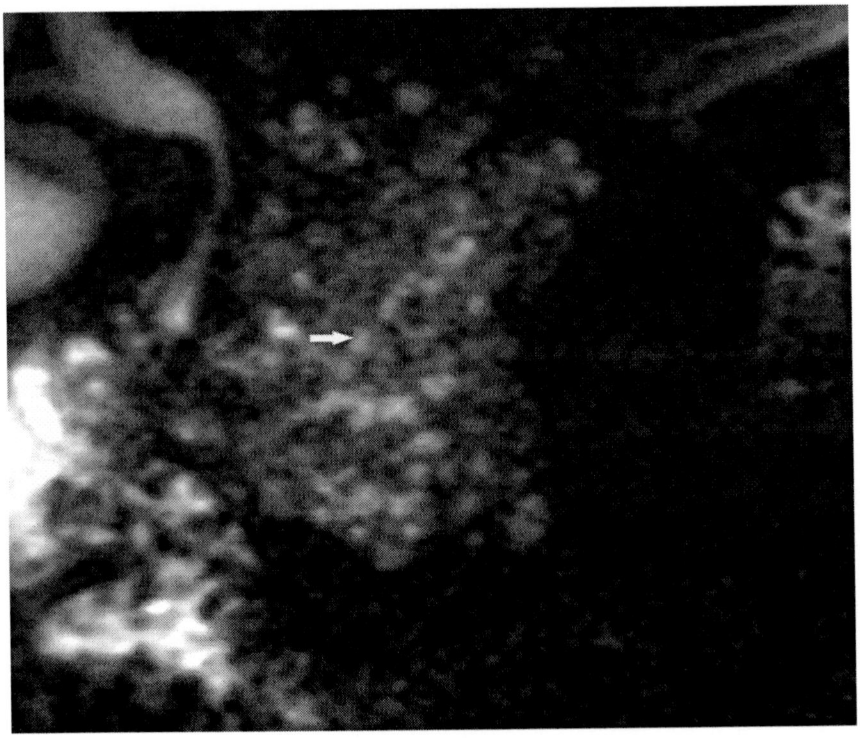

Figure 4h. MRCP-sequence again nicely displays some dilated side branches (white arrows) in the pathologic area. Also note the presence of a pancreatogram.

Magnetic Resonance Imaging in the Differentiation of Focal Chronic Pancreatitis and Pancreatic Adenocarcinoma

MRI is generally considered a valuable tool in the assessment of the full spectrum of pancreatic diseases. Relatively specific morphologic and signal intensity features permit characterization of CP and pancreatic duct adenocarcinoma in many cases but certainly not always. MRI studies can be considered in the following settings in patients with prior CT imaging who have focal enlargement of the pancreas with no definable mass or in patients in whom clinical history is worrisome for malignancy and in whom findings on CT imaging are equivocal or difficult to interpret and in situations requiring distinction between CP with focal enlargement and pancreatic cancer.[116] Still, differentiation between focal CP and a focal solid pancreatic cancer can be very difficult.

When findings of CP are identified in a patient without a prior history of CP or of ethanol abuse, an obstructing lesion should be suspected (Figure 5) [117]. Pancreatic duct adenocarcinoma is the usual cause of chronic obstructive pancreatitis and comprises 75% to 90% of all pancreatic adenocarcinomas (Figure 6).[118] Differentiating between an inflammatory mass due to CP and pancreatic adenocarcinoma on the basis of imaging criteria remains difficult. Irregularity of the pancreatic duct, intraductal or parenchymal calcifications, diffuse pancreatic involvement, and normal or smoothly stenotic pancreatic duct penetrating through the mass ("duct penetrating sign") favor the diagnosis of CP over pancreatic adenocarcinoma (Figure 7, Figure 8).[110] In distinction, a smoothly dilated pancreatic duct with an abrupt interruption, dilatation of both biliary and pancreatic ducts ("double-duct sign"), and obliteration of the perivascular fat planes favor the diagnosis of cancer. MRI may be superior to CT for the evaluation of pancreatic adenocarcinoma, especially if the lesion is small and non-contour-deforming. The tumor is often best delineated on unenhanced T1w FS images and multiphasic contrast-enhanced sequences [32]. However, as mentioned, even when using MRI, differentiating (early) pancreatic adenocarcinoma from mass-forming focal CP remains difficult. Typically, the chronically inflamed pancreas will enhance more than will pancreatic adenocarcinoma on immediate postgadolinium images, particularly those tumors arising in the head. Unfortunately, the degree of contrast-enhancement cannot be used to reliably distinguish these entities because abundant fibrosis is seen in both CP and adenocarcinoma, accounting for their similar appearances [110].

A study of Kim T. et al. [119] revealed two different enhancement patterns in pancreatic masses due to focal CP as seen on two-phase helical CT and on dynamic MRI: pancreatic masses due to CP appeared as hypoenhanced demarcated masses or as isoenhancing nondemarcated masses on pancreatic phase images. The two different enhancement patterns in masses due to CP might be explained by the difference in the degree of fibrosis between the mass and the nonenlarged portion of the pancreas. Fibrosis was pathologically identified in the nonenlarged portion of the pancreas in patients with nondemarcated masses on CT scans or MRI images, whereas fibrosis was not found in the nonenlarged portion of the pancreas in patients with demarcated masses. Fibrosis is one of the main pathologic changes characteristic of CP.[2] Therefore, when CP occurs focally, the inflammatory mass is visibly demarcated on CT scans or on MRI images.

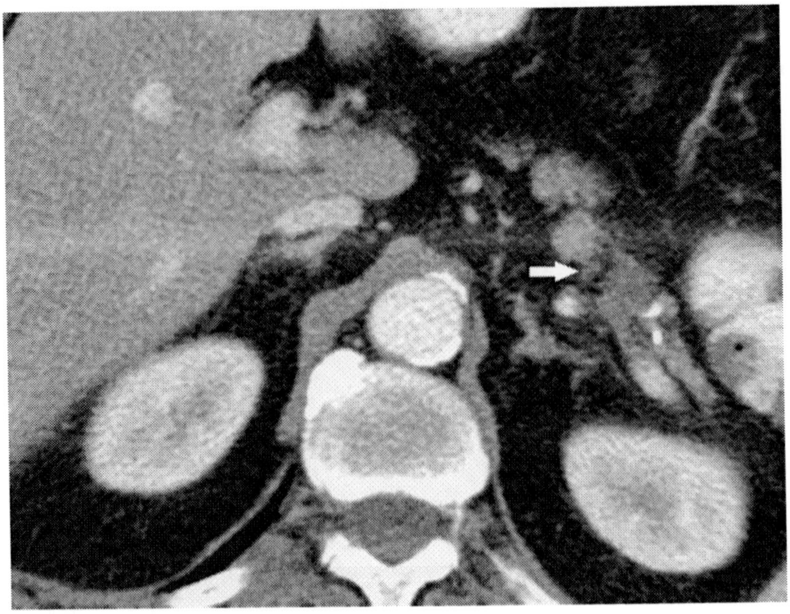

Figure 5a. CT-scan in a delayed venous phase (2 minutes post IV injection of contrast agent) displaying a persisting hypodense area (white arrow) at the level of the pancreatic tail. More proximally, the pancreatic tail shows signs of hypodensity caused by obstructive inflammation of the pancreatic parenchyma.

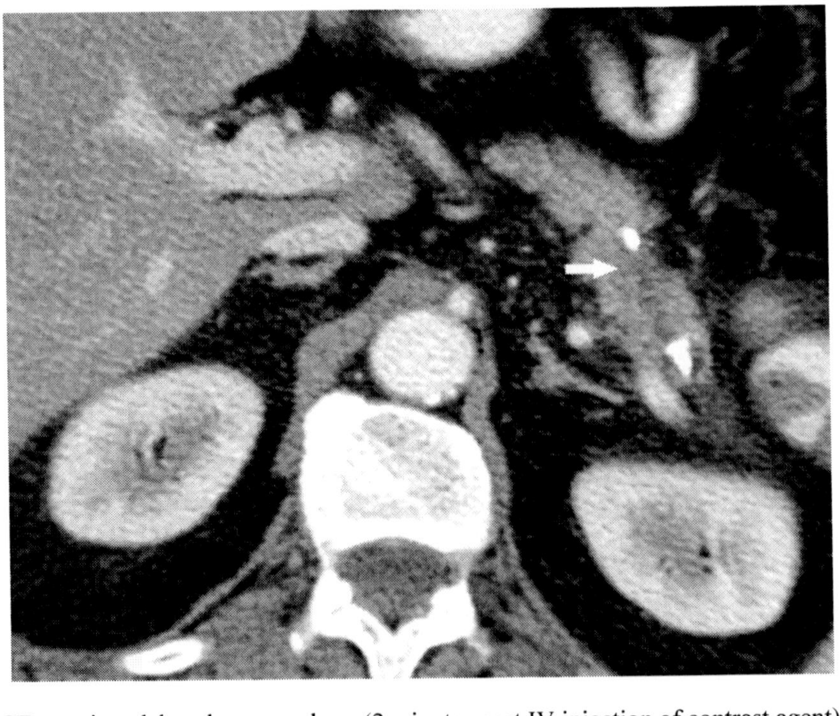

Figure 5b. CT-scan in a delayed venous phase (2 minutes post IV injection of contrast agent) displaying the earlier mentioned persisting hypodense area (white arrow) and some nearby calcifications at the level of the pancreatic tail.

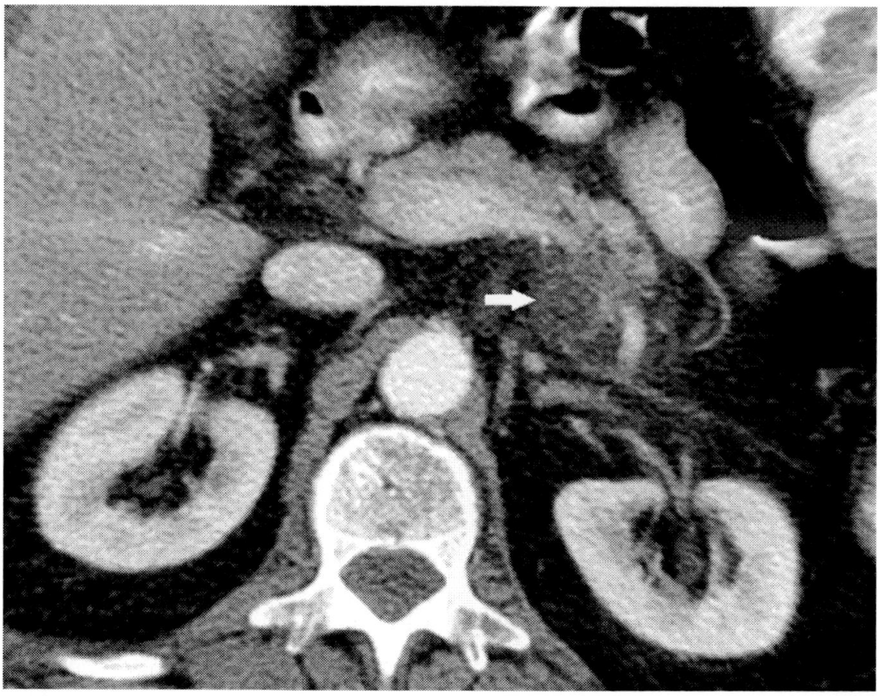

Figure 5c. CT-scan in a delayed venous phase (2 minutes post IV injection of contrast agent) displaying the earlier mentioned persisting hypodense area (white arrow) associated with an area of focal inflammation of the peripancreatic fatty tissue.

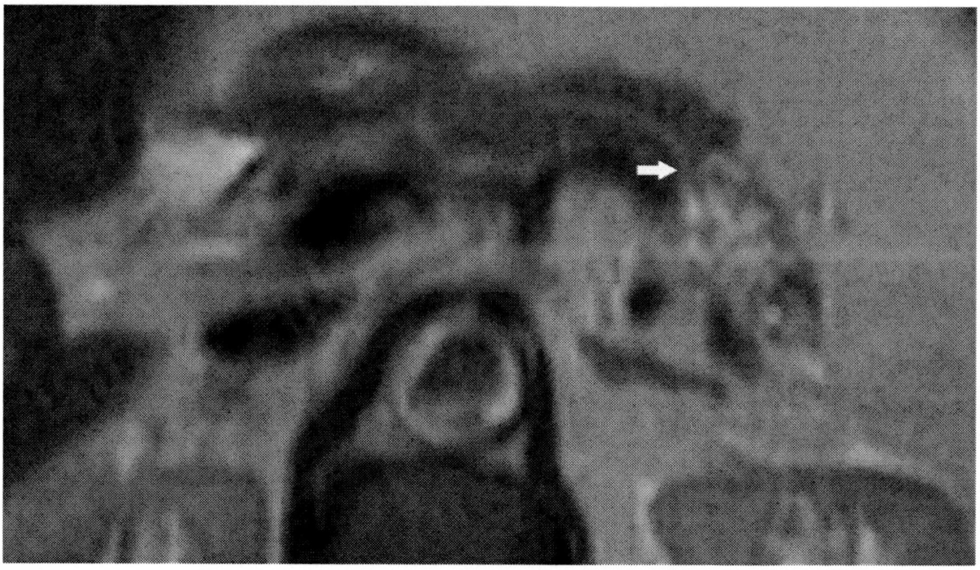

Figure 5d. T2w TSE (short TE) MRI-sequence displaying a clearly distinctive border (white arrow) between normal and pathologic (proximal part of pancreatic tail) pancreatic parenchyma. The pathologic pancreatic parenchyma is clearly more hyperintense due to edema at some dilated side branches at this level.

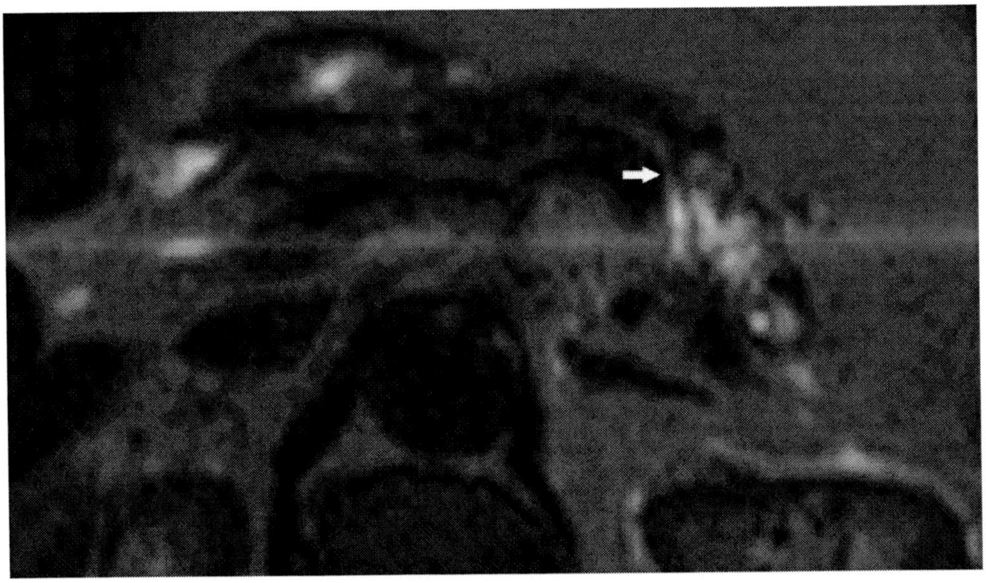

Figure 5e. T2w TSE (long TE) MRI-sequence displaying the above mentioned clearly distinctive border (white arrow) between normal and pathologic (proximal part of pancreatic tail) pancreatic parenchyma. The pathologic pancreatic parenchyma is clearly more hyperintense due to edema at some dilated side branches at this level.

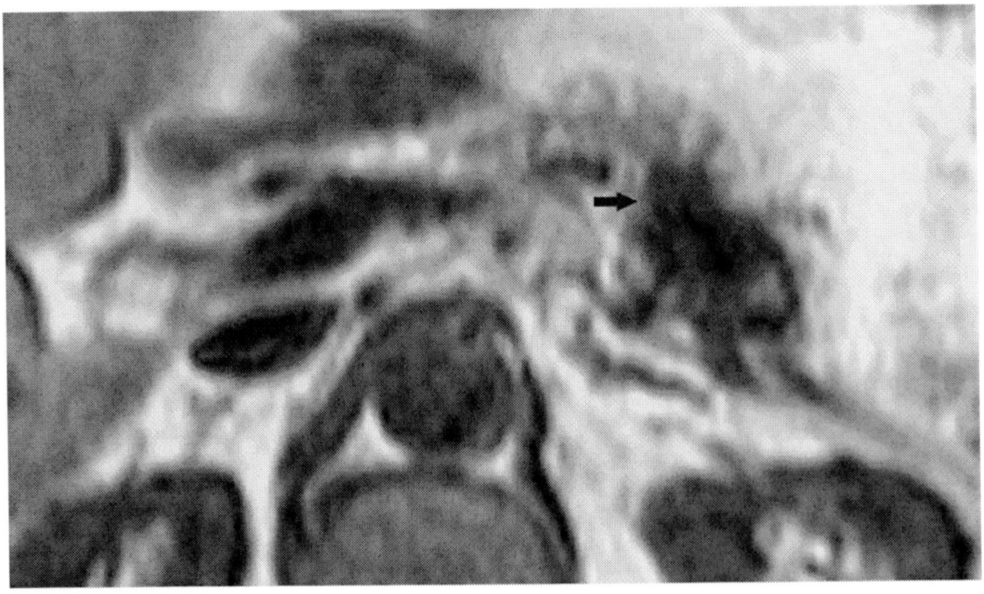

Figure 5f. T1w GE MRI-sequence before IV injection of contrast agent and without fat suppression also displays the above mentioned clearly distinctive border (black arrow) between normal and pathologic (proximal part of pancreatic tail) pancreatic parenchyma. The pathologic pancreatic parenchyma is clearly more hypointense on T1w imaging due to edema and decrease of protein-rich pancreatic juice. The normal part of the pancreatic parenchyma is clearly hyperintense due to the high protein concentration of the pancreatic juice.

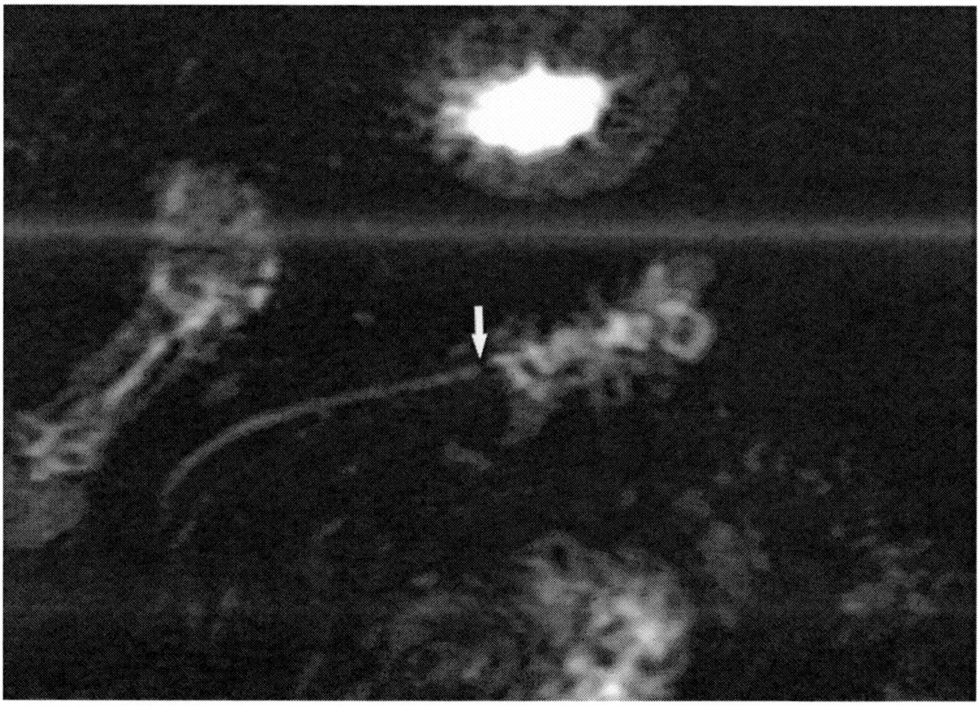

Figure 5g

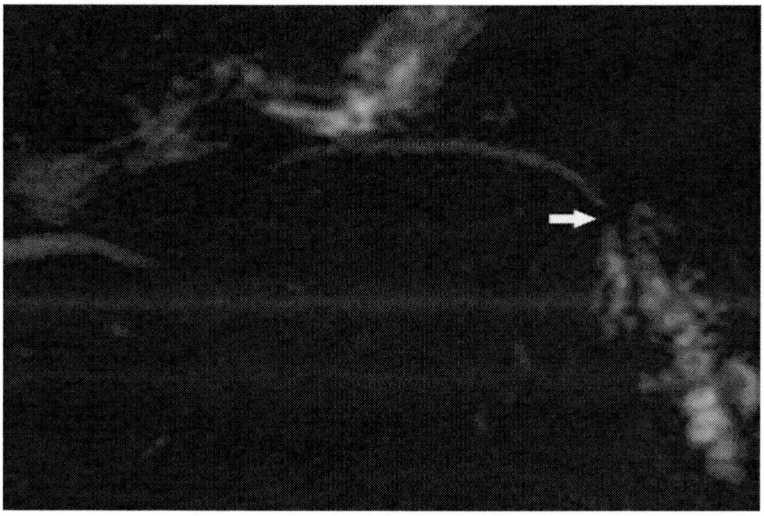

Figure 5h

Figure 5g, 5h. MRCP-sequence again displaying a clearly distinctive border (white arrow) between normal and pathologic (proximal part of pancreatic tail) pancreatic parenchyma. The pathologic pancreatic parenchyma is clearly more hyperintense due to edema at some dilated side branches at this level. Also notice a focal distinctive narrowing of the main pancreatic duct (white arrow) necessitating the search for or the exclusion of a focal pancreatic cancer.

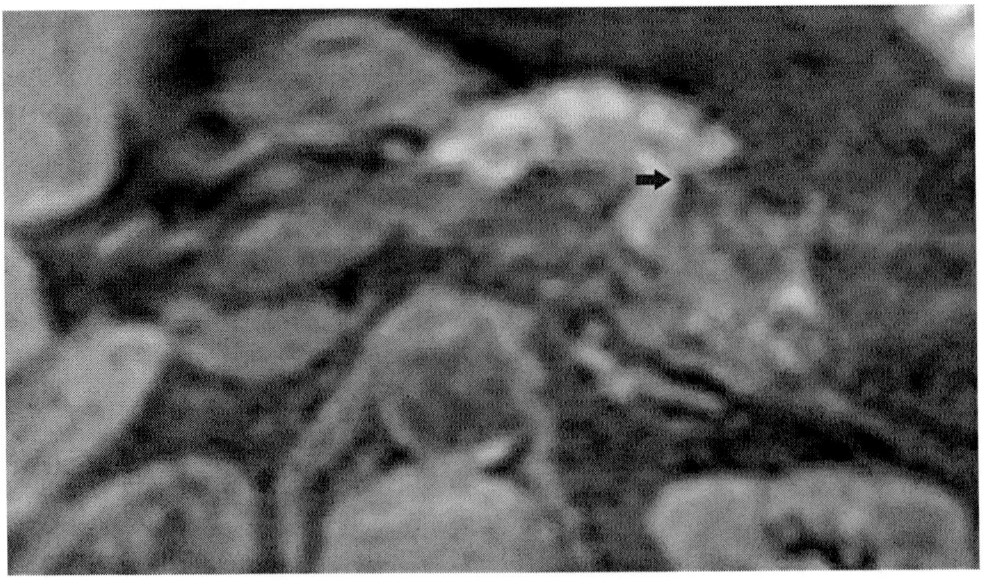

Figure 5i. T1w GE MRI-sequence with fat suppression before IV injection of contrast agent displaying the above mentioned clearly distinctive border (black arrow) between normal and pathologic (proximal part of pancreatic tail) pancreatic parenchyma.

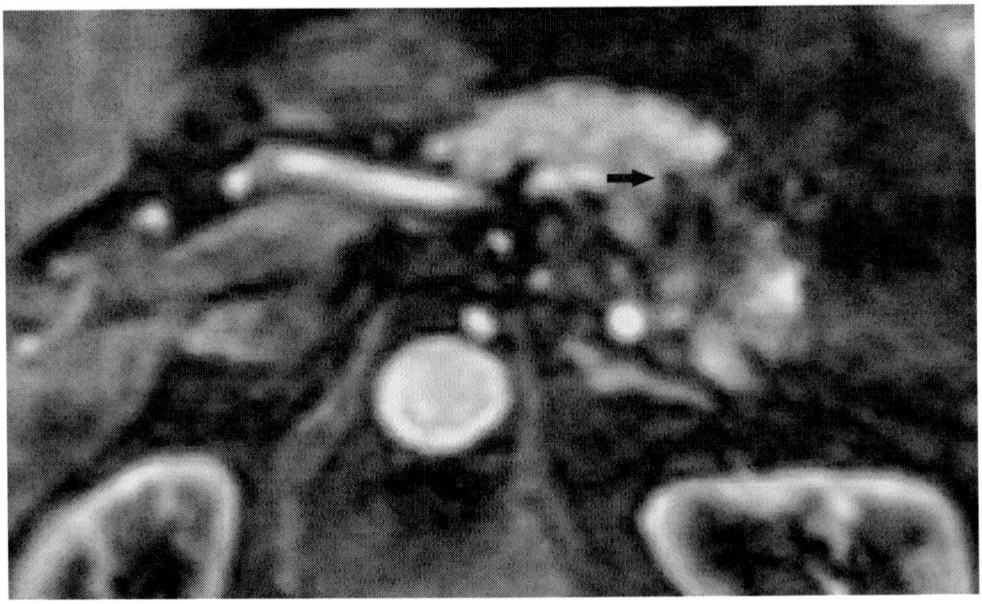

Figure 5j. T1w GE MRI-sequence with fat suppression in the dynamic late arterial phase after IV injection of contrast agent displaying the above mentioned clearly distinctive border (black arrow) between normal and pathologic (proximal part of pancreatic tail) pancreatic parenchyma. The pathologic pancreatic parenchyma is clearly less contrast-enhancing when compared with the normal pancreatic parenchyma.

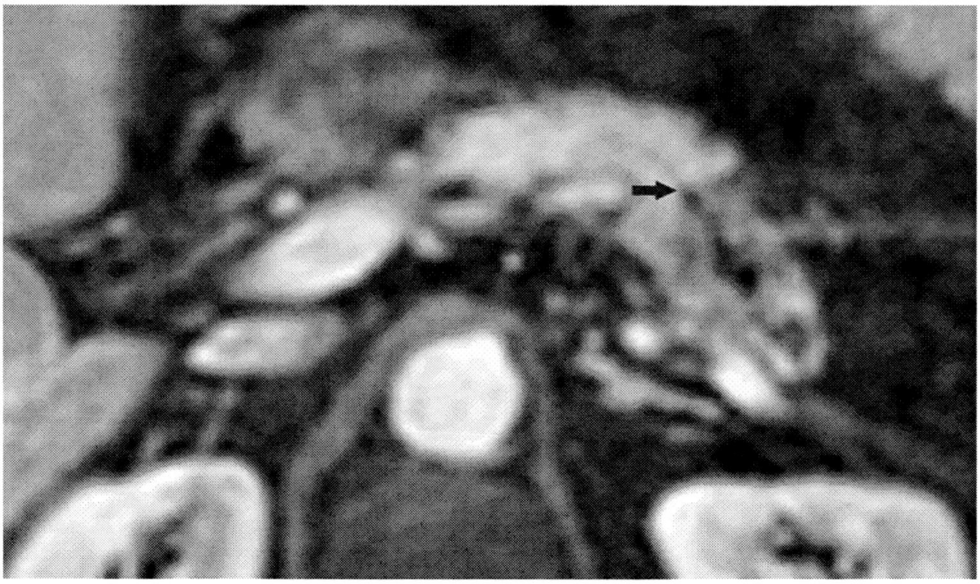

Figure 5k. T1w GE MRI-sequence with fat suppression in the early venous phase after IV injection of contrast agent displaying the above mentioned clearly distinctive border (black arrow) between normal and pathologic (proximal part of pancreatic tail) pancreatic parenchyma. The pathologic pancreatic parenchyma is clearly less contrast-enhancing when compared with the normal pancreatic parenchyma.

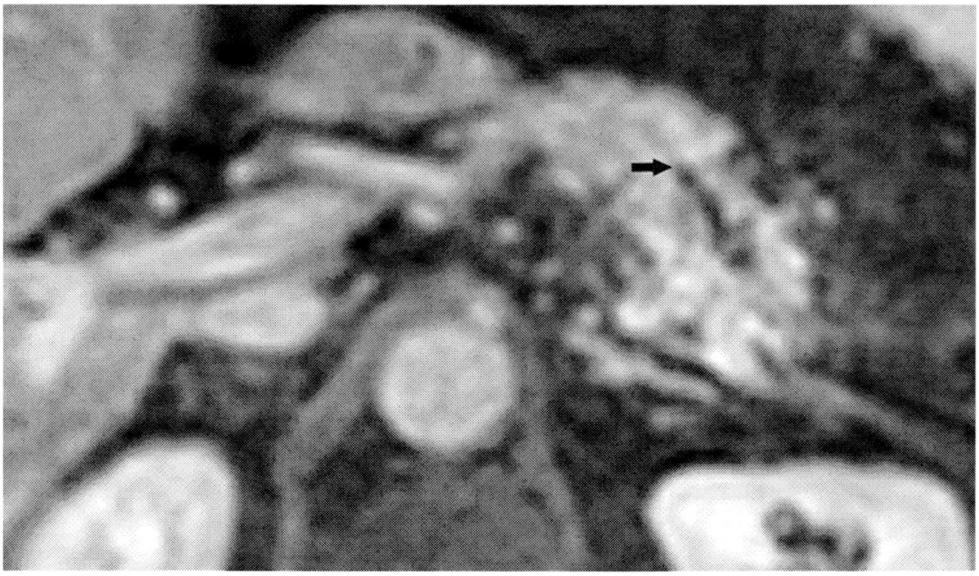

Figure 5l. T1w GE MRI-sequence with fat suppression in the delayed venous phase 5 minutes after IV injection of contrast agent. The border (black arrow) between normal and pathologic (proximal part of pancreatic tail) pancreatic parenchyma is hard to discriminate. This border can mainly be detected by an abrupt narrowing of the main pancreatic duct (black arrow) at this level. No underlying pancreatic cancer/solid mass can be detected.

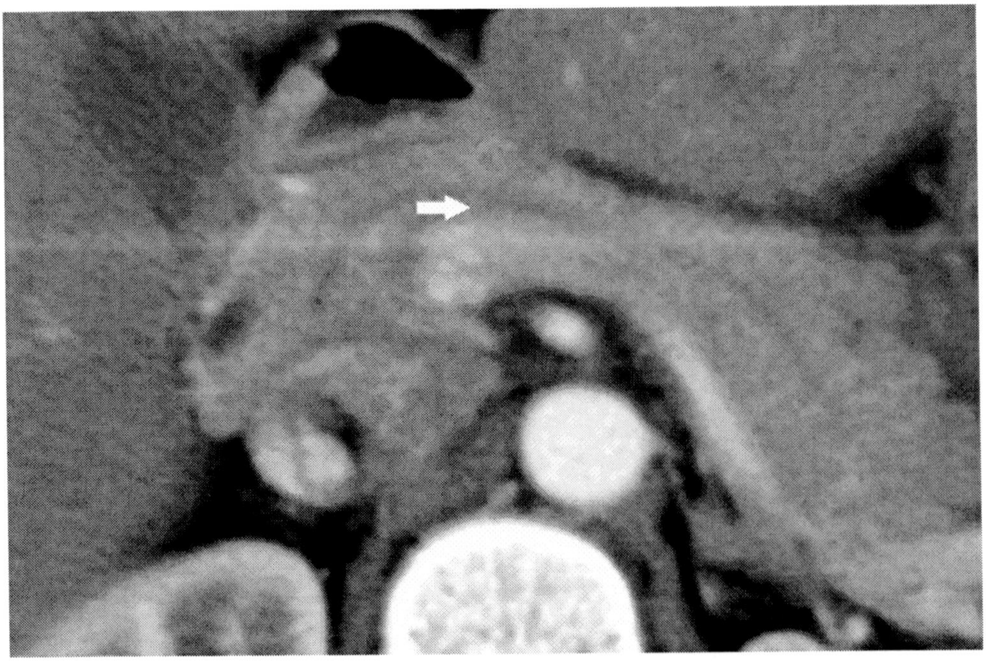

Figure 6a

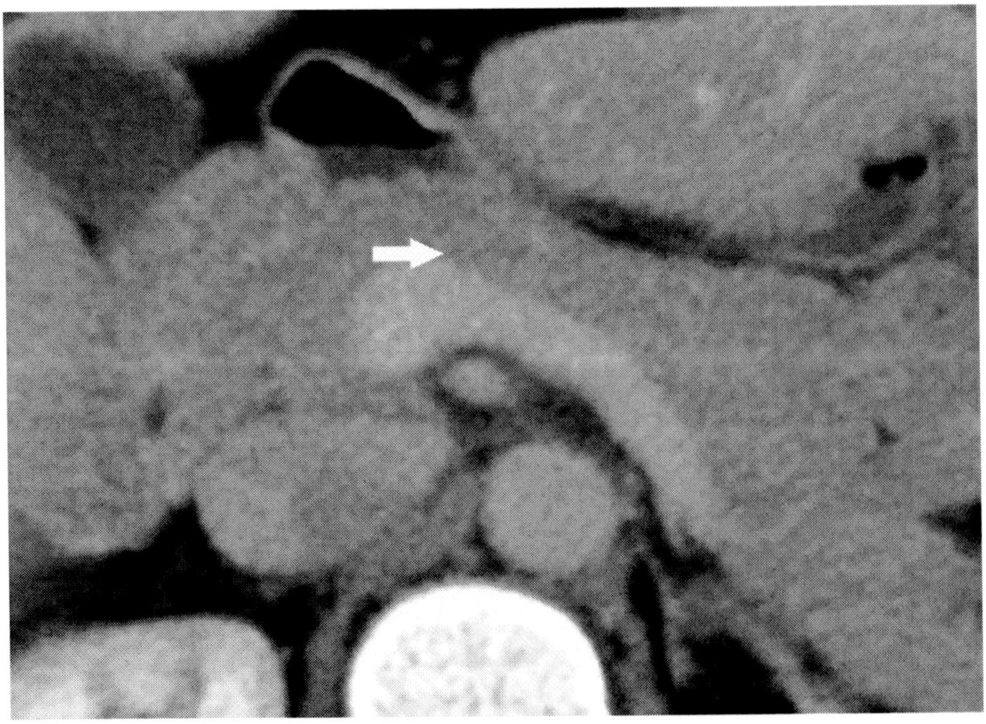

Figure 6b

Figure 6a, 6b. CT-scan in the dynamic late arterial phase after IV injection of contrast agent displaying an enlarged main pancreatic duct. No solid mass is seen at the level of the white arrow.

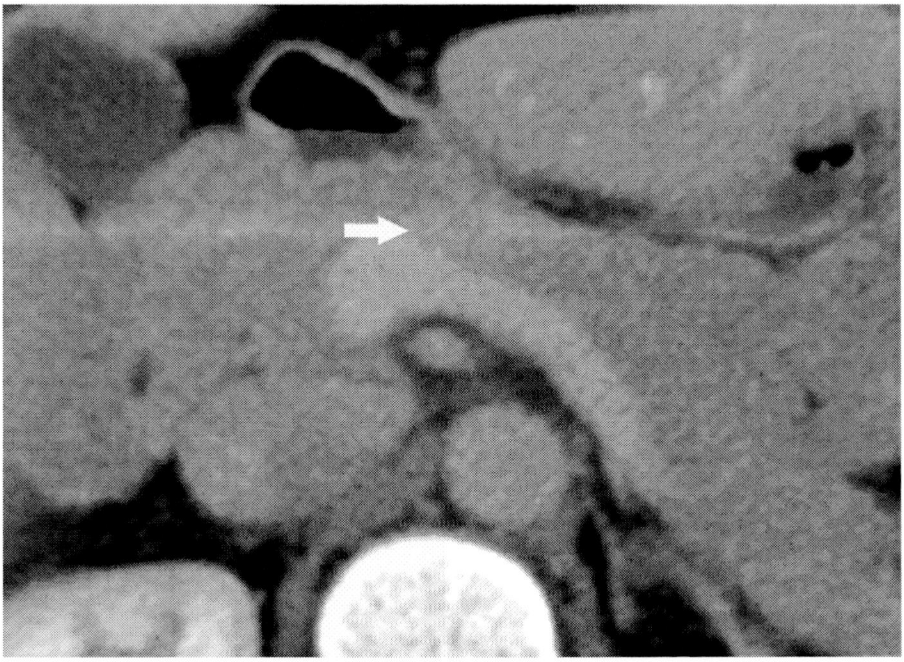

Figure 6c. BlackBlood Single Shot Spin Echo Echo Planar Imaging (BB SS SE-EPI) using a low diffusion gradient ($b=10s/mm^2$) in the transverse plane clearly displays one focal hyperintensity (white arrow) at the level of the pancreatic body. This finding is very suggestive of an underlying solid mass.

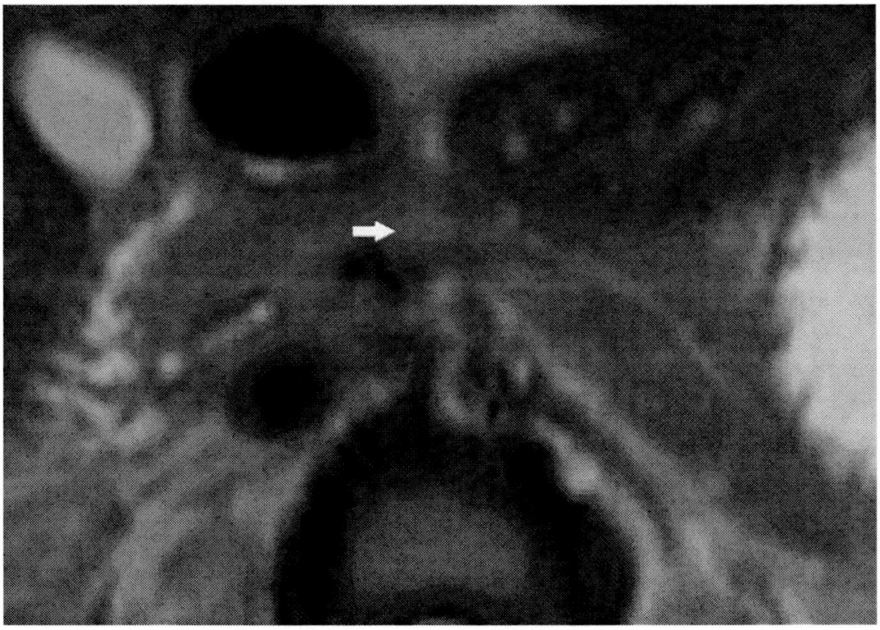

Figure 6d. T2w TSE (short TE) MRI-sequence in the transverse plane displaying an enlarged main pancreatic duct. A slight hyperintense area might be identified retrospectively.

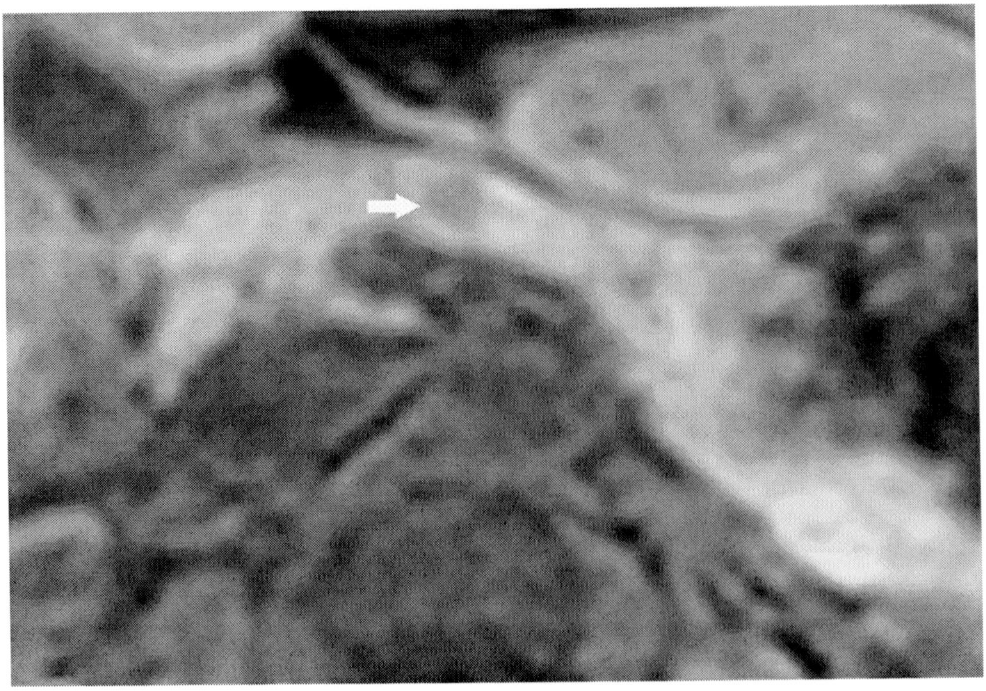

Figure 6e. T1w GE MRI-sequence before IV injection of contrast agent and with fat suppression displays a discrete hypointensity (white arrow) at the level of the pancreatic body.

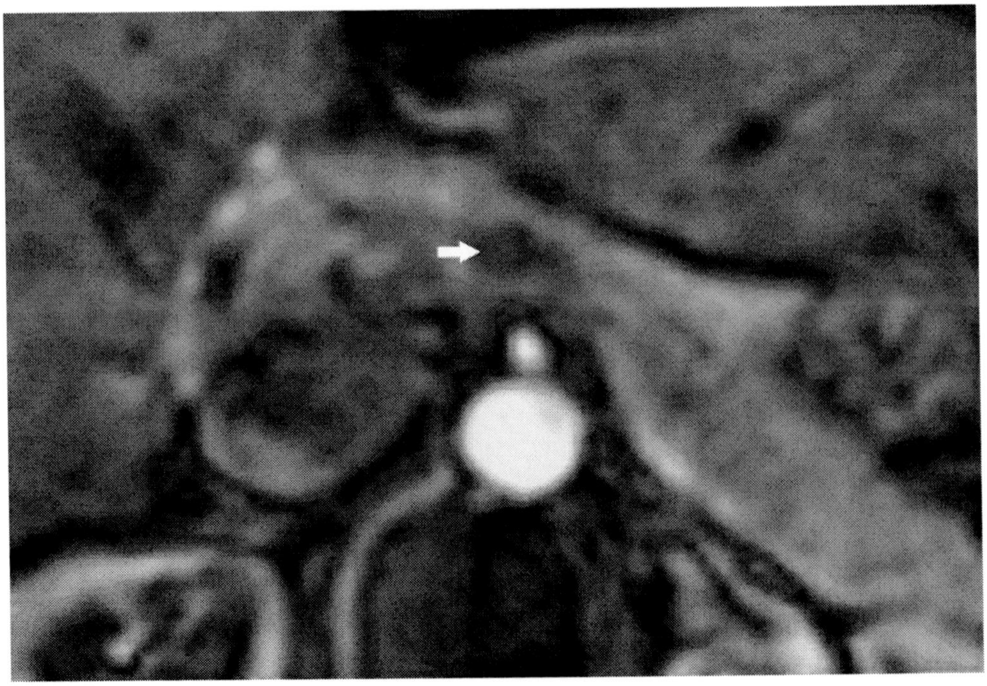

Figure 6f. T1w GE MRI-sequence with fat suppression in the dynamic late arterial phase after IV injection of contrast agent displays the above mentioned hypointensity (white arrow) more clearly.

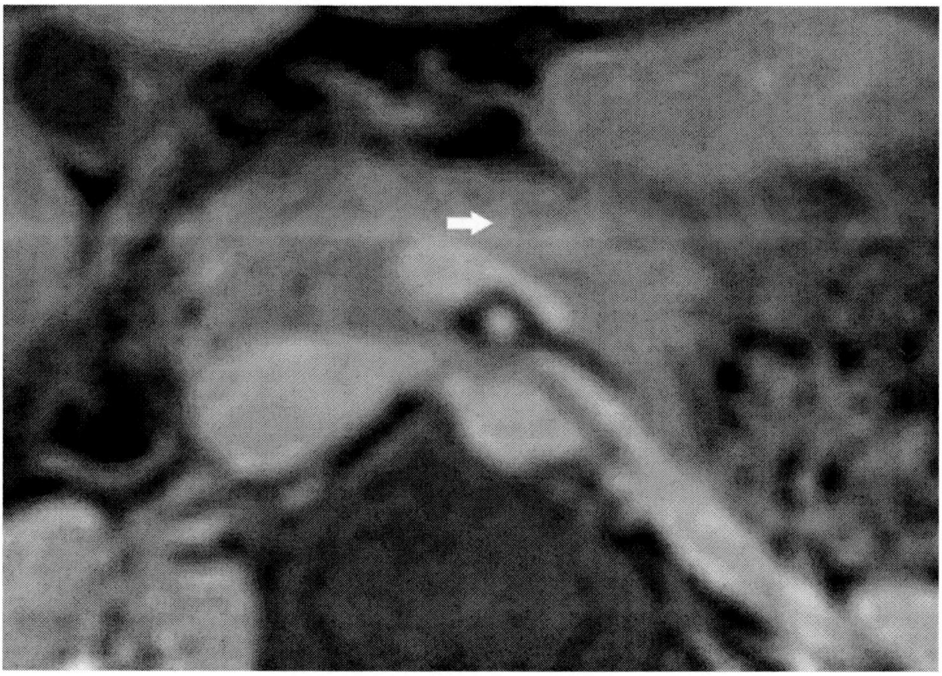

Figure 6g. T1w GE MRI-sequence with fat suppression in the delayed venous phase 5 minutes after IV injection of contrast agent displays the above mentioned hypointensity (white arrow) less clearly. This finding is rather suggestive for chronic pancreatitis.

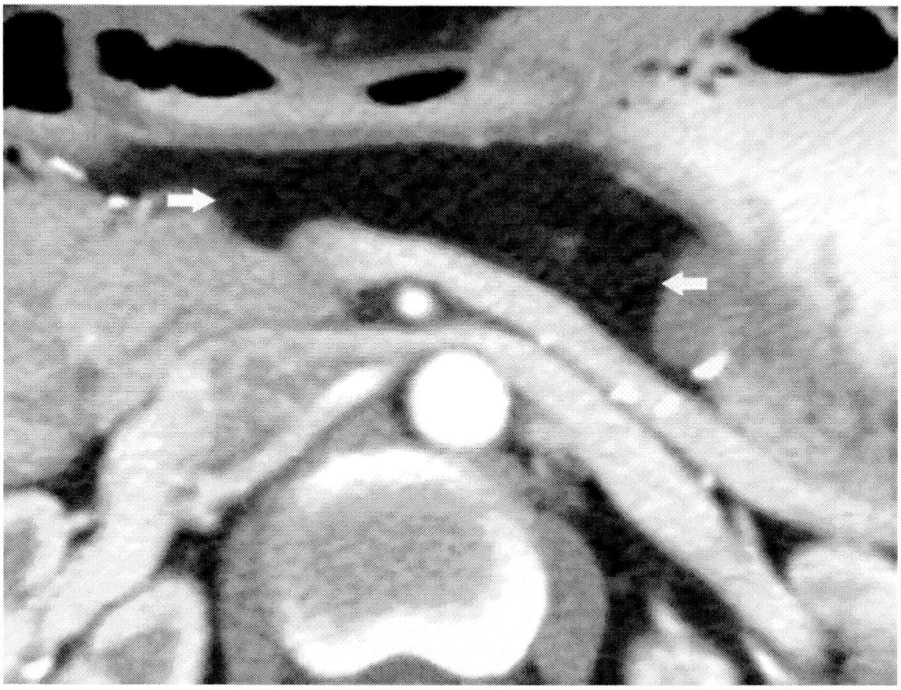

Figure 6h. CT-scan in the dynamic late arterial phase after IV injection of contrast agent displaying the remaining pancreatic parenchyma post-resection. A small focal pancreatic cancer was confirmed histopathologically.

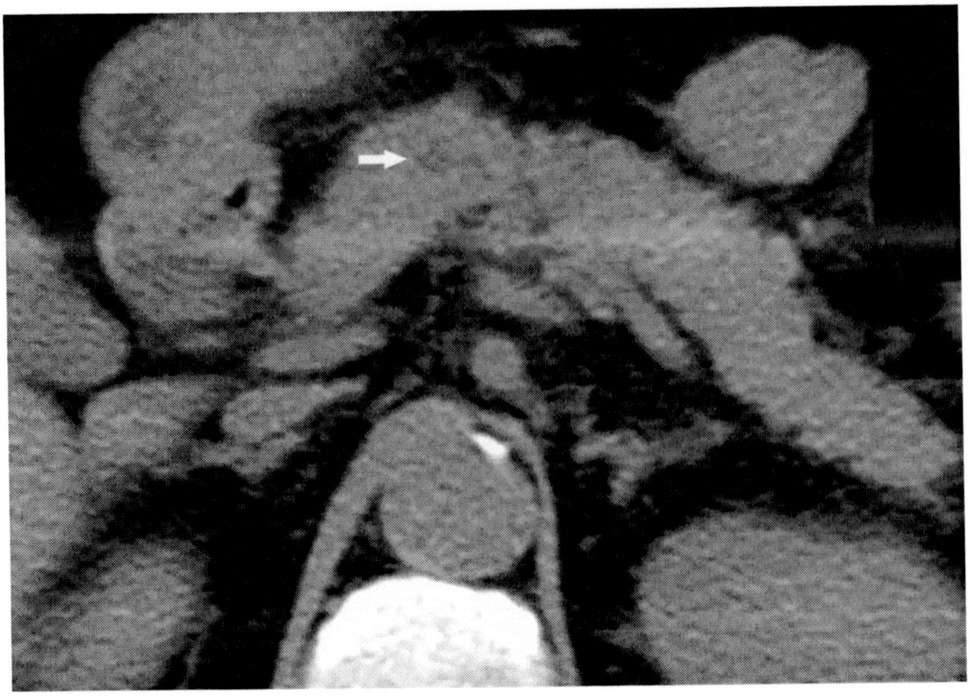

Figure 7a. CT-scan before IV injection of contrast agent displaying a discrete hypodense area (white arrow) at the level of the pancreatic neck. No further signs of pathology are seen.

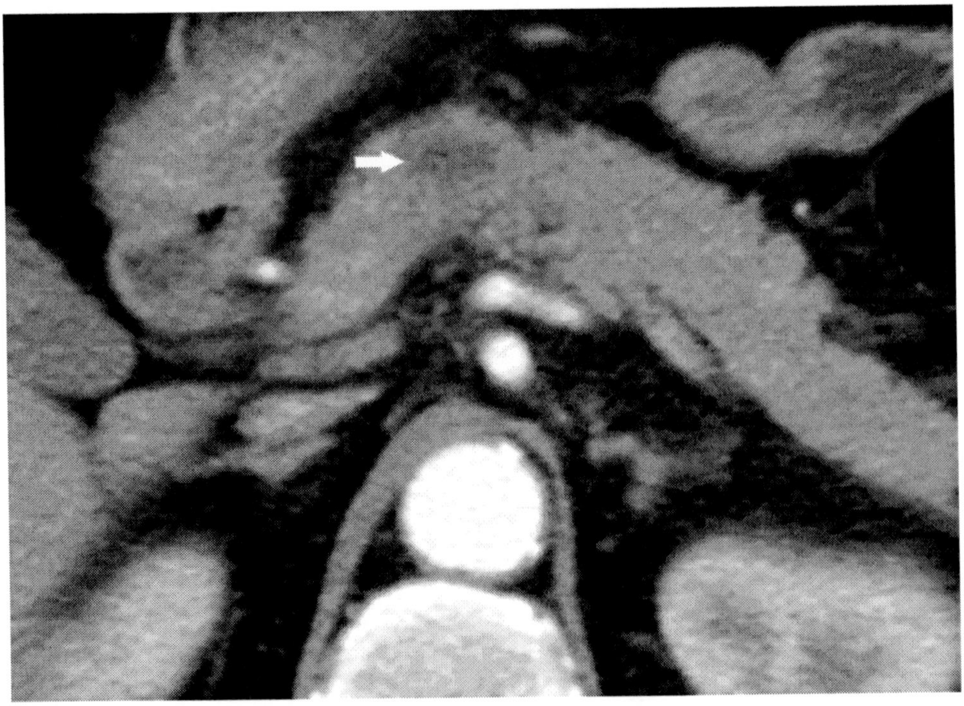

Figure 7b. CT-scan in the dynamic late arterial phase after IV injection of contrast agent more clearly displaying the above mentioned hypodense area (white arrow) at the level of the pancreatic neck. No further signs of pathology are seen.

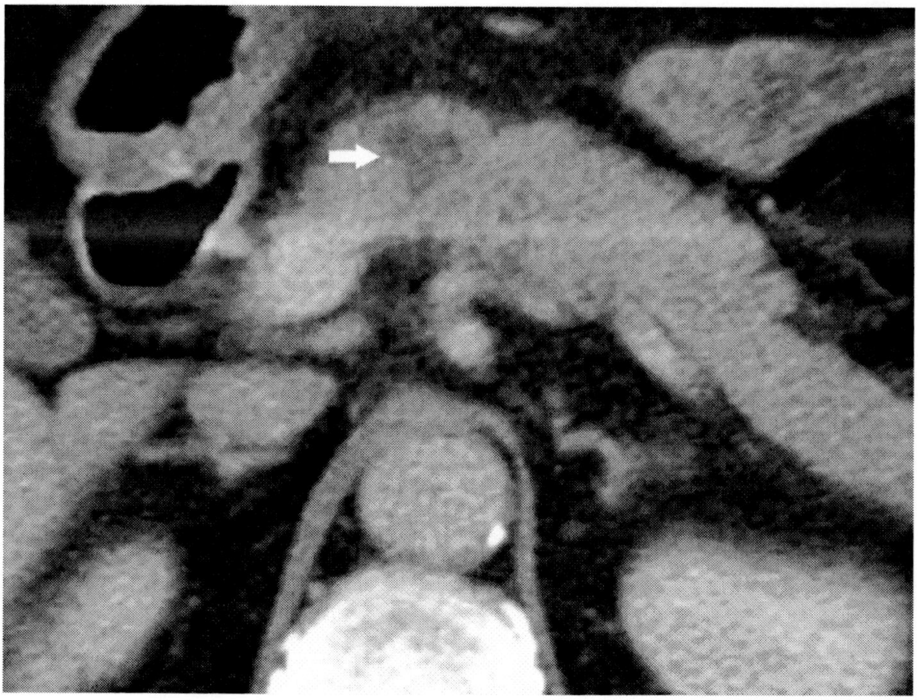

Figure 7c. CT-scan in the dynamic early venous phase after IV injection of contrast agent clearly displaying the above mentioned hypodense area (white arrow) at the level of the pancreatic neck. No further signs of pathology are seen. Using CT-scan in this case, the differential diagnosis between focal chronic pancreatitis and focal pancreatic cancer was very difficult.

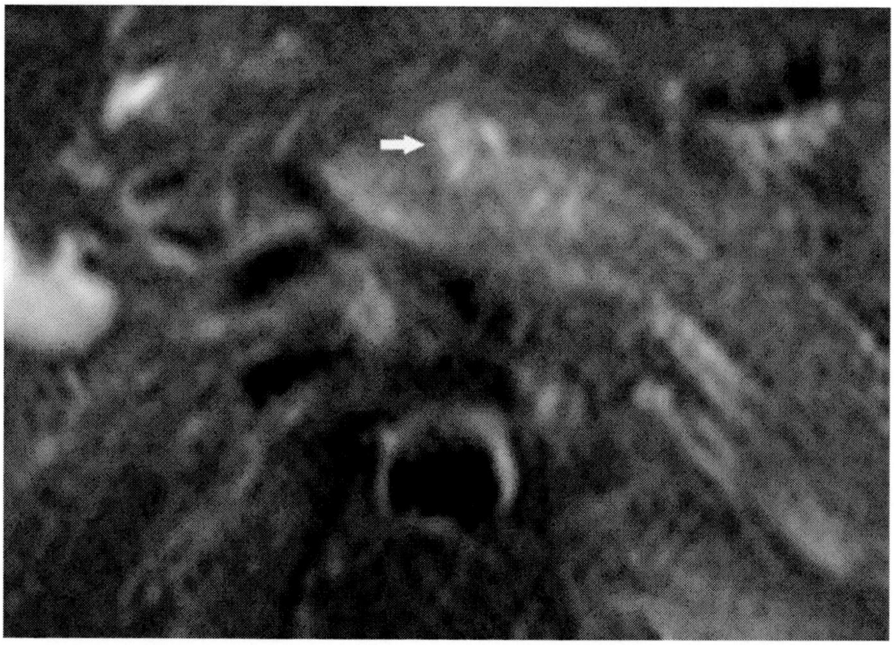

Figure 7d. T2w TSE (short TE) MRI-sequence displaying a moderate to frank hyperintense area (white arrow) at the level of the pancreatic neck. An abutting pathologically dilated side branch , indicative for chronic pancreatitis, is also depicted.

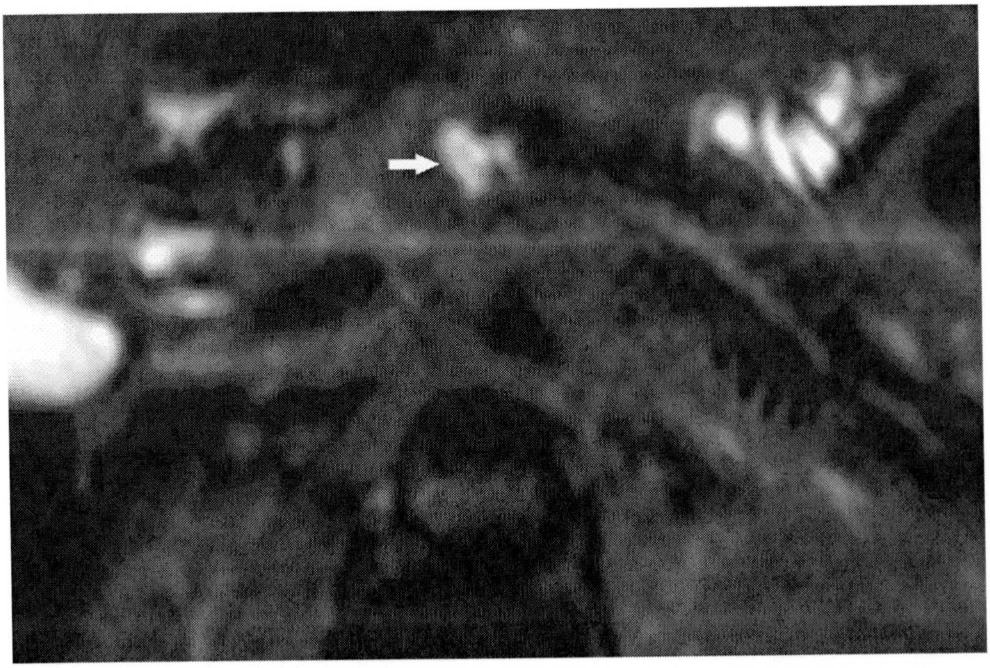

Figure 7e. T2w TSE (long TE) MRI-sequence still displaying the above mentioned area as hyperintense (white arrow) indicative for fluid (cyst). An abutting pathologically dilated side branch , indicative for chronic pancreatitis, is also depicted.

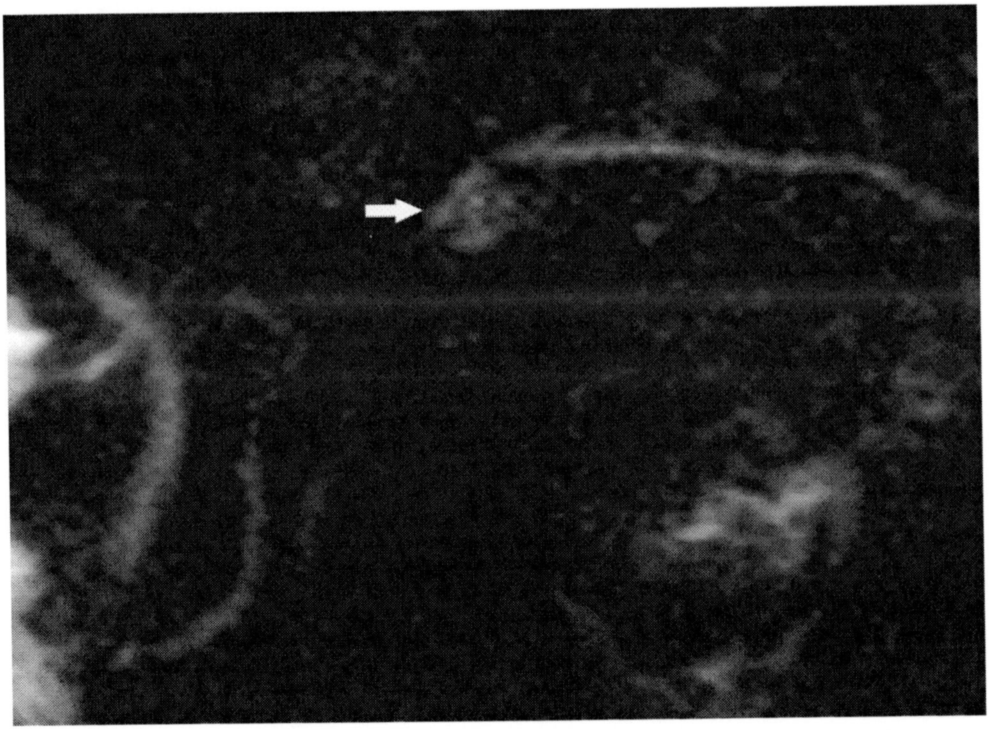

Figure 7f. MRCP-sequence displaying the above mentioned area as hyperintense (white arrow). An abutting pathologically dilated side branch, indicative for chronic pancreatitis, is also depicted.

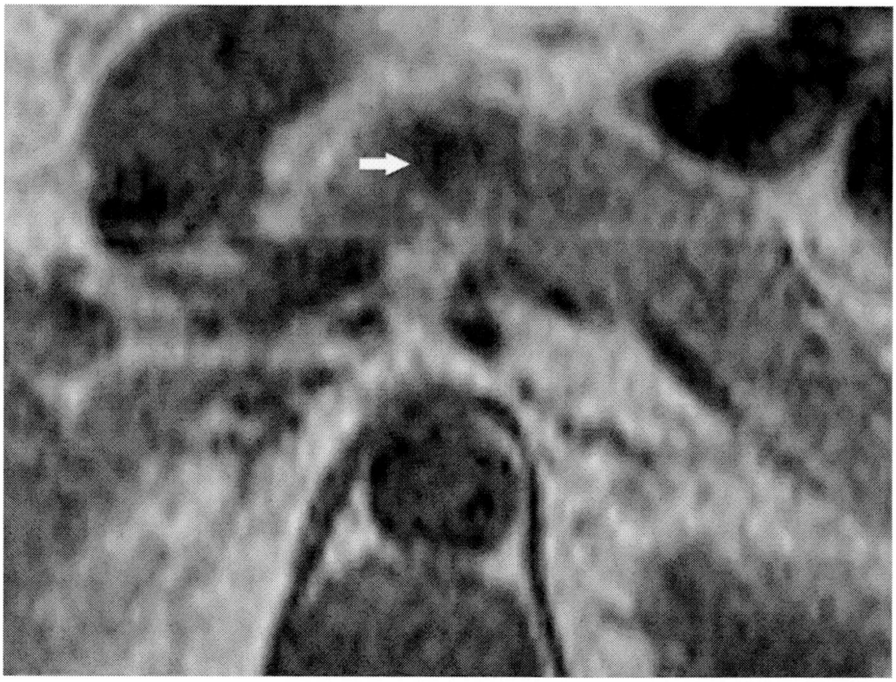

Figure 7g. T1w GE MRI-sequence before IV injection of contrast agent and without fat suppression displays the above mentioned area as hypointense (white arrow). Furthermore, the signal intensity of the remaining pancreatic parenchyma is too low, suggestive of pancreatitis.

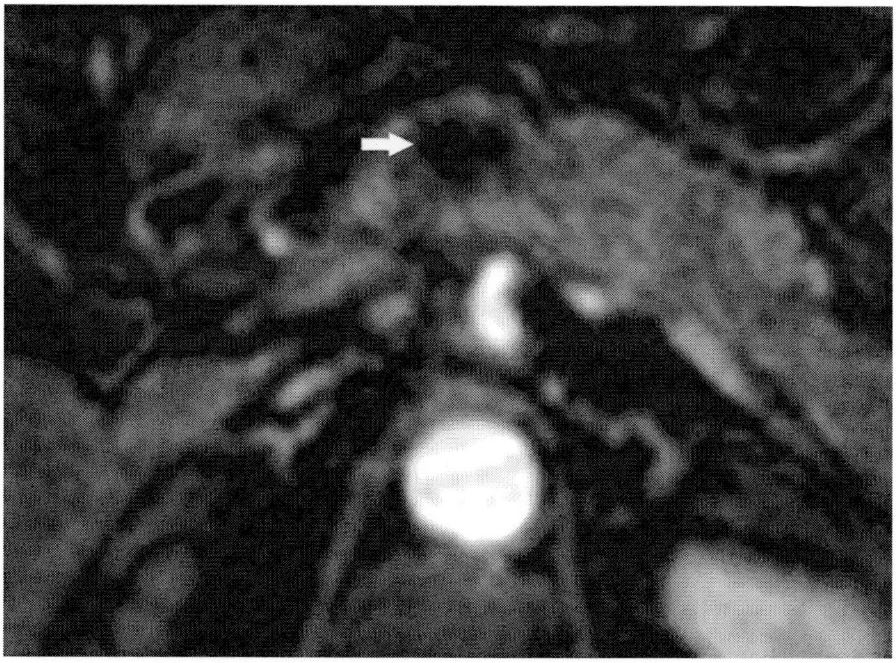

Figure 7h. T1w GE MRI-sequence with fat suppression in the dynamic late arterial phase after IV injection of contrast agent displaying the above mentioned area as hypointense (white arrow). No contrast-enhancement is seen at this level. The remaining pancreatic parenchyma displays heterogenous contrast-enhancement.

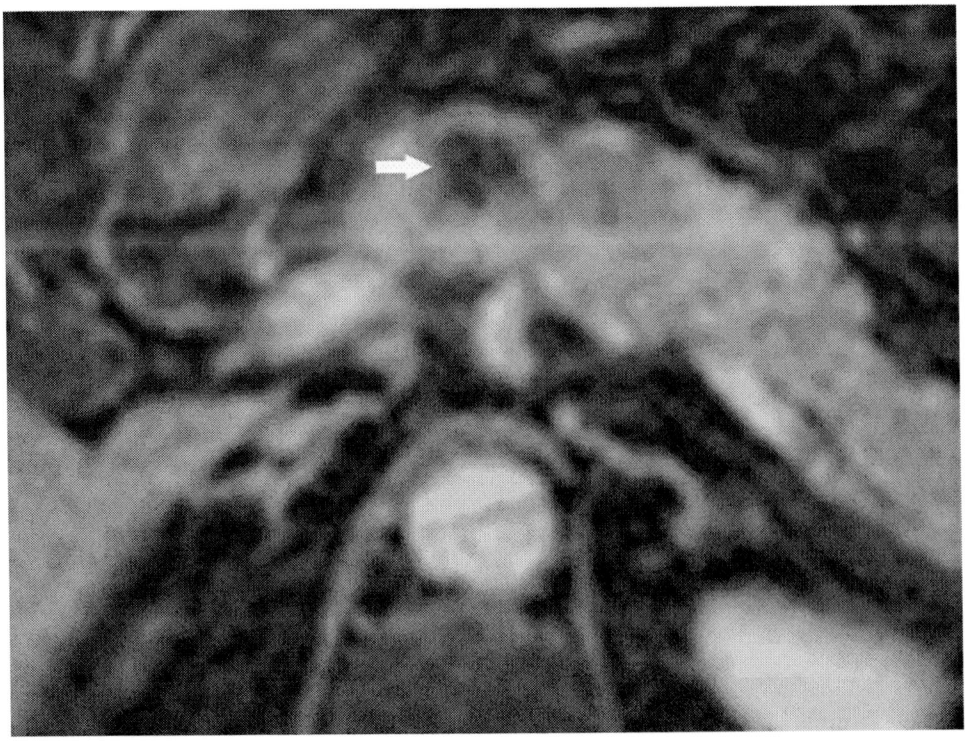

Figure 7i. T1w GE MRI-sequence with fat suppression in the delayed venous phase 5 minutes after IV injection of contrast agent displaying the above mentioned area as hypointense (white arrow). No contrast-enhancement is seen at this level. The remaining pancreatic parenchyma displays heterogenous contrast-enhancement.

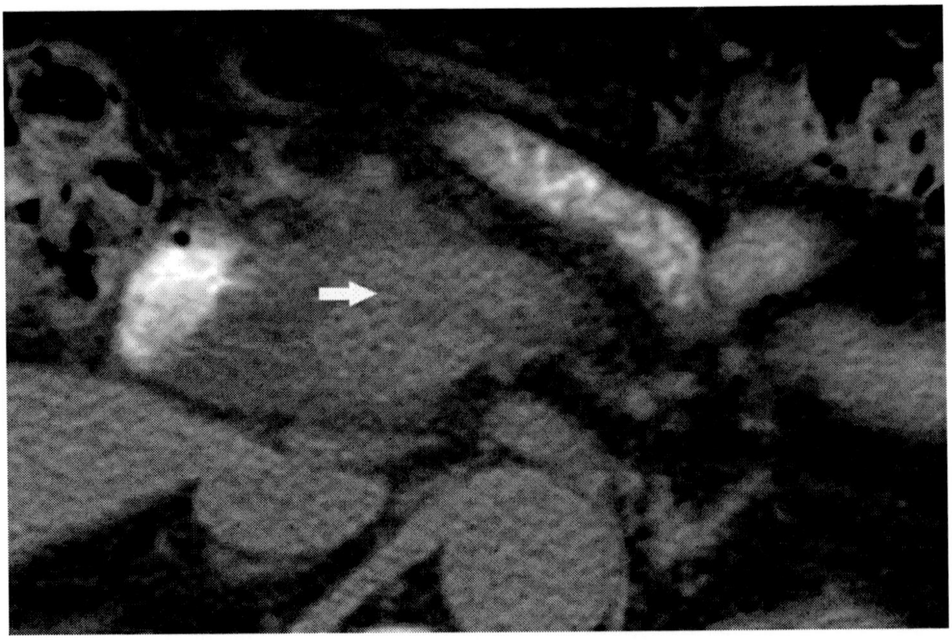

Figure 8a. CT-scan before IV injection of contrast agent displaying a hypodense area (white arrow) at the level of the pancreatic head.

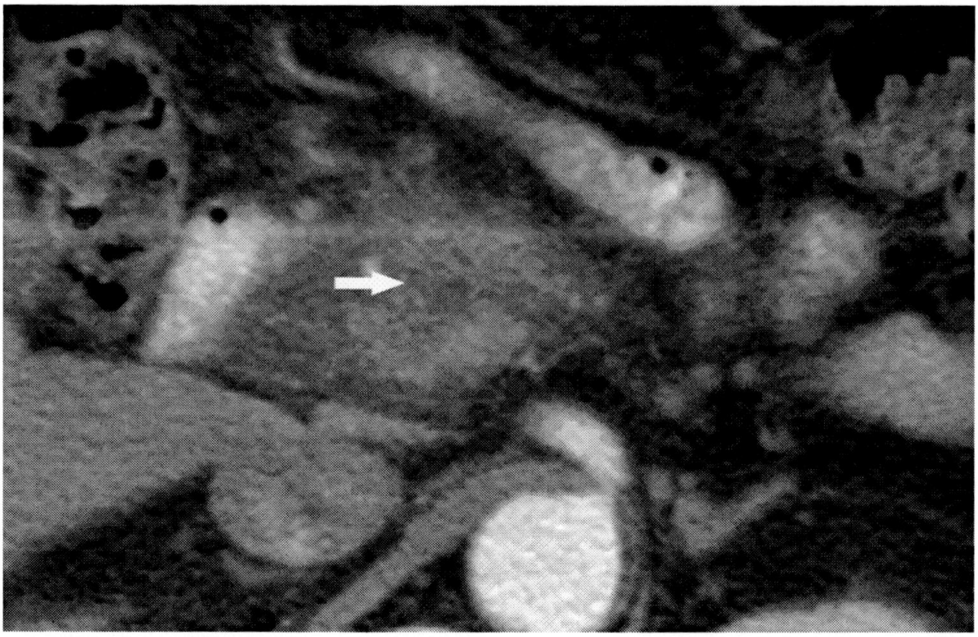

Figure 8b. CT-scan in the dynamic late arterial phase after IV injection of contrast agent more clearly displaying the above mentioned hypodense area (white arrow) at the level of the pancreatic head. Infiltration of the surrounding pancreatic fatty tissue is seen.

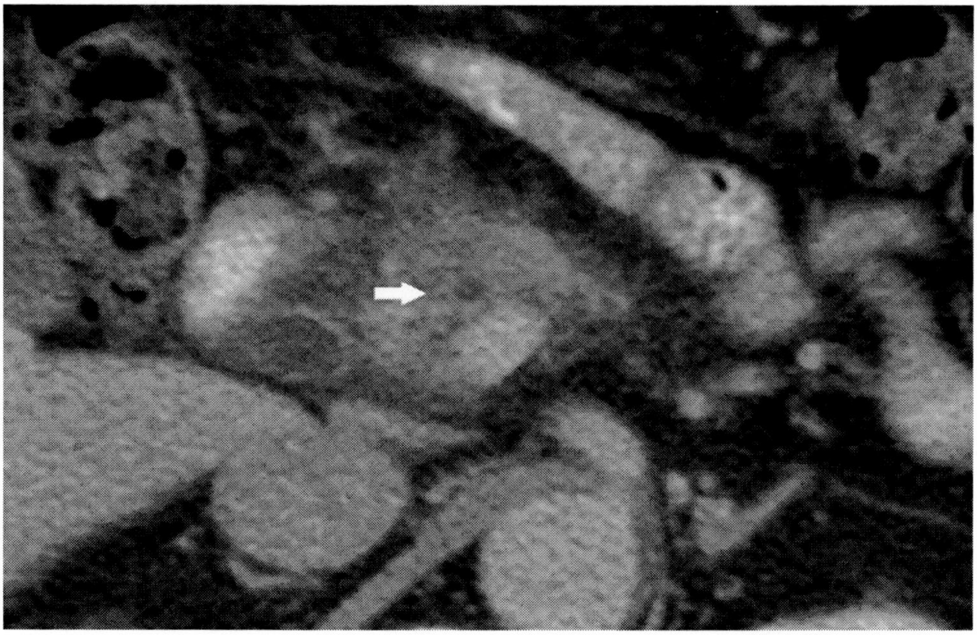

Figure 8c. CT-scan in the dynamic early venous phase after IV injection of contrast agent clearly displaying the above mentioned hypodense area (white arrow) at the level of the pancreatic head. An atypical hypodensity is seen in the center of this area.

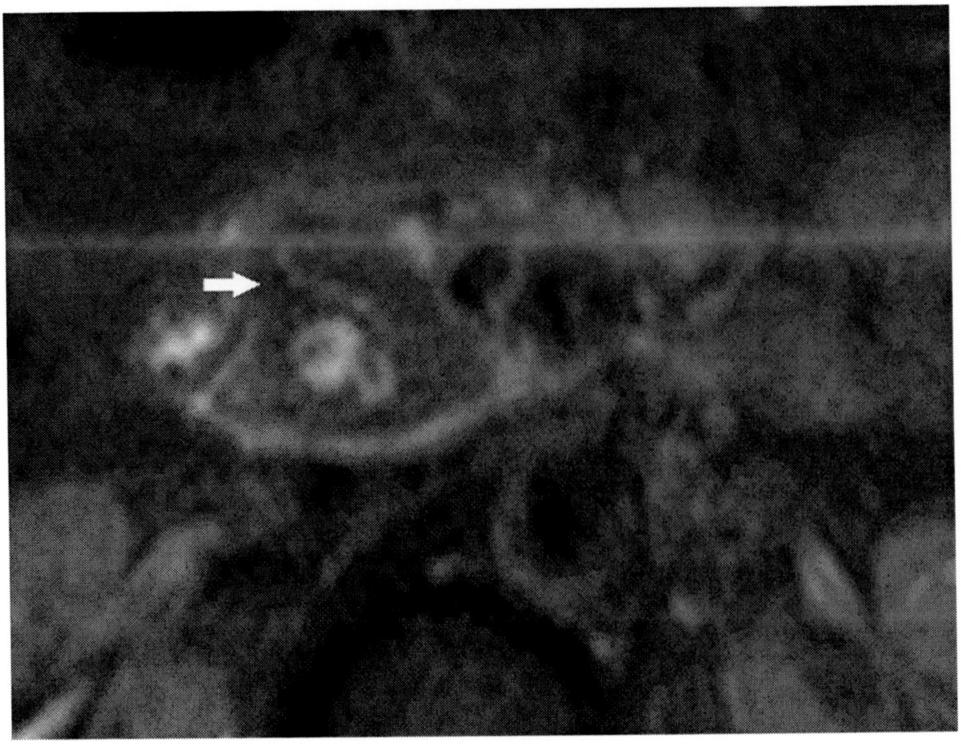

Figure 8d

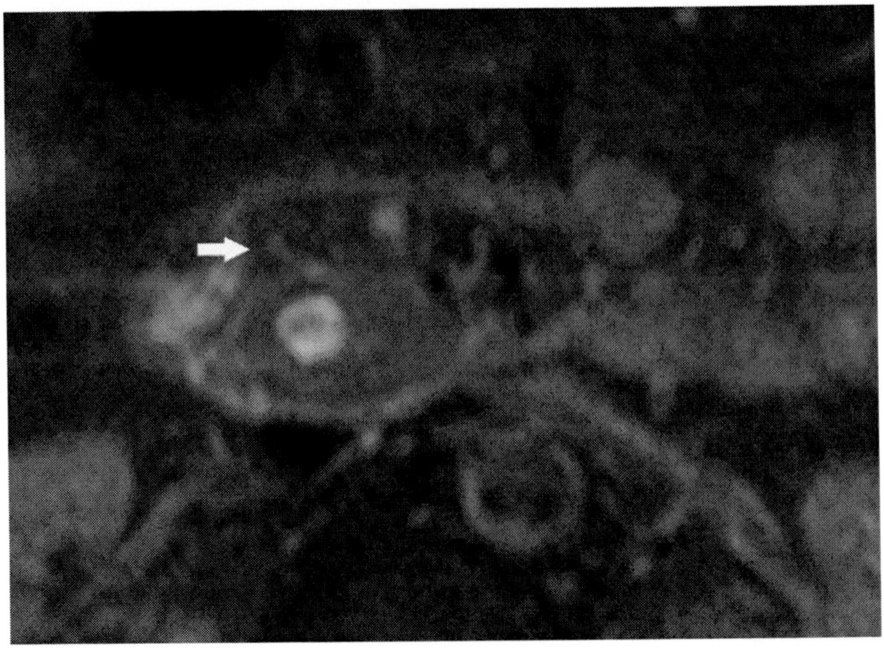

Figure 8e

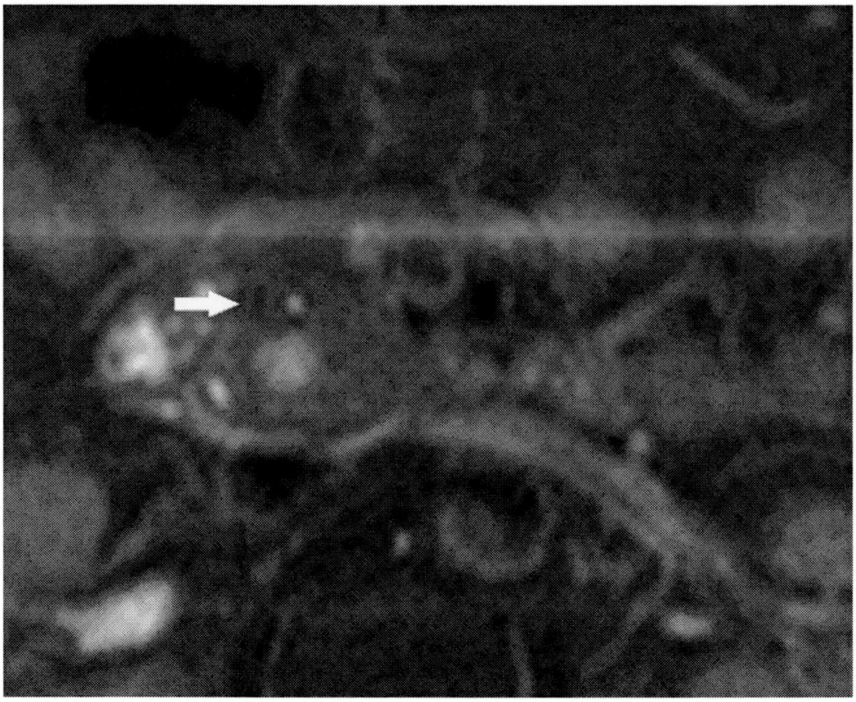

Figure 8f

Figure 8d, 8e, 8f. T2w TSE (long TE) MRI-sequence in the transverse plane displays a dilated side branch ("duct-penetrating" sign) in the pathologic area (white arrow).

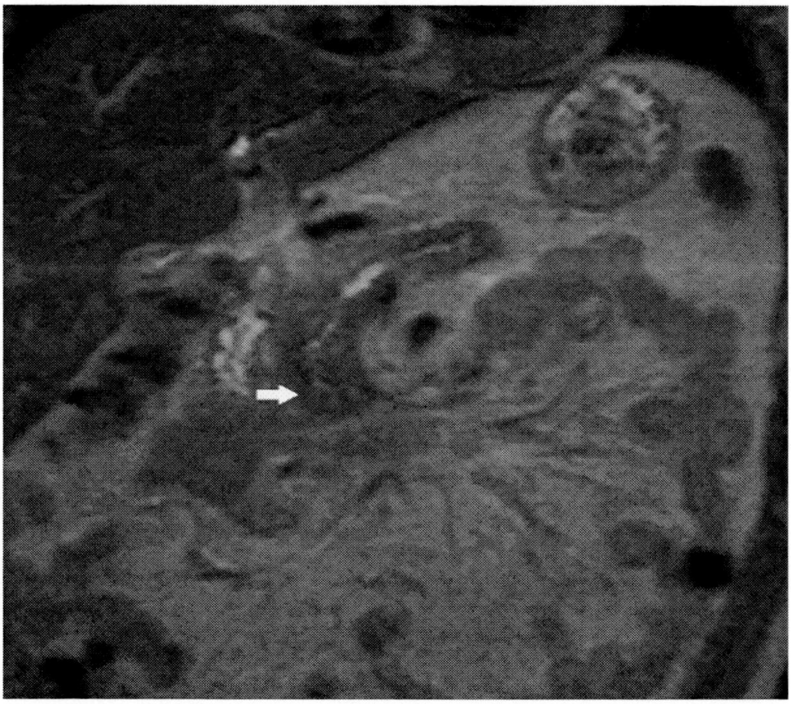

Figure 8g. T2w TSE (long TE) MRI-sequence in the coronal plane nicely displays some dilated side branches in the pathologic area (white arrow) indicative of the so-called "duct-penetrating" sign.

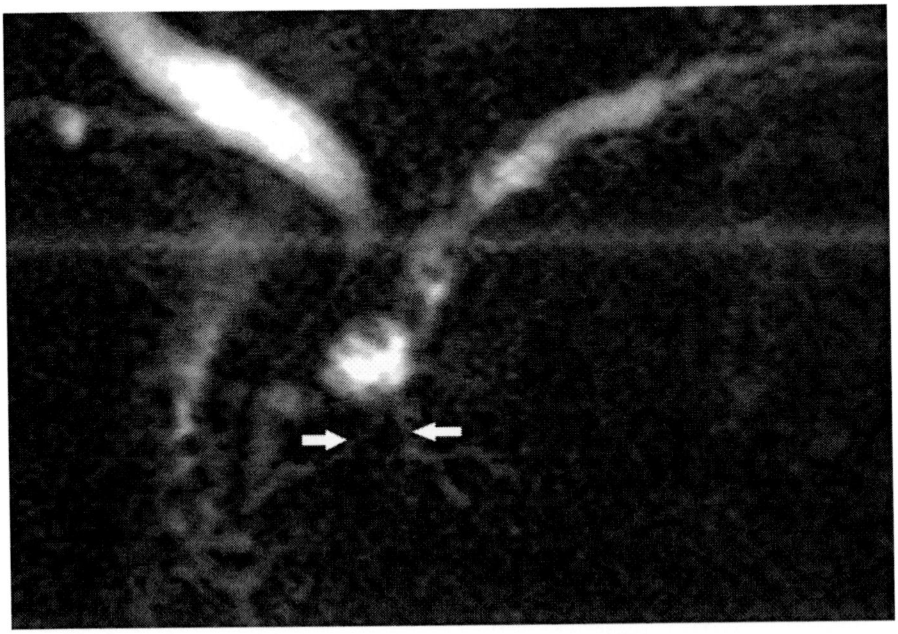

Figure 8h. MRCP-sequence again nicely displays some dilated side branches (white arrows) in the pathologic area.

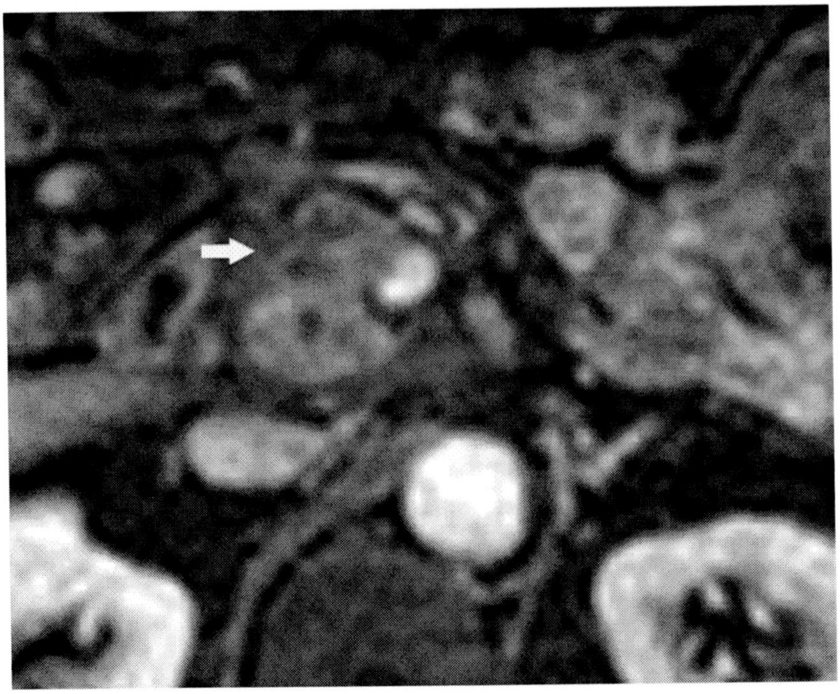

Figure 8i. T1w GE MRI-sequence with fat suppression in the delayed venous phase 5 minutes after IV injection of contrast agent displaying the above mentioned area as hypointense (white arrow). In this case, the diagnosis of focal chronic pancreatitis rather than pancreatic cancer is mainly made on the basis of the T2w sequences ("duct-penetrating" sign). T1w sequences were not useful in this case.

On the other hand, when CP occurs throughout the pancreas, the mass is not demarcated. It is thought that the hypoenhanced and demarcated pancreatic mass due to CP on pancreatic phase contrast-enhanced helical CT or MRI is not distinguishable from pancreatic adenocarcinoma, whereas the isoenhanced and nondemarcated masses may be distinguishable from hypovascular pancreatic adenocarcinoma or other hypervascular pancreatic tumors. However, histologic examination or close interval follow-up is needed for such isoenhanced and nondemarcated pancreatic masses. Tumor-free pancreatic parenchyma located proximally to a pancreatic adenocarcinoma obstructing the pancreatic duct may undergo atrophy and fibrosis and thus may show the same gradual enhancement pattern as pancreatic adenocarcinoma [110], whereas pancreatic adenocarcinoma located in the pancreatic head may show isoenhancement and no demarcation. In their study, two different enhancement patterns on two-phase helical CT and dynamic MRI were identified in masses due to CP. When histologic fibrosis is uniformly present through the gland in patients with CP, there is no demarcation of masses due to CP. When there is a greater degree of histologic fibrosis in the masslike part of the gland, the mass is often demarcated from the remaining pancreas, and the enhancement pattern on two-phase helical CT and dynamic gadolinium-enhanced MRI mimics that of pancreatic adenocarcinoma. Further work is needed to improve the rate of correct diagnosis of masses due to focal CP. Following our own experience, unenhanced T1w GE FS sequence (in combination with T2w imaging) often is a very accurate radiologic sequence allowing to detect a focal pancreatic adenocarcinoma appearing more hypointense compared with the surrounding pancreatic parenchyma (even in the presence of more proximally located obstructive CP). Comparable findings were published by Sica GT et al. using unenhanced T1w FS spin-echo [64].

MRCP may be helpful to aid in this differentiation, because chronic alcoholic pancreatitis, compared with chronic obstructive pancreatitis due to adenocarcinoma, is more frequently associated with an irregularly dilated duct with intraductal calcification.[120] The ratio of duct caliber to pancreatic gland width is higher in patients with adenocarcinoma.[121] Also, the "duct-penetrating sign," seen in 85% of CP and in only 4% of patients with cancer, helps to distinguish an inflammatory pancreatic mass from pancreatic adenocarcinoma. The "duct-penetrating sign" refers to a non-obstructed main pancreatic duct penetrating an inflammatory pancreatic mass, unlike its usual obstruction by pancreatic adenocarcinoma.[122] Furthermore, MRCP can depict the classic "double-duct sign" of pancreatic adenocarcinoma (enlargement and non-communication of the pancreatic and common bile ducts).[123] A normal-sized pancreatic duct is present in up to 20% of patients with adenocarcinoma, however, and should not dissuade its diagnosis in the setting of common bile duct dilation. MRI detection of early pancreatic cancer without pancreatic duct involvement has not been adequately studied [124].

Positron Emission Tomography in the Differentiation of Focal Chronic Pancreatitis and Pancreatic Adenocarcinoma

Positron Emission Tomography (PET) with 2-fluoro-2-deoxy-D-glucose (FDG) was recently introduced into clinical oncology because of its ability to demonstrate metabolic changes associated with various disease processes. Some studies investigated the possibility of identifying pancreatic cancer in CP with FDG-PET. [125, 126]

Tissue Diagnosis in the Differentiation of Focal Chronic Pancreatitis and Pancreatic Adenocarcinoma

Tissue diagnosis (cytologic or histologic examination) is mostly performed in the differential diagnosis between focal CP and pancreatic cancer. EUS-FNA is becoming the standard for obtaining cytologic diagnosis, although the sensitivity of EUS-FNA for the differential diagnosis of pancreatic masses is variable in the literature, being as low as 75% in some studies.[105] Moreover, the sensitivity was reported to be unacceptably lower (54%) in the context of CP, whereas surgical resection was still necessary to confirm the diagnosis.[106] Consequently, EUS-FNA in patients with pancreatic masses has a low negative predictive value, and its ability to differentiate between pancreatic cancer and pseudotumoral CP is limited.[127] The 10–20% false negative rate using EUS-FNA for resectable pancreatic cancer should not prohibit a patient from a potentially curative surgical procedure.[128] Sampling errors of EUS with EUS-FNA can occur because of the scant cellularity of specimens due to the small size of the lesions or the presence of CP. Other tumor-related factors may also decrease cellularity of samples, including extensive fibrosis (desmoplastic reaction) and necrosis, as well as the degree of differentiation (well-differentiated tumors require a larger number of needle passes then moderately or poorly differentiated tumors) [129, 130, 131, 132, 133, 134].

Power Doppler EUS in the Differentiation of Focal Chronic Pancreatitis and Pancreatic Adenocarcinoma

Power Doppler EUS also can provide useful information for the differential diagnosis of pancreatic masses. Saftoiu A et al. [127] included 42 consecutive patients with pancreatic tumor masses (27 men and 15 women) examined by EUS between January 2002 and August 2004. EUS procedures included power Doppler EUS as well as EUS-FNA in all patients. Final diagnosis of pancreatic cancer was confirmed in 29 patients on the basis of a combination of information provided by imaging tests, follow-up of at least 6 months, and laparotomy in 18 patients for diagnostic or palliative reasons. The results were in concordance with previous studies that showed a hypovascular pattern of pancreatic adenocarcinoma, as well as the formation of collaterals in advanced cases due to the invasion of the splenic or portal veins. Nonetheless, further studies of dynamic EUS with contrast agents are necessary to better characterize pancreatic masses. In their study [127], the ability of imaging methods (EUS with power Doppler imaging) was similar to that of EUS-FNA for the differential diagnosis of pancreatic cancer and pseudotumoral inflammatory masses. The addition of the information provided by the appearance of collaterals enhanced the diagnostic value of power Doppler ultrasonography, with better accuracy and a higher negative predictive value. Consequently, EUS with power Doppler imaging can provide information about the etiology of the tumor mass, even in the absence of tissue confirmation that may occur in patients with CP and pseudotumoral inflammatory masses. According to Saftoiu A et al. [127] the ability of power Doppler EUS to differentiate pancreatic masses has to be viewed as an adjunct to the other imaging techniques rather than a replacement of tissue confirmation. Currently, there is no imaging method that can reliably provide this capability in patients with pancreatic masses, especially in the setting of CP. Nevertheless, categorizing the risk of malignancy is very important for the clinical decision-making process and subsequent treatment (follow-up CT and EUS, repeated EUS-FNA, or surgery), especially in the cases with negative EUS-FNA findings, in which a diagnosis of pancreatic cancer cannot be excluded. Dynamic imaging is increasingly used for the differential diagnosis of pancreatic masses.[135] Pancreatic adenocarcinoma was described as usually hypovascular compared with the rest of the parenchyma, whereas inflammatory masses are isovascular or hypervascular. CE-EUS was also used for the differential diagnosis of pancreatic tumor masses for a better assessment of perfusion in the pancreatic tissue and inside the mass [136,137]. Pancreatic adenocarcinoma was shown to be relatively hypovascular compared with surrounding pancreatic tissue, whereas markedly hypervascular lesions were inflammatory masses. Although collaterals might also appear in CP because of segmentary portal hypertension, the relative frequency is inferior to the frequency of collateral appearance in patients with pancreatic cancer.[138] Consequently, combining the information provided by the absence of power Doppler signals and the presence of pancreatic collaterals yielded the best accuracy for the differential diagnosis between pseudotumoral CP and pancreatic adenocarcinoma.[127] Studies have shown comparable results with cytopathologic results (percutaneously or EUS-guided) with high sensitivity and specificity [137].

4. Dorsal Extension of Resectable Pancreatic Cancer

The main role of staging pancreatic adenocarcinoma is to offer the most appropriate and stage-specific treatment strategy to the individual patient. The most critical issue is the accurate identification of patients that are eligible for complete resection, being those with no evidence of involvement of the superior mesenteric artery or celiac axis and of the superior mesenteric and portal venous (SMPV) confluence, in the absence of metastatic disease.

Important as well is the pre-operative assessment of the retroperitoneal margin (the soft tissue margin directly adjacent to the proximal 3-4 cm of the superior mesenteric artery) which is nearly always close and often positive. Its involvement, either by direct extension of the tumour or from retroperitoneal ExtraPancreatic Neural Invasion (EPNI) will in large part determine the likelihood of subsequent local recurrence in the pancreatic bed. Following intrapancreatic neural involvement cancer cells spread within the perineural space along the nerves, even as they branch, and infiltrate into surrouding connective tissue and likewise in the retroperitoneal space.[139, 140, 141, 142] EPNI clearly has to be distinguished from macroscopic invasion of adjacent neural tissue by the primary tumour, which overgrows neural tissues. It is not revealed by imaging studies like MRI and EUS, and in the clinicopathologic study of Nakao et al. EPNI independently and significantly correlated with a shortened postoperative survival.[140, 143] Levy and colleagues recently reported on the identification of microscopic EPNI by EUS-guided aspiration or biopsy examination in 2 patients with pancreatic adenocarcinoma. They stated that, although not a criterion considered in the current American Joint Committee on Cancer staging system, the preoperative finding of EPNI has the potential to alter patient management because it might influence the decision to resect, the extent of resection, and the administration of targeted adjuvant therapy to treat this hidden focus of disease [144].

5. Future Developments in the Diagnosis of Pancreatic Disease

In the future, age-related changes of the pancreatic parenchyma and its possible influence on the perfusion parameters need further investigation to optimise differentiation between different severities of CP and a "normal" higher age pancreatic parenchyma. In the elderly, pancreatic changes comparable to those occurring in patients with CP have been described. Further perfusion-based MRI studies are required to determine optimal models, and new software tools should be developed for clinical studies. Also, perfusion-based MRI has been used for the study of the pancreatic parenchyma [51] but has never been used in the differentiation between focal pancreatitis and a solid pancreatic tumor.

Ongoing developments in linear endoscopic ultrasound allowing better 3D view of the vessels near the pancreas might make early diagnosis and staging of pancreatic tumors more reliable. In a pilot study of 22 patients, the additional 3D reconstructions provided using linear EUS appeared to improve the evaluation of vessel-tumor relationships in pancreatic cancer, especially in case of CP. 3D imaging using linear EUS might have other applications but the acquisition system needs to be improved [145].

Other promising techniques are under development hopefully improving early differentiation between focal CP and pancreatic cancer. In vivo ^{1}H-MR spectra have been used showing significantly less lipid in focal CP than in pancreatic adenocarcinoma. The mean metabolite-to-lipid ratios were significantly different between pancreatic adenocarcinoma and focal CP; there was an overlap in the distribution of ratios between these 2 disease entities. This means that a misclassification should have existed. Further studies with larger sample sizes are needed to determine more specific criteria to predict each disease entity. Another possible limitation is the similarity of the assigned frequencies of the lipids and the lactate peaks on ^{1}H-MR spectra and the abundance of lipid molecules in the abdomen. For this reason, the application of MRS can be limited to the cases with a lesion large enough to contain the localization voxel. Further research to develop the new techniques of MRS that use the smaller localization voxel is required to eliminate this limitation [146].

Optical coherence tomography (OCT) using infrared light to produce two-dimensional images (1-2 mm in depth) analogous to ultrasound provides an exciting alternative means to identify ductal malignancy and comparative studies are eagerly awaited [147, 148, 149].

Conclusion

For the time being, differentiating between early CP and early pancreatic cancer still can be very difficult and sometimes impossible. Hopefully, many cases of unnecessary operation or delayed adequate treatment can be avoided by future developments allowing optimized diagnosis of pancreatic disease in an early stage.

References

[1] Sarner M. Pancreatitis: definitions and classification. In: Go V, editor. *The exocrine pancreas: biology, pathobiology, and diseases.* 2nd ed. New York: Raven; 1986; 459-464.

[2] Ritchie A. Pancreas. In: Ritchie A, editor. *Boyd's textbook of pathology.* 9th ed. Philadelphia: Lea and Febiger; 1990; 1202-1234.

[3] DiMagno E, Layer P, Clain J. Chronic pancreatitis. In: Go V, editor. *The pancreas: biology, pathology, and disease.* 2nd ed. New York: Raven; 1993; 665-706.

[4] DiMagno M, DiMagno E. Chronic Pancreatitis. *Curr. Opin. Gastroenterol.,* 2006; 22: 487-497.

[5] Sarles H. Proposal adopted unanimously by the participants of the Symposium, Marseilles 1963. *Bibl. Gastroenterol,* 1965; 7: 7-8.

[6] Sarner M, Cotton P. Classification of pancreatitis. *Gut,* 1984; 25: 756-759.

[7] Singer M, Gyr K, Sarles H. Revised classification of pancreatitis: report of the Second International Symposium on the Classification of Pancreatitis in Marseille, France, March 28-30, 1984. *Gastroenterology,* 1985; 89: 683-685.

[8] Sarles H, Adler G, Dani R, Frey C, Gullo L, Harada H, Martin E, Norohna M, Scuro L. The pancreatitis classification of Marseilles, Rome 1988. *Scand. J. Gastroenterol.,* 1989; 24: 641-642.

[9] Chari S, Singer M. The problem of classification and staging of chronic pancreatitis: proposal based on current knowledge and its natural history. *Scand. J. Gastroenterol.,* 1994; 29: 949-960.

[10] Ammann R. A clinically based classification system for alcoholic chronic pancreatitis: summary of an international workshop on chronic pancreatitis. *Pancreas,* 1997; 14: 215-221.

[11] Ramesh H. Proposal for a New Grading System for Chronic Pancreatitis. *J. Clin. Gastroenterol.,* 2002; 35: 67-70.

[12] Etemad B, Whitcomb D. Chronic pancreatitis: diagnosis, classification, and new genetic developments. *Gastroenterology,* 2001; 120: 682-707.

[13] Tandon R, Sato N, Carg P. For the consensus study group. Chronic pancreatitis: Asia-Pacific consensus report. *J. Gastroenterol Hepatol.,* 2002; 17: 508-518.

[14] Mallery J, Centeno B, Hahn P, Chang Y, Warshaw A, Brugge W. Pancreatic tissue sampling guided by EUS, CT/US, and surgery: a comparison of sensitivity and specificity. *Gastrointest Endosc.,* 2002; 56: 218-224.

[15] Kloppel G, Maillet B. A morphological analysis of 57 resection specimens and 9 autopsy pancreata. *Pancreas,* 1991; 6: 266-274.

[16] Lähr J. What are the useful biological and functional markers of early-stage chronic pancreatitis? *J. Gastroenterol.*, 2007; 42(Suppl 17): 66-71.

[17] Ito T. Can measurement of chemokines become useful biological and functional markers of early-stage chronic pancreatitis? *J. Gastroenterol.,* 2007; 42(Suppl 17): 72-77.

[18] Steer M, Waxman I, Freedman S. Chronic pancreatitis. *N. Engl. J. Med.*, 1995; 332:1482-1490.

[19] Catalano M, Lahoti S, Geenen J, Hogan W. Prospective evaluation of endoscopic ultrasonography, endoscopic retrograde pancreatography, and secretin test in the diagnosis of chronic pancreatitis. *Gastrointest Endosc.*, 1998; 48:11-17.

[20] Wiersema M, Hawes R, Lehman G, Kochman M, Sherman S, Kopecky K. Prospective evaluation of endoscopic ultrasonography and endoscopic retrograde cholangiopancreatography in patients with chronic abdominal pain of suspected pancreatic origin. *Endoscopy,* 1993; 25: 555-564.

[21] Feldman M, Friedman L, Sleisenger M. Pathophysiology, Diagnosis, Management. In: Saunders W, editor. *Sleisenger and Fordtran's Gastrointestinal and Liver Disease.* 7th ed. Philadelphia; 2002; 465-478.

[22] Niederau C, Grendell J. Diagnosis of chronic pancreatitis. *Gastroenterology,* 1985; 88: 1973-1995.

[23] Bastid C, Sahel J, Filho M, Sarles H. Diameter of the main pancreatic duct in chronic calcifying pancreatitis. Measurement by ultrasonography versus pancreatography. *Pancreas,* 1990; 5: 524-527.

[24] Raimondo M, Wallace M. Diagnosis of Early Chronic Pancreatitis by Endoscopic Ultrasound. Are We There Yet? *J. Pancreas*, 2004; 5: 1-7.

[25] Rajan E, Clain J, Levy M, Norton I, Wang K, Wiersema M, Vazquez-Sequeiros E, Nelson B, Jondal M, Kendall R, Harmsen S, Zinsmeister A. Age-related changes in the pancreas identified by EUS: a prospective evaluation. *Gastrointest Endosc.,* 2005; 61: 401-406.

[26] Ly J, Miller F. MR imaging of the pancreas: a practical approach. *Radiol. Clin. N. Am.,* 2002; 40: 1289-1306.

[27] Semelka R, Shoenut J, Kroeker M, Micflikier A. Chronic pancreatitis: MR imaging features before and after administration of gadopentetate dimeglumine. *JMRI,* 1993; 3: 79-82.

[28] Sica G, Braver J, Cooney M, Miller F, Chai J, Adams D. Comparison of endoscopic retrograde cholangiopancreatography with MR cholangiopancreatography in patients with pancreatitis. *Radiology*, 1999; 210: 605-610.

[29] Takehara Y, Ichijo K, Tooyama N, Kodaira N, Yamamoto H, Tatami M, Saito M, Watahiki H, Takahashi M. Breath-hold MR cholangiopancreatography with a long-echo-train fast spin-echo sequence and a surface coil in chronic pancreatitis. *Radiology,* 1994; 192: 73-78.

[30] Soto J, Barish M, Yucel E, Clarke P, Siegenberg D, Chuttani R, Ferrucci J. Pancreatic duct: MR cholangiopancreatography with a three-dimensional fast spin-echo technique. *Radiology,* 1995; 196: 459-464.

[31] Bret P, Reinhold C, Taourel P, Guibaud L, Atri M, Barkun A. Pancreas divisum: evaluation with MR cholangiopancreatography. *Radiology,* 1996; 199: 99-103.

[32] Miller F, Keppke A, Wadhwa A, Ly J, Dalal K, Kamler V. MRI of Pancreatitis and Its Complications: Part 2, Chronic Pancreatitis. *AJR,* 2004; 183: 1645-1652.

[33] Matos C, Metens T, Devière J, Niçaise N, Braude P, Van Yperen G, Cremer M, Struyven J. Pancreatic duct: morphologic and functional evaluation with dynamic MR pancreatography after secretin stimulation. *Radiology,* 1997; 203: 435-441.

[34] Cappeliez O, Delhaye M, Devière J, Le Moine O, Metens T, Niçaise N, Cremer M, Struyven J, Matos C. Chronic Pancreatitis: Evaluation of Pancreatic Exocrine Function with MR Pancreatography after Secretin Stimulation. *Radiology,* 2000; 215: 358-364.

[35] Geenen J, Hogan W, Dodds W, Stewart E, Arndorfer R. Intraluminal pressure recording from the human sphincter of Oddi. *Gastroenterology,* 1980; 78: 317-324.

[36] Ochi K, Harada H, Mizushima T, Tanaka J, Matsumoto S. Intraductal secretin test is as useful as duodenal secretin test in assessing exocrine pancreatic function. *Dig. Dis. Sci.,* 1997; 42: 492-496.

[37] Wada K, Yamadera K, Yokoyama K, Goto M, Makino I. Application of pure pancreatic juice collection to the pancreatic exocrine function test. *Pancreas*, 1998; 16: 124-128.

[38] Gullo L, Costa P, Fontana G, Labo G. Investigation of exocrine pancreatic function by continuous infusion of caerulein and secretin in normal subjects and in chronic pancreatitis. *Digestion,* 1976; 14: 97-107.

[39] Gyr H, Agrawal N, Felsenfeld O, Font R. Comparative study of secretin and Lundh tests. *Am. J. Dig. Dis.*, 1975; 20: 506-512.

[40] Devière J, Gulbis B, Delhaye M, Quenon M, Cremer M. A study of the relationship between the canalar morphology and the exocrine function of the pancreas: a new method of linear estimation of the pancreatic function. *Acta Endosc.*, 1985; 15: 403-414.

[41] Hayakawa T, Kondo T, Shibata T, Noda A, Suzuki T, Nakano S. Relationship between pancreatic exocrine function and histological changes in chronic pancreatitis. *Am. J. Gastroenterol.*, 1992; 87: 1170-1174.

[42] Bozkurt T, Braun U, Leferink S, Gilly G, Lux G. Comparison of pancreatic morphology and exocrine functional impairment in patients with chronic pancreatitis. *Gut,* 1994; 35: 1132-1136.

[43] Malfertheiner P, Büchler M, Stanescu A, Ditschuneit H. Exocrine pancreatic function in correlation to ductal and parenchymal morphology in chronic pancreatitis. *Hepatogastroenterology,* 1986; 33: 110-114.

[44] Braganza J, Hunt L, Warwick F. Relationship between pancreatic exocrine function and ductal morphology in chronic pancreatitis. *Gastroenterology,* 1982; 82: 1341-1347.

[45] Otte M. Pankreasfunktionsdiagnostik. *Internist,* 1979; 20: 331-340.

[46] Matos C, Devière J, Cremer M, Niçaise N, Struyven J, Metens T. Acinar filling during secretin-stimulated MR pancreatography. *AJR,* 1998; 171: 165-169.

[47] Laugier R. Dynamic endoscopic manometry of the response to secretin in patients with chronic pancreatitis. *Endoscopy,* 1994; 26: 222-227.

[48] Karanjia N, Singh S, Widdison A, Lutrin F, Reber H. Pancreatic ductal and interstitial pressures in cats with chronic pancreatitis. *Dig. Dis. Sci.,* 1992; 37: 268-273.

[49] Reber H, Karanjia N, Alvarez C, Widdison A, Leung F, Ashley S, Lutrin F. Pancreatic blood flow in cats with chronic pancreatitis. *Gastroenterology*, 1992; 103: 652-659.

[50] Adler G, Schmid R. Chronic pancreatitis: still puzzling? *Gastroenterology,* 1997; 112: 1762-1765.

[51] Coenegrachts K, Van Steenbergen W, De Keyzer F, Vanbeckevoort D, Bielen D, Chen F, Dockx S, Maes F, Bosmans H. Dynamic contrast-enhanced MRI of the pancreas: initial results in healthy volunteers and patients with chronic pancreatitis. *JMRI*, 2004; 20: 990-997.

[52] Reber H, Karanjia N, Alvarez C, Widdison A, Leung F, Ashley S, Lutrin F. Pancreatic blood flow in cats with chronic pancreatitis. *Gastroenterology*, 1992; 103: 652-659.

[53] Patel A, Toyama M, Alvarez C, Nguyen T, Reber P, Ashley S, Reber H. Pancreatic interstitial pH in human and feline chronic pancreatitis. *Gastroenterology*, 1995; 109: 1639-1645.

[54] Lewis M, Lo S, Reber P, Patel A, Gloor B, Todd K, Toyama M, Sherman S, Ashley S, Reber H. Endoscopic measurement of pancreatic tissue perfusion in patients with chronic pancreatitis and control patients. *Gastrointest Endosc.*, 2000; 51: 195-199.

[55] Schilling M, Redaelli C, Reber P, Friess H, Signer C, Stoupis C, Buchler M. Microcirculation in chronic alcoholic pancreatitis: a laser Doppler flow study. *Pancreas*, 1999; 19: 21-25.

[56] Patel A, Reber P, Toyama M, Ashley S, Reber H. Effect of pancreaticojejunostomy on fibrosis, pancreatic blood flow, and interstitial pH in chronic pancreatitis. A feline model. *Ann Surg*, 1999; 230: 672-679.

[57] Verstraete K, Achten E, Dierick A. Dynamic contrast enhanced MRI of musculoskeletal neoplasms: different types and slopes of time-intensity curves (abstract). In: *Proceedings of the Society of Magnetic Resonance in Medicine;* Berkeley, California: Society of Magnetic Resonance in Medicine; 1992; 2609.

[58] Vaupel P, Kallinowski F, Okunieff P. Blood flow, oxygen and nutrient supply, and metabolic microenvironment of human tumors: a review. *Cancer Res.,* 1989; 49: 6449-6465.

[59] Kucharczyk J, Mintorovitch J, Asgari H, Moseley M. Diffusion/perfusion MR imaging of acute cerebral ischemia. *MRM,* 1991; 19: 311-315.

[60] Saeed M. Value of blood pool MR contrast agents in imaging of the heart and blood vessels. *Drugs Today*, 1999; 35: 879-892.

[61] Semelka R, Kroeker M, Shoenut J, Kroeker R, Yaffe C, Micflikier A. Pancreatic disease: prospective comparison of CT, ERCP, and 1.5-T MR imaging with dynamic gadolinium enhancement and fat suppression. *Radiology*, 1991; 181: 785-791.

[62] Winston C, Mitchell D, Outwater E, Ehrlich S. Pancreatic signal intensity on T1-weighted fat-saturation MR images: clinical correlation. *JMRI*, 1995; 5: 267-271.

[63] Zhang X-M, Shi H, Parker L, Dohke M, Holland G, Mitchell D. Suspected early or mild chronic pancreatitis: enhancement patterns on Gadolinium chelate dynamic MRI. *JMRI*, 2003; 17: 86-94.

[64] Sica G, Miller F, Rodriguez G, McTavish J, Banks P. Magnetic resonance imaging in patients with pancreatitis: evaluation of signal intensity and enhancement changes. *JMRI*, 2002; 15: 275-284.

[65] Prasad P, Wittmann J, Pereira S. Endoscopic Ultrasound of the Upper Gastrointestinal Tract and Mediastinum: Diagnosis and Therapy. *CVIR*, 2006; 29: 947-957.

[66] Sahai A, Zimmerman M, Aabakken L, Tarnasky P, Cunningham J, van Velse A, Hawes R, Hoffman B. Prospective assessment of the ability of endoscopic ultrasound to diagnose, exclude, or establish the severity of CP found by endoscopic retrograde cholangiopancreatography. *Gastrointest Endosc.*, 1998; 48:18-25.

[67] Sahai A. EUS and chronic pancreatitis. *Gastrointest Endosc.*, 2002; 56: S76-81.

[68] Vandervoort J, Soetikno R, Tham T, Wong R, Ferrari A, Montes H, Roston A, Slivka A, Lichtenstein D, Ruymann F, Van Dam J, Hughes M, Carr-Locke D. Risk factors for complications after performance of ERCP. *Gastrointest Endosc.*, 2002; 56: 652-656.

[69] Freeman M, DiSario J, Nelson D, Fennerty M, Lee J, Bjorkman D, Overby C, Aas J, Ryan M, Bochna G, Shaw M, Snady H, Erickson R, Moore J, Roel J. Risk factors for post-ERCP pancreatitis: a prospective, multicenter study. *Gastrointest Endosc.*, 2001; 54: 425-434.

[70] Wiersema M, Wiersema L. Endosonography of the pancreas: normal variation versus changes of early chronic pancreatitis. *Gastrointest Endosc. Clin. N. Am.*, 1995; 5: 487-496.

[71] Byrne M, Jowell P. Gastrointestinal imaging: endoscopic ultrasound. *Gastroenterology*, 2002; 122: 1631-1648.

[72] Lightdale C. Indications, contraindications, and complications of endoscopic ultrasonography. *Gastrointest Endosc*, 1996; 43: S15-19.

[73] Sahai A, Mishra G, Penman I, Williams D, Wallace M, Hadzijahic N, Pearson A, Vanvelse A, Hoffman B, Hawes R. EUS to detect evidence of pancreatic disease in patients with persistent or nonspecific dyspepsia. *Gastrointest Endosc.*, 2000; 52:153-159.

[74] Bhutani M. Endoscopic ultrasonography: changes of chronic pancreatitis in asymptomatic and symptomatic alcoholic patients. *J. Ultrasound Med.*, 1999; 18: 455-462.

[75] Kahl S, Glasbrenner B, Leodolter A, Pross M, Schulz H, Malfertheiner P. EUS in the diagnosis of early chronic pancreatitis: a prospective follow-up study. *Gastrointest Endosc.*, 2002; 55: 507-511.

[76] Yusoff I, Sahai A. A prospective, quantitative assessment of the effect of ethanol and other variables on the endosonographic appearance of the pancreas. *Clin. Gastroenterol. Hepatol*, 2004; 2: 405-409.

[77] Thuler F, da Costa P, de Paulo G, Nakao F, Ardengh J, Ferrari A. Endoscopic Ultrasonography and Alcoholic Patients: Can One Predict Early Pancreatic Tissue Abnormalities? *J. Pancreas*, 2005; 6: 568-574.

[78] Walsh T, Rode J, Theis B, Russell R. Minimal change chronic pancreatitis. *Gut*, 1992; 33: 1566-1571.

[79] Wallace M, Hawes R, Durkalski V, Chak A, Mallery S, Catalano M, Wiersema M, Bhutani M, Ciaccia D, Kochman M, Gress F, Van Velse A, Hoffman B. The reliability of EUS for the diagnosis of chronic pancreatitis: interobserver agreement among experienced endosonographers. *Gastrointest Endosc.*, 2001; 53: 294-299.

[80] Zimmermann M, Mishra G, Lewin D. Comparison of EUS findings with Histopathology in chronic pancreatitis [abstract]. *Gastrointest Endosc.*, 1997; 45: AB185.

[81] Hollerbach S, Klamann A, Topalidis T, Schmiegel W. Endoscopic ultrasonography (EUS) and fine-needle aspiration (FNA) cytology for diagnosis of chronic pancreatitis. *Endoscopy*, 2001; 33: 824-831.

[82] Hastier P, Buckley M, Francois E, Peten E, Dumas R, Caroli-Bosc F, Delmont J. A prospective study of pancreatic disease in patients with alcoholic cirrhosis: comparative diagnostic value of ERCP and EUS and long-term significance of isolated parenchymal abnormalities. *Gastrointest Endosc.*, 1999; 49: 705-709.

[83] Parada K, Peng R, Erickson R, Hawes R, Sahai A, Ziogas A, Chang K. A resource utilization projection study of EUS. *Gastrointest Endosc.*, 2002; 55: 328-334.

[84] Draganov P, Toskes P. Chronic pancreatitis. *Current opinion gastroenterol*, 2002; 18: 558-562.

[85] Jemal A, Murray T, Ward E, Samuels A, Tiwari R, Ghafoor A, Feuer E, Thun M. Cancer statistics, 2005. *CA Cancer J. Clin.*, 2005; 55: 10-30.

[86] Wiersema M. Accuracy of endoscopic ultrasound in diagnosing and staging pancreatic carcinoma. *Pancreatology*, 2001; 1: 625-632.

[87] Gress F, Gottlieb K, Sherman S, Lehman G. Endoscopic ultrasonography-guided fine-needle aspiration biopsy of suspected pancreatic cancer. *Ann Intern Med*, 2001; 134: 459-464.

[88] Moossa A, Gamagami R. Diagnosis and staging of pancreatic neoplasms. *Surg. Clin. North Am.*, 1995; 75: 871-890.

[89] DiMagno E, Reber H, Tempero M. AGA technical review on the epidemiology, diagnosis, and treatment of pancreatic ductal adenocarcinoma. American Gastroenterological Association. *Gastroenterology*, 1999; 117: 1464-1484.

[90] Trede M, Schwall G, Saeger H. Survival after pancreatoduodenectomy. 118 consecutive resections without an operative mortality. *Ann. Surg.*, 1990; 211: 447-458.

[91] Hawes R, Xiong Q, Waxman I, Chang K, Evans D, Abbruzzese J. A multispecialty approach to the diagnosis and management of pancreatic cancer. *Am. J. Gastroenterol.*, 2000; 95:17-31.

[92] Ahmad N, Lewis J, Ginsberg G, Haller D, Morris J, Williams N, Rosato E, Kochman M. Long term survival after pancreatic resection for pancreatic adenocarcinoma. *Am. J. Gastroenterol*, 2001; 96:2609-2615.

[93] Cameron J, Crist D, Sitzmann J, Hruban R, Boitnott J, Seidler A, Coleman J. Factors influencing survival after pancreaticoduodenectomy for pancreatic cancer. *Am. J. Surg.*, 1991; 161: 120-124.

[94] Sohn T, Yeo C, Cameron J, Koniaris L, Kaushal S, Abrams R, Sauter P, Coleman J, Hruban R, Lillemoe K. Resected adenocarcinoma of the pancreas-616 patients: results, outcomes, and prognostic indicators. *J. Gastrointest Surg.*, 2000; 4: 567-579.

[95] Richter A, Niedergethmann M, Sturm J, Lorenz D, Post S, Trede M. Long-term results of partial pancreaticoduodenectomy for ductal adenocarcinoma of the pancreatic head: 25-year experience. *World J. Surg.*, 2003; 27: 324-329.

[96] Pedrazzoli S, DiCarlo V, Dionigi R, Mosca F, Pederzoli P, Pasquali C, Kloppel G, Dhaene K, Michelassi F. Standard versus extended lymphadenectomy associated with pancreatoduodenectomy in the surgical treatment of adenocarcinoma of the head of the pancreas: a multicenter, prospective, randomized study. Lymphadenectomy Study Group. *Ann. Surg.*, 1998; 228: 508-517.

[97] Yeo C, Cameron J, Lillemoe K, Sohn T, Campbell K, Sauter P, Coleman J, Abrams R, Hruban R. Pancreaticoduodenectomy with or without distal gastrectomy and extended retroperitoneal lymphadenectomy for periampullary adenocarcinoma, part 2: randomized controlled trial evaluating survival, morbidity, and mortality. *Ann. Surg.*, 2002; 236: 355-366.

[98] DeWitt J, Devereaux B, Chriswell M, McGreevy K, Howard T, Imperiale T, Ciaccia D, Lane K, Maglinte D, Kopecky K, LeBlanc J, McHenry L, Madura J, Aisen A, Cramer H, Cummings O, Sherman S. Comparison of endoscopic ultrasonography and multidetector computed tomography for detecting and staging pancreatic cancer. *Ann. Intern. Med.*, 2004; 141: 753-763.

[99] Li D, Jiao L. Molecular Epidemiology of Pancreatic Cancer. *International Journal of Gastrointestinal Cancer*, 2003; 33: 3-13.

[100] Maitra A, Kern S, Hruban R. Molecular pathogenesis of pancreatic cancer. *Best Pract Res. Clin. Gastroenterol.*, 2006; 20: 211-226.

[101] Kloppel G. Pancreatic non-endocrine tumors. In: Kloppel G, Heitz PU, eds. *Pancreatic pathology*. Edinburgh: Churchill Livingstone; 1984; 87-88.

[102] Hosoki T. Dynamic CT of pancreatic tumors. *AJR*, 1983; 140: 959-965.

[103] Robbins S, Cotran R. The pancreas. In: Robbins SL, Cotran RS, eds. *Pathologic basis of disease*, 2nd ed. Philadelphia: Saunders; 1979: 1101-1102.

[104] Koito K, Namieno T, Nagakawa T, Morita K. Inflammatory Pancreatic Masses: Differentiation from Ductal Carcinomas with Contrast-Enhanced Sonography Using Carbon Dioxide Microbubbles. *AJR*, 1997; 169:1263-1267.

[105] Eloubeidi M, Chen V, Eltoum l, Jhala D, Chhieng DC, Jhala N, Vickers SM, Wilcox CM. Endoscopic ultrasound-guided fine-needle aspiration biopsy of patients with suspected pancreatic cancer: diagnostic accuracy and acute and 30-day complications. *Am. J. Gastroenterol.*, 2003; 98: 2663-2668.

[106] Fritscher-Ravens A, Brand L, Knofel W, Bobrowski C, Topalidis T, Thonke F, de Werth A, Soehendra N. Comparison of endoscopic ultrasound-guided fine needle aspiration for focal pancreatic lesions in patients with normal parenchyma and chronic pancreatitis. *Am. J. Gastroenterol.*, 2002; 97: 2768-2775.

[107] Farrell J. Diagnosing pancreatic malignancy in the setting of chronic pancreatitis: is there room for improvement? *Gastrointest Endosc.* 2005; 62: 737-741.

[108] Luetmar P, Stephens D, Ward E. Chronic pancreatitis: reassessment with current CT. *Radiology,* 1989; 171: 353–357.

[109] Müller M, Meyenberger C, Bertschinger P, Schaer R, Marincek B. Pancreatic tumors: evaluation with endoscopic US, CT, and MR imaging. *Radiology*, 1994; 190: 745–751.

[110] Johnson P, Outwater E. Pancreatic carcinoma versus chronic pancreatitis: dynamic MR imaging. *Radiology,* 1999; 212: 213-218.

[111] Lu D, Reber H, Krasny R, Kadell B, Sayre J. Local staging of pancreatic cancer: criteria for unresectability of major vessels as revealed by pancreatic-phase, thin section helical CT. *AJR*, 1997; 168: 1439-1443.

[112] Gabata T, Matsui O, Kadoya M, Yoshikawa J, Miyayama S, Takashima T, Nagakawa T, Kayahara M, Nonomura A. Small pancreatic adenocarcinomas: efficacy of MR imaging with fat suppression and gadolinium enhancement. *Radiology*, 1994; 193: 683-688.

[113] Van Hoe L, Gryspeerdt S, Marchal G, Baert A, Mertens L. Helical CT for the preoperative localization of islet cell tumors of the pancreas: value of arterial and parenchymal phase images. *AJR,* 1995; 165: 1437-1439.

[114] Elmas N. The role of diagnostic radiology in pancreatitis. *Eur. J. Radiol.,* 2001; 38:120-132.

[115] Friedman A. Pancreatic neoplasms and cysts. In: Friedman A, Dachman A, eds. *Radiology of the Liver, Biliary Tract, and Pancreas*. 1st ed. St. Louis: Mosby-Year Book; 1994; 807-934.

[116] Pamuklar E, Semelka R. MR imaging of the pancreas. *Magn. Reson. Imaging Clin. N. Am.*, 2005; 13: 313-330.

[117] Fayad L, Kowalski T, Mitchell D. MR cholangiopancreatography: evaluation of common pancreatic diseases. *Radiol. Clin. N. Am.*, 2003; 41: 97-114.

[118] Arslan A, Buanes T, Geitung J. Pancreatic carcinoma: MR, MR angiography and dynamic helical CT in the evaluation of vascular invasion. *Eur. J. Rad.,* 2001; 38: 151-159.

[119] Kim T, Murakami T, Takamura M, Hori M, Takahashi S, Nakamori S, Sakon M, Tanji Y, Wakasa K, Nakamura H. Pancreatic mass due to chronic pancreatitis: correlation of CT and MR imaging features with pathologic findings. *AJR*, 2001; 177: 367-371.

[120] Karawasa E, Goldberg H, Moss A, Federle M, London S. CT pancreatogram in carcinoma of the pancreas and chronic pancreatitis. *Radiology*, 1983; 148: 489-493.

[121] Ehnas N, Yoruhnaz I, Oran I, Oyar 0, Ozutemiz 0, Ozer H. A new criterion in differentiation of pancreatitis and pancreatic adenocarcinoma: artery-to-vein ratio using the superior mesenteric vessels. *Abdom. Imaging,* 1996; 21: 331-333.

[122] Ichikawa T, Sou H, Araki T, Arbab A, Yoshikawa T, Ishigame K, Haradome H, Hachiya J. Duct-penetrating sign at MRCP: usefulness for differentiating inflammatory pancreatic mass from pancreatic carcinomas. *Radiology*, 2001; 221: 107-116.

[123] Freeny P, Bilbao M, Katon R. Blind evaluation of endoscopic retrograde cholangiopancreatography (ERCP) in the diagnosis of pancreatic adenocarcinoma: the "double duct" and other signs. *Radiology*, 1976; 119: 271-274.

[124] Matos C, Bali M, Delhaye M, Devière J. Magnetic resonance imaging in the detection of pancreatitis and pancreatic neoplasms. *Best Pract. Res. Clin. Gastroenterol,* 2006; 20: 157-178.

[125] Remer E, Baker M. Imaging of chronic pancreatitis. *Radiol. Clin. North Am.,* 2002; 40:1229-1242.

[126] Lankish P. Function tests in the diagnosis of CP. *Int. J. Pancreatol.,* 1993; 14: 9-20.

[127] Saftoiu A, Popescu C, Cazacu S, Dumitrescu D, Georgescu C, Popescu M, Ciurea T, Gorunescu F. Power Doppler Endoscopic Ultrasonography for the Differential Diagnosis Between Pancreatic Cancer and Pseudotumoral Chronic Pancreatitis. *J. Ultrasound Med.,* 2006; 25: 363-372.

[128] Fickling W, Wallace M. Endoscopic ultrasound and upper gastrointestinal disorders. *J. Clin. Gastroenterol.,* 2003; 36: 103-110.

[129] Eloubeidi M, Jhala D, Chhieng D, Chen V, Eltoum I, Vickers S, Mel Wilcox C, Jhala N. Yield of endoscopic ultrasound-guided fine-needle aspiration biopsy in patients with suspected pancreatic carcinoma. *Cancer,* 2003; 99: 285-292.

[130] Vilmann P, Hancke S. A new biopsy handle instrument for endoscopic ultrasound guided biopsy. *Gastrointest Endosc.,* 1996; 43: 238-242.

[131] Erickson R. EUS-guided FNA. *Gastrointest Endosc.,* 2004; 60: 267-279.

[132] Itoi T, Itokawa F, Sofuni A, Nakamura K, Tsuchida A, Yamao K, Kawai T, Moriyasu F. Puncture of solid pancreatic tumors guided by endoscopic ultrasonography: A pilot study series comparing Trucut and 19-gauge and 22-gauge aspiration needles. *Endoscopy,* 2005; 37: 362-366.

[133] Wittmann J, Kocjan G, Sgouros S, Deheragoda M, Pereira S. Endoscopic ultrasound-guided tissue sampling by combined fine needle aspiration and trucut needle biopsy: A prospective study. *Cytopathology,* 2006; 17: 27-33.

[134] Ylagan L, Edmundowicz S, Kasal K, Walsh D, Lu D. Endoscopic Ultrasound Guided Fine-Needle Aspiration Cytology of Pancreatic Carcinoma. A 3-Year Experience and Review of the Literature. *Cancer,* 2002; 96: 362-369.

[135] Takhar A, Palaniappan P, Dhinga R, Lobo D. Recent developments in diagnosis of pancreatic cancer. *BMJ,* 2004; 329: 668-673.

[136] Bhutani M, Hoffman B, van Velse A, Hawes R. Contrast-enhanced endoscopic ultrasonography with galactose microparticles: SHU508A (Levovist). *Endoscopy,* 1997; 29: 635-639.

[137] Becker D, Strobel D, Bernatik T, Hahn E. Echo-enhanced and power Doppler EUS for the discrimination between focal pancreatitis and pancreatic carcinoma. *Gastrointest Endosc,* 2001; 53: 784-789.

[138] Eloubeidi M, Iseman D, Chen V, Vickers SM, Wilcox CM. Prevalence and significance of periduodenal venous collaterals in patients evaluated for pancreaticobiliary disorders by endosonography. *Endoscopy* 2003; 35:1015-1019.

[139] Ozaki H, Hiraoka T, Mizumoto R, Matsuno S, Matsumoto Y, Nakayama T, Tsunoda T, Suzuki T, Monden M, Saitoh Y, Yamauchi H, Ogata Y. The prognostic significance of lymph node metastasis and intrapancreatic perineural invasion in pancreatic cancer after curative resection. *Surg. Today,* 1999; 29: 16-22.

[140] Nagakawa T, Kayahara M, Ueno K, Ohta T, Konishi I, Ueda N, Miyazaki I. A clinicopathologic study on neural invasion in cancer of the pancreatic head. *Cancer*, 1992; 69: 930-935.

[141] Kayahara M, Nagakawa T, Futagami F, Kitagawa H, Ohta T, Miyazaki I. Lymphatic flow and neural plexus invasion associated with adenocarcinoma of the body and tail of the pancreas. *Cancer,* 1996; 78: 2485-2491.

[142] Takahashi T, Ishikura H, Kato H, Tanabe T, Yoshiki T. Intra-pancreatic, extra-tumoral perineural invasion. An indicator for the presence of retroperitoneal neural plexus invasion by pancreatic adenocarcinoma. *Acta Pathol. Japonica*, 1992; 42: 99-103.

[143] Nakao A, Harada A, Nonami T, Kaneko T, Takagi H. Clinical significance of adenocarcinoma invasion of the extrapancreatic nerve plexus in pancreatic cancer. *Pancreas,* 1996; 12: 357-361.

[144] Levy M, Topazian M, Keeney G, Clain J, Gleeson F, Rajan E, Wang K, Wiersema M, Farnell M, Chari S. Preoperative Diagnosis of Extrapancreatic Neural Invasion in Pancreatic Cancer. *Clin. Gastroenterol. Hepatol,* 2006; 4: 1479-1482.

[145] Fritscher-Ravens A, Knoefel W, Krause C, Swain C, Brandt L, Patel K. Three-Dimensional Linear Endoscopic Ultrasound-Feasibility of a Novel Technique Applied for the Detection of Vessel Involvement of Pancreatic Masses. *Am. J. Gastroenterol.*, 2005; 100: 1296-1302.

[146] Cho S, Lee D, Lee K, Ji H, Lee K, Ros P, Suh C. Differentiation of Chronic Focal Pancreatitis From Pancreatic Carcinoma by In Vivo Proton Magnetic Resonance Spectroscopy. *JCAT,* 2005; 29: 163-169.

[147] Singh P, Chak A, Willis J, Rollins A, Sivak M. In vivo optical coherence tomography imaging of the pancreatic and biliary ductal system. *Gastrointest. Endosc., 2005;* 62: 970-974.

[148] Testoni P, Mangiavillano B, Albarello L, Arcidiacono P, Mariani A, Masci E, Doglioni C. Optical coherence tomography to detect epithelial lesions of the main pancreatic duct: an ex vivo study. *Am. J. Gastroenterol.*, 2005; 100: 2777-2783.

[149] Kwon R, Scheiman J. New Advances in Pancreatic Imaging. *Curr. Opin. Gastroenterol.*, 2006; 22: 512-519.

In: Pancreatitis Research Advances
Editor: William C. Langley, pp. 149-177
ISBN: 978-1-60021-883-5

Chapter IV

Current Concepts of the Molecular Biology of Tumor Necrosis Factor-Alpha in Experimental Acute Pancreatitis

Giuseppe Malleo[1,2], *Emanuela Mazzon*[1], *Ajith K. Siriwardena*[2] *and Salvatore Cuzzocrea*[1]
[1] Department of Clinical, Experimental Medicine and Pharmacology, University of Messina, Italy
[2] Department of Surgery, Hepatobiliary Unit, University of Manchester, United Kingdom.

Abstract

Acute pancreatitis is an emerging disease with great variability in severity. Whereas it runs a mild, self-limiting course in most patients, in others it can take a severe form characterized by extensive necrosis and in-hospital mortality rate in excess of 25%. It has been shown that many individuals facing severe pancreatitis develop multiple organ dysfunction syndrome (MODS), and much effort has been spent to improve understanding of the mechanism of disease progression from acinar cell injury to an overwhelming, life-threatening condition. Although the pathophysiology of acute pancreatitis has not been clearly established, emerging evidence suggests that dysregulation in immune response and interactions between leukocytes, soluble mediators (such as cytokines) and vascular endothelium contribute to the generalization of the inflammatory response.

The pleiotropic cytokine tumor necrosis factor (TNF)-α is considered one of the major mediators associated to the local and systemic tissue damage, being a key regulator of pro-inflammatory genes and a priming activator of immune and endothelial cells. Thus, investigators have regarded blocking its production or action as an attractive treatment option for pancreatitis, and various non-specific and specific anti-TNF-α agents have been tested in animal models with promising results. Our group contributed to the present research line in the light of recent findings, which evidenced an early up-regulation of the cytokine both in acinar and immune cells in the course of the disease. In addition, significantly elevated plasma levels have been demonstrated in patients with worse prognosis and outcome. Accordingly, we assessed in two studies the effects of thalidomide (an immunomodulatory agent which suppresses TNF-α biosynthesis and angiogenesis) and of Etanercept (a soluble TNF-α receptor construct which neutralizes the circulating cytokine) on the development of cerulein-induced acute pancreatitis in mice. We also evaluated, in the same model, the effects of genetic deletion of TNF-receptor I. In all our studies we observed a substantial amelioration of histological and biochemical features of pancreatitis, a decrease in the expression of pro-inflammatory cytokines, VEGF and adhesion molecules, a diminished neutrophil infiltration and pancreas apoptosis. Although a full extrapolation of experimental data has to be made with caution, acute pancreatitis may represent a suitable disease for TNF-α antagonism: timing of intervention and a careful selection of inclusion and exclusion criteria may aid in better defining the population most likely to benefit in future clinical trials.

Introduction

Acute pancreatitis is an inflammatory process of the pancreas with variable involvement of other regional or remote organ systems. Most episodes of pancreatitis are mild, self-limiting and characterized histologically by moderate acinar compromise, interstitial oedema, and inflammatory cell infiltration. Spontaneous and complete recovery usually occurs in few days. In 10–20% of the cases, however, severe disease develops and parts of the pancreas and surrounding tissue may become necrotic. Patients with severe disease require prolonged in-hospital stay and critical care treatment. In this group, morbidity and mortality rates are in excess of 10% and even greater (25-30%) in infected necrosis with multiple organ dysfunction syndrome [1,2].

The essential point in the concept of acute pancreatitis is the initiation of a local inflammatory infiltration through intrapancreatically activated digestive enzymes; systemic progression may follow with variable degrees. Rapid production and release of pro-inflammatory mediators such as cytokines and chemokines and their subsequent interactions with vascular endothelium and leukocytes are integral to this process [3].

Being a key-regulator of pro-inflammatory genes and a priming activator of immune and endothelial cells, tumor necrosis factor (TNF)-α represents one of the most prominent inflammatory mediators associated with acute pancreatitis [4]. This has been confirmed by different experimental approaches such as direct plasma measurement [5] and gene targeting techniques [6]. Therefore, a better insight into the kinetics, regulation and effects of this mediator may help in comprehending the sequence of pathophysiological changes at the acinar level and at distant sites during the course of acute pancreatitis.

There is also evidence that TNF-α blockade may be beneficial in experimental pancreatitis [7]. However, to date, no clinical studies have been conducted in human disease due to variety of reasons including the disappointing results obtained in trials of TNF-monoclonal antibody in sepsis.

Here, we outline the recent findings on the involvement of TNF-α in the pathogenesis of acute pancreatitis, and we review our results on pharmacological and genetic inhibition of this cytokine in pre-clinical models of the disease.

An Overview of the Molecular Biology of TNF-α and TNF-Receptor Superfamily

TNF-α is the prototypic member of a gene superfamily that regulates essential biologic functions such as immune response, cell proliferation, survival, differentiation and apoptosis. These biological activities encompass beneficial effects in immune response against several pathogens and in organogenesis of lymphoid structures as well as host damaging effects in sepsis, cachexia, autoimmune, and inflammatory diseases [8].

Primarily produced by immune cells such as monocytes and macrophages, TNF-α can also be released by other cell types, including acinar cells. The protein product is initially synthesized as a 26-kD cell surface-associated molecule anchored by an N-terminal hydrophobic domain. A specific matrix metalloproteinase protein, TNF-converting enzyme (TNFCE), cleaves the 26-kD form into a soluble 17-kD form which self-assembles in non-covalent bound homotrimers and interacts with membrane bound or soluble TNF-receptors (TNFR) [9.10].

Receptor activation by TNF family ligands causes recruitment of various adaptor proteins with subsequent activation of downstream signaling pathways.

According to specific intracellular sequences and to signaling adaptors recruited, TNFR superfamily can be classified in three major groups [11].

The first group includes receptors, such as TNFR1 (p55 or 55-kD TNFR), Fas and various others, that share a highly conserved sequence of about 80 amino acids in the cytoplasmic region called the *death domain*. Activation of these receptors leads to homotypic interactions with adaptor proteins containing *death domains* such as Fas-associated death domain (FADD) and TNFR-associated death domain (TRADD) [12-14].

FADD and TRADD are the proximal transducers of apoptosis initiated by the FasL/Fas and TNF-α/TNFR1 interactions respectively. However, TRADD recruitment can also trigger downstream events related to inflammation [15] through further adaptor proteins including TNF receptor associated factors (TRAFs), receptor interacting protein (RIP) and mitogen-activated kinase-activating death domain (MADD) [12].

TRAFs, RIP and MADD mediate the activation of NF-kB and of mitogen activated protein kinases (MAPK) cascade [16-18].

The second group includes receptors, such as TNFR2 (p75 or 75-kD TNFR), CD30, CD40 and others, that contain in their cytoplasmic region specific amino-acid sequences called TNFR-associated factors (TRAFs)-interacting motifs (TIMs).

Activation of TIMs leads to recruitment of TRAF family members. These molecules share a highly conserved motif called TRAF domain and possess no enzymatic activity. As the recruitment of TRAFs is necessary for TRADD activation, it has been speculated that TNFR2 may serve to increase TNFR1 signalling through TRAFs recruitment or, alternatively, as a counter-regulatory to suppress TNF-α mediated signaling [19,20].

The third group includes decoy receptors such as DR1 and DR3 and others. To date, no specific signalling motifs have been observed in this group.

In conclusion, the extracellular domains of TNFR1 and TNFR2 are homologous and manifest similar affinity for TNF-α, but the cytoplasmic regions of the two receptors are distinct and mediate different downstream events: signalling via TNFR1 seems the major mechanism responsible for the effects of TNF-α [Figure 1].

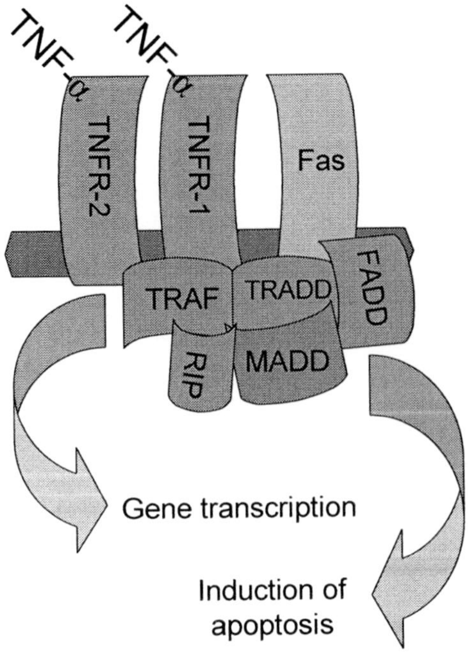

Figure 1. Model of TNF-α-mediated intracellular signalling. The interaction between TNF-α and its transmembrane receptors recruits different adaptor proteins and triggers downstream events leading – when deregulated – to an over-activation of inflammatory gene transcription and/or an enhanced apoptotic cell death. TRADD is the proximal transducer of apoptosis, and its interaction with FADD activates caspase-8. A complex association between TRADD, TRAFs, RIP and MADD promotes transcriptional activation of various pro-inflammatory genes. TRAFs = TNF receptor associated factors; RIP = Receptor interacting protein; TRADD = TNF receptor associated death domain; FADD = Fas associated death domain; MADD = Mitogen activated kinases death domain.

Role of TNF-α in Acinar Injury during Acute Pancreatitis

Acinar Cells as a Source of TNF-α

TNF-α is substantially up-regulated in the pancreas during the early phases of acute pancreatitis. Norman and colleagues first showed the increased expression of TNF-α mRNA in murine pancreatitis, and activated immune cells infiltrating the pancreas such as monocytes and macrophages were considered the most prominent source of the cytokine [21]. Soon after, Gukovskaya and colleagues shifted the focus to acinar cells, demonstrating that dispersed pancreatic acini produce, release and respond to TNF-α [22]. Although it remains to be elucidated whether activated acinar cells are able to produce a whole spectrum of pro-inflammatory cytokines, it is now clear that they promote the inflammatory process not only releasing active enzymes locally and lipids systemically, but – more surprisingly – behaving like genuine inflammatory cells [23]. This emerging concept has been very recently reinforced by the unexpected finding of the leukocyte-specific receptor-like protein CD45 within acinar cells. CD45 expression is down-regulated during acute pancreatitis by redox sensitive mechanisms, and acinar levels are inversely correlated with the production of TNF-α [24,25]. These observations support the notion that CD45 may negatively control TNF-α production, and – more extensively – the revolutionary concept of a function for acinar cells in immunocompetency.

Comparative *in vivo* kinetic studies evaluated by semi-quantitative analysis of mRNA expression [26] or – more recently – by flow cytometry [27,28] the time-course of TNF-α production in acinar cells and leukocytes after pancreatic injury. TNF-α up-regulation occurred in acinar cells soon after cerulein or lipopolysaccharide (LPS) administration in mice, with a peak at six hours; whereas no signal of TNF-α bioactivity was present in neutrophils infiltrating the pancreas until twelve hours from treatment.

Similarly, anti-inflammatory mediators such as IL-10 were up-regulated in pancreatic tissue in the early phases of acute pancreatitis and the ability of acinar cells to produce IL-10 has been recently demonstrated [28].

Another factor, which may contribute to acinar TNF-α production, is pancreatitis-associated ascitic fluid (PAAF), which accumulates in the abdominal cavity as a result of the microcirculatory impairment. Sterile PAAF obtained from rats with bile-pancreatic duct ligation pancreatitis enhanced TNF-α production in isolated acinar cells and – interestingly – neither heating nor pre-treating PAAF with anti-rat TNF-α monoclonal antibodies or trypsin inhibitors were able to suppress this cytokine up-regulation, suggesting that PAAF-stimulated TNF-α production is independent of TNF-α itself. In the same experiment, peripheral blood leukocytes failed to produce TNF-α after PAAF challenge and, similarly, agents stimulating cytokine production in monocytes (such as LPS) and lymphocytes had no effect on acinar cells [29]. These results may indicate that LPS and TNF-α, by themselves, are not physiological stimuli for TNF-α production in acinar cells and that PAAF may be involved in the pathophysiology of acute pancreatitis by TNF-α production. On the other hand, it has been shown that inflammatory mediators contained in PAAF may contribute to the progression of pancreatitis acting on monocytes in a "specific" fashion, thereby demonstrating the existence of selective patterns of cytokines activation in different cell types.

Therefore, acinar cells submitted to stress activate TNF-α gene expression as a part of a general response against aggression. The extent, the progress and the severity of acute pancreatitis may initially depend on the relative imbalance between pro- and anti-inflammatory responses at the acinar level. The subsequent up-regulation of pro-inflammatory genes may offer the first signal to attract immune cells to the damaged pancreas.

Molecular Pathways of Acinar TNF-α Production

TNF-α expression can be regulated at different levels. The two principal mechanisms identified are a transcriptional and a post-transcriptional regulation.

At the transcriptional level, the encoding of TNF-α gene and of other stress-related genes, such as genes for other cytokines, chemokines, cell adhesion molecules, cyclo-oxygenase-2 (COX-2) and inducible nitric oxide synthase (iNOS), is triggered by transcription factors and signalling cascades activated by a variety of stimuli ranging from cell damaging physical factors to mitogens and cytokines [30].

Nuclear factor (NF)-kB, protein kinases, Smad proteins, and the steroid hormone family peroxisome proliferators-activated receptors (PPARs) regulate gene transcription in acute pancreatitis [31, 32]. The activation of the pluripotent transcription factor NF-kB in response to acinar cells injury has been the most widely investigated [33-35], although the mechanisms and the signalling pathways involved still remain partially unclear.

Acinar NF-kB production in experimental pancreatitis demonstrates biphasic kinetics with a first peak at the onset and a second peak at three hours and onwards [33]. Early events leading to NF-kB activation and gene induction are dysregulation of digestive enzymes secretion, intracellular enzyme activation by CCK-8/cerulein, and elevated levels of oxygen free radicals [36-38].

TNF-α is a potent inducer of NF-kB: In acinar cells exposed to TNF-α, high levels of the p65 NF-kB subunit in the nucleus with DNA binding increased by sevenfold have been observed [39]. In this regard, Gukovsky et al showed that TNF-α blockage is associated with a marked inhibition of the second NF-kB peak, whereas it has no effects on the early peak [33].

The post-receptor events mediating NF-kB activation induced by TNF-α are now being elucidated, and protein kinases C (PKC), a family of serine/treonine kinases, appear to play an important role. PKC-δ/-ε isoforms are necessary for TNF-α induced NF-kB activation [36], and the signalling pathway involves the TNFR p55 death domain. PKC-δ and PKC-ε trigger a cascade involving IkB kinases, which leads to hyperphosphorylation and proteolytic degradation of IkB proteins [40]. Subsequently, NF-kB dimers translocate from the cytosol to the nucleus, where they bind to their consensus sequence on the promoter-enhancer region of inflammatory genes. Others and we demonstrated that interfering in this NF-kB pathway through antioxidants has beneficial effects on the inflammatory response in experimental acute pancreatitis [30, 41, 42].

However, NF-kB is not the only transcriptional factor regulating gene expression after acinar injury. A recent paper associated NF-kB inhibition only to a partial decrease of TNF-α production in acinar cells [29], and in another study no correlation between cytokine/chemokine concentrations and NF-kB activation was observed in human pancreatitis [43].

Protein kinases seem crucial in activating gene transcription through other pathways than NF-kB. Intracellular tyrosine kinases, for example, are involved in TNF-α-mediated inflammatory responses, and we have demonstrated that inhibition of tyrosine kinase-mediated cellular signalling reduces the severity of murine pancreatitis and the systemic release of TNF-α [44]. Furthermore, tyrosine kinase inhibitor treatment influences the phosphorylation of mitogen activated protein kinases (MAPK) through a mechanism still largely unknown.

MAPK are serine/treonine kinases, which include three sub-families: extracellular signal-regulated kinase (erk 1/2), c-Jun NH_2-terminal protein kinase (JNK) and p38. Their activation in the pancreas occurs through G-protein-coupled receptors and mediates different cellular events, including TNF-α expression [18, 45-47]. MAPK activation in acinar cells could be regulated by CD45. A CD45 reduction in response to stress may "switch on" MAPK cascade and TNF-α up-regulation [24].

In rat pancreatic acini challenged with cholecistokinin, erk 1/2 (p42, p44) and JNKs ($p46^{jnk}$, $p55^{jnk}$) peak within minutes after the induction and decrease approximately at one hour [48]. Their selective inhibition was associated with decreased TNF-α gene transcription, reduced intrapancreatic levels of TNF-α and resulted in a significant amelioration of acute pancreatitis in mice [49, 50].

p38 mediates the phosphorylation and activation of various transcription factors including CHOP, ATF-2 and Elk1 via MK-2, a member of MAPK-activated protein kinases (MAPKAPKs) [45,48]. Accumulating evidence suggests that MK-2 is essential for LPS-induced TNF-α biosynthesis [51]. Very recently Tietz and colleagues investigated the effects of MK-2 gene deletion showing that mice lacking MK-2 are unable to produce TNF-α and IL-6 and are protected against pancreatic/acinar injury [52]. Interestingly, the mechanism through which MK-2 regulates TNF-α does not involve TNFR-mediated signalling, TNF-α gene transcription or transcription factors mediating the p38/MK-2 pathway [51]. It is thus likely that MK-2 promotes TNF-α up-regulation at a post-transcriptional level. In this regard, it has been proposed that MK-2 targets the AU-rich 3'-untranslated elements (ARE) of TNF-α mRNA through the heterogeneous nuclear ribonucleoprotein A0 (hnRNP A0) [53,54]. However, hnRNP A0 has not thus far been localized in acinar cells.

Other acinar events stimulated by TNF-α include the activation of transcription factors of PPAR-α/γ, Smad and STAT family. PPAR are a family of nuclear receptors of ligand transcription factors related to retinoid, steroid and thyroid hormone receptors. We have recently investigated the role of PPAR-α and PPAR-γ in cerulein-induced pancreatitis, showing that they may act as down-regulators of the inflammatory process through a modulation of TNF-α production [32, 55].

The pathophysiology of Smad proteins in acinar cells is poorly understood. They seem to mediate signals from the transforming growth factor-β (TGF-β) superfamily and they may be involved in essential cellular functions such as differentiation, proliferation and death [56] through negative regulation of target genes, which are still largely unknown.

Very recently, Robinson and colleagues reported that transcription factors STAT-1 and STAT-3 are substantially up-regulated in AR42J cells challenged with recombinant TNF-α, and that peptide YY (an inhibitory gastrointestinal hormone) may act as a broad spectrum transcriptional silencer in response to TNF-α stimulation in this cell line [31,57].

Pancreatitis associated protein 1 (PAP-1), whose expression may be enhanced by oxidative stress, is another factor thought to mediate TNF-α signalling in pancreatitis [58]. PAP-1 activation seems strongly induced by the transcription co-factor p8, as mice lacking p8 are not able to express PAP-1 and develop worse histological signs of pancreatitis than the correspondent wild type mice [59]. Similarly, PAP-1 inhibition in experimental pancreatitis was associated with significantly poor outcome, suggesting that this mediator possesses anti-inflammatory properties. Although a study showed that PAP-1 expression is strongly NF-kB-dependent [58], the interaction is complex as other studies show that it is able to inhibit NF-kB itself in response to TNF-α through a JAK/STAT-mediated mechanism [60].

In conclusion, TNF-α activity is regulated by an intricate intracellular network. Many of these cellular mechanisms are not unique to the pancreatic acinar cell but represent a generic response mechanism to inflammation. However, key findings to emerge are that the acinar cell behaves as an inflammatory stimulus via a series of TNF-dependent and also TNF-independent pathways.

TNF-α- Mediated Acinar Cell Responses

i) Cytoskeletal Disorganization

An intact actin cytoskeleton is essential for physiological enzyme secretion in acinar cells. It has been demonstrated that secretagogues and oxidative stress [61-63] induce concentration-dependent reorganization of actin microfilaments and changes in acinar cell shape. In particular, supramaximal stimulation with secretagogues was associated with reduction or loss of cell polarity, dramatic blebbing and decrease in apical filamentous actin, clear signs of disruption of the actin cytoskeleton, stress fiber formation and enlarged acinar lumina [64].

A major regulator of the homeostasis of the actin cytoskeleton is heat shock protein 27 (Hsp-27), whose up-regulation is significantly increased under stress conditions [63,65]. Activation of proline-rich tyrosine kinase 2 (Pyk2) and the p38 MAPK/MK-2 pathway are involved in this process [66].

Overexpression of Hsp-27 may preserve the actin cytoskeleton at the apical pole of acinar cells and maintain efficient zymogen exocytosis [67]. Thus, it would be predicted that MK-2 inhibition worsen the course of pancreatitis, but it has been shown that MK-2 knockout mice have normal levels of Hsp-27, although they lack the ability to phosphorylate the protein [52].

TNF-α may play a role in cytoskeletal modification following acinar cell injury. Satoh and colleagues demonstrated that acinar cells responding to TNF-α show an increase of filamentous actin along the basolateral membrane and a marked decrease at the apical pole [68]. Of note, TNF-α alone did not provoke enzyme activation and secretion or cytoplasmic blebs. The deleterious effects on the cytoskeleton induced by TNF-α are mediated by Pyk2, which is phosphorylated by PKC-δ/-ε isoforms and Src kinases. Further studies are required to distinguish the differences between cytoskeletal modifications induced by secretagogues and TNF-α, which may depend on the differential phospholipase-C activation and on cytosolic Ca^{2+} levels.

ii) Cell Death

Both necrosis and apoptosis occur in experimental pancreatitis. It is now well known that the severity of the disease is related to the type and the degree of cell death: severe pancreatitis is associated with extensive acinar cell necrosis, while mild pancreatitis reveals extensive apoptotic cell death and a minimal amount of necrosis [69]. Thus, apoptosis has been interpreted as a beneficial cell response to injury, and inducing apoptosis as a potentially effective strategy to decrease the severity of experimental pancreatitis [70,71]. Initiation of apoptosis can be signalled through two major pathways, (which interact or cross-talk abundantly): the extrinsic pathway is promoted by transmembrane death receptors such as TNFR and Fas, whereas the intrinsic pathway seems to be critically regulated by alterations in mitochondrial permeability [72]. Both result in the activation of initiator and effector caspases.

To date, the mechanisms through which acinar cells are directed into apoptotic or necrotic pathways are still unclear. Different regulating events, a delicate balance of mediators and of pro- and antiapoptotic members of the bcl-2 gene family acts in an intricate network, which finally determines the pattern of cell death [73]. Cell energy status is thought to be a critical factor regulating the apoptosis/necrosis ratio. Apoptosis requires ATP for activating caspases, whereas necrosis does not seem to require an energy investment. Thus, severe mitochondrial dysfunction may influence ATP levels, leading to a fail in caspase activation and to necrosis [74]. Another mechanism involved ATP depletion is the "PARP suicide hypothesis" [75].

TNF-α is capable of stimulating acinar cell death through necrosis and/or apoptosis. An interaction with TNFR1 can activate signalling complexes leading to the apoptotic arm or to NF-kB/MAPKs pathways [22,76]. These events are influenced at various levels, including regulation of receptor/ligand expression and induction of anti-apoptotic molecules. One key regulator of TNF-α induced cell death is NF-kB that – apart from its role in promoting the inflammatory response (and indirectly necrosis) – has been shown to down-regulate apoptosis. NF-kB neutralization results in a marked potentiation of caspase activity, which inhibits necrosis and intra-acinar enzyme activation [77]. The anti-apoptotic effects of NF-kB activation involve the expression of newly synthesized proteins such as cellular inhibitors of apoptosis (IAP-1/2, XIAP), which inactivate downstream caspases [78]. Moreover, NF-kB promotes the expression of the caspase-8 inhibitor FLIP and of adaptor proteins TRAF1/2 [79, 80].

Another candidate for mediating antiapoptotic effects is PAP I which apart from its anti-inflammatory effects has been demonstrated to induce a significant decrease in apoptosis in rat acinar cells exposed to TNF-α [81].

Recent findings indicated that death receptors such as TNFR1, Fas and TRAIL can also mediate an alternative and coordinated form of non-accidental necrosis separate from the "classic" necrosis triggered by cellular stress and ATP depletion [82]. This newly discovered cell death mechanism has been called "programmed necrosis" or "necrosis-like programmed cell death", and its physiological significance as well as the signalling pathways involved are largely unknown. To date, the only proven mediator of this alternative pathway is the adaptor protein RIP, deficiency of which protects against TNF-α-induced programmed necrosis [82]. Mareninova and colleagues shed light into RIP-mediated death signals in experimental pancreatitis: RIP degradation by caspases correlates with low necrosis and a high degree of apoptosis demonstrating that RIP signals programmed necrosis and that caspases may exert a protective effect in pancreatitis [83].

Also, it was reported that lipid rafts translocation following TNFR1 activation is a critical event in NF-kB up-regulation and that inhibiting the formation of lipid rafts switches TNF-α signalling from NF-kB to apoptotic activation [84].

In conclusion, the determination of cell death pathways in pancreatitis and identification of strategies to switch necrosis to apoptosis may have a therapeutic value. Besides its well-defined pro-inflammatory activities in the early stages of the disease, TNF-α mediates pro-apoptotic effects, (especially when NF-kB is blocked) as well as programmed necrosis. Given the central role of TNF-α in determining cell death, further studies are required to better clarify the intracellular events involved and the consequences of therapeutic strategies on cytokine inhibition.

Role of TNF-α in Pancreatitis-Associated Inflammatory Response

Adhesion Cascade, Neutrophils, Oxidative Stress and TNF- α in the Pancreas

In response to pro-inflammatory stimuli arising from acinar cells, an intricate sequence of events involving tissue vasculature and inflammatory cells occurs. TNF-α and oxygen free radicals (OFR) cause an uncontrolled up-regulation of endothelial adhesion molecules, which in turn promote rolling, adhesion, aggregation and transmigration of leukocytes into inflamed tissues [75]. In particular, the recruitment of neutrophils, key cells in mediating organ injury, is triggered by an adhesion cascade involving selectins and ICAM-1 [85]. While selectins account for the initial low-energy neutrophils rolling along vessels wall, ICAM-1 is responsible for their firm adhesion. ICAM-1 was also localized in rat pancreatic acinar cells and up-regulated by cerulein [86], and ICAM-1 knockout mice displayed decreased neutrophil infiltration and improved outcome in experimental pancreatitis [87].

Telek and colleagues demonstrated that OFR may give the earliest signal to attract inflammatory cells to damaged pancreas: NF-kB up-regulation, strong P-selectin and mild ICAM-1 expression were first detected at the sites of acinar oxidative stress, together with moderate neutrophil margination [37]. Subsequently, massive P-selectin/E-selectin/ICAM-1 expression and a large number of adherent neutrophils were observed [88-90]. It has been speculated that acinar oxidative stress may mediate the mobilization of preformed P-selectin from Weibel-Palade bodies in response to noxious stimuli, whereas a *de novo* synthesis of P-/E-selectin and ICAM-1 occurs in response to augmented TNF-α production and increased levels of OFR in the pancreas [91]. Thus, OFR formation "switches" from acinar cells to neutrophils, where the activation of inducible nitric oxide synthase (iNOS) and the release of elastase (which hydrolyzes elastin, fibronectin, proteoglycans and collagen) represent the major contributor of tissue injury [85,92]. In this regard, we showed that the absence of iNOS, as well as the administration of superoxide dismutase mimetics, reduces the development of cerulein-induced pancreatitis in mice [93, 94].

Moreover, neutrophils infiltrating the pancreas have also been recently shown to contribute via OFR to a further pathologic activation of digestive enzymes in acinar cells as well as to the activation of nuclear enzyme PARP (poly (ADP-ribose) polymerase) through strand breaks in DNA [95]. Growing evidence suggests that PARP-1 inhibition modulates the inflammatory process in the pancreas through mechanisms involving TNF-α: it was recently demonstrated in our laboratory that TNF-α levels were significantly reduced in mice treated with 3-Aminobenzamide, a PARP-1 inhibitor [75].

TNF-α may also intensify oxidative stress converting xanthine dehydrogenase to xanthine oxidase in the endothelial cells of the pancreatic micro-vasculature [96] and enhancing chemotaxis and activation of neutrophils [97].

Overall, a complex cross-talk between oxidative stress and TNF-α generates in the course of pancreatic injury a vicious circle that amplifies the local inflammatory response. We propose a pathway shown in figure 2, which summarizes the self-perpetuating loop involving oxidative stress and TNF-α during pancreas injury.

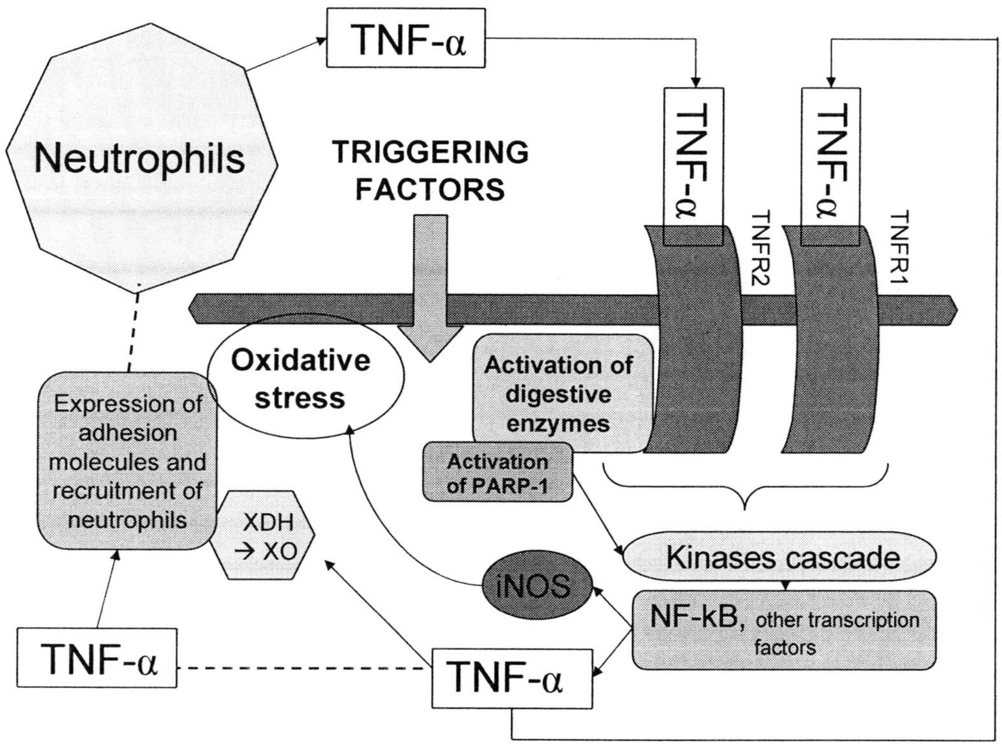

Figure 2. Cross-talk between TNF-α and oxidative stress. TNF-α promotes the expression of leukocyte adhesion molecules in endothelial cells, and neutrophils migrate into the inflamed pancreas. Furthermore, it activates neutrophils and converts xanthine dehydrogenase into xanthine oxidase in endothelial cells. Injured acinar cells, endothelial cells and neutrophils over-produce reactive oxygen species (ROS), which enhance the activation of the nuclear enzyme PARP-1 and of MAPK. PARP-1 and MAPK account for further production of TNF-α.. NF-kB = Nuclear factor kB; iNOS = Inducible nitric oxide synthase; MAPK = Mitogen activated protein kinases; PARP-1 = Poly(ADP-ribose) polymerase; X-DH = xanthine dehydrogenase; XO = xanthine oxidase.

Monocytes/Macrophages and TNF-α

TNF-α is considered one of the major mediators associated with systemic tissue injury. In this regard, circulating monocytes and resident macrophages play a primary role [98,99]. Their activation may be triggered by early signals released from the pancreas that gain access to the systemic circulation: specific pancreatic enzymes such as elastase, carboxypeptidase A and lipase were shown to induce TNF-α in a rat alveolar macrophage cell line via NF-kB [100]. However, recent reports suggest that pancreatic elastase free from contaminating endotoxin fails to activate murine macrophages to release TNF-α [101]. Another mechanism activating macrophages may derive from signals provided by injured cells that alerts the immune system to danger [102]. Accumulating evidence showed that tissue damage is recognized at the cell level via toll-like receptor-mediated detection of intracellular molecules (known as "alarmins") released by dying cells [103,104]. Endogenous alarmins would be the equivalent of the exogenous pathogen-associated molecular pattern (PAMPs), conveying similar messages and eliciting similar responses: alarmins and PAMPs can be therefore considered subgroups of a larger set, the damage associated molecular pattern (DAMPs); and this finding would provide a further molecular link between cell injury, inflammation and immunity.

Peripheral Blood Monocytes

Circulating monocytes spontaneously over-express TNF-α in experimental pancreatitis. The kinetic of these cells and of TNF-α production was investigated in a rat pancreatic duct obstruction model. A marked increase in monocyte plasma levels has been observed in the early stages of pancreatitis, followed by a substantial drop toward baseline levels and a second elevation thereafter. This behaviour may be determined by a massive expression of the adhesion molecule CD11b, which induces monocytes/macrophage homing and enhanced TNF-α tissue production [90].

Peritoneal Macrophages

Peritoneal mononuclear cells, which are involved in the defence of the abdominal cavity against infection, are responsible for excessive production of TNF-α in pancreatitis. PAAF and trypsin are known to modulate the function of peritoneal macrophages, resulting in augmented TNF-α levels, apoptotic cytotoxitcity and end-organ damage [105-108]. Experimental necrotizing pancreatitis was associated with a marked decrease of peritoneal macrophages [109].

Kupffer Cells

Pancreatitis-associated liver injury is dependent on dysregulation of Kupffer cells, the largest resident macrophage population [110,111]. Using *in vitro* elastase challenging and *in situ* liver perfusion, it has been reported that Kupffer cells respond to injury by up-regulating MAPK, NF-kB and TNF-α gene expression [112,113]. Gene targeting strategies suggested that TNF-α and FasL in turn may enhance both Kupffer cells and hepatocyte apoptotic death [114-116], and NF-kB may play a role in death receptor/ligands regulation [117].

Lung Injury and TNF-α

The main pancreatitis-associated end-organ dysfunction is acute lung injury, which is indistinguishable both clinically and pathologically from the adult respiratory distress syndrome (ARDS). This is a common early complication of acute pancreatitis leading to death in approximately one third of patients with severe disease.

Lung injury is mediated by an over-activation of alveolar macrophages, which release several substances (such as nitric oxide (NO), chemokines, arachidonic acid metabolites and TNF-α) and recruit neutrophils [118,119] . P38 MAPK has been implicated in TNF-α up-regulation within lungs in rat pancreatitis [120].

The liver plays a major role in inducing lung inflammation in response to pancreatitis. Inhibition of Kupffer cells was associated with a decrease in TNF-alpha levels, neutrophil infiltration, and to an amelioration of lung injury in several experimental models of pancreatitis [121,122]. Finally, it has been reported that pancreatitis associated protein-1 (PAP-1) induces lung inflammation in rat taurocholate pancreatitis through activation of TNF-α expression in hepatocytes and a subsequent increase in circulating TNF-α protein [123].

Recently, Lundberg and colleagues reported a temporal correlation between TNF-α release, up-regulation of pulmonary ICAM-1/VCAM-1, neutrophils sequestration and lung injury in diet-induced pancreatitis in mice [147]. A temporal delay between the onset of acute pancreatitis, lung injury and other organ dysfunction was also shown in other animal models [124].

TNF-α as a Therapeutic Target in Acute Pancreatitis

There are still no specific therapies for acute pancreatitis and treatment remains largely supportive, although in the last few years, studies have shown a reduction in mortality in patients receiving prophylactic antibiotics [125] and also in individuals undergoing endoscopic sphincterotomy for severe gallstone-related disease [126].

In view of the central role of TNF-α in the innate host inflammatory response, investigators have regarded blocking the production or the action of this cytokine as an attractive treatment option for a variety of conditions associated with excessive or poorly controlled inflammation. Several strategies have been developed for neutralizing TNF-α, including polyclonal antibodies, monoclonal antibodies, soluble receptors constructs, and non-specific agents (e.g. thalidomide, phosphodiesterase inhibitors, metalloproteinase inhibitors and others) [127] [Table 2]. In the last decade more than one hundred forty pre-clinical studies have been conducted to assess the effects of TNF-α neutralization in models of acute infection or inflammation (especially sepsis) and to identify appropriate patient populations for therapeutic intervention [128]. Subsequently, twelve completed phase II and III randomized clinical trials have been carried out in human sepsis showing only a very modest impact on mortality, although in a highly heterogeneous population of patients [129-131].

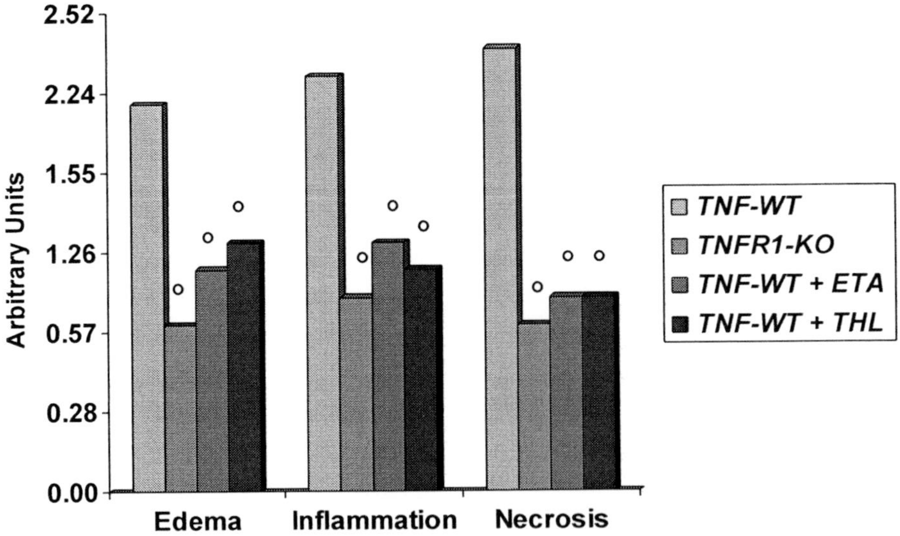

Figure 3. Effects of the anti-TNF-α agents Etanercept and Thalidomide on edema formation, inflammatory cell infiltration and acinar necrosis in cerulein-induced acute pancreatitis in TNF-α wild type (WT) mice. TNFR1-knockout (KO) mice were used as control. °$p < 0.05$ *versus* cerulein-treated WT mice.

Few experimental studies and no clinical trials have been conducted on TNF-α neutralization in acute pancreatitis so far. Selective inhibitors of cytokine production have been reported to prevent histological changes and to improve the survival rate in closed duodenal loop pancreatitis in rats [132]. Denham and colleagues – by administering an inhibitor of macrophage production of TNF-α and IL-1 – showed a dramatic reduction in tissue damage and in pancreatitis severity in mice [133].

Another anti-cytokine agent with rheologic properties which significantly reduced histological score, biochemical manifestations and glutathione depletion in different experimental models of pancreatitis was the methylxanthine derivative pentoxifylline [134,135]. The simultaneous inhibition of TNF-α and xanthine oxidase, with pentoxifylline and oxypurinol respectively abolished the inflammatory changes associated with taurocholate pancreatitis [136]. Anti TNF-α antibodies have been initially used to evaluate the temporal relationship between induction of pancreatitis and the rise of TNF-α in serum. In particular, pre-treatment with polyclonal anti-TNF-α antibodies in experimental pancreatitis inhibits the early burst of TNF-α activity and significantly improved the course of the disease as well as overall survival in rats, thereby demonstrating that an early selective blockage of TNF-α may be of value [137-139]. Very recently, Oruc and colleagues reported that infliximab, a monoclonal anti-TNF-α antibody, ameliorates the course of both oedematous and severe necrotizing pancreatitis in rats, although in severe disease it did not influence neutrophil activity, pancreatic oedema or mortality [7].

The first study evaluating the early and delayed effects of a recombinant dimeric form of soluble TNFR1 (p55) was conducted in rat choline-deficient diet pancreatitis. A marked amelioration of biochemical parameters, histological score, lung-associated injury and overall survival were observed either in prophylactic or delayed treatment, whereas mortality rate was significantly diminished in the latter group [140].

Novel Strategies for TNF-α Inhibition in Experimental Pancreatitis

Etanercept

Recently, Denham et al. have demonstrated that knockout mice for TNF-α receptor 1 are protected against acute pancreatitis and pancreatitis-associated lung injury [141]. In addition, Douni et al. showed that the production of the human TNF-α receptor 1 in transgenic mice results in a severe systemic inflammatory syndrome [142]. These results suggested that antagonizing TNFR functions by blocking interactions with circulating TNF-α may down-regulate the inflammatory response. Physiologically, this may occur by means of soluble receptors.

Soluble TNF-α receptors (sTNFR) directly derive from proteolytic cleavage of membrane TNF-α receptor 1 (p55) and TNF-α receptor 2 (p75); their shedding from cell membrane is markedly enhanced during inflammation, and elevated levels have been evaluated as predictors for the development of multiple organ failure [5].

The biologic significance of TNF-α receptor shedding is, however, still under debate. As physiological neutralizing capacity of sTNFR seems relatively low (so that in theory a 30- to 300-fold molar excess would be necessary to block elevated concentrations of circulating TNF-α) [143], in low concentrations, sTNFR may serve as TNF-α carriers into the circulation.

Recently, recombinant sTNFR constructs with enhanced binding capacity, such as Etanercept, have proven to be effective in neutralizing TNF-α during inflammatory conditions. Etanercept is a humanized dimeric soluble form of TNFR2, it binds to two TNF-α molecules blocking their interaction with cell surface TNF-α receptors and rendering TNF-α biologically inactive. TNF-α inactivation is a thousand times stronger than inactivation by p75 monomeric TNF-α receptor [144]. Etanercept inhibits the activity of TNF-α *in vitro* and its effects have been examined *in vivo* in different animal model systems of inflammatory and autoimmune diseases [145]. In the clinical setting, it has been recently approved for the treatment of rheumatoid arthritis, juvenile rheumatoid arthritis [146,147], ankylosing spondylitis [148], psoriatic arthritis [149] and plaque psoriasis [150].

Therefore, we investigated the effects of this recombinant TNFR2 construct on the inflammatory response and apoptosis in a murine model of necrotizing acute pancreatitis induced by cerulein, in comparison with genetic deletion of TNF receptor 1 (TNFR1). The degree of pancreatic injury, amylase and lipase levels ($p<0.05$), TNF-α, TGF-β and VEGF formation ($p<0.01$), the expression of adhesion molecules ($p<0.01$), neutrophil infiltration ($p<0.01$) and the induction of apoptosis (assessed by immunostaining for FasL, Bax, Bcl-2 ($p<0.01$) and by TUNEL assay) in the pancreas were significantly reduced in a similar degree in Etanercept-treated and TNFR1-KO mice [151]. Our study provided the first evidence that pharmacological treatment with Etanercept significantly ameliorates the development of cerulein-induced acute pancreatitis in mice. In parallel, the genetic approach directly supported the view that TNF-α plays an integral role in the development of murine pancreatitis.

Thalidomide

Dysregulation in immune response represent a major aspect of acute pancreatitis. Interactions of cellular and protein components with vascular endothelium contribute to the pathogenesis of the disease, resulting in changes in haemostatic balance, increased leukocyte adhesion, loss of barrier function, increased permeability, migration, proliferation and successive angiogenesis [152]. In particular, acute pancreatitis was associated with markedly positive immunostaining for VEGF (an endothelial cell-specific mitogen) and TGF-β (a cytokine involved in tissue repair and fibrogenesis) in acinar and ductal epithelial cells as well as in inflammatory infiltration cells and granulation tissue.

Thalidomide is an anti-inflammatory and immunomodulatory drug that, forty years after the withdrawal for its devastating teratogenic effects, is gaining popularity for cancer therapy and for treating autoimmune diseases [153]. It inhibits TNF-α production by enhancing TNF mRNA degradation [154], but also modulates the adhesiveness in microvascular beds (through the modification of surface cell adhesion molecules) [155] and suppresses the nuclear transcription factor NF-kB activity [156]. In addition, thalidomide was found to suppress angiogenesis possibly through the inhibition of endothelial cell proliferation [157].

To verify that thalidomide has beneficial therapeutic properties by interfering with the release of pro-inflammatory mediators, neutrophil infiltration and angiogenesis; we have investigated its effects on the development of cerulein-induced acute pancreatitis in mice.

Treatment of mice with thalidomide significantly reduced the histologic degree of pancreatic injury, edema ($p<0.01$), amylase and lipase plasma levels ($p<0.01$), intra-pancreatic and plasma levels of TNF-alpha and IL-1 ($p<0.01$), immunostaining for p-selectin and ICAM-1 ($p<0.01$), neutrophil accumulation ($p<0.01$), immunostaining for TGF-beta and VEGF ($p<0.01$), the degree of pancreatic apoptosis (assessed by TUNEL) and immunostaining for FasL and Bax ($p<0.01$) [158].

Therefore, thalidomide exerts beneficial effects on the development of acute pancreatitis induced by cerulein in mice. Our observations may help to clarify the therapeutic actions of thalidomide and the role of anti-TNF-α and immunomodulatory agents in acute pancreatitis.

Future Directions

Much effort has been spent to clarify the pathophysiology of TNF-α and develop a new medical treatment strategy for acute pancreatitis. Others and we showed that pre-clinical studies on TNF-α inhibition are promising, but a full extrapolation of experimental data has to be made with caution.

In the last decade, more than 2.000 papers on the treatment of experimental acute pancreatitis have been published, but only a few of the strategies tested have translated to clinical practice. Although animal models mimic some aspects of human pancreatitis, overall they may fail to reproduce accurately the disease and they are may not be completely predictive for the pathophysiology or treatment [159]. Moreover, in human pancreatitis the majority of organ failure occurs before initiation of treatment, and novel compounds, which attenuate the development of experimental pancreatitis, may be less effective when administered in humans several hours or days after the onset of disease [160].

TNF-α biology *in vivo* is complex. Although TNF-α neutralization attenuates the systemic inflammatory response, it does so at the cost of impairing innate antimicrobial defenses, especially against intracellular pathogens. Opportunistic infections and hepatotoxicity were reported [128]. Thus, anti TNF-α therapy could be even harmful in those conditions, such as sepsis, in which microbial growth contributes the disease pathogenesis. On the contrary, blocking TNF-α could be useful in conditions where microbial proliferation does not occur, and this is in accordance with the results obtained neutralizing TNF-α in experimental models of endotoxiemia [161]. Acute pancreatitis may represent a suitable disease for TNF-α antagonism, being - especially in the early phases - a condition in which the inflammatory response is not initiated and driven forward by an infection. However, three clinical trials of TNF-α inhibition in congestive heart failure were prematurely halted for lack of benefit or adverse outcomes (including increased mortality) [162,163]. In addition, meta-analyses of anti-TNF-α trials in patients with rheumatoid arthritis demonstrate a significant dose-dependent risk of infections and malignancies [164].

What are, then, the factors that may influence a future trial on anti-TNF-α therapy in pancreatitis? It seems critical that the temporal course of events such as changes in serum TNF-α levels is related to trial intervention [160]. On one hand, an early TNF-α neutralization could be able at least to decrease the cytokine burst and the induction of further cytokine production by inflammatory cells, but – as seen – in clinical settings it may not be easy to observe patients within one or two hours from the onset of the disease, when TNF-α peaks in the circulation. Therefore, a potential trial needs to record the time from onset of symptoms to intervention in addition to the more conventionally recorded delay between hospital admission and intervention. On the other hand, delayed intervention, mostly using TNF-α receptor constructs, has proven to be moderately effective in LPS challenging in human volunteers and septic shock, in a dose-dependent fashion [128]. Although delayed trials would interfere with a multi-systemic TNF-α secretion, it must be remembered that the TNF-α responsible for tissue injury may not be the free circulating form, but rather the cell-associated protein. Moreover, at this stage there is an activation of downstream events in different organs, and TNF-α over-production is only an aspect of that intricate cytokine network that characterizes host response in acute pancreatitis.

In conclusion, it should be kept in mind that experimental studies are of paramount importance and have dramatically improved our knowledge on the role of TNF-α in pancreatitis. However, pre-clinical studies may increase the apparent efficacy of TNF-α antagonism, generating unreasonable expectations as the strategy is translated to clinical settings. Finally, timing of antagonism and careful selection of inclusion and exclusion criteria may aid in better defining the optimal population in potential, future trials.

References

[1] Working Party of the British Society of Gastroenterology: Association of Surgeons of Great Britain and Ireland: Pancreatic Society of Great Britain and Ireland: Association of Upper GI Surgeons of Great Britain and Ireland. UK guidelines for the management of acute pancreatitis. *Gut*. 2005; 54 Suppl 3:iii1-9.

[2] Bradley EL 3rd. A clinically based classification system for acute pancreatitis. Summary of the International Symposium on Acute Pancreatitis, Atlanta, Ga, September 11 through 13, 1992. *Arch Surg*. 1993; 128:586-90.

[3] Granger J and Remick D. Acute pancreatitis: models, markers, and mediators. *Shock*. 2005; 24 Suppl 1:45-51.

[4] Bhatia M, Wong FL, Cao Y, Lau HY, Huang J, Puneet P, Chevali L. Pathophysiology of acute pancreatitis. *Pancreatology*. 2005; 5:132-144.

[5] Hirota M, Nozawa F, Okabe A, Shibata M, Beppu T, Shimada S, Egami H, Yamaguchi Y, Ikei S, Okajima T, Okamoto K, Ogawa M. Relationship between plasma cytokine concentration and multiple organ failure in patients with acute pancreatitis. *Pancreas*. 2000; 21:141-146.

[6] Schafer C, Tietz AB, Goke B: Pathophysiology of acute experimental pancreatitis: lessons from genetically engineered animal models and new molecular approaches. *Digestion*. 2005; 71:162-172.

[7] Oruc N, Ozutemiz O, Yukelsen V, Nart D, Celik HA, Yuce G and Batur Y. Infliximab: a new therapeutic agent in acute pancreatitis? *Pancreas*. 2004; 28:1-8.

[8] Hehlgans T, Pfeffer K. The intriguing biology of the tumour necrosis factor/tumour necrosis factor receptor superfamily: players, rules and the games. *Immunology*. 2005; 115:1-20.

[9] Idriss HT, Naismith JH. TNF alpha and the TNF receptor superfamily: structure-function relationship(s). *Microsc Res Tech*. 2000; 50:184-195.

[10] Peschon JJ, Slack JL, Reddy P, Stocking KL, Sunnarborg SW, Lee DC, Russell WE, Castner BJ, Johnson RS, Fitzner JN, Boyce RW, Nelson N, Kozlosky CJ, Wolfson MF, Rauch CT, Cerretti DP, Paxton RJ, March CJ, Black RA. An essential role for ectodomain shedding in mammalian development. *Science*. 1998; 282:1281-1284.

[11] Dempsey PW, Doyle SE, He JQ, Cheng G. The signaling adaptors and pathways activated by TNF superfamily. *Cytokine Growth Factor Rev*. 2003; 14:193-209.

[12] Bazzoni F, Beutler B. The tumor necrosis factor ligand and receptor families. *N. Engl. J. Med*. 1996; 334:1717-1725.

[13] Chinnaiyan AM, Tepper CG, Seldin MF, O'Rourke K, Kischkel FC, Hellbardt S, Krammer PH, Peter ME, Dixit VM. FADD/MORT1 is a common mediator of CD95 (Fas/APO-1) and tumor necrosis factor receptor-induced apoptosis. *J. Biol. Chem*. 1996; 271:4961-4965.

[14] Kischkel FC, Lawrence DA, Chuntharapai A, Schow P, Kim KJ, Ashkenazi A. Apo2L/TRAIL-dependent recruitment of endogenous FADD and caspase-8 to death receptors 4 and 5. *Immunity*. 2000; 12:611-620.

[15] Legler DF, Micheau O, Doucey MA, Tschopp J, Bron C. Recruitment of TNF receptor 1 to lipid rafts is essential for TNFalpha-mediated NF-kappaB activation. *Immunity.* 2003; 18:655-664.

[16] Stanger BZ, Leder P, Lee TH, Kim E, Seed B. RIP: a novel protein containing a death domain that interacts with Fas/APO-1 (CD95) in yeast and causes cell death. *Cell.* 1995; 81:513-523.

[17] Hsu H, Huang J, Shu HB, Baichwal V, Goeddel DV. TNF-dependent recruitment of the protein kinase RIP to the TNF receptor-1 signaling complex. *Immunity.* 1996; 4:387-396.

[18] Dong C, Davis RJ, Flavell RA. MAP kinases in the immune response. *Annu. Rev. Immunol.* 2002; 20:55-72.

[19] Tartaglia LA, Pennica D, Goeddel DV. Ligand passing: the 75-kDa tumor necrosis factor (TNF) receptor recruits TNF for signaling by the 55-kDa TNF receptor. *J Biol Chem.* 1993; 268:18542-18548.

[20] Peschon JJ, Torrance DS, Stocking KL, Glaccum MB, Otten C, Willis CR, Charrier K, Morrissey PJ, Ware CB, Mohler KM. TNF receptor-deficient mice reveal divergent roles for p55 and p75 in several models of inflammation. *J. Immunol.* 1998; 160:943-952.

[21] Norman JG, Fink GW, Franz MG. Acute pancreatitis induces intrapancreatic tumor necrosis factor gene expression. *Arch Surg.* 1995; 130:966-970.

[22] Gukovskaya AS, Gukovsky I, Zaninovic V, Song M, Sandoval D, Gukovsky S and Pandol SJ. Pancreatic acinar cells produce, release, and respond to tumor necrosis factor-alpha. Role in regulating cell death and pancreatitis. *J. Clin. Invest.* 1997; 100:1853-1862.

[23] Mayer JM. Shifting the focus from leukocyte to acinar cell: which is the more important mediator of pancreatic inflammation? *Crit. Care Med.* 2005; 33:248.

[24] De Dios I, Ramudo L, Alonso JR, Recio JS, Garcia-Montero AC, Manso MA. CD45 expression on rat acinar cells: involvement in pro-inflammatory cytokine production. *FEBS Lett.* 2005; 579:6355-6360.

[25] De Dios I, Ramudo L, Garcia-Montero A, Manso M: Redox-sensitive modulation of CD45 expression in pancreatic acinar cells during acute pancreatitis. *J. Pathol.* 2006; 210:234-239.

[26] Vaccaro MI, Ropolo A, Grasso D, Calvo EL, Ferreria M, Iovanna JL, Lanosa G. Pancreatic acinar cells submitted to stress activate TNF-alpha gene expression. *Biochem. Biophys. Res. Commun.* 2000; 268:485-90.

[27] Ramudo L, Manso MA, Sevillano S, de Dios I. Kinetic study of TNF-alpha production and its regulatory mechanisms in acinar cells during acute pancreatitis induced by bile-pancreatic duct obstruction. *J. Pathol.* 2005; 206:9-16.

[28] Ramudo L, Manso MA, Vicente S, De Dios I. Pro- and anti-inflammatory response of acinar cells during acute pancreatitis. Effect of N-acetylcysteine. *Cytokine.* 2005; 32:125-31.

[29] Ramudo L, Manso MA, De Dios I. Biliary pancreatitis-associated ascitic fluid activates the production of tumor necrosis factor-alpha in acinar cells. *Crit. Care Med.* 2005; 33:143-148.

[30] Virlos I, Mazzon E, Serraino I, Di Paola R, Genovese T, Britti D, Thiemerman C, Siriwardena AK, and Cuzzocrea S. Pyrrolidine dithiocarbamate reduces the severity of cerulein-induced murine acute pancreatitis. *Shock*. 2003; 20:544-550.

[31] Vona-Davis L, Yu A, Magabo K, Evans T, Jackson B, Riggs D, McFadden D. Peptide YY attenuates transcription factor activity in tumor necrosis factor-alpha-induced pancreatitis. *J. Am. Coll. Surg.* 2004; 199:87-95.

[32] Genovese T, Mazzon E, Di Paola R, Muià C, Crisafulli C, Malleo G and Cuzzocrea S. Role of endogenous Peroxisome Proliferators Activated Receptors alpha (PPAR-α) ligands in the development of acute pancreatitis induced by cerulein. *Immunology*. 2006; 118:559-570.

[33] Gukovsky I, Gukovskaya AS, Blinman TA, Zaninovic V, Pandol SJ. Early NF-kappaB activation is associated with hormone-induced pancreatitis. *Am. J. Physiol.* 1998; 275:1402-1414.

[34] Vaquero E, Gukovsky I, Zaninovic V, Gukovskaya AS, Pandol SJ. Localized pancreatic NF-kappaB activation and inflammatory response in taurocholate-induced pancreatitis. *Am. J. Physiol Gastrointest Liver Physiol.* 2001; 280:1197-1208.

[35] Steinle AU, Weidenbach H, Wagner M, Adler G, Schmid RM. NF-kappaB/Rel activation in cerulein pancreatitis. *Gastroenterology*. 1999; 116:420-430.

[36] Satoh A, Gukovskaya AS, Nieto JM, Cheng JH, Gukovsky I, Reeve JR Jr, Shimosegawa T, Pandol SJ. PKC-delta and -epsilon regulate NF-kappaB activation induced by cholecystokinin and TNF-alpha in pancreatic acinar cells. *Am. J. Physiol. Gastrointest Liver Physiol.* 2004; 287:582-591.

[37] Telek G, Scoazec JY, Chariot J, Ducroc R, Feldmann G, Roz C. Cerium-based histochemical demonstration of oxidative stress in taurocholate-induced acute pancreatitis in rats. A confocal laser scanning microscopic study. *J. Histochem. Cytochem.* 1999; 47:1201-1212.

[38] Sevillano S, de la Mano AM, Manso MA, Orfao A, De Dios I. N-acetylcysteine prevents intra-acinar oxygen free radical production in pancreatic duct obstruction-induced acute pancreatitis. *Biochim. Biophys Acta.* 2003 ;1639:177-184.

[39] Wulczyn FG, Krappmann D, Scheidereit C. The NF-kappa B/Rel and I kappa B gene families: mediators of immune response and inflammation. *J. Mol. Med.* 1996; 74:749-769.

[40] Siebenlist U, Franzoso G, Brown K. Structure, regulation and function of NF-kappa B. *Annu. Rev. Cell Biol.* 1994; 10:405-455.

[41] Virlos I, Mazzon E, Serraino I, Genovese T, Di Paola R, Thiemerman C, Siriwardena AK, Cuzzocrea S. Calpain I inhibitor ameliorates the indices of disease severity in a murine model of cerulein-induced acute pancreatitis. *Intensive Care Med.* 2004; 30:1645-1651.

[42] Letoha T, Somlai C, Takacs T, Szabolcs A, Rakonczay Z Jr, Jarmay K, Szalontai T, Varga I, Kaszaki J, Boros I, Duda E, Hackler L, Kurucz I, Penke B. The proteasome inhibitor MG132 protects against acute pancreatitis. *Free Radic Biol. Med.* 2005; 39:1142-1151.

[43] O'Reilly D, Roberts JR, Cartmell MT, Demaine AG, Kingsnorth AN. Heat shock factor-1 and nuclear factor-kappaB are systemically activated in human acute pancreatitis. *JOP*. 2006; 7:174-184.

[44] Balachandra S, Genovese T, Mazzon E, Di Paola R, Thiemerman C, Siriwardena AK, Cuzzocrea S. Inhibition of tyrosine-kinase-mediated cellular signaling by tyrphostins AG 126 and AG556 modulates murine experimental acute pancreatitis. *Surgery*. 2005; 138:913-923.

[45] Blinman TA, Gukovsky I, Mouria M, Zaninovic V, Livingston E, Pandol SJ, Gukovskaya AS. Activation of pancreatic acinar cells on isolation from tissue: cytokine upregulation via p38 MAP kinase. *Am. J. Physiol. Cell Physiol.* 2000; 279:1993-2003.

[46] Duan RD, Williams JA. Cholecystokinin rapidly activates mitogen-activated protein kinase in rat pancreatic acini. *Am. J. Physiol.* 1994; 267:401-408.

[47] Grady T, Dabrowski A, Williams JA, Logsdon CD. Stress-activated protein kinase activation is the earliest direct correlate to the induction of secretagogue-induced pancreatitis in rats. *Biochem. Biophys Res. Commun.* 1996; 227:1-7.

[48] Schafer C, Ross SE, Bragado MJ, Groblewski GE, Ernst SA, Williams JA. A role for the p38 mitogen-activated protein kinase/Hsp 27 pathway in cholecystokinin-induced changes in the actin cytoskeleton in rat pancreatic acini. *J Biol Chem.* 1998; 273:24173-24180.

[49] Minutoli L, Altavilla D, Marini H, Passaniti M, Bitto A, Seminara P, Venuti FS, Famulari C, Macri A, Versaci A, Squadrito F. Protective effects of SP600125 a new inhibitor of c-jun N-terminal kinase (JNK) and extracellular-regulated kinase (ERK1/2) in an experimental model of cerulein-induced pancreatitis. *Life Sci.* 2004; 75:2853-2866.

[50] Wagner AC, Mazzucchelli L, Miller M, Camoratto AM, Goke B. CEP-1347 inhibits caerulein-induced rat pancreatic JNK activation and ameliorates caerulein pancreatitis. *Am. J. Physiol. Gastrointest Liver Physiol.* 2000; 278:165-172.

[51] Kotlyarov A, Neininger A, Schubert C, Eckert R, Birchmeier C, Volk HD, Gaestel M. MAPKAP kinase 2 is essential for LPS-induced TNF-alpha biosynthesis. *Nat Cell Biol.* 1999; 1:94-97.

[52] Tietz AB, Malo A, Diebold J, Kotlyarov A, Herbst A, Kolligs FT, Brandt-Nedelev B, Halangk W, Gaestel M, Goke B, Schafer C. Gene deletion of MK2 inhibits TNF-alpha and IL-6 and protects against cerulein-induced pancreatitis. *Am. J. Physiol. Gastrointest. Liver Physiol.* 2006; 290:1298-1306.

[53] Neininger A, Kontoyiannis D, Kotlyarov A, Winzen R, Eckert R, Volk HD, Holtmann H, Kollias G, Gaestel M. MK2 targets AU-rich elements and regulates biosynthesis of tumor necrosis factor and interleukin-6 independently at different post-transcriptional levels. *J. Biol. Chem.* 2002; 277:3065-3068.

[54] Rousseau S, Morrice N, Peggie M, Campbell DG, Gaestel M, Cohen P. Inhibition of SAPK2a/p38 prevents hnRNP A0 phosphorylation by MAPKAP-K2 and its interaction with cytokine mRNAs. *EMBO J.* 2002; 21:6505-6514.

[55] Cuzzocrea S, Pisano B, Dugo L, Ianaro A, Britti D, Patel NS, Di Paola R, Genovese T, Di Rosa M, Caputi AP, Thiemermann C. Rosiglitazone, a ligand of the peroxisome

proliferator-activated receptor-gamma, reduces acute pancreatitis induced by cerulein. *Intensive Care Med.* 2004; 30:951-956.

[56] Moustakas A, Souchelnytskyi S, Heldin CH. Smad regulation in TGF-beta signal transduction. *J. Cell Sci.* 2001; 114:4359-4369.

[57] Robinson K, Vona-Davis L, Riggs D, Jackson B, McFadden D. Peptide YY attenuates STAT1 and STAT3 activation induced by TNF-alpha in acinar cell line AR42J. *J. Am. Coll. Surg.* 2006; 202:788-796.

[58] Ortiz EM, Dusetti NJ, Vasseur S, Malka D, Bodeker H, Dagorn JC, Iovanna JL.The pancreatitis-associated protein is induced by free radicals in AR4-2J cells and confers cell resistance to apoptosis. *Gastroenterology.* 1998; 114:808-816.

[59] Vasseur S, Folch-Puy E, Hlouschek V, Garcia S, Fiedler F, Lerch MM, Dagorn JC, Closa D, Iovanna JL. p8 improves pancreatic response to acute pancreatitis by enhancing the expression of the anti-inflammatory protein pancreatitis-associated protein I. *J. Biol. Chem.* 2004; 279:7199-7207.

[60] Folch-Puy E, Granell S, Dagorn JC, Iovanna JL, Closa D. Pancreatitis-associated protein I suppresses NF-kappa B activation through a JAK/STAT-mediated mechanism in epithelial cells. *J. Immunol.* 2006; 176:3774-3779.

[61] O'Konski MS, Pandol SJ. Cholecystokinin JMV-180 and caerulein effects on the pancreatic acinar cell cytoskeleton. *Pancreas.* 1993; 8:638-646.

[62] Muallem S, Kwiatkowska K, Xu X, Yin HL. Actin filament disassembly is a sufficient final trigger for exocytosis in nonexcitable cells. *J. Cell Biol.* 1995; 128:589-598.

[63] Schafer C, Clapp P, Welsh MJ, Benndorf R, Williams JA. HSP27 expression regulates CCK-induced changes of the actin cytoskeleton in CHO-CCK-A cells. *Am. J. Physiol.* 1999; 277:1032-43.

[64] Jungermann J, Lerch MM, Weidenbach H, Lutz MP, Kruger B, Adler G. Disassembly of rat pancreatic acinar cell cytoskeleton during supramaximal secretagogue stimulation. *Am. J. Physiol.* 1995; 268:328-338.

[65] Tashiro M, Schafer C, Yao H, Ernst SA, Williams JA. Arginine induced acute pancreatitis alters the actin cytoskeleton and increases heat shock protein expression in rat pancreatic acinar cells. *Gut.* 2001; 49:241-450.

[66] Tapia JA, Ferris HA, Jensen RT, Garcia LJ. Cholecystokinin activates PYK2/CAKbeta by a phospholipase C-dependent mechanism and its association with the mitogen-activated protein kinase signaling pathway in pancreatic acinar cells. *J. Biol. Chem.* 1999 ;274:31261-31271.

[67] Kubisch C, Dimagno MJ, Tietz AB, Welsh MJ, Ernst SA, Brandt-Nedelev B, Diebold J, Wagner AC, Goke B, Williams JA, Schafer C. Overexpression of heat shock protein Hsp27 protects against cerulein-induced pancreatitis. *Gastroenterology.* 2004; 127:275-286.

[68] Satoh A, Gukovskaya AS, Edderkaoui M, Daghighian MS, Reeve JR Jr, Shimosegawa T, Pandol SJ. Tumor necrosis factor-alpha mediates pancreatitis responses in acinar cells via protein kinase C and proline-rich tyrosine kinase 2. *Gastroenterology.* 2005; 129:639-651.

[69] Kaiser AM, Saluja AK, Sengupta A, Saluja M, Steer ML. Relationship between severity, necrosis, and apoptosis in five models of experimental acute pancreatitis. *Am. J. Physiol.* 1995; 269:1295-1304.

[70] Saluja A, Hofbauer B, Yamaguchi Y, Yamanaka K, Steer M. Induction of apoptosis reduces the severity of caerulein-induced pancreatitis in mice. *Biochem. Biophys. Res. Commun.* 1996; 220:875-878.

[71] Bhatia M, Wallig MA, Hofbauer B, Lee HS, Frossard JL, Steer ML, Saluja AK. Induction of apoptosis in pancreatic acinar cells reduces the severity of acute pancreatitis. *Biochem. Biophys. Res. Commun.* 1998; 246:476-483.

[72] Guzman EA, Rudnicki M. Intricacies of host response in acute pancreatitis. *J. Am. Coll. Surg.* 2006; 202:509-519.

[73] Gomez G, Lee HM, He Q, Englander EW, Uchida T, Greeley GH Jr.Acute pancreatitis signals activation of apoptosis-associated and survival genes in mice. *Exp. Biol. Med.* 2001; 226:692-700.

[74] Lemasters JJ. V. Necrapoptosis and the mitochondrial permeability transition: shared pathways to necrosis and apoptosis. *Am. J. Physiol.* 1999; 276:1-6.

[75] Mazzon E, Genovese T, Di Paola R, Muià C, Crisafull C, Malleo G, Esposito E, Meli R, Sessa E, Cuzzocrea S. Effects of 3-aminobenzamide, an inhibitor of poly (ADP-ribose) polymerase, in a mouse model of acute pancreatitis induced by cerulein. *Eur. J. Pharmacol.* 2006; 549:149-156.

[76] Yasuda H, Kataoka K, Ichimura H, Mitsuyoshi M, Iida T, Kita M, Imanishi J. Cytokine expression and induction of acinar cell apoptosis after pancreatic duct ligation in mice. *J. Interferon Cytokine Res.* 1999; 19:637-644.

[77] Gukovsky I, Reyes CN, Vaquero EC, Gukovskaya AS, Pandol SJ. Curcumin ameliorates ethanol and nonethanol experimental pancreatitis. *Am. J. Physiol. Gastrointest Liver Physiol.* 2003; 284:85-95.

[78] Gukovskaya AS, Pandol SJ. Cell death pathways in pancreatitis and pancreatic cancer. *Pancreatology.* 2004; 4:567-586.

[79] Aggarwal BB. Apoptosis and nuclear factor-kappa B: a tale of association and dissociation. *Biochem Pharmacol.* 2000; 60:1033-1039.

[80] Karin M, Lin A. NF-kappaB at the crossroads of life and death. *Nat. Immunol.* 2002; 3:221-227.

[81] Malka D, Vasseur S, Bodeker H, Ortiz EM, Dusetti NJ, Verrando P, Dagorn JC, Iovanna JL. Tumor necrosis factor alpha triggers antiapoptotic mechanisms in rat pancreatic cells through pancreatitis-associated protein I activation. *Gastroenterology.* 2000; 119:816-828.

[82] Holler N, Zaru R, Micheau O, Thome M, Attinger A, Valitutti S, Bodmer JL, Schneider P, Seed B, Tschopp J. Fas triggers an alternative, caspase-8-independent cell death pathway using the kinase RIP as effector molecule. *Nat. Immunol.* 2000; 1:489-495.

[83] Mareninova OA, Sung KF, Hong P, Lugea A, Pandol SJ, Gukovsky I, Gukovskaya AS. Cell death in pancreatitis: caspases protect from necrotizing pancreatitis. *J. Biol. Chem.* 2006; 281:3370-3381.

[84] Legler DF, Micheau O, Doucey MA, Tschopp J, Bron C. Recruitment of TNF receptor 1 to lipid rafts is essential for TNFalpha-mediated NF-kappaB activation. *Immunity.* 2003; 18:655-664.

[85] Genovese T, Mazzon E, Di Paola R, Muia C, Crisafulli C, Menegazzi M, Malleo G, Suzuki H, Cuzzocrea S. Hypericum perforatum attenuates the development of cerulein-induced acute pancreatitis in mice. *Shock.* 2006; 25:161-167.

[86] Zaninovic V, Gukovskaya AS, Gukovsky I, Mouria M, Pandol SJ. Cerulein upregulates ICAM-1 in pancreatic acinar cells, which mediates neutrophil adhesion to these cells. *Am. J. Physiol. Gastrointest Liver Physiol.* 2000; 279:666-676.

[87] Frossard JL, Saluja A, Hofbauer B, Lee HS, Bhatia M, Bhagat L, Steer ML. The role of intercellular adhesion molecule 1 and neutrophils in acute pancreatitis and pancreatitis-associated lung injury. *Gastroenterology.* 1999; 116:694-701.

[88] Telek G, Ducroc R, Scoazec JY, Pasquier C, Feldmann G, Roze C. Differential upregulation of cellular adhesion molecules at the sites of oxidative stress in experimental acute pancreatitis. *J. Surg Res.* 2001; 96:56-67.

[89] Kimura Y, Hirota M, Okabe A, Inoue K, Kuwata K, Ohmuraya M, Ogawa M. Dynamic aspects of granulocyte activation in rat severe acute pancreatitis. *Pancreas.* 2003; 27:127-132.

[90] de Dios I, Perez M, de La Mano A, Sevillano S, Orfao A, Ramudo L, Manso MA. Contribution of circulating leukocytes to cytokine production in pancreatic duct obstruction-induced acute pancreatitis in rats. *Cytokine.* 2002; 20:295-303.

[91] Lundberg AH, Granger DN, Russell J, Sabek O, Henry J, Gaber L, Kotb M, Gaber AO. Quantitative measurement of P- and E-selectin adhesion molecules in acute pancreatitis: correlation with distant organ injury. *Ann. Surg.* 2000; 231:213-222.

[92] Cuzzocrea S, Rossi A, Serraino I, Di Paola R, Dugo L, Genovese T, Britti D, Sciarra G, De Sarro A, Caputi AP, Sautebin L. 5-lipoxygenase knockout mice exhibit a resistance to acute pancreatitis induced by cerulein. *Immunology.* 2003; 110:120-130.

[93] Cuzzocrea S, Mazzon E, Dugo L, Serraino I, Centorrino T, Ciccolo A, Van de Loo FA, Britti D, Caputi AP, Thiemermann C. Inducible nitric oxide synthase-deficient mice exhibit resistance to the acute pancreatitis induced by cerulein. *Shock.* 2002; 17:416-422.

[94] Cuzzocrea S, Genovese T, Mazzon E, Di Paola R, Muia C, Britti D, Salvemini D. Reduction in the development of cerulein-induced acute pancreatitis by treatment with M40401, a new selective superoxide dismutase mimetic. *Shock.* 2004; 22:254-261.

[95] Mota RA, Sanchez-Bueno F, Saenz L, Hernandez-Espinosa D, Jimeno J, Tornel PL, Martinez-Torrano A, Ramirez P, Parrilla P, Yelamos J. Inhibition of poly(ADP-ribose) polymerase attenuates the severity of acute pancreatitis and associated lung injury. *Lab. Invest.* 2005; 85:1250-1262.

[96] Friedl HP, Till GO, Ryan US, Ward PA. Mediator-induced activation of xanthine oxidase in endothelial cells. *FASEB J.* 1989; 3:2512-2518.

[97] Kusske AM, Rongione AJ, Reber HA. Cytokines and acute pancreatitis. *Gastroenterology.* 1996; 110:639-642.

[98] de Beaux AC, Ross JA, Maingay JP, Fearon KC, Carter DC. Proinflammatory cytokine release by peripheral blood mononuclear cells from patients with acute pancreatitis. *Br J. Surg.* 1996; 83:1071-1075.

[99] McKay CJ, Gallagher G, Brooks B, Imrie CW, Baxter JN. Increased monocyte cytokine production in association with systemic complications in acute pancreatitis. *Br J. Surg.* 1996; 83:919-923.

[100] Jaffray C, Mendez C, Denham W, Carter G, Norman J. Specific pancreatic enzymes activate macrophages to produce tumor necrosis factor-alpha: role of nuclear factor kappa B and inhibitory kappa B proteins. *J. Gastrointest Surg.* 2000; 4:370-377.

[101] Geisler F, Algul H, Riemann M, Schmid RM. Questioning current concepts in acute pancreatitis: endotoxin contamination of porcine pancreatic elastase is responsible for experimental pancreatitis-associated distant organ failure. *J. Immunol.* 2005; 174:6431-6439.

[102] Matzinger P. The danger model: a renewed sense of self. *Science.* 2002; 296:301-305.

[103] Shy Y, Evans JE, Rock KL. Molecular identification of a danger signal that alerts the immune system to danger. *Nature.* 2003; 425:516-521.

[104] Bianchi ME. DAMPs, PAMPs and alarmins: all we need to know about danger. *J. Leukoc. Biol.* 2007; 81:1-5.

[105] Satoh A, Shimosegawa T, Masamune A, Fujita M, Koizumi M, Toyota T. Ascitic fluid of experimental severe acute pancreatitis modulates the function of peritoneal macrophages. *Pancreas.* 1999; 19:268-275.

[106] Lundberg AH, Eubanks JW 3rd, Henry J, Sabek O, Kotb M, Gaber L, Norby-Teglund A, Gaber AO. Trypsin stimulates production of cytokines from peritoneal macrophages in vitro and in vivo. *Pancreas.* 2000; 21:41-51.

[107] Takeyama Y, Nishikawa J, Ueda T, Hori Y, Yamamoto M, Kuroda Y. Involvement of peritoneal macrophage in the induction of cytotoxicity due to apoptosis in ascitic fluid associated with severe acute pancreatitis. *J. Surg Res.* 1999; 82:163-171.

[108] Mikami Y, Takeda K, Shibuya K, Qiu-Feng H, Shimamura H, Yamauchi J, Egawa S, Sunamura M, Yagi H, Endo Y, Matsuno S. Do peritoneal macrophages play an essential role in the progression of acute pancreatitis in rats? *Pancreas.* 2003; 27:253-260.

[109] Mikami Y, Takeda K, Shibuya K, Qiu-Feng H, Egawa S, Sunamura M, Matsuno S. Peritoneal inflammatory cells in acute pancreatitis: Relationship of infiltration dynamics and cytokine production with severity of illness. *Surgery.* 2002; 132:86-92.

[110] Yang J, Denham W, Carter G, Tracey KJ, Norman J. Macrophage pacification reduces rodent pancreatitis-induced hepatocellular injury through down-regulation of hepatic tumor necrosis factor alpha and interleukin-1beta. *Hepatology.* 1998; 28:1282-1288.

[111] Murr MM, Yang J, Fier A, Kaylor P, Mastorides S, Norman JG. Pancreatic elastase induces liver injury by activating cytokine production within Kupffer cells via nuclear factor-Kappa B. *J. Gastrointest. Surg.* 2002; 6:474-480.

[112] Jaffray C, Yang J, Norman J. Elastase mimics pancreatitis-induced hepatic injury via inflammatory mediators. *J. Surg. Res.* 2000; 90:95-101.

[113] Murr MM, Yang J, Fier A, Gallagher SF, Carter G, Gower WR Jr, Norman JG. Regulation of Kupffer cell TNF gene expression during experimental acute

pancreatitis: the role of p38-MAPK, ERK1/2, SAPK/JNK, and NF-kappaB. *J. Gastrointest. Surg.* 2003; 7:20-25.

[114] Yang J, Gallagher SF, Haines K, Epling-Burnette PK, Bai F, Gower WR Jr, Mastorides S, Norman JG, Murr MM. Kupffer cell-derived Fas ligand plays a role in liver injury and hepatocyte death. *J. Gastrointest. Surg.* 2004; 8:166-174.

[115] Gallagher SF, Yang J, Baksh K, Haines K, Carpenter H, Epling-Burnette PK, Peng Y, Norman J, Murr MM. Acute pancreatitis induces FasL gene expression and apoptosis in the liver. *J. Surg. Res.* 2004; 122:201-209.

[116] Gallagher SF, Peng Y, Haines K, Baksh K, Epling-Burnette PK, Yang J, Murr MM. Fas/FasL play a central role in pancreatitis-induced hepatocyte apoptosis. *J. Gastrointest. Surg.* 2005; 9:467-474.

[117] Peng Y, Gallagher SF, Haines K, Baksh K, Murr MM. Nuclear factor-kappaB mediates Kupffer cell apoptosis through transcriptional activation of Fas/FasL. *J Surg Res.* 2006; 130:58-65.

[118] Closa D, Sabater L, Fernandez-Cruz L, Prats N, Gelpi E, Rosello-Catafau J.Activation of alveolar macrophages in lung injury associated with experimental acute pancreatitis is mediated by the liver. *Ann. Surg.* 1999; 229:230-236.

[119] Bhatia M, Brady M, Zagorski J, Christmas SE, Campbell F, Neoptolemos JP, Slavin J. Treatment with neutralising antibody against cytokine induced neutrophil chemoattractant (CINC) protects rats against acute pancreatitis associated lung injury. *Gut.* 2000; 47:838-844.

[120] Denham W, Yang J, Wang H, Botchkina G, Tracey KJ, Norman J. Inhibition of p38 mitogen activate kinase attenuates the severity of pancreatitis-induced adult respiratory distress syndrome. *Crit. Care Med.* 2000; 28:2567-2572.

[121] Folch E, Prats N, Hotter G, Lopez S, Gelpi E, Rosello-Catafau J, Closa D. P-selectin expression and Kupffer cell activation in rat acute pancreatitis. *Dig. Dis. Sci.* 2000; 45:1535-1544.

[122] Gloor B, Blinman TA, Rigberg DA, Todd KE, Lane JS, Hines OJ, Reber HA. Kupffer cell blockade reduces hepatic and systemic cytokine levels and lung injury in hemorrhagic pancreatitis in rats. *Pancreas.* 2000; 21:414-420.

[123] Folch-Puy E, Garcia-Movtero A, Iovanna JL, Dagorn JC, Prats N, Vaccaro MI, Closa D. The pancreatitis-associated protein induces lung inflammation in the rat through activation of TNFalpha expression in hepatocytes. *J. Pathol.* 2003; 199:398-408.

[124] Lundberg AH, Granger N, Russell J, Callicutt S, Gaber LW, Kotb M, Sabek O, Gaber AO. Temporal correlation of tumor necrosis factor-alpha release, upregulation of pulmonary ICAM-1 and VCAM-1, neutrophil sequestration, and lung injury in diet-induced pancreatitis. *J. Gastrointest Surg.* 2000; 4:248-257.

[125] Berger HG, Rau B, Isenmann R, Schwarz M, Gansauge F, Poch B. Antibiotic prophylaxis in severe acute pancreatitis. *Pancreatology.* 2005; 5:10-19.

[126] Neoptolemos JP, Carr-Locke DL, London NJ, Bailey IA, James D, Fossard DP. Controlled trial of urgent endoscopic retrograde cholangiopancreatography and endoscopic sphincterotomy versus conservative treatment for acute pancreatitis due to gallstones. *Lancet.* 1988; 2:979-983.

[127] Malleo G, Mazzon E, Siriwardena AK, Cuzzocrea S. Role of tumor necrosis factor-alpha in acute pancreatitis: from biological basis to clinical evidence. *Shock*. 2007, *in press*.

[128] Lorente JA, Marshall JC. Neutralization of tumor necrosis factor in preclinical models of sepsis. *Shock*. 2005; 24:107-19.

[129] Abraham E, Wunderink R, Silverman H, Perl TM, Nasraway S, Levy H, Bone R, Wenzel RP, Balk R, Allred R, et al. Efficacy and safety of monoclonal antibody to human tumor necrosis factor alpha in patients with sepsis syndrome. A randomized, controlled, double-blind, multicenter clinical trial. TNF-alpha MAb Sepsis Study Group. *JAMA*. 1995; 273:934-941.

[130] Dhainaut JF, Vincent JL, Richard C, Lejeune P, Martin C, Fierobe L, Stephens S, Ney UM, Sopwith M. CDP571, a humanized antibody to human tumor necrosis factor-alpha: safety, pharmacokinetics, immune response, and influence of the antibody on cytokine concentrations in patients with septic shock. CPD571 Sepsis Study Group. *Crit. Care Med*. 1995; 23:1461-1469.

[131] Reinhart K, Wiegand-Lohnert C, Grimminger F, Kaul M, Withington S, Treacher D, Eckart J, Willatts S, Bouza C, Krausch D, Stockenhuber F, Eiselstein J, Daum L, Kempeni J. Assessment of the safety and efficacy of the monoclonal anti-tumor necrosis factor antibody-fragment, MAK 195F, in patients with sepsis and septic shock: a multicenter, randomized, placebo-controlled, dose-ranging study. *Crit. Care Med*. 1996; 24:733-742.

[132] Hirano T. Cytokine suppressive agent improves survival rate in rats with acute pancreatitis of closed duodenal loop. *J. Surg. Res*. 1999; 81:224-229.

[133] Denham W, Fink G, Yang J, Ulrich P, Tracey K, Norman J. Small molecule inhibition of tumor necrosis factor gene processing during acute pancreatitis prevents cytokine cascade progression and attenuates pancreatitis severity. *Am. Surg*. 1997; 63:1045-1049.

[134] Gomez-Cambronero L, Camps B, de La Asuncion JG, Cerda M, Pellin A, Pallardo FV, Calvete J, Sweiry JH, Mann GE, Vina J, Sastre J. Pentoxifylline ameliorates cerulein-induced pancreatitis in rats: role of glutathione and nitric oxide. *J Pharmacol Exp Ther*. 2000; 293:670-676.

[135] Marton J, Farkas G, Takacs T, Nagy Z, Szasz Z, Varga J, Jarmay K, Balogh A, Lonovics J. Beneficial effects of pentoxifylline treatment of experimental acute pancreatitis in rats. *Res. Exp. Med*. 1998; 197:293-299.

[136] Pereda J, Sabater L, Cassinello N, Gòmez-Cambronero L, Closa D, Folch-Puy E, Aparisi L, Calvete J, Cerdà M, Lledò S, Viña J and Sastre J. Effect of simultaneous inhibition of TNF- alpha production and xanthine oxidase in experimental acute pancreatitis: the role of mitogen activated protein kinases. *Ann. Surg*. 2004; 240:108-116.

[137] Grewal HP, Mohey el Din A, Gaber L, Kotb M, Gaber AO. Amelioration of the physiologic and biochemical changes of acute pancreatitis using an anti-TNF-alpha polyclonal antibody. *Am. J. Surg*. 1994; 167:214-218.

[138] Hughes CB, Gaber LW, Mohey el-Din AB, Grewal HP, Kotb M, Mann L, Gaber AO. Inhibition of TNF alpha improves survival in an experimental model of acute pancreatitis. *Am. Surg.* 1996;62(1):8-13.

[139] Hughes CB, Grewal HP, Gaber LW, Kotb M, Mohey el-Din AB, Mann L, Gaber AO. Anti-TNFalpha therapy improves survival and ameliorates the pathophysiologic sequelae in acute pancreatitis in the rat. *Am. J. Surg.* 1996; 171:274-280.

[140] Norman JG, Fink GW, Messina J, Carter G, Franz MG. Timing of tumor necrosis factor antagonism is critical in determining outcome in murine lethal acute pancreatitis. *Surgery.* 1996; 120:515-521.

[141] Denham W, Yang J, Fink G, Denham D, Carter G, Ward K, Norman J. Gene targeting demonstrates additive detrimental effects of interleukin 1 and tumor necrosis factor during pancreatitis. *Gastroenterology.* 1997; 113:1741-1476.

[142] Douni E, Kollias G. A critical role of the p75 tumor necrosis factor receptor (p75TNF-R) in organ inflammation independent of TNF, lymphotoxin alpha, or the p55TNF-R. *J. Exp. Med.* 1998; 188:1343-1352.

[143] Van Zee KJ, Kohno T, Fischer E, Rock CS, Moldawer LL, Lowry SF. Tumor necrosis factor soluble receptors circulate during experimental and clinical inflammation and can protect against excessive tumor necrosis factor alpha in vitro and in vivo. *Proc. Natl. Acad. Sci. USA.* 1992; 89:4845-4849.

[144] Yung RL. Etanercept Immunex. *Curr. Opin. Investig Drugs.* 2001; 2:216-221.

[145] Pugsley MK. Etanercept Immunex. *Curr Opin Investig Drugs.* 2001; 2:1725-1731.

[146] Moreland LW, Baumgartner SW, Schiff MH, Tindall EA, Fleischmann ER, Weaver AL, Ettlinger RE, Cohen S, Koopman WJ, Mohler K, Widmer MB, Blosch CM. Treatment of rheumatoid arthritis with a recombinant human tumor necrosis factor receptor (p75)-Fc fusion protein. *N. Engl. J. Med.* 1997; 337:141-147.

[147] Moreland LW, Schiff MH, Baumgartner SW, Tindall EA, Fleischmann ER, Bulpitt KJ, Weaver AL, Keystone EC, Furst DE, Mease PJ, Ruderman EM, Horwitz DA, Arkfeld DG, Garrison L, Burge DJ, Blosch CM, Lange ML, McDonnell ND, Weinblatt ME. Etanercept therapy in rheumatoid arthritis. A randomized, controlled trial. *Ann. Intern. Med.* 1999; 130:478-486.

[148] Gorman JD, Sack KE, Davis JC Jr. Treatment of ankylosing spondylitis by inhibition of tumor necrosis factor alpha. *N. Engl. J. Med.* 2002; 346:1349-1356.

[149] Mease PJ, Goffe BS, Metz J, Van der Stoep A, Finck B, Burge DJ .Etanercept in the treatment of psoriatic arthritis and psoriasis: a randomised trial. *Lancet.* 2000; 356:385-390.

[150] Papp KA, Tyring S, Lahfa M, Prinz J, Griffiths CE, Nakanishi AM, Zitnik R, van de Kerkhof PC, Melvin L; Etanercept Psoriasis Study Group .A global phase III randomized controlled trial of etanercept in psoriasis: safety, efficacy, and effect of dose reduction. *Br. J. Dermatol.* 2005; 152:1304-1312.

[151] Malleo G, Mazzon E, Genovese T, Di Paola R, Muià C, Centorrino T, Siriwardena AK, Cuzzocrea S: Etanercept attenuates the development of cerulein-induced acute pancreatitis in mice. A comparison with TNF-α genetic deletion. *Shock.* 2007; in press.

[152] Kadl A, Leitinger N: The role of endothelial cells in the resolution of acute inflammation. *Antioxid Redox. Signal.* 2005; 7:1744-1754.

[153] Laffitte E, Reviz J: Thalidomide: and old drug with new clinical applications. *Expert Opin. Drug Saf.* 2004; 3:47-56.

[154] Moreira AL, Sampaio EP, Zmuidzinas A, Frindt P, Smith KA, Kaplan G: Thalidomide exerts its inhibitory actions on tumor necrosis factor α by enhancing mRNA degradation. *J. Exp. Med.* 1993; 177:1675-1680.

[155] Yasui K, Kobayashi N, Yamazaki T, Agematsu K: Thalidomide as an immunotherapeutic agent: the effects on neutrophil-mediated inflammation. *Curr. Pharm. Des.* 2005; 11:395-401.

[156] Keifer JA, Guttridge DC, Ashburner BP, Baldwin AS Jr: Inhibition of NF-kappa B activity by thalidomide through suppression of IkappaB kinase activity. *J. Biol. Chem.* 2001; 276:22382-22387.

[157] Raje N, Anderson KC: Thalidomide and immunomodulatory drugs as cancer therapy. *Curr. Opin. Oncol.* 2002; 14:635-640.

[158] Malleo G, Mazzon E, Genovese, Di Paola, Muià C, Crisafulli C, Siriwardena AK, Cuzzocrea S. Effects of thalidomide in a mouse model of cerulein-induced acute pancreatitis. *Shock.* 2007; in press.

[159] Malleo G, Shah KJ, Siriwardena AK. In: *Association of Surgeons in training (Thirtieth Anniversary) Yearbook.* pp 84-86, 2006.

[160] Mason J, Siriwardena AK. Designing future clinical trials in acute pancreatitis. *Pancreatology.* 2005; 5:113-115.

[161] Jin H, Yang R, Marsters SA, Bunting SA, Wurm FM, Chamow SM, Ashkenazi A. Protection against rat endotoxic shock by p55 tumor necrosis factor (TNF) receptor immunoadhesin: comparison with anti-TNF monoclonal antibody. *J. Infect. Dis.* 1994; 170:1323-1326.

[162] Mann DL, McMurray JJ, Packer M, Swedberg K, Borer JS, Colucci WS, Djian J, Drexler H, Feldman A, Kober L, Krum H, Liu P, Nieminen M, Tavazzi L, van Veldhuisen DJ, Waldenstrom A, Warren M, Westheim A, Zannad F, Fleming T. Targeted anticytokine therapy in patients with chronic heart failure: results of the Randomized Etanercept Worldwide Evaluation (RENEWAL). *Circulation.* 2004; 109:1594-1602.

[163] Chung ES, Packer M, Lo KH, Fasanmade AA, Willerson JT; Anti-TNF Therapy Against Congestive Heart Failure Investigators. Randomized, double-blind, placebo-controlled, pilot trial of infliximab, a chimeric monoclonal antibody to tumor necrosis factor-alpha, in patients with moderate-to-severe heart failure: results of the anti-TNF Therapy Against Congestive Heart Failure (ATTACH) trial. *Circulation.* 2003; 107:3133-3140.

[164] Bongartz T, Sutton AJ, Sweeting MJ, Buchan I, Matteson EL, Montori V. Anti-TNF antibody therapy in rheumatoid arthritis and the risk of serious infections and malignancies: systematic review and meta-analysis of rare harmful effects in randomized controlled trials. *JAMA.* 2006; 295:2275-2285.

In: Pancreatitis Research Advances
Editor: William C. Langley, pp. 179-199

ISBN: 978-1-60021-883-5

Chapter V

Prevention of Life-Threatening Complications in Severe Acute Pancreatitis: Results of Our Research

Takeo Yasuda[*,1], *Takashi Ueda*[1], *Yoshifumi Takeyama*[2], *Makoto Shinzeki*[1], *Hidehiro Sawa*[1], *Takahiro Nakajima*[1] *and Yoshikazu Kuroda*[1]

[1] Department of Gastroenterological Surgery,
Kobe University Graduate School of Medical Sciences,
Kobe 650-0017, Japan

[2] Department of Surgery, Kinki University School of Medicine,
Osaka-sayama 589-8511, Japan

Abstract

In severe acute pancreatitis (SAP), multiple organ dysfunction syndrome (MODS) in the early phase and infectious complications in the late phase are contributors to high mortality. MODS is a consequence of the systemic inflammatory response syndrome, and infectious complication is thought to be a result of bacterial translocation from the gastrointestinal tract. We are researching these two major complications. Here we introduce our results.

Introduction

Despite recent advances of diagnosis and treatment modalities, the mortality rate in severe acute pancreatitis (SAP) is still high [1]. Multiple organ dysfunction syndrome

[*] Correspondence to: Takeo Yasuda, Department of Gastroenterological Surgery, Kobe University Graduate School of Medical Sciences, 7-5-2 Kusunoki-cho, Chuo-ku, Kobe 650-0017, Japan. Telephone: +81-78-382-5925. Facsimile: +81-78-382-5939. E-mail: yasudatk@med.kobe-u.ac.jp

(MODS) in the early phase [2, 3] and infectious complications (infected pancreatic necrosis and sepsis) in the late phase [4-7] are contributors to high mortality in this disease. MODS is a consequence of the systemic inflammatory response syndrome (SIRS), and it is conceivable that release of humoral mediators from the excessive activated macrophages/monocytes and neutrophils may lead to the remote organ injury. Infectious complication is thought to be a result of bacterial translocation (BT) from the gastrointestinal tract, and breakdown of intestinal integrity is considered to be implicated in the mechanism [8-12]. We are researching the mechanism of these two major complications. Here we review the literature and introduce our research results.

1. Investigation of Early Phase Complications

A. Participation of Apoptosis in Multiple Organ Dysfunction Syndrome

Abstract

Apoptosis occurred in the renal tubular cells and hepatocytes, and was involved in organ dysfunction with experimental SAP. Inhibition of apoptosis improved organ injury in some experimental models. Pancreatitis-associated ascitic fluid (PAAF) contains apoptosis-inducing factor, and PAAF increases intracellular Na^+ and Ca^{2+} concentration on hepatocytes. Transforming growth factor-β and hematin in PAAF are two major factors for hepatocellular injury.

Apoptosis was initially recognized as "programmed cell death", a type of cell death distinct from necrosis, which eliminates excessive or unwanted cells in the course of organ development. Recently, apoptosis has been shown to be involved in cellular injury associated with many pathological conditions such as inflammatory diseases. Moreover, it has been reported that many cytokines (e.g., interleukin (IL)-1β, tumor necrosis factor (TNF)-α, and transforming growth factor (TGF)-β) and free radicals (e.g., nitric oxide) induce apoptotic cell death in various cell systems. Similarly, SAP is considered to be a typical pathological condition complicating a systemic inflammatory response with a "cytokine storm" [13]. Therefore, it is conceivable that apoptosis is involved in the systemic manifestations (remote organ injuries) of SAP. We first disclosed that pancreatitis-associated ascitic fluid (PAAF) had the ability to induce apoptotic cell death in Madin-Darby canine kidney (MDCK) cells in 1995 [14]. Next, we demonstrated in 1998 that thymic atrophy was caused by thymocyte apoptosis in rat experimental SAP [15], and thereafter we successively disclosed the participation of apoptosis in systemic complications with SAP. In this chapter, we mainly introduce our research results about the significance of apoptosis in MODS.

Pancreas

Concerning apoptosis in the pancreas itself, Kaiser et al. found that the severity of acute pancreatitis was inversely related to the degree of apoptosis, suggesting that apoptosis might be a beneficial response to acinar cell injury in acute pancreatitis [16]. This observation led to the next data that the severity of pancreatitis was significantly reduced by prior induction of apoptosis [17, 18]. Hahm et al. also reported the same finding [19], indicating that apoptosis could be a favorable response to acinar cells and that induction of apoptotic acinar cell death might reduce the severity of acute pancreatitis.

Kidney

In clinical SAP, acute renal failure occurs within a few days from the onset in spite of satisfactory resuscitation, and sometimes it becomes lethal [20]. Some investigators reported that renal failure was simply due to hypovolemia (renal hypoperfusion) [21], but others said that PAAF from a canine SAP model caused acute renal failure suggesting that PAAF contained nephrotoxic substances [22]. We first demonstrated that PAAF contained the substances inducing apoptotic cell death in MDCK cells, an established cell line from canine renal tubular epithelium [14].

Subsequently, we first disclosed that apoptosis was detected on the renal tubules 6 hours after induction of rat SAP, and that similar tubular apoptosis was induced by the injection of PAAF into the peritoneal cavities of healthy rats [23]. Moreover, we found that the PAAF induced apoptosis on the isolated renal tubules and normal rat kidney cells (NRK52E cells) and that anti-TNF-α neutralizing antibody did not affect the apoptosis-inducing activity of the PAAF. These observations suggest that renal cell injury by apoptosis is involved in renal failure in the early stage of SAP and that PAAF contained the apoptosis-inducing factor.

Liver

The liver has an important role in the systemic response to critical illness, and progressive liver dysfunction may lead to the failure of other organs such as the lung and kidney. Apoptosis of hepatocytes was reported to be involved in liver failure complicated with systemic manifestations such as endotoxemia [24]. Next to renal tubular cell apoptosis, we showed that apoptosis was detected in hepatocytes in the rats both with SAP and with the intraperitoneal injection of PAAF, and that apoptotic cell injury and hepatic dysfunction were ameliorated by administration of IL-1β-converting enzyme inhibitor [25]. Furthermore, we clarified that the PAAF exhibited cytocidal activity in rat primary hepatocyte culture via apoptosis, and that anti-TGF-β neutralizing antibody partially blocked the apoptosis. These results suggest that apoptotic cell injury of hepatocytes is possibly involved in the mechanism of hepatic failure.

In the next study, we demonstrated that strong expression of TGF-β1 was detected in the liver and the peritoneal macrophages in the course of SAP, and that TGF-β1 levels were also elevated in plasma, in PAAF, and in the liver homogenate [26]. Moreover, the macrophage depletion partially inhibited the elevation of TGF-β1 protein levels, hepatocyte apoptosis, and the serum alanine aminotransferase (ALT) elevation. These results indicate that macrophages are responsible for hepatocellular injury in SAP by means of apoptosis, and that macrophage-derived TGF-β1 is one of the major factors inducing the hepatocyte apoptosis.

Thereafter, we demonstrated that hematin (hem oxidative) is one of the cytotoxic (apoptosis-inducing) factors in PAAF that causes hepatocellular injury [27]. PAAF contained a lot of hematin, and intraperitoneal injection of hematin into healthy rats caused hepatocyte apoptosis and the elevation of serum aspartate aminotransferase (AST) and lactate dehydrogenase (LDH) levels. In vitro, hematin decreased hepatocyte viability and increased hepatocyte apoptosis, similar to the effects of PAAF. Fractionation of PAAF and hematin by gel column chromatography revealed that the first peak of cytotoxic activity of PAAF corresponded to that of hematin, which is responsible for about 30% of the cytotoxic activity of PAAF. We speculate that the second peak of cytotoxic activity of PAAF includes TGF-β1 (responsible for about 30-50% of the activity) and other unknown components (responsible for about 20-40% of the activity).

Lung

During SAP, the respiratory dysfunction occurred ranging from mild hypoxia to an adult respiratory distress syndrome (ARDS)-like pulmonary injury, which needs respiratory support. Concerning the lung apoptosis in SAP, Wang et al. first reported in 1998 [28]. In this report, they found the apoptosis in type II pneumocytes 12 hours and 24 hours after the onset in rat SAP, confirmed dysfunction of the pulmonary endothelial barrier, and assumed the involvement of TNF. Subsequently, Yuan et al. demonstrated that apoptosis was induced in alveolar epithelial cells 5 hours after the induction of SAP in rat [29]. Their results suggest that apoptosis of alveolar epithelial cells may be involved in pancreatitis-associated lung injury, and that the mechanism of apoptosis probably correlates with the expression of apoptosis-regulated gene bax and p53 but is not related with the expression of TGFβ-1.

Significance of PAAF

During SAP, increasing permeability of vascular epithelial cells resulted huge ascitic fluid and pleural effusion. PAAF has been shown to play an important role in the progression of SAP. Frey et al. showed that the PAAF from canine SAP had a lethal effect on the rats when administered into their abdominal cavity [30]. Coticchia et al. demonstrated that clinical PAAF blocked the respiration of the liver mitochondria isolated from rats in vitro [31]. Bielecki et al. showed the same effect of PAAF in both canine model and human cases [32]. Satake et al. reported that PAAF from canine SAP caused acute renal failure [22]. As described above, we demonstrated that PAAF had apoptosis-inducing activity in renal tubules and hepatocytes in vitro and in vivo [14, 23, 25]. In this field, we further clarified several findings about the effects of PAAF and the involvement of PAAF-induced cellular injury in the mechanism of organ failure.

In 1999, we identified the importance of peritoneal macrophages as a source of apoptosis-inducing factors in PAAF. We demonstrated that peritoneal macrophage depletion by peritoneal lavage deleted apoptosis-inducing activity in PAAF collected from rats with SAP, suggesting that peritoneal macrophages secreted apoptosis-inducing factors into PAAF [33]. Subsequently, we disclosed that macrophage-derived TGF-β1 and hematin were two major apoptosis-inducing factors in PAAF that caused hepatocellular injury [26, 27]. We also demonstrated that PAAF increased the cellular activity of caspase-3, key enzyme in the signaling pathway of apoptosis, in MDCK cells [34].

On the other hand, in vivo rat liver NMR spectroscopy revealed that SAP caused severe hepatocellular acidosis, profound intracellular sodium accumulation, and bioenergy (ATP) depletion early in the course, and that these effects were as severe as those induced by total liver ischemia [35]. Furthermore, intraperitoneal injection of PAAF into healthy rats also induced severe hepatocellular acidosis, rapid accumulation of hepatic intracellular sodium, impaired hepatic cytosolic phosphorylation potential, and increased hepatic utilization of

ATP [36]. These effects may account for the eventual development of liver dysfunction associated with SAP.

In the next study, we investigated the effect of PAAF on hepatocytes intracellular Ca^{2+} concentration ($[Ca^{2+}]_i$) [37]. We demonstrated that $[Ca^{2+}]_i$ increased from 1 minute after the addition of PAAF, and that the fraction of PAAF with molecular weight $\geq 5 \times 10^4$ possessed both $[Ca^{2+}]_i$ elevation activity and cytotoxic activity. Platelet-activating factor antagonist blocked the PAAF-elicited $[Ca^{2+}]_i$ elevation. These results suggest that the dramatic elevation of hepatocyte $[Ca^{2+}]_i$ due to PAAF may be closely related to the hepatocellular injury in SAP and that platelet-activating factor may play a pivotal role in increasing hepatocyte $[Ca^{2+}]_i$. PAAF also increased $[Ca^{2+}]_i$ on MDCK cells in a dose-dependent manner, suggesting that elevation of $[Ca^{2+}]_i$ in various cells may be involved in the mechanism of MODS in SAP.

Norman and colleagues found multiple pathways for PAAF-induced apoptosis in hepatocytes. They identified the existence of heat-stable factors in PAAF that elicited apoptosis in cultured hepatocytes [38], and they found that PAAF induced liver injury and hepatocyte apoptosis by activating p38-MAPK and caspase-3 dependent pro-apoptotic pathways [39].

B. Mediators Involved in Inflammation and Organ Injury

Abstract

Blood levels of hepatocytes growth factor (HGF), vascular endothelial growth factor (VEGF), high-mobility group box chromosomal protein 1 (HMGB1), and tissue factor were significantly elevated in patients with SAP, and had correlation with disease severity. This shows some possibility of new therapeutic approach. For example, blockade of HMGB1, and supply of HGF and VEGF improved organ injury in experimental models.

Hepatocyte Growth Factor (HGF)

Hepatocyte growth factor (HGF) is a potent mitogen for parenchymal liver cells and functions as a hepatotrophic factor for liver regeneration after hepatic injury. Furthermore, HGF is found to target a wide variety of cells and act as a mitogen, motogen, morphogen, and tumor suppressor. Thus HGF is now considered to be a cytokine that plays multifunctional and critical roles in tissue repair and organogenesis. We first demonstrated that serum HGF levels on admission were elevated in patients with acute pancreatitis and that serum HGF levels were significantly higher in patients with SAP, in patients with organ dysfunction, and in the non-survivors [40]. Therefore, it is conceivable that serum human HGF levels may reflect the severity, organ dysfunction, and prognosis in acute pancreatitis.

In the following study, we compared the clinical utility of HGF for the detection of SAP and for predicting prognosis, infection, and organ dysfunction during the clinical course of acute pancreatitis with the clinical utility of C-reactive protein (CRP) and IL-6. HGF was more useful than CRP or interleukin IL-6 for predicting prognosis, renal dysfunction, and respiratory dysfunction, suggesting that serum HGF levels on admission may be a useful clinical parameter for determining the prognosis of acute pancreatitis and that HGF may be closely related to the organ dysfunction of acute pancreatitis [41].

Then, we clarified the role of HGF in rat experimental SAP [34]. Plasma HGF levels were elevated in rat SAP, and the degree of elevation was correlated with the severity and the organ dysfunctions. In rats SAP, HGF protein and mRNA levels significantly increased in the liver, kidney, and lung, which were injured organs. When anti-HGF neutralizing antibody was administered, liver dysfunction worsened, and apoptotic cells increased in the kidney. Recombinant HGF inhibited the cytocidal activity of PAAF on MDCK cells, and prevented the caspase-3 activation and apoptotic cell death induced by PAAF. These results suggest that HGF is produced in injured organs and may function as an organotrophic and anti-apoptotic factor against the organ injuries in SAP.

Vascular Endothelial Growth Factor (VEGF)

Vascular endothelial growth factor (VEGF), also known as vascular permeability factor, is a heparin-binding glycoprotein with potent angiogenic, mitogenic and vascular permeability-enhancing activities specific for endothelial cells. VEGF can also stimulate cell migration and inhibit apoptosis. VEGF has been suggested to be important mediators for inflammation and during normal and pathological angiogenesis. We determined serum VEGF concentrations in patients with SAP and investigated the effects of VEGF in experimental SAP [42].

Serum VEGF levels were significantly elevated in patients with SAP, but were not related to severity or prognosis. Serum VEGF levels with organ dysfunction (liver and kidney) were higher than those without organ dysfunction. In rat SAP, serum VEGF levels were significantly elevated. Recombinant VEGF did not affect the lung water content, volume of ascitic fluid, hematocrit, or serum amylase, but improved hepatic and renal dysfunctions. Apoptosis of liver and kidney was significantly inhibited by the administration of VEGF. These results suggest that VEGF is closely related to organ dysfunction in SAP, and that VEGF may function as not a vascular permeability factor, but a protective factor via the anti-apoptotic effect against organ injuries. In the following study, we recently found that VEGF inhibits intestinal epithelial cell apoptosis and following BT in rat SAP as described below [43].

High-Mobility Group Box Chromosomal Protein 1 (HMGB1)

High mobility group box chromosomal protein 1 (HMGB1), originally discovered 30 years ago as a nuclear DNA binding protein, was recently identified as a late-acting mediator of endotoxin lethality. Injection of HMGB1 itself was lethal, and serum levels of HMGB1 increased after the administration of endotoxin. Antibodies to HMGB1 attenuated mortality associated with endotoxemia. HMGB1 was also found to have the capacity to induce cytokines and activate inflammatory cells when it was applied extracellularly, implicating HMGB1 as a proinflammatory mediator. We first demonstrated that serum HMGB1 levels were significantly elevated in patients with SAP and were significantly positively correlated with the Japanese severity score and Glasgow score [44]. The HMGB1 levels were higher in patients with organ dysfunction and infection during the clinical course and in non-survivors. These results suggest that HMGB1 may act as a key mediator for inflammation and organ failure in SAP.

Subsequently, we also disclosed the participation of HMGB1 in rat and mouse SAP models. Serum HMGB1 levels were increased in rat SAP and were correlated with the disease severity [45]. The expressions of HMGB1 protein in the pancreas, liver, kidney, lung, and small intestine were increased maximally 6, 12, 12, 18, and 12 hours after the induction of SAP, respectively. In mice SAP, anti-HMGB1 neutralizing antibody significantly improved the elevation of serum amylase level and the histological alterations of the pancreas and lung [46]. Anti-HMGB1 antibody also significantly ameliorated the elevations of serum ALT and creatinine. Therefore, blockade of HMGB1 attenuated the development of SAP and associated organ dysfunction, indicating that HMGB1 acted as a key mediator for inflammatory response and organ injury in SAP.

Tissue Factor (TF)

Coagulative disorders are known to occur in SAP, and they are related to its severity and organ dysfunctions. Serious complications such as MODS and disseminated intravascular coagulation result from microcirculatory disturbances and microvascular thrombosis, which are caused by vascular endothelial cell injuries and hypercoagulation. Tissue factor (TF) is a transmembrane glycoprotein that activates the extrinsic pathway of the blood coagulation cascade. Monocytes/macrophages and endothelial cells can be stimulated to express TF transiently by inflammatory and immunological reactions. Plasma TF levels increase in patients with sepsis and acute coronary syndrome. We first demonstrated that plasma TF levels significantly increased in patients with SAP [47]. Plasma TF level in alcoholic SAP with pancreatic necrosis was significantly higher than that in alcoholic SAP without pancreatic necrosis and non-alcoholic SAP with pancreatic necrosis, respectively. Incidence of abnormal high value was 64% in alcoholic SAP with pancreatic necrosis. Utility of plasma TF for detection of pancreatic necrosis in alcoholic SAP was superior to those of Japanese severity score and LDH. These results suggest that TF may be closely related to the development of pancreatic necrosis in alcoholic SAP and that plasma TF level may be a useful marker for it.

Simple Prognostic Score in Clinical SAP

In human SAP, it is important clinically to predict the prognosis at the time of admission. Various biochemical parameters were evaluated for the assessment of severity and prognosis of acute pancreatitis, but there were few useful markers as a single parameter. For this reason, it is now accepted widely that scoring systems such as Ranson score [48], Glasgow score [49], and APACHE II score [50] are reliable severity indexes. In Japan, Japanese severity score (JSS) is used generally [51]. We clarified many markers for the evaluation of severity and the prediction of prognosis as mentioned above, but they were insufficient to replace these conventional scoring systems independently. However, these scoring systems consist of multiple factors and they are complicated. Thus, we recently proposed a simple scoring system for the prediction of the prognosis of SAP [52]. We evaluated prognostic factors by receiver operator characteristic (ROC) curve analyses and multivariate analysis from data that were obtained on admission of 137 patients with SAP in our department, and determined 3 most useful factors. Three prognostic factors were blood urea nitrogen (BUN) $\geq$25 mg/dL, LDH $\geq$900 IU/L, and dynamic contrast-enhanced computed tomography (CE-CT) finding with pancreatic necrosis. On admission, 137 patients were classified from 0 to 3 by the number of positive items (simple prognostic score [SPS]). Mortality rates for patients whose SPS was 0, 1, 2, and 3 were 2%, 18%, 48%, and 67%, respectively. Furthermore, when usefulness of SPS was compared with conventional scoring systems, the area under the curve by ROC curve analyses in SPS was 0.83; Ranson score was 0.83; JSS was 0.83; APACHE II score was 0.81, and Glasgow score was 0.75. This scoring system that comprised 3 items is simple, is feasible for the prediction of prognosis as equally as conventional scoring systems, and is useful for the selection of the extremely severe patients with SAP on admission.

2. Investigation of Late Phase Complications

A. Bacterial and Endotoxin Translocation during Severe Acute Pancreatitis

Abstract

The mechanism of bacterial translocation (BT) is not well known. From our experimental data, apoptosis in gut epithelial cells is implicated in BT. Breakdown of intestinal mucosa via accelerated apoptosis increased intestinal permeability, and caused BT and endotoxemia. Maintenance of gut integrity by caspase inhibitor, oxygenated perfluorochemical, and VEGF significantly improved the increase of apoptosis and permeability, and thereby reduced BT or endotoxemia.

Sepsis resulting from infected pancreatic necrosis is the most serious complication in the late phase of SAP [4-7]. Infected pancreatic necrosis occurs commonly more than 2-3 weeks after admission. Patients with infected necrosis had more organ failures and higher mortality rate compared with those with sterile necrosis. Thus, conquest of infection is a prime problem in the treatment strategy. This complication is thought to be a result of the bacterial translocation (BT) and endotoxin translocation from the gastrointestinal tract [8-12]. Breakdown of gut barrier integrity, systemic and local immunosuppression since early phase, and bacterial overgrowth due to the decrease of gut motility are postulated as important factors in such translocation. Especially, disruption of intestinal mucosal integrity, accompanied by increase in permeability, is believed to play a pivotal role in the mechanism of BT [53-57].

Intestinal Epithelial Apoptosis and Intestinal Permeability

It is suggested that increase in intestinal permeability is correlated with the changes of tight junction and/or apoptosis in intestinal epithelial cells. So, we investigated the changes of intestinal mucosa and its permeability in SAP [58]. Permeability of ileum was significantly increased 6 hours after induction of rat SAP. Blood endotoxin level was significantly elevated and BT occurred 18 hours after induction of SAP. Six hours after induction of SAP, expressions of tight junction proteins (ZO-1 and Occludin) were not altered, but apoptosis of ileum mucosa was significantly accelerated. Addition of PAAF to T84 cells (an intestinal cell line) did not affect expressions of ZO-1 or Occludin, but significantly increased the apoptosis and significantly decreased the transepithelial electric resistance (integrity of monolayer cells). These results suggest that breakdown of intestinal mucosa via accelerated apoptosis may increase in intestinal permeability in SAP and that PAAF contains factor(s) which accelerates the apoptosis of intestinal epithelial cells. Wang et al. also demonstrated that apoptosis was accelerated on ileal intestinal epithelial cells in rat with necrotizing pancreatitis, and that growth hormone down-regulated the excessive apoptosis, maintained the integrity of intestinal mucosal barrier, and reduced BT [59, 60].

Effect of Caspase Inhibitor

It is believed that cascade of caspase activation plays central roles in the signaling pathway of apoptosis. There are two major signal transduction pathways in caspase-dependent apoptosis: death receptor pathway (e.g., Fas, TNF-α) and mitochondrial (intrinsic) pathway. Caspase-10 is an initiator in death receptor pathway. Caspase-9 is an initiator in mitochondrial pathway. Caspase-3 is an effector in both pathway s . In the following study, first, to clarify the molecular mechanism of the intestinal epithelial cell apoptosis in SAP, involvement of caspases was examined. Since we found caspases (caspase-10, -9, and –3) activation in the intestinal epithelial cells in the early phase (2 hours after induction) of rat SAP, effects of polycaspase inhibitor on intestinal integrity (apoptosis, permeability, and villous height) and endotoxin/bacterial translocation in SAP were investigated [61]. Polycaspase inhibitor (Z-VAD-fmk) significantly improved the increasing apoptosis and permeability. Caspase inhibitor did not prevent BT, but improved the disorder of intestinal mucosa (villous height) and elevation of blood endotoxin 18 hours after induction of SAP. Moreover, caspase inhibitor significantly improved the 24-hour mortality rate. Z-VAD-fmk indeed inhibited the caspase-3 activation in intestinal mucosa of SAP. These results suggest that caspase activation makes a key role in accelerated apoptosis of intestinal epithelial cells in SAP and that breakdown of intestinal mucosa via accelerated apoptosis causes the increase of intestinal permeability and following endotoxin translocation in SAP.

Effect of Oxygenated Perfluorochemical

Ischemic changes and microcirculatory disturbances of the gut also have been reported to play important roles for the development of BT in SAP [55, 62-64]. In this field, we examined the effect of oxygenation of intestinal mucosa to BT [65]. Perfluorochemicals are biologically inert liquids in which oxygen is remarkably soluble, and can dissolve 40% or more oxygen by volume under hyperoxygenation. They have the ability to bind oxygen reversibly, and their usefulness as oxygen carrier to tissues or organs has been demonstrated without apparent biological toxicity. In rat models, intraperitoneal administration of oxygenated perfluorochemical did not improve the mortality rate, but reduced the incidence of BT to the mesenteric lymph nodes from 60% to 37% 12 hours after the induction of SAP, and significantly reduced the number of bacterial colonies detected after 24 hours. The apoptotic changes of intestinal mucosa were significantly suppressed by the treatment. These results indicate that sufficient oxygenation inhibits apoptosis of intestinal epithelium and BT induced in SAP.

Effect of Vascular Endothelial Growth Factor (VEGF)

As described above, we demonstrated that serum vascular endothelial growth factor (VEGF) levels were significantly elevated in clinical and experimental SAP, and that administration of VEGF significantly inhibited the apoptosis of the liver and kidney and improved hepatic and renal dysfunctions in rat [42]. In the following study, we found that VEGF inhibited intestinal epithelial cell apoptosis and following BT in rat SAP [43]. Injection of recombinant rat VEGF did not affect the degree of SAP (serum amylase/lipase levels or histological findings) or the permeability changes (hematocrit or pancreatic water content), but significantly reduced the apoptosis of ileal mucosa 8 hours after the induction of SAP. VEGF significantly improved the decrease of villous height, and significantly reduced the incidence of BT. Moreover; VEGF significantly increased the microvessel counts, and significantly improved the elevation of plasma plasminogen activator inhibitor-1 levels (an index of vascular endothelial cell injury). Concerning the mechanism of inhibitory effect of VEGF on intestinal epithelial cell apoptosis, two possible mechanisms are postulated. First, VEGF may promote the repair of microvessels in injured mucosa by stimulating angiogenesis, improve the microcirculation and ischemic changes, and suppress the intestinal epithelial cell apoptosis. Second, VEGF may inhibit the vascular endothelial cell apoptosis itself, and may improve vascular endothelial cell injury and microcirculatory disturbance of intestinal mucosa.

Treatment Strategy against Infection

It is conceivable that maintenance of gut barrier integrity reduces the systemic inflammatory response and prevents BT due to an atrophic and leaky gut. Therefore, significance of bowel treatment attracted attention against infectious complications, and selective digestive decontamination (SDD) and enteral nutrition (EN) therapies were introduced in patients with SAP. Luiten et al. reported that SDD reduced gram-negative colonization of the digestive tract and prevented subsequent pancreatic infection in SAP [66]. On the other hand, a meta-analysis of seven randomized controlled trials revealed that EN reduced the incidence of infection and the length of hospital stay [67]. So, we analyzed the treatment outcome of SDD and EN in 90 patients with SAP in our department [68]. SDD reduced the incidence of organ dysfunction (70% to 59%) and mortality rate (40% to 28%). EN further reduced the incidence of infected pancreatic necrosis (31% to 21%), frequency of surgery for pancreas (28% to 18%), and mortality rate (28% to 16%). Results in this study raised the possibility that SDD and EN might decrease the complications and reduce the mortality rate.

In the following study, we investigated the clinical outcome of continuous regional arterial infusion of protease inhibitor and antibiotics (CRAI) in 84 patients with acute necrotizing pancreatitis and EN in 145 patients with SAP [69]. CRAI and EN are now generally utilized in Japan as prevention therapies against infection in SAP [70]. Takeda et al. first introduced CRAI clinically [71]. The theory of CRAI is to carry the high dose of protease inhibitor and antibiotics even when the microcirculation of the pancreas is damaged. Recent experimental study has revealed that CRAI of an antibiotic via the superior mesenteric artery (SMA) is effective in mitigating intestinal mucosal damage and preventing BT, thereby improving survival in SAP [72]. In our department, when the pancreatic necrosis was detected by CE-CT on admission (within 72 hours after the onset), angiography was undertaken and the catheter was placed at the celiac artery (CA) and the SMA. The protease inhibitor (nafamostat mesilate: 150 mg/day via the CA, 100 mg/day via the SMA), and the antibiotic (imipenem: 0.5g/day via the CA, 0.5 g/day via the SMA) were administered by CRAI for 5-7 days after admission. EN (ELENTAL^{TM}) was performed through the naso-jejunal tube after the recovery of gut motility (within 3-7 days after admission). CRAI reduced the incidence of infection (51% to 34%), the frequency of surgery (63% to 27%), and the mortality rate (54% to 37%). EN reduced the frequency of surgery (32% to 23%) and the mortality rate (35% to 19%). These results suggest that CRAI and EN may improve the clinical outcome of SAP, with the effects of reducing the infection and avoiding the surgery for pancreas.

B. Immunosuppression during Severe Acute Pancreatitis

Abstract

In patients with SAP, immunosuppression occurs from the early phase and peripheral lymphocyte reduction due to apoptosis is linked to the development of subsequent infection. In experimental SAP, thymic atrophy and splenic atrophy occurs, and Th1 (T helper cell type 1)/Th2 (T helper cell type 2) balance tends to Th1 suppression. Serum levels of IL-18, one of Th1 cytokines, are significantly elevated in patients with SAP, and are correlated with CD4/8 rate of lymphocyte, suggesting that IL-18 may be closely related to helper T cell response. Immunostimulation may be a new treatment strategy against the infectious complications.

Immunologic impairment in the early phase may be linked to the increased susceptibility to subsequent infection and the development of septic complications. Several investigators have reported the reduction of peripheral lymphocyte count in acute pancreatitis [73-77], and it may reflect the immunologic impairment. Therefore, it is conceivable that immunosuppression occurs from the early phase in patients with SAP, but the immunologic impairment in SAP has not yet been analyzed in detail. Moreover, the relationship between immunosuppression (lymphocyte reduction) and subsequent infection was not investigated. In this chapter, we review our research results about them.

Thymic Atrophy

Concerning the immunosuppression in SAP, first we investigated the alterations of thymus to clear the impairment of cellular immunity in rat SAP [15]. Both thymus weight and number of thymocytes decreased significantly 20 hours after induction of SAP. Neither thymus atrophy nor thymocyte reduction was observed in rats with mild pancreatitis. This thymic atrophy in SAP is due to the thymocyte apoptosis. Apoptotic change was confirmed by in situ nick-end labeling, DNA agarose gel electrophoresis, and cell cycle analysis.

Peripheral Lymphocyte Reduction

Curley et al. reported a significant decrease in the proportion of CD4-positive lymphocytes (T helper cells) in SAP [74]. Recent reports demonstrated a significant decrease in CD4- and CD8-positive lymphocytes in SAP [75-77]. We examined the significance of decreased lymphocytes in patients with SAP and the role of apoptosis [78]. In 48 patients with SAP, the peripheral lymphocyte count on admission was significantly decreased in patients with subsequent infection in comparison to those without infection. Analysis of lymphocyte subsets revealed that both B and T lymphocytes were decreased in peripheral circulation in the patients with infection, and that it was primarily CD8-positive lymphocytes that decreased in these subsets. Cell cycle analysis of lymphocytes indicated that apoptotic changes occurred in lymphocytes from patients with SAP but not in lymphocytes from healthy control subjects. In rat SAP, total peripheral lymphocytes and T lymphocytes were significantly decreased 5 hours after induction of SAP. These results suggest that peripheral lymphocytes are eliminated from systemic circulation possibly as a result of apoptosis.

Splenic Atrophy

The spleen is a major immune organ as well as the thymus, and is involved not only in the clearance of particulate antigens and injured or old cells within the host, but also in the regulation of cell-mediated immune processes and the production of opsonins. Thus, we next examined the alterations of spleen in rat SAP [79]. Both splenic weights and numbers of splenocytes were significantly decreased 12 and 24 hours after induction of SAP. Apoptosis was not detected in splenocytes from rats with SAP 6, 12, and 24 hours after the induction, but apoptosis was detected in peripheral lymphocytes from rats with SAP 6 hours after the induction. Peripheral lymphocytes were significantly decreased 6, 12, and 24 hours after the induction. With antecedent splenectomy, peripheral lymphocyte counts 12 hours after the induction of SAP were significantly lower than those in rats who had not undergone splenectomy. These results suggest that splenic atrophy resulting from splenocyte reduction occurs in rat SAP, and that splenocytes are recruited into systemic circulation in response to peripheral lymphocyte reduction as a result of apoptosis.

Functional Alterations of Splenocytes

There were several reports regarding the quantitative changes of lymphocytes as described above, however few works have been done concerning the functional changes of lymphocytes in SAP. It is possible that lymphocyte hyporesponsiveness occurs in the early stage of SAP. Recently, the concept of "Th1 (T helper cell type 1)/Th2 (T helper cell type 2) balance was introduced for understanding the pathophysiologic response during septic or preseptic conditions such as severe burn or trauma. Th1 cells produce IL-2 and interferon (IFN)-γ, activate cytotoxic T cells, and initiate cellular immunity. Th2 cells secrete IL-10 and IL-4, activate B cells, and stimulate production of certain antibodies. Thus, we investigated the functional alterations of splenocytes in rat SAP to clarify the Th1/Th2 balance during SAP [80]. In splenocytes harvested 24 hours after induction of SAP, proliferative capacity with concanavalin A (con A) stimulation was significantly reduced. IL-2 release with con A stimulation and IFN-γ release with or without con A stimulation were significantly decreased. IL-10 release with con A stimulation was also significantly decreased. The IL-2/IL-10 concentration ratio secreted by the splenocytes was significantly reduced. These results suggest that splenocyte function is markedly suppressed in experimental SAP and that Th1/Th2 balance tends to Th1 suppression as a whole. Dysfunction of lymphocytes including splenocytes may play a certain role in the development of subsequent septic complications in SAP.

Immunosuppression in Patients with SAP

As clinical research, we analyzed the various immunologic parameters at the time of admission in 101 patients with SAP, and clarified the predictable factors of subsequent infection. Furthermore, chronologic change of lymphocyte count was investigated, and utility of lymphocyte count for predicting infection was compared with conventional scoring systems [81]. Serum immunoglobulin (Ig)G, serum IgM, lymphokine–activated killer cell activity, and natural killer cell activity were low, and incidence of abnormal low value was 50%, 65%, 46% and 42%, respectively. Serum C3 was significantly negatively correlated with the APACHE II score. The lymphocyte count was decreased below the normal range, and was significantly negatively correlated with the APACHE II score. CD4-, CD8-, and CD20-positive lymphocyte counts were below the normal range, and CD4- and CD8-positive lymphocyte counts were significantly lower in the infection group. The lymphocyte count on day 14 after admission was significantly lower in the infection group and was more useful for predicting infection than conventional scoring systems. These results suggest that immunosuppression occurs from the early phase in SAP, and that quantitative impairment of lymphocytes, mainly T lymphocytes, may be closely related to infectious complications during SAP. CD4- and CD8-positive lymphocyte counts on admission and the lymphocyte count on day 14 after admission may be useful for predicting infection.

IL-18

IL-18 is a cytokine produced from Kupffer cells and activated macrophages, and IL-18 acts on Th1 cells and in combination with IL-12 strongly induces production of IFN-γ. IL-18 has many other functions, including induction of proinflammatory cytokines, upregulation of adhesion molecules, and activation of natural killer (NK) cell activity. Thus, IL-18 is now considered to be an important regulator of inflammation, immunological reactions, and tissue injury. We determined the serum IL-18 concentrations in patients with SAP at the time of admission, and relationships between their serum IL-18 levels and various clinical factors for SAP were analyzed [82]. Serum IL-18 levels were significantly elevated in patients with SAP, and were significantly positively correlated with the Ranson score and JSS. Serum IL-18 levels were significantly negatively correlated with base excess and total protein, and were significantly positively correlated with the CD4/CD8 rate of lymphocytes, serum IL-6 levels, and serum IL-8 levels. On day 7 after admission, the CD4/CD8 rate of lymphocytes and the rate of CD4-positive lymphocytes were significantly positively correlated with serum IL-18 levels. Furthermore, serum IL-18 levels in patients with hepatic dysfunction were significantly higher than those without hepatic dysfunction. These results suggest that serum IL-18 levels are significantly elevated and are correlated with severity in patients with SAP and that IL-18 may be closely related to helper T cell response and hepatic dysfunction in this disease.

Immunosuppressive Acidic Protein (IAP)

Immunosuppressive acidic protein (IAP) is an immunosuppressive factor to be present in serum and ascites of cancer patients, and it is utilized as a tumor marker. It is suggested that IAP is also an acute-phase reactant that has a correlation with the impairment of host's immunity. Now IAP is utilized as not only a tumor marker but also an index of immune status of the hosts. Therefore, it is conceivable that IAP may be associated with immunosuppression in SAP. So, we determined serum IAP levels in patients with SAP at the time of admission, and relationships between their serum IAP levels and various clinical factors were analyzed [83]. Serum IAP level increased on admission and we recognized abnormally high levels in 88% of patients. Serum IAP level was significantly lower in patients of Stage 3 and 4 (JSS ≥9) than that in patients of Stage 2 (2≤ JSS ≤8). It was also significantly lower in patients whose Ranson score was ≥5 than that in patients whose Ranson score was ≤4. Moreover, it was significantly lower in patients with pancreatic necrosis than that in patients without pancreatic necrosis. Serum IAP was significantly negatively correlated with hematocrit, serum lipase, and serum IFN-γ, and was significantly positively correlated with serum total protein. Serum IAP levels in patients of Stage 2 reached a higher peak 7 days after admission and decreased more rapidly than those in patients of Stage 3 and 4. Thus, we first demonstrated that serum IAP levels were elevated in patients with SAP, but were significantly lower in patients with a higher grade of severity or pancreatic necrosis. These results suggest that serum IAP levels may be related to systemic inflammatory response and reflect the immunoresponsiveness in patients with SAP.

Toll-Like Receptor (TLR)

The innate immune system recognizes pathogen-associated molecular patterns (PAMPs) that are expressed on infectious agents, but not on the host. Toll-like receptors (TLRs) recognize microorganisms as the innate immune system, and are involved in the host defense mechanism. Activation of TLRs leads not only to the induction of inflammatory responses but also to the development of antigen-specific adaptive immunity. TLR2 recognizes lipoteichoic acid (LTA) of gram-positive bacteria, and TLR4 recognizes lipopolysaccharide (LPS) of gram-negative bacilli. Since the innate immune system operates mainly via TLRs on macrophages, it is conceivable that expression of TLRs on macrophages and their responsiveness to the agonists are of great importance for inflammatory response and the host defense mechanism in SAP. Thus, we recently investigated the expression of TLRs on macrophages and their TLRs-mediated cytokine production in rat SAP [84]. Macrophages were isolated from bronchoalveolar lavage fluid 6 hours after induction of SAP. The expression of TLR2 (mRNA and protein) and LTA-mediated TNF-α production were significantly decreased in SAP. The expression of TLR4 (mRNA and protein) and LPS-mediated TNF-α production was also significantly decreased in SAP. These results suggest that the impaired responsiveness to LTA and LPS of macrophages is derived from decreased expression of TLR2 and TLR4, respectively. This suppression of immune response in the early phase may be implicated in the mechanism of infection.

As to the local immune response, we investigated the expression of TLR2 and TLR4 in intestinal mucosa in rat SAP [85]. TLR2 and TLR4 proteins were increased 2 and 6 hours after induction of SAP, and were decreased 12 and 18 hours after induction of SAP. Immunoreactivities for them were detected at the top of villi and crypt in control rats. They were increased (especially at Paneth cells) 6 hours after the induction, and were diminished 12 hours after the induction. Activated nuclear factor (NF)-κB was increased 6 hours after the induction, and was decreased 18 hours after the induction. BT occurred 18 hours after the induction. These results suggest that intestinal immune response enhances in the early phase and suppresses in the late phase of SAP, and TLRs may be implicated in the mechanism of BT.

In the following study, to clarify the role of TLR4 in the pathophysiology of SAP, we investigated the effects of TLR4-deficiency on SAP using wild-type (C3H/HeN) and TLR4-deficient (C3H/HeJ) mice [86]. C3H/HeJ mice have been demonstrated to have a missense mutation in the third exon of TLR4, yielding a nonfunctional TLR4, and it is known that TLR4-deficient C3H/HeJ mice are hyporesponsive to the biological effects of LPS. Severity of SAP was similar in TLR4-deficient and wild-type mice. Serum AST, ALT, BUN and creatinine were significantly lower in TLR4-deficient mice. Apoptosis of liver and kidney was reduced in TLR4-deficient mice. Positive rate of gram-negative bacterial culture of pancreas was significantly higher in TLR4-deficient mice. Serum IL-1β and TNF-α levels were significantly lower in TLR4-deficient mice. TLR4 protein expressions in the liver, kidney, and small intestine were increased 4 hours after induction of SAP and were decreased 12 hours after induction of SAP. These results suggest that TLR4 is implicated in the mechanism of organ dysfunction and BT in SAP, and that TLR4 may facilitate the inflammatory response and function defensively against infection.

3. Conclusion

Abstract

In spite of various efforts, the clinical outcome of SAP is not satisfactory. Further investigations are needed.

In spite of various efforts, the clinical outcome of SAP is not satisfactory. In the light of the above-mentioned lines of evidence, numerous factors such as apoptotic cell death, a lot of mediators (cytokines), immunosuppression, and TLRs are involved in the systemic manifestations in SAP. As future outlook, we would like to develop a novel approach for the treatment of SAP based upon our research results. Control of apoptosis, blockade of aggravation mediator or supply of protective mediator, immunomodulation, and targeted antagonization or agonization of TLRs may be useful as new therapeutic strategy against the life-threatening complications in SAP. Especially, we think that control of intestinal epithelial cell and vascular endothelial cell apoptosis, improvement of microcirculation, and immunostimuation are promising. However, it is postulated that these strategies cannot always achieve the satisfactory effects, because the mechanisms responsible for the life-threatening complications are multifactorial and differ among various organs and various complications. Now, it is clinically hopeful that CRAI and EN may reduce the life-threatening complications and thereby improve the mortality rate in SAP. The efficacy of CRAI and EN should be verified by large-scale randomized controlled trial. Furthermore, we expect that new beneficial treatments will be added in the near future. Further investigations are needed to improve the clinical outcome of SAP.

References

[1] Nathens, A. B.; Curtis, J. R.; Beale, R. J.; Cook, D. J.; Moreno, R. P.; Romand, J. A.; Skerrett, S. J.; Stapleton, R. D.; Ware, L. B.; Waldmann, C. S. Management of the critically ill patient with severe acute pancreatitis. *Crit. Care Med.*, 2004, 32, 2524-36.

[2] Tenner, S.; Sica, G.; Hughes, M.; Noordhoek, E.; Feng, S.; Zinner, M.; Banks, P. A. Relationship of necrosis to organ failure in severe acute pancreatitis. *Gastroenterology*, 1997, 113, 899-903.

[3] Buter, A.; Imrie, C. W.; Carter, C. R.; Evans, S.; McKay, C. J. Dynamic nature of early organ dysfunction determines outcome in acute pancreatitis. *Br. J. Surg*, 2002, 89, 298-302.

[4] Beger, H. G.; Bittner, R.; Block, S.; Buchler, M. Bacterial contamination of pancreatic necrosis. A prospective clinical study. *Gastroenterology*, 1986, 91, 433-8.

[5] Farkas, G.; Marton, J.; Mandi, Y.; Szederkenyi, E. Surgical strategy and management of infected pancreatic necrosis. *Br. J. Surg.*, 1996, 83, 930-3.

[6] Isenmann, R.; Rau, B.; Beger, H. G. Bacterial infection and extent of necrosis are determinants of organ failure in patients with acute necrotizing pancreatitis. *Br. J. Surg.*, 1999, 86, 1020-4.

[7] Buchler, M. W.; Gloor, B.; Muller, C. A.; Friess, H.; Seiler, C. A.; Uhl, W. Acute necrotizing pancreatitis: treatment strategy according to the status of infection. *Ann. Surg.*, 2000, 232, 619-26.

[8] Kivilaakso, E.; Valtonen, V. V.; Malkamaki, M.; Palmu, A.; Schroder, T.; Nikki, P.; Makela, P. H.; Lempinen, M. Endotoxaemia and acute pancreatitis: correlation between the severity of the disease and the anti-enterobacterial common antigen antibody titre. *Gut*, 1984, 25, 1065-70.

[9] Runkel, N. S.; Moody, F. G.; Smith, G. S.; Rodriguez, L. F.; LaRocco, M. T.; Miller, T. A. The role of the gut in the development of sepsis in acute pancreatitis. *J. Surg. Res.*, 1991, 51, 18-23.

[10] Medich, D. S.; Lee, T. K.; Melhem, M. F.; Rowe, M. I.; Schraut, W. H.; Lee, K. K. Pathogenesis of pancreatic sepsis. *Am. J. Surg.*, 1993, 165, 46-50.

[11] Gianotti, L.; Munda, R.; Alexander, J. W.; Tchervenkov, J. I.; Babcock, G. F. Bacterial translocation: a potential source for infection in acute pancreatitis. *Pancreas*, 1993, 8, 551-8.

[12] Widdison, A. L.; Karanjia, N. D.; Reber, H. A. Routes of spread of pathogens into the pancreas in a feline model of acute pancreatitis. *Gut*, 1994, 35, 1306-10.

[13] Makhija, R.; Kingsnorth, A. N. Cytokine storm in acute pancreatitis. *J. Hepatobiliary Pancreat Surg.*, 2002, 9, 401-10.

[14] Nishikawa, J.; Takeyama, Y.; Ueda, T.; Hori, Y.; Ueno, N.; Yamamoto, M.; Saitoh, Y. Induction of apoptotic cell death by pancreatitis-associated ascitic fluid in Madin-Darby canine kidney cells. *FEBS Lett*, 1995, 373, 19-22.

[15] Takeyama, Y.; Nishikawa, J.; Ueda, T.; Hori, Y. Thymic atrophy caused by thymocyte apoptosis in experimental severe acute pancreatitis. *J. Surg. Res.*, 1998, 78, 97-102.

[16] Kaiser, A. M.; Saluja, A. K.; Sengupta, A.; Saluja, M.; Steer, M. L. Relationship between severity, necrosis, and apoptosis in five models of experimental acute pancreatitis. *Am. J. Physiol.*, 1995, 269, 1295-304.

[17] Saluja, A.; Hofbauer, B.; Yamaguchi, Y.; Yamanaka, K.; Steer, M. Induction of apoptosis reduces the severity of caerulein-induced pancreatitis in mice. *Biochem. Biophys. Res. Commun.*, 1996, 220, 875-8.

[18] Bhatia, M.; Wallig, M. A.; Hofbauer, B.; Lee, H. S.; Frossard, J. L.; Steer, M. L.; Saluja, A. K. Induction of apoptosis in pancreatic acinar cells reduces the severity of acute pancreatitis. *Biochem. Biophys. Res. Commun.*, 1998, 246, 476-83.

[19] Hahm, K. B.; Kim, J. H.; You, B. M.; Kim, Y. S.; Cho, S. W.; Yim, H.; Ahn, B. O.; Kim, W. B. Induction of apoptosis with an extract of Artemisia asiatica attenuates the severity of cerulein-induced pancreatitis in rats. *Pancreas*, 1998, 17, 153-7.

[20] Tran, D. D.; Oe, P. L.; de Fijter, C. W.; van der Meulen, J.; Cuesta, M. A. Acute renal failure in patients with acute pancreatitis: prevalence, risk factors, and outcome. *Nephrol Dial Transplant*, 1993, 8, 1079-84.

[21] Levy, M.; Geller, R.; Hymovitch, S. Renal failure in dogs with experimental acute pancreatitis: role of hypovolemia. *Am. J. Physiol.*, 1986, 251, 969-77.

[22] Satake, K.; Kanazawa, G.; Hiura, A.; Nishiwaki, H.; Ha, S. S.; Chung, Y. S.; Umeyama, K.; Yukimura, T. Renal function in experimentally induced acute pancreatitis in dogs: how it is affected by the nephrotoxic substance in pancreatic exudate from ascitic fluid. *Jpn. J. Surg.* 1991, 21, 88-95.

[23] Takase, K.; Takeyama, Y.; Nishikawa, J.; Ueda, T.; Hori, Y.; Yamamoto, M.; Kuroda, Y. Apoptotic cell death of renal tubules in experimental severe acute pancreatitis. *Surgery,* 1999, 125, 411-20.

[24] Bohlinger, I.; Leist, M.; Gantner, F.; Angermuller, S.; Tiegs, G.; Wendel, A. DNA fragmentation in mouse organs during endotoxic shock. *Am. J. Pathol.*, 1996, 149, 1381-93.

[25] Takeyama, Y.; Hori, Y.; Takase, K.; Ueda, T.; Yamamoto, M.; Kuroda, Y. Apoptotic cell death of hepatocytes in rat experimental severe acute pancreatitis. *Surgery*, 2000, 127, 55-64.

[26] Hori, Y.; Takeyama, Y.; Ueda, T.; Shinkai, M.; Takase, K.; Kuroda, Y. Macrophage-derived transforming growth factor-beta1 induces hepatocellular injury via apoptosis in rat severe acute pancreatitis. *Surgery*, 2000, 127, 641-9.

[27] Ueda, T.; Takeyama, Y.; Takase, K.; Hori, Y.; Kuroda, Y.; Ho, H. S. Hematin is one of the cytotoxic factors in pancreatitis-associated ascitic fluid that causes hepatocellular injury. *Surgery,* 2002, 131, 66-74.

[28] Wang, X. D.; Borjesson, A.; Sun, Z. W.; Wallen, R.; Deng, X. M.; Zhang, H. Y.; Hallberg, E.; Andersson, R. The association of type II pneumocytes and endothelial permeability with the pulmonary custocyte system in experimental acute pancreatitis. *Eur. J. Clin. Invest.*, 1998, 28, 778-85.

[29] Yuan, Y. Z.; Gong, Z. H.; Lou, K. X.; Tu, S. P.; Zhai, Z. K.; Xu, J. Y. Involvement of apoptosis of alveolar epithelial cells in acute pancreatitis-associated lung injury. *World J. Gastroenterol.*, 2000, 6, 920-24.

[30] Frey, C. F.; Wong, H. N.; Hickman, D.; Pullos, T. Toxicity of hemorrhagic ascitic fluid associated with hemorrhagic pancreatitis. *Arch. Surg.*, 1982, 117, 401-4.

[31] Coticchia, J. M.; Lessler, M. A.; Carey, L. C.; Gower, W. R.; Mayer, A. D.; McMahon, M. J. Peritoneal fluid in human acute pancreatitis blocks hepatic mitochondrial respiration. *Surgery*, 1986, 100, 850-6.

[32] Bielecki, J. W.; Dlugosz, J.; Pawlicka, E.; Gabryelewicz, A. The effect of pancreatitis associated ascitic fluid on some functions of rat liver mitochondria. A possible mechanism of the damage to the liver in acute pancreatitis. *Int. J. Pancreatol.*, 1989, 5, 145-56.

[33] Takeyama, Y.; Nishikawa, J.; Ueda, T.; Hori, Y.; Yamamoto, M.; Kuroda, Y. Involvement of peritoneal macrophage in the induction of cytotoxicity due to apoptosis in ascitic fluid associated with severe acute pancreatitis. *J. Surg. Res.*, 1999, 82, 163-71.

[34] Ueda, T.; Takeyama, Y.; Hori, Y.; Shinkai, M.; Takase, K.; Goshima, M.; Yamamoto, M.; Kuroda, Y. Hepatocyte growth factor increases in injured organs and functions as an organotrophic factor in rats with experimental acute pancreatitis. *Pancreas*, 2000, 20, 84-93.

[35] Ho, H. S.; Ueda, T.; Liu, H. The impacts of experimental necrotizing pancreatitis on hepatocellular ion homeostasis and energetics: an in vivo nuclear magnetic resonance study. *Surgery*, 1998, 124, 372-9.

[36] Ueda, T.; Ho, H. S.; Anderson, S. E.; Takeyama, Y. Pancreatitis-induced ascitic fluid and hepatocellular dysfunction in severe acute pancreatitis. *J. Surg. Res.*, 1999, 82, 305-11.

[37] Ueda, T.; Takeyama, Y.; Hori, Y.; Takase, K.; Goshima, M.; Kuroda, Y. Pancreatitis-associated ascitic fluid increases intracellular Ca(2+) concentration on hepatocytes. *J. Surg. Res.*, 2000, 93, 171-6.

[38] Murr, M. M.; Yang, J.; Fier, A.; Foulis, P. R.; Loughorn, T. P., Jr.; Epling-Burnette, P. K.; Norman, J. G. Pancreatitis-associated ascitic fluid induces hepatocyte death independent of local cytokines. *J. Surg. Res.*, 2002, 106, 308-13.

[39] Yang, J.; Fier, A.; Carter, Y.; Liu, G.; Epling-Burnette, P. K.; Bai, F.; Loughran, T. P., Jr.; Mastorides, S.; Norman, J. G.; Murr, M. M. Liver injury during acute pancreatitis: the role of pancreatitis-associated ascitic fluid (PAAF), p38-MAPK, and caspase-3 in inducing hepatocyte apoptosis. *J Gastrointest Surg*, 2003, 7, 200-7.

[40] Ueda, T.; Takeyama, Y.; Toyokawa, A.; Kishida, S.; Yamamoto, M.; Saitoh, Y. Significant elevation of serum human hepatocyte growth factor levels in patients with acute pancreatitis. *Pancreas*, 1996, 12, 76-83.

[41] Ueda, T.; Takeyama, Y.; Hori, Y.; Nishikawa, J.; Yamamoto, M.; Saitoh, Y. Hepatocyte growth factor in assessment of acute pancreatitis: comparison with C-reactive protein and interleukin-6. *J. Gastroenterol.*, 1997, 32, 63-70.

[42] Ueda, T.; Takeyama, Y.; Yasuda, T.; Matsumura, N.; Sawa, H.; Nakajima, T.; Kuroda, Y. Vascular endothelial growth factor increases in serum and protects against the organ injuries in severe acute pancreatitis. *J. Surg. Res.*, 2006, 134, 223-30.

[43] Nakajima, T; Ueda, T; Takeyama, Y; Yasuda, T; Shinzeki, M; Sawa, H; Kuroda, Y. Protective effects of vascular endothelial growth factor on intestinal epithelial apoptosis

and bacterial translocation in experimental severe acute pancreatitis. *Pancreas*, 2007, in press.

[44] Yasuda, T.; Ueda, T.; Takeyama, Y.; Shinzeki, M.; Sawa, H.; Nakajima, T.; Ajiki, T.; Fujino, Y.; Suzuki, Y.; Kuroda, Y. Significant increase of serum high-mobility group box chromosomal protein 1 levels in patients with severe acute pancreatitis. *Pancreas*, 2006, 33, 359-63.

[45] Yasuda, T; Ueda, T; Shinzeki, M; Sawa, H; Nakajima, T; Takeyama, Y; Kuroda, Y. Increase of high mobility group box chromosomal protein 1 in blood and injured organs in experimental severe acute pancreatitis. *Pancreas*, 2007, in press.

[46] Sawa, H.; Ueda, T.; Takeyama, Y.; Yasuda, T.; Shinzeki, M.; Nakajima, T.; Kuroda, Y. Blockade of high mobility group box-1 protein attenuates experimental severe acute pancreatitis. *World J. Gastroenterol.*, 2006, 12, 7666-70.

[47] Sawa, H.; Ueda, T.; Takeyama, Y.; Yasuda, T.; Matsumura, N.; Nakajima, T.; Ajiki, T.; Fujino, Y.; Suzuki, Y.; Kuroda, Y. Elevation of plasma tissue factor levels in patients with severe acute pancreatitis. *J. Gastroenterol.*, 2006, 41, 575-81.

[48] Ranson, J. H.; Rifkind, K. M.; Roses, D. F.; Fink, S. D.; Eng, K.; Spencer, F. C. Prognostic signs and the role of operative management in acute pancreatitis. *Surg. Gynecol. Obstet.*, 1974, 139, 69-81.

[49] Blamey, S. L.; Imrie, C. W.; O'Neill, J.; Gilmour, W. H.; Carter, D. C. Prognostic factors in acute pancreatitis. *Gut*, 1984, 25, 1340-6.

[50] Knaus, W. A.; Draper, E. A.; Wagner, D. P.; Zimmerman, J. E. APACHE II: a severity of disease classification system. *Crit. Care Med.*, 1985, 13, 818-29.

[51] Ogawa, M.; Hirota, M.; Hayakawa, T.; Matsuno, S.; Watanabe, S.; Atomi, Y.; Otsuki, M.; Kashima, K.; Koizumi, M.; Harada, H.; Yamamoto, M.; Nishimori, I. Development and use of a new staging system for severe acute pancreatitis based on a nationwide survey in Japan. *Pancreas*, 2002, 25, 325-30.

[52] Ueda, T.; Takeyama, Y.; Yasuda, T.; Matsumura, N.; Sawa, H.; Nakajima, T.; Ajiki, T.; Fujino, Y.; Suzuki, Y.; Kuroda, Y. Simple scoring system for the prediction of the prognosis of severe acute pancreatitis. *Surgery*, 2007, 141, 51-8.

[53] Ryan, C. M.; Schmidt, J.; Lewandrowski, K.; Compton, C. C.; Rattner, D. W.; Warshaw, A. L.; Tompkins, R. G. Gut macromolecular permeability in pancreatitis correlates with severity of disease in rats. *Gastroenterology*, 1993, 104, 890-5.

[54] Wang, X. D.; Wang, Q.; Andersson, R.; Ihse, I. Alterations in intestinal function in acute pancreatitis in an experimental model. *Br. J. Surg.*, 1996, 83, 1537-43.

[55] Hotz, H. G.; Foitzik, T.; Rohweder, J.; Schulzke, J. D.; Fromm, M.; Runkel, N. S.; Buhr, H. J. Intestinal microcirculation and gut permeability in acute pancreatitis: early changes and therapeutic implications. *J. Gastrointest. Surg.*, 1998, 2, 518-25.

[56] Ammori, B. J.; Leeder, P. C.; King, R. F.; Barclay, G. R.; Martin, I. G.; Larvin, M.; McMahon, M. J. Early increase in intestinal permeability in patients with severe acute pancreatitis: correlation with endotoxemia, organ failure, and mortality. *J. Gastrointest. Surg.*, 1999, 3, 252-62.

[57] Juvonen, P. O.; Alhava, E. M.; Takala, J. A. Gut permeability in patients with acute pancreatitis. *Scand. J. Gastroenterol.*, 2000, 35, 1314-8.

[58] Yasuda, T.; Takeyama, Y.; Ueda, T.; Shinzeki, M.; Sawa, H.; Nakajima, T.; Kuroda, Y. Breakdown of intestinal mucosa via accelerated apoptosis increases intestinal permeability in experimental severe acute pancreatitis. *J. Surg. Res.*, 2006, 135, 18-26.

[59] Wang, X.; Wang, B.; Wu, J.; Wang, G. Beneficial effects of growth hormone on bacterial translocation during the course of acute necrotizing pancreatitis in rats. *Pancreas*, 2001, 23, 148-56.

[60] Wang, X.; Wang, B.; Wu, K.; Xu, M.; Gong, Z. Growth hormone downregulated the excessive apoptosis of ileal intestinal epithelial cells in rats during the early course of acute necrotizing pancreatitis. *Pancreas,* 2002, 25, 205-9.

[61] Yasuda, T.; Takeyama, Y.; Ueda, T.; Shinzeki, M.; Kishi, S.; Sawa, H.; Nakajima, T.; Kuroda, Y. Protective Effect of Caspase Inhibitor on Intestinal Integrity in Experimental Severe Acute Pancreatitis. *J. Surg. Res.*, 2007, Epub ahead of print

[62] Foitzik, T.; Eibl, G.; Hotz, B.; Hotz, H.; Kahrau, S.; Kasten, C.; Schneider, P.; Buhr, H. J. Persistent multiple organ microcirculatory disorders in severe acute pancreatitis: experimental findings and clinical implications. *Dig. Dis. Sci.*, 2002, 47, 130-8.

[63] Rahman, S. H.; Ammori, B. J.; Holmfield, J.; Larvin, M.; McMahon, M. J. Intestinal hypoperfusion contributes to gut barrier failure in severe acute pancreatitis. *J. Gastrointest. Surg.*, 2003, 7, 26-35.

[64] Yamenel, L.; Mas, M. R.; Comert, B.; Isik, A. T.; Aydin, S.; Mas, N.; Deveci, S.; Ozyurt, M.; Tasci, I.; Unal, T. The effect of activated protein C on experimental acute necrotizing pancreatitis. *Crit. Care*, 2005, 9, 184-90.

[65] Shinzeki, M.; Takeyama, Y.; Ueda, T.; Yasuda, T.; Kishi, S.; Kuroda, Y. Intraperitoneal administration of oxygenated perfluorochemical inhibits bacterial translocation associated with severe acute pancreatitis. *Kobe J. Med. Sci.*,. 2003, 49, 17-24.

[66] Luiten, E. J.; Hop, W. C.; Lange, J. F.; Bruining, H. A. Controlled clinical trial of selective decontamination for the treatment of severe acute pancreatitis. *Ann. Surg.*, 1995, 222, 57-65.

[67] McClave, S. A.; Chang, W. K.; Dhaliwal, R.; Heyland, D. K. Nutrition support in acute pancreatitis: a systematic review of the literature. *J. Parenter Enteral. Nutr.*, 2006, 30, 143-56.

[68] Sawa, H; Ueda, T; Takeyama, Y; Yasuda, T; Shinzeki, M; Matsumura, N; Nakajima, T; Matsumoto, I; Fujita, T; Ajiki, T; Fujino, Y; Kuroda, Y. Treatment outcome of selective digestive decontamination and enteral nutrition in patients with severe acute pancreatitis. *J. Hepatobiliary Pancreat. Surg.*, 2007, in press.

[69] Yasuda, T; Ueda, T; Takeyama, Y; Shinzeki, M; Sawa, H; Nakajima, T; Matsumoto, I; Fujita, T; Sakai, T; Ajiki, T; Fujino, Y; Kuroda, Y. Treatment strategy against infection: clinical outcome of continuous regional arterial infusion, enteral nutrition, and surgery in severe acute pancreatitis. Manuscript, submitted.

[70] Takeda, K.; Takada, T.; Kawarada, Y.; Hirata, K.; Mayumi, T.; Yoshida, M.; Sekimoto, M.; Hirota, M.; Kimura, Y.; Isaji, S.; Koizumi, M.; Otsuki, M.; Matsuno, S. JPN Guidelines for the management of acute pancreatitis: medical management of acute pancreatitis. *J. Hepatobiliary Pancreat Surg.*, 2006, 13, 42-7.

[71] Takeda, K.; Matsuno, S.; Sunamura, M.; Kakugawa, Y. Continuous regional arterial infusion of protease inhibitor and antibiotics in acute necrotizing pancreatitis. *Am. J. Surg.*, 1996, 171, 394-8.

[72] Isaji, S.; Mizuno, S.; Tabata, M.; Yamagiwa, K.; Yokoi, H.; Uemoto, S. Bacterial analysis of infected pancreatic necrosis and its prevention. *J. Hepatobiliary Pancreat Surg.*, 2003, 10, 419-24.

[73] Christophi, C.; McDermott, F.; Hughes, E. S. Prognostic significance of the absolute lymphocyte count in acute pancreatitis. *Am. J. Surg.*, 1985, 150, 295-6.

[74] Curley, P. J.; McMahon, M. J.; Lancaster, F.; Banks, R. E.; Barclay, G. R.; Shefta, J.; Boylston, A. W.; Whicher, J. T. Reduction in circulating levels of CD4-positive lymphocytes in acute pancreatitis: relationship to endotoxin, interleukin 6 and disease severity. *Br. J. Surg.*, 1993, 80, 1312-5.

[75] Pezzilli, R.; Billi, P.; Beltrandi, E.; Maldini, M.; Mancini, R.; Morselli Labate, A. M.; Miglioli, M. Circulating lymphocyte subsets in human acute pancreatitis. *Pancreas*, 1995, 11, 95-100.

[76] Widdison, A. L.; Cunningham, S. Immune function early in acute pancreatitis. *Br. J. Surg.*, 1996, 83, 633-6.

[77] Uehara, S.; Gothoh, K.; Handa, H.; Tomita, H.; Tomita, Y. Immune function in patients with acute pancreatitis. *J. Gastroenterol Hepatol.*, 2003, 18, 363-70.

[78] Takeyama, Y.; Takas, K.; Ueda, T.; Hori, Y.; Goshima, M.; Kuroda, Y. Peripheral lymphocyte reduction in severe acute pancreatitis is caused by apoptotic cell death. *J. Gastrointest Surg.*, 2000, 4, 379-87.

[79] Yasuda, T.; Takeyama, Y.; Ueda, T.; Takase, K.; Nishikawa, J.; Kuroda, Y. Splenic atrophy in experimental severe acute pancreatitis. *Pancreas*, 2002, 24, 365-72.

[80] Ueda, T.; Takeyama, Y.; Yasuda, T.; Takase, K.; Nishikawa, J.; Kuroda, Y. Functional alterations of splenocytes in severe acute pancreatitis. *J. Surg. Res.*, 2002, 102, 161-8.

[81] Ueda, T.; Takeyama, Y.; Yasuda, T.; Shinzeki, M.; Sawa, H.; Nakajima, T.; Ajiki, T.; Fujino, Y.; Suzuki, Y.; Kuroda, Y. Immunosuppression in patients with severe acute pancreatitis. *J. Gastroenterol.*, 2006, 41, 779-84.

[82] Ueda, T.; Takeyama, Y.; Yasuda, T.; Matsumura, N.; Sawa, H.; Nakajima, T.; Ajiki, T.; Fujino, Y.; Suzuki, Y.; Kuroda, Y. Significant elevation of serum interleukin-18 levels in patients with acute pancreatitis. *J. Gastroenterol.*, 2006, 41, 158-65.

[83] Shinzeki, M; Ueda, T; Takeyama, Y; Yasuda, T; Sawa, H; Nakajima, T; Matsumoto, I; Fujita, T; Ajiki, T; Fujino, Y; Kuroda, Y. Serum immunosuppressive acidic protein levels in patients with severe acute pancreatitis. *Pancreas*, 2007, in press.

[84] Matsumura, N; Takeyama, Y; Ueda, T; Yasuda, T; Shinzeki, M; Sawa, H; Nakajima, T; Kuroda, Y. Decreased expression of toll-like receptor 2 and 4 on macrophages in experimental severe acute pancreatitis. *Kobe J. Med. Sci.*, 2007, in press.

[85] Sawa, H; Ueda, T; Takeyama, Y; Yasuda, T; Shinzeki, M; Matsumura, N; Nakajima, T; Kuroda, Y. Expression of toll-like receptor 2 and 4 in intestinal mucosa in experimental severe acute pancreatitis. *Hepatogastroenterology*, 2007, in press.

[86] Sawa, H; Ueda, T; Takeyama, Y; Yasuda, T; Shinzeki, M; Nakajima, T; Kuroda, Y. Role of toll-like receptor 4 in the pathophysiology of mice severe acute pancreatitis. *Surg. Today*, 2007, in press.

In: Pancreatitis Research Advances
Editor: William C. Langley, pp. 201-231

ISBN: 978-1-60021-883-5

Chapter VI

Diagnosis of Autoimmune Pancreatitis

***Takahiro Nakazawa**[*,1], **Hirotaka Ohara**[1], **Hitoshi Sano**[2], **Tomoaki Ando**[1], **Kazuki Hayashi**[1], **Haruhisa Nakao**[1] and **Takashi Joh**[1]*

[1]Nagoya City University Graduate School of Medical Sciences,
Department of Internal Medicine and Bioregulation,
Nagoya, Japan
[2]Gifu Prefectual Tajimi Hospital,
Department of Gastroenterology, GIFU, Japan

Abstract

Characteristic imaging features of AIP are diffuse narrowing of the main pancreatic duct with an irregular wall, enlargement of the pancreas. However, with the increasing number of AIP cases, various imaging findings atypical to the classical definition of AIP are being encountered. First, we examined the imaging findings of 37 AIP cases and also examined misdiagnosed cases to determine their reasons for misdiagnosis. Only 7 cases showed typical AIP findings. Six cases were misdiagnosed with pancreatic cancer and two with bile duct cancer. Seven cases were surgically treated. Five cases were misdiagnosed due to non-existence of or unfamiliarity with the concept of AIP and of sclerosing cholangitis with AIP. Another three cases were diagnosed with pancreatic cancer because of segmental stenosis of the main pancreatic duct and no or focal enlargement of the pancreas. We also review characteristic imaging findings of AIP.

Second, AIP is often associated with systemic extrapancreatic lesions. Sclerosing cholangitis associated with AIP are different clinical entities from primary sclerosing cholangitis. Cholangiographic findings, clinical courses, effectiveness of steroid therapy, pathological findings are different. Similarly, sialadenitis associated with AIP are different clinical entities from Sjögren Syndrome. Pathological studies of AIP patients

* Address for correspondence: Takahiro Nakazawa, M.D. Nagoya City University Graduate School of Medical Sciences, Department of Internal Medicine and Bioregulation, Nagoya, Japan 1 Kawasumi, Mizuho-cho, Mizuho-ku Nagoya 467-8601, Japan. Phone:052-853-8211, Fax:052-852-0952.

disclosed that plasma cells stained for anti-IgG4 antibody were seen mainly in the pancreas, biliary tract, salivary gland, and large intestine, and antibodies to the pancreas, biliary tract, salivary gland exist in the serum of patients with AIP. In addition, Inflammatory pseudotumors of liver, lung show similar pathologic findings to those of AIP. Inflammatory pseudotumors and AIP are closely related clinical entities in the category of IgG4-related autoimmune diseases.

From these results, we prepare new diagnostic criteria by modifying the Japanese version and propose the concept of "autoimmune sclerosing cholangiopancreatitis."

Introduction

Chronic pancreatitis is a progressive inflammatory disease characterized by abdominal pain, irreversible morphological change, and insufficiency of exocrine and endocrine. While most common forms of chronic pancreatitis are related to alchol ingestion, some cases of unknown origins have been called idiopathic pancreatitis. In 2001, Etemad et al. categorized the major predisposing factors to chronic pancreatitis as (i) toxic-metabolic, (ii) idiopathic, (iii) genetic, (iv) autoimmune, (v) recurrent and severe acute pancreatitis, and (vi) obstructive (TIGAR-O system) [1].

Sarles et al. first reported the phenomenon of pancreatitis with hypergammaglobulinaemia and its possible relation to the phenomena of self-immunization [2]. Since the term "autoimmune pancreatitis (AIP)" was coined in 1995[3], a number of reports have been published [4-5].

AIP should be diagnosed currently based on the characteristic imaging findings such as irregular narrowing of the main pancreatic duct and enlargement of whole pancreas. Hypergammaglobulinaemia or high serum IgG levels are observed in AIP patients. Anti-nuclear antibodies were positive in some of the AIP patients, which strongly suggests that they have an autoimmune disease. The characteristic histological findings in AIP are peripancreatic duct inflammatory cell infiltration, pancreatic acinar cell atrophy, pancreatic parenchymal fibrosis, and obstructive phlebitis. The diagnostic criteria for AIP has been first proposed by the Japan Pancreatic Society [6]. The criteria are summarized as follows. (1) Pancreatic imaging studies show diffuse narrowing of the main pancreatic duct with irregular wall (more than 1 / 3 length of the entire pancreas) and enlargement of the pancreas. (2) Laboratory data demonstrate abnormally elevated levels of serum □-globulin and / or IgG, or the presence of autoantibodies. (3) Histopathological examination of the pancreas shows fibrotic changes with lymphocyte and plasma cell infiltration. For diagnosis, criterion 1 must be present, together with at least one of criteria 2 and 3.

In this chapter, we explained the difficulty in diagnosing AIP by imaging findings based on our experiences. Then, we demonstrated the sytemic extrapancreatic lesions associated with AIP, mainly sclerosing cholangitis. Last, from these results, we prepare a new diagnostic criteria by modifying the Japanese version and propose the concept of" autoimmune sclerosing cholangiopancreatitis."

Imaging Findings

We examined the imaging findings of 37 AIP cases and also examined misdiagnosed cases to determine their reasons for misdiagnosis [7]. A total of 37 patients with AIP have reported to our hospital or its affiliate over the past 17 years (from 1989 to May 2005). Diagnosis was given based on the criteria for AIP determined by the Japanese Pancreatic Society in 2000 as mentioned above [6].

Pancreatic Changes on ERP (Table 1)

Twenty-two AIP cases showed typical diffuse narrowing of the main pancreatic duct with an irregular wall. Nine AIP cases showed segmental narrowing of the main pancreatic duct, and of these, six showed upstream dilation. Six cases showed head-tail narrowing of the main pancreatic duct.

Horiuchi et al. reported that 7 of 27 AIP cases showed segmental irregular narrowing of the main pancreatic duct in the head of the pancreas, while 4 and 3 cases showed segmental stenosis in both the head and tail and body and tail, respectively [8]. Wakabayashi et al. reported that chronic pancreatitis with focal narrowing of the main pancreatic duct is part of the same clinical spectrum as chronic pancreatitis with diffuse narrowing of the main pancreatic duct, and examined whether diffuse and focal distribution are related to the stage or extent of the disease [9].

Table 1. Pancreatic changes on ERP ***(Gastrointest Endosc 2007, 65: 99-108)***

Extent of irregular narrowing of the main pancreatic duct	Upstream dilation	No. cases
Diffuse (>1/3)		22
Segmenal (<1/3)		9
Head	+	4
	-	3
Body	+	2
	-	0
Tail	+	0
	-	0
Head-tail		6

+, Present -, absent.

Pancreatic Findings on CT and US (Table 2)

Twenty-seven AIP cases showed typical diffuse enlargement of the pancreas. Six cases showed localized enlargement, one showed head-tail enlargement and three showed no enlargement. Abdominal US showed multiple low echoic masses in one case and a single low echoic mass in three cases. Localized enlargement of the pancreas associated with AIP sometimes presents as a low-density mass lesion in the pancreas head. Such cases are often misdiagnosed with pancreatic cancer and surgically treated [10-11]. A low echoic mass on US and localized enlargement of the pancreas on US and CT presented as homogeneous delayed enhancement of the pancreas on CT. These findings can help distinguish AIP from pancreatic cancer [12-13].

Three cases showed calcification of the pancreas in our cases; two showed multiple calcification and one showed single calcification. Yoshida et al. reported that the characteristic features of AIP are the absence of pancreatic cysts and stones [3]. During clinical onset of AIP, calcification spots are thought to be a rare finding. Eight of 42 AIP patients previously showed stone formation in their clinical courses [14].

Pancreatic cysts were detected in two cases. Few reports have documented cases of AIP complicated by the formation of pseudocysts in the pancreas. Nishimura et al. reported a patient with AIP in whom pseudocyst formation existed in the pancreas [15]. The pancreatic cyst in one of our cases naturally disappeared before steroid therapy. In another case, the pancreatic cyst disappeared after steroid therapy but recurred with enlargement of the pancreas after reduction of the steroid dosage, disappearing again after increased steroid dosage. We speculated that severe stenosis of the pancreatic duct was responsible for pancreatic cyst formation and considered these cysts as retention cysts.

Table 2. Pancreatic findings on CT and US

Findings	Number of cases
Extent of enlargement	
Diffuse (>1/3)	27
Locarized (<1/3)	
head	6
body	0
tail	0
Head-tail)	1
No enlargement	3
Calcification	3
Pancreatic cyst	2
Low echoic mass	
multiple	1
single	3

(Gastrointest Endosc 2007, 65: 99-108)

Bile Duct Changes on ERC (Table 3)

No biliary stenosis was detected in three cases. We used our classification of biliary involvement (see "*SCLEROSING CHOLANGITIS*"). Stenosis was located in the lower part of the common bile duct only in Type 1; diffusely distributed in the intra and extrahepatic bile duct in Type 2; in both the hilar hepatic lesion and lower part of the common bile duct in Type 3; and as stricture of the bile duct in the hilar hepatic lesion only in Type 4. Stenosis of intrapancreatic bile duct was detected in 18 cases. 17 cases showed stenosis in extrapancreatic bile ducts.

Table 3. Bile duct changes on ERC

Type of cholangiographic changes	Number of cases
No changes	3
Type I	18
Type II	9
Type III	4
Type IV	3

(Gastrointest Endosc 2007, 65: 99-108)

Summary of the Imaging Findings of 37 AIP Cases

Only 7 of the 37 AIP cases showed typical AIP findings: diffuse narrowing of the main pancreatic duct with an irregular wall (more than 1/3 the length of the entire pancreas), enlargement of the pancreas, common bile duct stricture in the pancreas with dilation of the bile duct upstream, no pancreatic calcification and no pancreatic cysts. The other 30 cases showed a variety of imaging features atypical of AIP.

The Reason for Misdiagnosis

Six cases were misdiagnosed with pancreatic cancer and 2 with bile duct cancer. Seven cases were surgically treated. The reason for misdiagnosis in 5 cases was unfamiliarity with the concept of AIP and sclerosing cholangitis with AIP (SC with AIP). The two cases were diagnosed in 1992 and 1993, respectively, before the concept of AIP was established. Another three cases were misdiagnosed with pancreatic cancer because of segmental stenosis of the main pancreatic duct and no or localized enlargement of the pancreas. In addition, dilation of the proximal pancreatic duct affected discrimination from pancreatic cancer in one case.

Extrapancreatic Lesions

Recently, cases of primary or isolated AIP without other autoimmune diseases have been reported. In contrast, the occasional coexistence of pancreatitis with other systemic exocrinopathy has led to the concept of a syndrome complex, idiopathic fibrosclerosis, multifocal fibrosclerosis because of the diversity of systemic autoimmune disease [16-18]. Autoimmunity was categorized as one of the 6 risk factors in the TIGAR-O risk factor classification system of chronic pancreatitis, which are roughly divided into two groups—isoloated and systemic autoimmune pancreatitis [1].

Associated Diseases

We summarized the systemic extrapancreatic lesions of 51 AIP case in our hospital or its affiliate over the past 18 years (Table 4). Diverse systemic extra-pancreatic lesions were observed as follows: enlargement of the submandibular gland (n=8 patients), retroperitoneal fibrosis (n=5), mediastinal lymph node swelling (n=2), allergic purpura (Shönlein-Henoch purpura, immune thrombocytopenic purpura; n=1, respectively), lung fibrosis (n=1), autoimmune sensorineural hearing loss (n=1), cervical lymph node enlargement (n=1), hypothyroidism (n=1), and tubulorinterstitial nephritis (n=1).

In 15 cases of AIP with associated systemic extra-pancreatic lesions, the clinical manifestations of the extra-pancreatic lesions occurred with those of AIP synchronously (n=10) and at different times (n=5). On the other hand, the clinical course of case 3 was quite different. Two years prior to the diagnosis of autoimmune pancreatitis, case 3 suffered from bilateral sclerosing submaxillaritis, and 4 years after cessation of steroid therapy for a pancreatic lesion, autoimmune sensorineural hearing loss developed. At that time, CT and MRCP detected no abnormal findings in the pancreas. Following this, the patient suffered from allergic purpura and arthritis with an elevated IgG level. On retrospect, to spare unnecessary surgical procedures, we should have realized that all these conditions stemmed from a single systemic disease. As illustrated in this case, however, symptoms can appear non-simultaneously making it difficult to determine their association. In addition, by detecting the common causes of systemic conditions, we should be able to make a more precise diagnosis of AIP.

Table 4. Summary of AIP Patients with Systemic Extrapancreatic Lesions

case No	age	gender	chief complaint	associated disease	Time of diagnosis
1	61	Male	obstructive jaundice	Schonlein-Henoch purpura	simultaneouslly
2	70	Male	obstructive jaundice	interstitial pneumoniae immune thrombocytopenic purpura	simultaneouslly
3	62	Female	obstructive jaundice	Sclerosing sialadenitis allergic purpura autoimmune sensorineural hearing loss	before after //
4	62	Male	No symptom	Sclerosing sialadenitis	simultaneouslly
5	76	Male	obstructive jaundice	Sclerosing sialadenitis	simultaneouslly
6	49	Male	abdominal pain	mediastinal lymph node swelling cervical lymph node swelling Sclerosing sialadenitis	simultaneouslly
7	68	Male	abdominal pain	retroperitorium fibrosis	simultaneouslly
8	66	Female	abdominal pain	retroperitorium fibrosis	before
9	59	Male	Body weight loss	Sclerosing sialadenitis	before
10	69	Female	No symptom	Hypothyroidism	before
11	56	Male	No symptom	mediastinal lymph node swelling Sclerosing sialadenitis retroperitorium fibrosis	before // simultaneouslly
12	76	Male	obstructive jaundice	Sclerosing sialadenitis	simultaneouslly
13	54	Male	obstructive jaundice	Sclerosing sialadenitis Tublointerstitial nephritis	simultaneouslly
14	76	Male	obstructive jaundice	retroperitorium fibrosis	simultaneouslly
15	75	Male	obstructive jaundice	retroperitorium fibrosis	simultaneouslly

Comparison of Clinical and Laboratory Date between Patients with AIP with and without Systemic Extrapancreatic Lesions

We have reported already the character of AIP with systemic extra-pancreatic lesions in 31 AIP patients [19]. There were no significant differences between the two groups age, gender, and extent of narrowing of the main pancreatic duct or enlargement of the pancreas. Gamma globulin levels were significantly higher in AIP patients with systemic extra pancreatic lesions than those without (3.0±1.2 vs. 1.8±1.2, $P<0.05$). IgG levels were also significantly higher among those with systemic extra-pancreatic lesions than those without (3032±975 vs. 2010±1244, $P<0.05$) as were IgG4 levels (727±813 vs. 227±197, $P<0.05$).

We restudied 51 AIP patients and compared the IgG value and IgG4 value between patients with AIP with and without systemic extrapancreatic lesions. IgG levels were significantly higher among those with systemic extra-pancreatic lesions than those without (3167±1097 vs. 2040±1099, $P<0.01$) as were IgG4 levels (1089±824 vs. 491±594, $P<0.05$).

The results of this study revealed that AIP patients with systemic extra-pancreatic lesions exhibit higher levels of gamma globulins, IgG and IgG4, all of which are considered hallmarks of autoimmune abnormality. These patients required maintenance therapy with doses of immunosuppressive medication higher than those required for AIP patients without systemic extra-pancreatic lesions. When encountering cases of AIP with elevated gamma globulins, IgG and IgG4 levels, the possible coexistence of other systemic extra-pancreatic lesions should therefore be considered.

Steroid therapy is effective in treating AIP; however, it has also been reported that in some patients with diffuse lesions narrowing the pancreatic duct, chronic pancreatitis improves during the natural clinical course without the aid of steroids or biliary drainage [20]. It is not certain, therefore, whether all patients with AIP should receive steroid therapy. Nevertheless, this study showed that some cases with systemic extra-pancreatic lesions should receive steroid therapy, because in the absence of steroid therapy the prognosis might be rather poor for cases of immune thrombocytopenic purpura, autoimmune sensorineural hearing loss and interstitial lung fibrosis. Cases of AIP with systemic extra-pancreatic lesions showed high gamma globulin, IgG and IgG4 levels and required maintenance steroid therapy. If patients with systemic extra-pancreatic lesions are encountered, we should therefore not focus on any particular aspect but rather on the possibility of a syndrome complex. In managing patients with AIP with high gamma globulin, IgG and IgG4 levels, an attempt should also be made to detect the existence of other systemic extra-pancreatic lesions that require steroid treatment.

Literature Review of AIP Cases with Systemic Extrapancreatic Lesions (Excluding Involvement of Biliary Tract)

We have also reviewed documentation of the systemic extra-pancreatic lesions associated with cases of AIP in Japanese and English literature (Table 5) [19]. Sjögren's syndrome, ulcerative colitis, retroperitoneal fibrosis, sialadenitis, thyroiditis, and idiopathic thrombocytopenic purpura were frequently cited. However, Sjögren's syndrome was more frequently noted in Japan, whereas IBD made a more frequent appearance in Western literature. Enlargement of the submandibular gland and sclerosing sialadenitis associated with AIP is different from typical Sjögren's syndrome. Sclerosing sialadenitis associated with AIP have been considered as Küttner's tumor [21] or Mikulicz's diseae [22]. In our study [23], the salivary gland of three patients showed abundant IgG4+ plasma cell infiltration. However, five patients with Sjögren's syndrome showed no infiltration by IgG4+ plasma cells. 90% of patients with Sjögren's syndrome are middle-aged women, whereas AIP is common in elderly men. Anti-Ro [SS-A] and anti-La [SS-B] antibodies are negative in AIP patients. The sera from AIP patients strongly reacted with the normal salivary gland epithelium [23]. Thus, AIP may affect the salivary gland by a mechanism different from that of Sjögren's syndrome.

Of the cases presented here, none had AIP associated with inflammatory bowel disease. Zamoni et al. [24] and Notohara et al [25] showed a high prevalence of inflammatory bowel disease with AIP and proved that the pathological findings of AIP associated with inflammatory bowel disease were different from those of AIP without inflammatory bowel disease.

Retroperitoneal fibrosis is also frequently associated disease with AIP. Hamno et al have reported dense infiltration of IgG-4 positive plasma cells and obliterative phlebitis [26]. A case with retroperitoneal and mediastinal fibrosis in the absence of AIP was reported [27].

Table 5. Review of AIP Cases with Systemic Etrapancreatic Lesions

		Western countries n=172	Japan n=132	Total n=304	
Sjögren's syndrome		13	24	37	P<0.01
IBD	UC	14	5	19	NS
	CD	4	0	4	NS
	Total	18	5	23	P<0.05
Retroperitoneal fibrosis		9	8	17	NS
Sialadenitis		5	1	6	NS
Thyroid disease		4	1	5	NS
ITP		2	3	5	NS
RA		2	1	3	NS
Interstitial pneumonia		1	2	3	NS
Tubulointerstitial nephritis		1	2	3	NS
SLE		0	2	2	NS
AIH		0	2	2	NS
Orbital pseudotumor		2	0	2	NS
Malignant lymphoma		2	0	2	NS

IBD, inflammatory bowel disease; UC, ulcerative colitis; CD, Crohn's disease; ITP, idiopathic thrombocytopenic purpura.

RA, reumatoid arthritis; SLE, systemic lupus erythematosus; AIH, autoimmune hepatitis; NS., not significant.

(Pancreas 2005, 31: 232-237).

Immune thrombocytopenic purpura [28], interstitial pneumonia [29], tubulointestinal nephritis [30], high prevalence of hypothyroidism [31] and hilar accumulation of gallium-67 [32] are also reported.

Pathological Study

The pathogenesis of AIP remains unknown. An autoimmune mechanism has been postulated, and pancreatic duct epithelium-derived carbonic anhydrase II and lactoferrin have been reported to be potential target antigens [33-35]. Pathological studies of AIP tissue demonstrated infiltration of CD4-positive T lymphocytes around the main pancreatic duct [33], expression of HLA-DR antigen in the pancreatic duct cells [33]. Hamano *et al.* [36] found that AIP patients had significantly higher serum IgG4 levels than patients with other pancreatic or biliary system diseases. In addition, they reported patients with AIP complicated by retroperitoneal fibrosis [26]. Their histological study showed infiltration of IgG4-positive plasma cells in ureteral and pancreatic lesions. Kamisawa *et al.* [37] reported diffuse infiltration of CD4- or CD8-positive T lymphocytes and IgG4-positive plasma cells in the peripancreatic tissue, extrahepatic bile duct and gallbladder as well as in the pancreas, suggesting that AIP affects not only the pancreas but also extrapancreatic organs. From these observations, we postulated the presence of autoantibody to various tissues in the serum of

AIP patients. However, there has been no histological proof as to the presence of such autoantibodies in AIP patients' serum.

We investigated what extrapancreatic organs are affected in AIP, and whether autoantibody to such organs was present in the serum [23]. First, we immunohistochemically studied not only the pancreas but also extrapancreatic tissues/organs derived from AIP patients. Second, we immunohistochemically analyzed with what components of normal tissue the patients' serum specifically reacted, using the organs extracted for other diseases. In addition, since glucocorticoid therapy has been reported to dramatically improve pancreatic and bile duct lesions, the reactions of the patients' serum to theses tissues were examined before and after glucocorticoid therapy.

Immunohistochemical Analysis of Patients' Tissues

Tissues from various organs (pancreas, liver, bile duct, stomach, duodenum, large intestine and salivary gland) obtained from 19 AIP patients were examined for infiltration of IgG4-positive plasma cells. Infiltration of the plasma cells positive for IgG4 was evaluated by counting the number of the positive plasma cells in the 10 high power fields (HPFs) and dividing the value by 10. The degrees of infiltration were categorized in the following four scores; Score 0 = 0 per 1 HPF, Score 1 = less than 20 per 1 HPF, Score 2 = 20 to 50 per 1 HPF, and Score 3 = more than 50 per 1 HPF.

The results of immunohistochemical examination are summarized in Table 6. Infiltration of IgG4-positive plasma cells in and around the pancreatic duct walls was observed in 4 of the 5 AIP patients. In the liver of 7 of the 9 patients, the limiting plates were destroyed, and bridging fibrosis was noted in 4 patients. In all patients, infiltration of lymphocytes and plasma cells was seen around the intrahepatic bile duct in the portal areas. The degree of infiltration of IgG4-positive plasma cells was score 2 or higher in all patients. IgG4-positive plasma cell infiltration was observed in and around the extrahepatic and intrapancreatic bile duct walls of 5 of the 9 patients, and 4 of them had score 2 or higher, with no damage to bile duct cells. IgG4-positive plasma cells infiltrated in the gastric mucosal layer of 2 of the 6 patients, but none of them had score 3. Similar plasma cells infiltrated in the duodenal mucosal layer of 4 of the 5 patients, but most of them had a low score. IgG4-positive plasma cells infiltrated in the colonic mucosal layer of 4 of the 5 patients, and 2 of them had score 3. In the salivary gland, 2 patients examined showed abundant IgG4-positive plasma cell infiltration with a score of 2 or 3.

Immunohistochemical Analysis Using Patients' Sera

Sera obtained from 6 AIP patients (5 male, one female, mean age 64 years, range 48-76 years) and 6 healthy volunteers (5 male, one female, mean age 64.4 years, range 60-67 years) were used. Surgically removed, formalin-fixed, and paraffin-embedded tissue sections obtained from the patients with other diseases, but with no autoimmune disease, were immunostained.

Table 6. Immunohistochemical analysis of tissuses of AIP patients and control groups

		Score 0	1	2	3	P Value *
Pancreatic duct walls	AIP (n=5)	1	1	1	2	p<0.05
	Chronic pancreatitis (n=6)	5	1	0	0	
Intrahepatic bile duct in the portal areas	AIP (n=11)	0	2	8	1	p<0.05
	PSC (n=10)	5	5	0	0	
Extrahepatic and intrapancreatic bile duct	AIP (n=8)	1	3	1	3	p<0.05
	PSC (n=4)	3	1	0	0	
Salivary gland	AIP (n=3)	0	0	1	2	p<0.05
	Sjögren's syndrom (n=5)	5	0	0	0	
Gastric mucosal layer	AIP (n=7)	5	1	1	0	NS
	Chronic gastritis (n=3)	3	0	0	0	
Duodenal mucosal layer	AIP (n=6)	2	3	1	0	NS
	PSC (n=3)	2	0	1	0	
Colonic mucosal layer	AIP (n=6)	2	2	0	2	NS
	PSC (n=7)	5	1	1	0	

Counting the number of the IgG4-positive plasma cells in the high power field.
*Score 0 = 0, Score 1<20; 20≦ Score 2 ≦50; or 50<Score 3.
The Mann-Whitney test was used to calculate two-sided P values.
(Histopathology 2005; 47:147–158).

The normal tissue sections (3 cases each from the pancreas, extrahepatic biliary duct, salivary gland, esophagus, stomach, small intestine, large intestine and lung) were obtained from patients having undergone pancreatoduodenectomy, hepatectomy, sialoadenectomy, esophagectomy, gastrectomy, enterectomy, colectomy and pneumonectomy, respectively. The 3-micrometer-thick sections were immunostained with the sera (dilution 1: 10) overnight. Then the sections were incubated with mouse anti-human IgG4 monoclonal antibody, followed by the standard streptavidin biotin-peroxidase method. The anti-human IgG4 monoclonal antibody lost the effect by the absorption test with IgG4. Ratios of positive cells were evaluated as following, Score 0 = 0, Score 1 = less than 20%, Score 2 = 20% to 50%, and Score 3 = more than 50%. The values were expressed as the mean ± the standard deviation.

Table 7 shows the reactivity of the patients' serum autoantibody to various tissues. Table 8 shows the effect of glucocorticoid therapy on tissues reactive with patients' sera.

In the pancreas, the duct epithelial cells positively reacted with serum IgG4 from 5 of the 6 AIP patients. No islets or acinar cells stained positively. Imaging of all the patients possessing positive serum showed an enlarged pancreas with diffuse narrowing of the main pancreatic duct. The stainability by the sera after glucocorticoid therapy of the patients was significantly decreased compared with that before the therapy (p=0.01).

In the liver, the hepatocytes were weakly stained diffusely. The intrahepatic bile duct epithelium was also positively stained with the sera from 4 of the 6 patients. Imaging showed intrahepatic bile duct stricture in 2 of the 4 positive-serum patients, but no abnormalities in the remaining 2 patients. Glucocorticoid therapy significantly decreased the stainability (p=0.031).

Table 7. IgG4 immunoreactivity of normal tissuses incubated with the serum of AIP patients and control group

	AIP (n=6)				Control (n=6)				P Value*
	0	1	2	3	0	1	2	3	
Duct epithelium in pancreas	0	5	1	0	6	0	0	0	p<0.05
Acinar cells in pancreas	6	0	0	0	6	0	0	0	NS
Islet cells in pancreas	6	0	0	0	6	0	0	0	NS
Hepatocytes	6	0	0	0	6	0	0	0	NS
Intrahepatic bile duct epithelium	1	4	1	0	6	0	0	0	p<0.05
Extrahepatic and intrapancreatic bile duct	0	1	4	1	6	0	0	0	p<0.05
Epithelium in gallbladder	0	1	4	1	6	0	0	0	p<0.05
Duct epithelium in salivary gland	0	1	0	5	6	0	0	0	p<0.05
Acinar cells in salivary gland	6	0	0	0	6	0	0	0	NS
Squamous epithelium in oesophagus	4	1	1	0	6	0	0	0	NS
Mucosal epithelium in stomach	3	3	0	0	6	0	0	0	NS
Mucosal epithelium in small intestine	6	0	0	0	6	0	0	0	NS
Mucosal epithelium in large intestine	6	0	0	0	6	0	0	0	NS
Epithelial cells in lung	5	1	0	0	6	0	0	0	NS

*IgG4-positive cells were evaluated as Score 0 = 0-5%, Score 1= 6-20%, Score 2= 21-50% or Score 3 = more than 50%. The Mann-Whitney test was used to calculate two-sided P values. *(Histopathology 2005; 47:147–158).*

The extrahepatic and intrapancreatic bile duct epithelium reacted with the sera from 5 of the 6 patients. Imaging showed extrahepatic bile duct stricture in 4 of these 5 patients, but no abnormalities in 1 patient. Glucocorticoid therapy significantly decreased the stainability (p=0.0093).

In the gallbladder, the epithelial cells were positively stained with the sera from all the patients. Imaging showed gallbladder wall thickening in 3 of them. Glucocorticoid therapy significantly decreased the stainability (p=0.0078).

The duct epithelium in the salivary gland was positive with the serum from each patient. The acinar cells were negative. Glucocorticoid therapy significantly decreased the stainability (p=0.035).

In the esophagus, the squamous epithelial cells and the accessory gland duct epithelium were weakly positive with the sera from 3 patients. The accessory gland acinar cells were negative. The stomach, small intestine and large intestine were negligibly stainable, and the lung was unstainable. Decreased stainability by glucocorticoid therapy was not apparent.

These findings suggest that AIP is a systemic disease in which IgG4 autoantibodies to various organ antigens are present in the serum of patients. In this study, to prove the presence of autoantibody to pancreas and/or extrapancreatic organs, the patients' serum was reacted with normal tissue, and the positive reaction was detected by staining with anti-IgG4 antibody. As a result, the epithelia of pancreatic duct, bile duct, gallbladder and salivary gland duct in particular showed a strong reaction, suggesting that the patients' sera contain autoantibody to the respective epithelial cells, inducing inflammatory cell infiltration.

Table 8. Effect of glucocorticoid therapy on tissues reactive with patients' sera

	Before Glucocorticoid Therapy			After Glucocorticoid Therapy			P Value*
	case 1	case 2	case 3	case 1	case 2	case 3	
Duct epithelium in pancreas	1	1	1	0	0	0	p<0.05
Acinar cells in pancreas	0	0	0	0	0	0	NS
Islet cells in pancreas	0	0	0	0	0	0	NS
Hepatocytes	0	0	0	0	0	0	NS
Intrahepatic bile duct epithelium	1	1	0	0	0	0	p<0.05
Extrahepatic and intrapancreatic bile duct epithelium	2	2	1	0	0	0	p<0.05
Epithelium in gallbladder	2	2	1	1	1	0	p<0.05
Duct epithelium in salivary gland	3	3	1	2	3	0	p<0.05
Acinar cells in salivary gland	0	0	0	0	0	0	NS
Squamous epithelium in oesophagus	1	0	0	0	0	0	NS
Mucosal epithelium in stomach	1	0	0	0	0	0	NS
Mucosal epithelium in small intestine	0	0	0	0	0	0	NS
Mucosal epithelium in large intestine	0	0	0	0	0	0	NS
Epithelial cells in lung	0	0	0	0	0	0	NS

IgG4-positive cells were evaluated as Score 0 = 0-5%, Score 1= 6-20%, Score 2= 21-50% or Score 3 = more than 50%

*The Wilcoxon's rank sum test for paired samples was used to calculate two-sided P values.

The extrahepatic and intrapancreatic bile duct epithelium reacted with the sera from 5 of the 6 patients. Imaging showed extrahepatic bile duct stricture in 4 of these 5 patients, but no abnormalities in 1 patient. Glucocorticoid therapy significantly decreased the stainability ($p=0.0093$).

In the gallbladder, the epithelial cells were positively stained with the sera from all the patients. Imaging showed gallbladder wall thickening in 3 of them. Glucocorticoid therapy significantly decreased the stainability ($p=0.0078$).

The duct epithelium in the salivary gland was positive with the serum from each patient. The acinar cells were negative. Glucocorticoid therapy significantly decreased the stainability ($p=0.035$).

In the esophagus, the squamous epithelial cells and the accessory gland duct epithelium were weakly positive with the sera from 3 patients. The accessory gland acinar cells were negative. The stomach, small intestine and large intestine were negligibly stainable, and the lung was unstainable. Decreased stainability by glucocorticoid therapy was not apparent.

These findings suggest that AIP is a systemic disease in which IgG4 autoantibodies to various organ antigens are present in the serum of patients. In this study, to prove the presence of autoantibody to pancreas and/or extrapancreatic organs, the patients' serum was reacted with normal tissue, and the positive reaction was detected by staining with anti-IgG4 antibody. As a result, the epithelia of pancreatic duct, bile duct, gallbladder and salivary gland duct in particular showed a strong reaction, suggesting that the patients' sera contain autoantibody to the respective epithelial cells, inducing inflammatory cell infiltration.

Sclerosing Cholangitis

Sclerosing cholangitis have been reportedly often associated with AIP [38]. We have reported cases of atypical sclerosing cholangitis in which the criteria for classic primary sclerosing cholangitis (PSC) were met but that the clinical course was better than anticipated in Japanese since 1996 [39]. In these cases, there was always an unusual associated pancreatitis, characterized by diffuse narrowing of the main pancreatic duct and enlargement of the pancreas. The sclerosing cholangitis, as well as the pancreatic changes, respond well to treatment with a corticosteroid or biliary drainage [39-40]. In contrast, PSC is a progressive disease, regardless of therapy, that involves the intra- and extrahepatic bile ducts and leads to biliary cirrhosis. The efficacy of corticosteroid therapy for PSC is questionable [41-42], and liver transplantation is the only effective treatment. Thus, it is necessary to discriminate between these two diseases before making therapeutic decisions. Chronic pancreatitis with diffuse narrowing of the main pancreatic duct also is known, based on its etiology, as AIP.

Accordingly, atypical sclerosing cholangitis with unusual pancreatitis also can be termed sclerosing cholangitis with autoimmune pancreatitis (SC with AIP), although it also has been called sclerosing pancreatocholangitis, based on imaging findings[40], and lymphoplasmacytic sclerosing pancreatitis with cholangitis, based on histopathologic findings[43].

We compared the presenting complaint or abnormality, associated disease, cholangiographic findings, pancreatic changes, treatment, and clinical course were studied for several cases of PSC (n = 32) and SC with AIP (n =40).

Clinical Differences between Primary Sclerosing Cholangitis and Sclerosing Cholangitis with Autoimmune Pancreatitis

Clinical features (Table 9): The number of SC with AIP cases was greater among men than women. However, there were no gender differences noted among those in the PSC group. The patient ages at clinical onset were significantly older for those with SC withAIP. The age at clinical onset of PSC is during the 30s in Western countries [44]. The average age for our PSC patients was 43.4±19.4 years, comparable with that of PSC in Western countries. However, the average age for SC with AIP patients was significantly higher, comparable with that of AIP [45].

Among the chief complaints, obstructive jaundice was most frequently observed in SC with AIP, reflecting marked concentric stenosis of the large bile duct. However, patients with PSC who came to the hospital without symptoms after liver injury were identified by a physical examination. Twenty-four of 40 SC with AIP patients (60%) showed obstructive jaundice, while only 1 of 32 PSC patients presented with obstructive jaundice.

Inflammatory bowel disease was only associated with PSC, and there was no chronic pancreatitis detected among PSC cases. Sclerosing sialadenitis and retroperitorium fibrosis were detected only in SC with AIP. These patients associated with inflammatory bowel disease exhibited ulcerative colitis and colitis with aphtha, erosion, and/or redness that could not be definitely diagnosed as ulcerative colitis or Crohn disease.

Table 9. Clinical Features

		SC with AIP (n=40)	PSC (n=32)
Gender (Male: Female)		29:11	17:15
Age		*62.7±10.7	42.4±19.5
Presenting complaint or abnormality	Obstructive jaundice	24	1
	Liver test abnormalities	5	23
	Esophageal varices rupture	0	2
Associated disease	Inflammatory bowel disease	0	15
	Chronic pancreatitis	40	0
	Sclerosing sialadenitis	6	0
	Retroperitorium fibrosis	2	0

*P<0.01

The character of associated ulcerative colitis was similar to that reported previously. The rectum was spared, and none of the patients had a severe clinical course [46]. In addition, we reported that they showed a characteristic distribution of inflammation. Colonoscopic findings revealed erosion and edematous mucosa mainly on the right side of the colon. Sequential biopsy also revealed more inflammatory cell infiltration in the right side of the colon [47]. Uchida et al. [48] reported that the main lesions that they observed also occurred here as well. Inflammatory bowel disease was not associated with SC with AIP in our study. However, there are some reports of AIP associated with ulcerative colitis [24, 25]. Zamboni et al. [24] and Notohara et al [25] showed a high prevalence of inflammatory bowel disease with AIP and proved that the pathological findings of AIP associated with inflammatory bowel disease were different from those of AIP without inflammatory bowel disease. There exists one problem where these pancreatitis cases associated with inflammatory bowel disease should be included into the category of AIP or not. Frulloni et al. [49] found that the most common disease associated with AIP is ulcerative colitis (35%), although the detailed characteristics of associated ulcerative colitis have not been determined. Colonoscopic and histologic findings for a case reported by Yoshida et al [50] showed total colonic involvement and intense of inflammation were more strongly observed in the rectum and left side of the colon, as is typical for ulcerative colitis. Characteristic findings of ulcerative colitis associated with PSC may be useful for a differential diagnosis between PSC and SC with AIP.

None of the PSC cases was associated with chronic pancreatitis in our cases. PSC is reportedly associated with chronic pancreatitis [51-53], and comparable recently published papers reported low incidences of these diseases [54,55]. In Japan, chronic pancreatitis is more commonly associated with PSC than inflammatory bowel disease [56]. However, this conclusion was reached in a report published before the concept of AIP was established. After investigating Japanese case reports of PSC with chronic pancreatitis [57,58], we suspect that most of these cases were SC with AIP.

Treatment and clinical course (Table10): Some SC with AIP patients underwent surgery based on the diagnosis of pancreatic cancer or cholangiocellularcarcinoma. Other patients had better clinical courses following drainage or steroid administration compared with the PSC patients. Nine patients were treated with biliary drainage only, 6 with surgery only, and 4 were observed. Fifteen patients were initially treated with steroids, and 6 received steroids later in their course. Despite UDCA or steroid administration, PSC patients had progressive cholangiographic or liver histologic findings. Some patients developed liver cirrhosis and died of liver failure, and 3 with liver failure received a liver transplant. The other patient who received a transplant died of sepsis after surgery.

Table 10. Treatment and Clinical Course

		SC with AIP (n=40)	PSC (n=32)
Treatment	steroid	21	5
	ursodeoxycholic acid	0	21
	biliary drainage	9	2
	surgical resection	6	0
	liver transplantation	0	4
	no treatment	4	0
Clinical course	no recurrence	31	0
	recurrence/progression	7	0
	liver failure	0	5
	cholangiocellular carcinoma	0	3

Blood chemistry data (Table 11): Bilirubin was significantly higher in SC with AIP cases, reflecting obstructive jaundice. IgG values did not differ between the 2 groups. However, IgG4 was significantly higher in those with SC with AIP. Antinuclear antibodies were detected at rates of 63.9% and 44.4%, respectively, in SC with AIP and PSC cases. Table 12 showed distribution of IgG4 value in SC with AIP and PSC cases. Twenty of 22 SC with AIP cases showed higher IgG4 value than cut-off value 135mg/dl. All 14 PSC cases showed lower value. Therefore, IgG4 value is useful marker in discrimination for SC with AIP and PSC.

Table 11. Blood Chemistry Data

	SC with AIP (n=40)	PSC (n=32)	
AST (< 50 IU/L)	156±233	121±118	n.s.
ALT (< 50 IU/L)	281±290	156±167	n.s.
T.Bilirubin (< 1.2 mg/dl)	6.0±6.9	2.3±3.2	P<0.01
ALP (< 230 U/L)	1118±818	1083±920	n.s.
Gamma GTP (< 85 U/L)	577±579	384±305	〃
Amylase (130< 450U/L)	137±146	120±124	〃
Eosinocyte (0.7< 6.0%)	4.2±3.6	7.3±6.0	P<0.05
Gamma globulins (< 1.25g/dl)	2.3±1.2	1.7±0.5	n.s.
IgG (< 1700 U/L)	2412±1284	2217±743	〃
IgA (< 1700 U/L)	270±113	367±160	〃
IgM (< 220 U/L)	124±106	219±144	〃
IgG4 (< 135 U/L)	718±693 (n=22)	32.5±29.0 (n=14)	P<0.01
Antinuclearantibodies (positive rate)	23/36(63.9%)	12/27(44.4%)	n.s.

Pathological Findings

The histologic findings for the SC with AIP cases were classified as stage I or II. However, some cases of PSC showed findings indicating stage III or IV. Lymphocyte infiltration was limited to the periportal area in those with SC with AIP. Also, fibrous tissue around the bile duct was seen in SC with AIP, but the degree of fibrosis was less severe, and an onion skin appearance was not observed compared with PSC (Table 12).

Infiltration of IgG4 positive plasma cells was seen around the intrahepatic bile duct in the portal areas and the extrahepatic bile duct walls in AIP significantly greater than PSC. Uehara et al have also reported that the IgG4-positive plasma cell/mononuclear cell ratio was significantly higher in SC with AIP than in PSC [59].

Table 12. Liver biopsy staging

	PSC (n=26)	SC with AIP (n=10)
Staging (Ludwig and LaRusso's)		
Stage I	6	3
II	10	7
III	3	0
IV	7	0

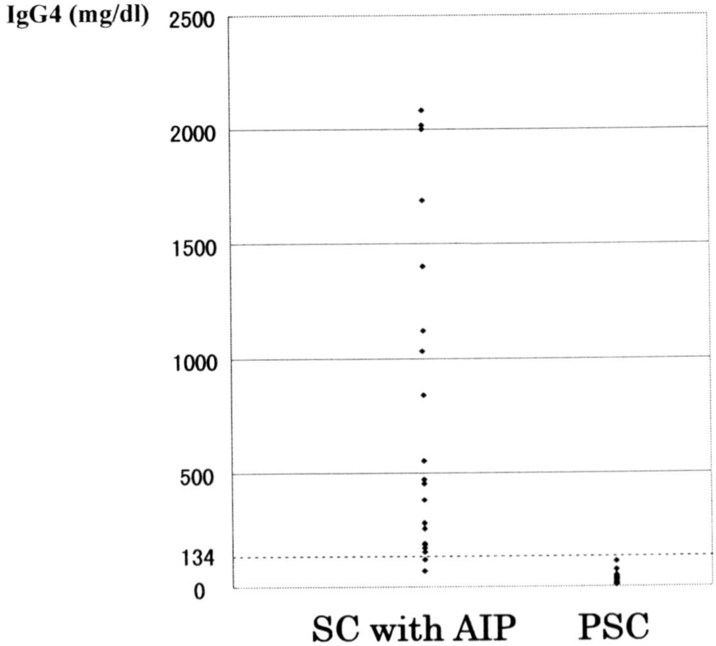

Figure 1. IgG4 value of SC with AIP and PSC.

Cholongiographic Differences between Primary Sclerosing Cholangitis and Sclerosing Cholangitis with Autoimmune Pancreatitis

PSC is a chronic syndrome of unknown cause characterized by diffuse inflammation and fibrosis, first described by Delbet in 1924 [60]. Cholangiography typically shows beading and irregularity of bile ducts. It was originally considered very rare, but development of ERCP in the early 1970's allowed improved diagnosis with a consequent increase in cases. The first criteria for diagnosis of PSC in 1964 included the absence of previous operative trauma to the biliary system, the absence of calculi in the gallbladder and common bile duct, sclerosis and stenosis involving all or most of the extrahepatic bike ducts and finally the exclusion of malignant disease involving the biliary system [61]. The criteria for diagnosis of PSC published by Mayo clinic group have been world-widely used [44, 62]. However, there are no specific criteria. The characteric cholangiograpy and excluding other causes of secondary cholangitis is essential for confirmation of the diagnosis of PSC; ERC is the method of choice. Adequate cholangiograms also can be obtained via a percutaneous transhepatic approach. The typical cholangiographic findings of PSC include multifocal beading of both the intrahepatic and the extrahepatic biliary tree. The intrahepatic bile ducts alone or of the extrahepatic bile ducts alone can be involved. Strictures are typically diffusely distributed and are short and annular, with intervening segments of normal or slightly dilated duct, the classic beaded appearance [61]. MacCarty et al. [63] noted band strictures, diverticula, and mural irregularities in 21%, 27%, and 44%, respectively, of cases, with the former two findings being characteristic of PSC. Majoie et al. [64] proposed that cholangiographic abnormalities can be subdivided into 3 intrahepatic and 4 extrahepatic patterns, and Craig et al. [65] found that high-grade intrahepatic duct strictures and diffuse intrahepatic strictures were statistically significant prognostic factors. In contrast to PSC, there are only a few reports concerning cholangiographic changes with AIP [66-68].

In this chapter, we show the characteristic findings for these two types of sclerosing cholangitis, PSC and SC with AIP based on our previous study. Cholangiograms from patients with primary sclerosing cholangitis (n = 29) and sclerosing cholangitis with autoimmune pancreatitis (n = 26) were studied with regard to length and region of stricture formation, and other characteristic findings [68].

Length of stricture. Length of stricture was defined as suggested by Craig et al. [65]. The term stricture with prestenotic dilatation was used instead of confluent stricture, because it is difficult to discriminate a long stricture from a pruned-tree appearance. Accordingly, long strictures were included only if accompanied by prestenotic simple dilatation. This finding pertained only to the intrahepatic ducts; all other findings pertained to both the intrahepatic and extrahepatic ducts. Strictures were classified as follows: band-like (1-2 mm) (0 = absent, 1+ = one region, 2+ = two or more regions); segmental stricture (>3 mm) (0 = absent, 1+ = one region, 2+ = two or more regions); long stricture with prestenotic dilatation (>10 mm) (0 = absent, 1+ = one region, 2+ = two or more regions).

Characteristic findings of PSC. Beaded appearance (short, annular strictures alternating with normal or minimally dilated segments; 0 = absent, 1+ = one region, 2+ = two or more regions); pruned-tree appearance (diminished arborization of intrahepatic ducts and pruning; 0 = absent, 1+ = one segment, 2+ = two or more regions); diverticulum-like formation (outpouchings resembling diverticula, often protruding between adjacent strictures; 0 = absent, 1+ = one region, 2+ = two or more regions); shaggy appearance (mural irregularities, producing a characteristic shaggy appearance without stenosis; 0 = absent, 1+ < 3 cm in length, 2+ = 3 cm or longer).

Region of stricture. Hilar hepatic region (0 = absent, 1+ > 25% narrowing of duct, 2+ = 0%-25% narrowing of duct); stricture of distal third of common bile duct (0 = absent, 1+ > 25% narrowing of duct, 2+ = 0%-25% narrowing of duct).

We restudied Cholangiographic findings for PSC (n=29) vs. SC with AIP (n=36) are compared in Table 13. Band-like stricture, beaded appearance, pruned-tree appearance, and diverticulum-like formation were only found in PSC. Long stenosis, segmental stricture, and long stricture with prestenotic dilatation were significantly more common in SC with AIP. In a few cases in both groups, shaggy appearance and stricture of the hilar region were present. Stricture of distal common bile duct also was observed in both groups but was significantly more frequent among patients with SC with AIP.

Based on these results, we made a schematic explanation for characteristic cholangiographic findings of PSC and SC with AIP (Figure 2) [69]. Basically, the presence of long strictures is suggestive of SC with AIP. Short strictures is suggestive of PSC. These differences can be explained from the pathological differences. Severe inflammation by infiltration of lymphoplasmacytes in AIP contributes to the wall thickness of bile duct and the compression of bile duct lumen in the longer length. In the cases of PSC, severe fibrosis around bile duct cotribute to the obstruction of bile duct in the short length showing beaded appearance.

Table 13. Comparison of cholangiogram between PSC and SC with AIP

1. Length of stricture

	band-like stricture		segmental stricture		dilation after confluent stricture	
score	PSC	SC with AIP	PSC	SC with AIP	PSC	SC with AIP
0	11	36	19	0	25	23
1+	6	0	5	22	3	4
2+	12	0	5	14	1	9
Pvalue	PSC>SCwithAIP, P<0.001		PSC<SCwithAIP, P<0.001		PSC<SCwithAIP, P<0.05	

2. Characteristic findings of PSC

	beaded appearance		pruned-tree appearance		diverticulum-like outpouching		shaggy appearance	
score	PSC	SC with AIP	PSC	SC with AIP	PSC	SC with AIP	PSC	SC with AIP
0	16	36	11	36	19	36	25	32
1+	4	0	5	0	9	0	2	2
2+	9	0	13	0	1	0	2	2
Pvalue	PSC>AIP, P<0.01		PSC>AIP, P<0.001		PSC>AIP, P<0.01		n.s.	

3. Region of stricture

	stricture of hepatic hilar region		stricture of lower CBD	
score	PSC	SC with AIP	PSC	SC with AIP
0	22	26	17	4
1+	4	3	6	2
2+	3	7	6	30
Pvalue	n. s.		PSC<SCwithAIP, P<0.001	

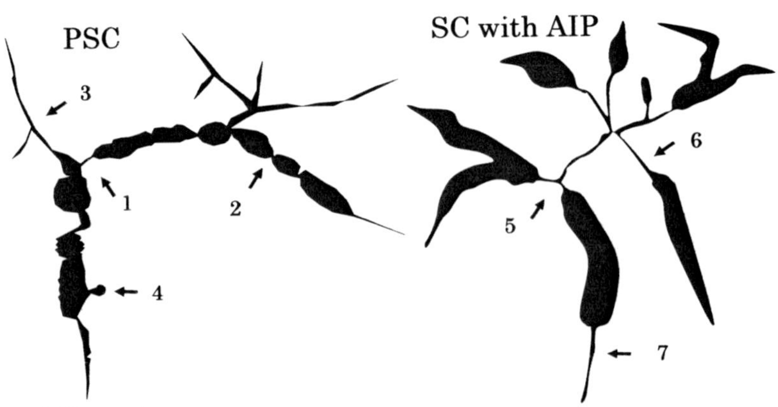

1. band-like stricture
2. beaded appearance
3. pruned-tree appearance
4. diverticulum-like outpouching
5. segmental stricture
6. long stricture with prestenotic dilation
7. stricture of lower CBD

Figure 2. Schematic illustration of comparison of cholangiographic findings –PSC VS. sclerosing cholangitis (SC) with AIP-.

Discriminant Analysis

Discriminant analysis was performed after selection of variables by the stepwise method (Table 14) [68]. Age was used as a variable to control for the contribution of age in the two groups. This affected the constant term in the discriminant function formula; therefore, before attempting to discriminate PSC instead of SC with AIP, in patients in other settings with this formula, specific attention should be given to the role of age in those settings. The stepwise method selected band-like stricture, pruned-tree appearance, and stricture of distal common bile duct as variables (Table 14). When the discriminant function formula was applied to all cases, median and 5th and 95th percentiles were 5.64, 0.016, 11.5 for PSC, respectively, and _5.73, _6.72, _0.10 for SC with AIP, respectively. Twentyseven of 28 cases of PSC and 25 of 26 of SC with AIP were correctly classified by the discriminant function (Figure 3).

Table 14. Discriminant analysis

Variables	Discriminant coefficients	Odds ratio	p Value
Age	- 0.0941976	0.910103	0.00620678
Band-like stricture	3.40993	30.2631	0.0000214291
Pruned-tree appearance	1.21525	3.37113	0.148121
Stricture of distal third of CBD	- 3.02868	0.0483797	0.00000961773

CBD: Common bile duct; PSC: primary sclerosing cholangitis; SC, sclerosing cholangitis; AIP, autoimmune pancreatitis.

The odds ratio for age estimates that for each additional year of age, the odds for being found with PSC, instead of SC with AIP, decreased by a factor of about 9%.

Discriminant p value = 0.954393; A discriminant function formula constant = 6.21049.

Z = 6.21049—0.0941976 × (age) + 3.40993 × (band-like stricture) +
1.21525 × (pruned-tree appearance)—3.02868 ×(stricture of distal third of CBD)
(Gastrointest Endosc 2004, 60: 937-944)

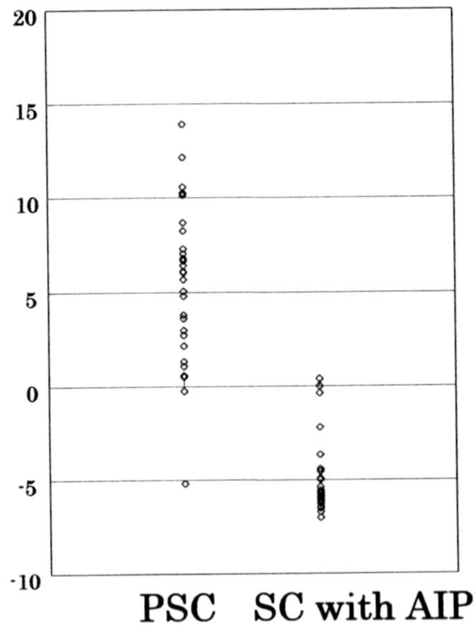

Figure 3. Score of PSC and SC with AIP by Discriminant analysis.

The Concept of "Autoimmune Sclerosing Cholangitis"

The discriminant score calculated by the discriminant function formula for one case of PSC was -5.21, far lower than that for the other cases of PSC (Figure 3). Cholangiography in this patient demonstrated stenosis in the both hilar region and distal common bile duct [68]. There was neither enlargement of the pancreas on CT nor diffuse narrowing of the main pancreatic duct on retrograde pancreatography. A diagnosis was made of cholangiocarcinoma, and right lobe hepatectomy was performed in this patient. Evaluation of the resection specimen revealed wall thickening with prominent fibrosis but no malignancy. Thus, the final diagnosis in this case was PSC. However, based on the results of the present study, the surgical specimen was re-examined. HandE stained sections revealed severe fibrosis and prominent infiltration of lymphocytes and plasma cells, and elastica van Gieson's solution stained sections demonstrated obliterative phlebitis of veins. A large number of plasma cells were positively stained by anti-IgG4 antibodies. Therefore, the pathological diagnosis was changed from PSC to lymphoplasmacytic sclerosing cholangitis without pancreatitis. This case was excluded from the PSC group. This case may be a new clinical entity within the AIP category, because the histopathologic findings were compatible with the biliary changes of lymphoplasmacytic sclerosing pancreatitis, characteristic of AIP[25,70], and plasma cells that stained positive with anti-IgG4 antibody were present.. This entity is called by us "*Autoimmune sclerosing cholangitis* (AISC) "for two reasons: first, the term "autoimmune cholangitis" already is used for another disease, a type of primary biliary cirrhosis that has the same clinical course as autoimmune hepatitis.; second, the term"sclerosing" is important because it reflects the pathological character. There is a report of a patient with sclerosing pancreatocholangitis with an atypical clinical course in which sclerosing cholangitis preceded the appearance of pancreatic lesions [71]. Thus, in the early stages of SC with AIP, patients might be given a diagnosis of PSC on the basis of clinical findings and imaging. Hamano et al. also reported similar three cases with biliary involvement and without pancreatic changes under the name of IgG4 related cholangitis [72]. Zen et al reported that sclerosing lesions identical to those of AIP can affect various levels of the biliary tree. Some of those cases present as SC, some as hepatic inflammatory pseudotumor [73].

Schematic Classification of SC with AIP by Cholangiograpy

We previously reported that the cholangiogram of SC with AIP can be classified into 4 types based on the region of the strictures. Here, a new schematic classification of SC with AIP by cholangiography was made based on both the regions of the strictures and the details of the cholangiographic findings (Figure 4) [74]. In this new classification of cholangiographic changes in SC withAIP, stenosis was located only in the lower part of the common bile duct in type 1; stenosis was diffusely distributed in the intrahepatic and extrahepatic bile ducts in type 2; stenosis was detected in both the hilar hepatic lesions and the lower part of the common bile ducts in type 3; and strictures of the bile duct were detected only in the hilar hepatic lesions in type 4. In our cases, there were 20, 8, 4, and 4 occurrences of types 1, 2, 3, and 4, respectively. Type 2 was further subdivided into 2 types. Extended narrowing of the intrahepatic bile ducts with prestenotic dilation was widely distributed in type 2a. Narrowing of the intrahepatic bile ducts without prestenotic dilation and reduced bile duct branches were widely distributed in type 2b, in which the cholangiograms showed a withered-tree appearance.

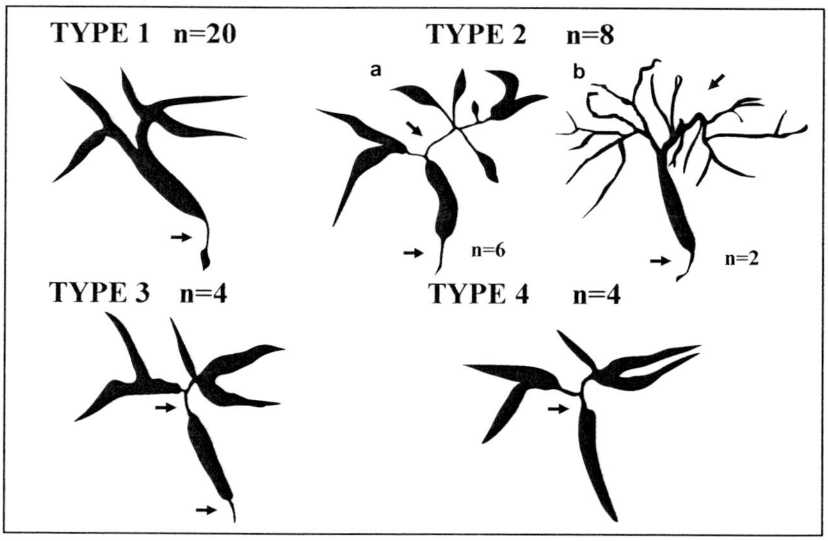

(Pancreas 2006, 32: 229)

Figure 4. Schematic Classification of SC with AIP by Cholangiograpy

However, they did not show the diminished bile duct branches, like the pruned-tree appearance, which is typical of cholangiographic findings for PSC. Cholangiographic findings in our classification often lead to a misdiagnosis of type 1 as pancreatic carcinoma, type 2 as PSC, and types 3 and 4 as cholangiocarcinoma.

Inflammatory Pseudotumors

Inflammatory pseudotumors (IPTs), also known as inflammatory myofibroblastic tumors (IMTs), are uncommon mass lesions whose origin and pathophysiology remain controversial. Hepatic IPTs are thought to be closely related to AIP because a large number of plasma cells stained for anti-IgG4 antibody are seen in both [73]. We reported that 1 pancreatic IPT and 3 extrapancreatic IPT (2 lung, 1 spleen) cases showed the histologic similarities to AIP. Immunohistochemical findings are summarized in (Table 15). Lymphoplasmacellular infiltration, Smooth muscle actin (SMA) -expressing spindle cells, and prominent fibrosis were observed in both groups. There were also a large number of IgG4-positive plasma cells in both groups. The percent value of IgG4-positive plasma cells/total plasma cells was 28.3 ±16.5 (mean ± SD) and 45.5± 12.0 in IPT and AIP, respectively.

Table 15. Histopathologic Similarities of Inflammatory Pseudotumor to AIP

Immunohistochemical study for AIP

case No.	Inflammatory Cell infiltration	plasma Cell infiltration	SMA	CD4	CD8	Obliterative phrebititis	IgG4+plasma cell /total plasma cells
1	+++	++	+	++	++	+	63.5%
2	+++	++	+++	++	++	+	44.5%
3	++	++	++	+	++	+	36.5%
4	++	++	+	-	++	+	49.9%
5	+++	++	+	++	++	+	33.1%
6	+++	++	+	++	++	+	43.7%

Immunohistochemical study for IPT

case	Inflammatory Cell infiltration	plasma Cell infiltration	SMA	CD4	CD8	Obliterative phrebititis	IgG4+plasma cell /total plasma cells
pancreas	+	+	+++	+	++	+	51.2%
spleen	+++	++	+++	−	++	+	25.8%
lung	++	++	+	−	++	+	11.6%
lung	+	+++	+	−	++	−	24.7%

(Pancreas 2006, 32: 115-116).

Obliterative phlebitis was seen in 3 of 4 cases of IPT and in all AIP cases. Lymphocytes mainly showed CD8 and not CD4 staining in IPT and both in AIP. No Epstein-Barr virus-encoded RNA (EBER)-positive cells were detected in both the IPT and AIP cases. The results suggest that IPT and AIP show similar pathologic findings and are closely related clinical entities in the category of IgG4-related autoimmune diseases. Zen et al reported nine cases with an inflammatory pseudotumor of the lung [75] and one case with an inflammatory pseudotumor of the brest [76].

The Concept of Autoimmune Sclerosing Cholangiopancreatitis and Diagnostic Criteria

From this study, AIP is associated with systemic extrapancreatic lesions. They show infiltration of abundant IgG4-positive plasma cells. Kamisawa et al propose the concept “IgG4-related sclerosing disease” [77].

In clinical practice, obstructive jaundice is most frequently observed among the chief complaits in AIP patients. After biliary drainage, differential diagnosis begins. The characteristic cholangiographic findings make a significant contribution to the diagnosis of AIP. For a diagnosis of biliary involvements, the most valuable finding is that which represents AIP. Therefore, we can make a precise diagnosis by referring to both biliary and pancreatic findings, and propose the concept of “autoimmune sclerosing cholangiopancreatitis”. “Sclerosing” is important because the cases with AIP and those with SC with AIP diagnosed in Japan show irregular narrowing of the bile and pancreatic ducts, in addition to the pathological features of lymphoplasmacytic sclerosing pancreatitis with cholangitis [43].

Table 16. Diagnostic Criteria for AIP

1. The pancreatic imaging studies show irregular narrowing of the main pancreatic duct with an equally irregular wall and *enlargement of the pancreas.
2. Laboratory data demonstrate abnormally elevated levels of serum gamma-globulin and/or IgG, and/or IgG4 or the presence of autoantibodies.
3. Histopathological examination of the pancreas shows fibrotic changes with lymphocyte and IgG4- positive plasma cell infiltration.
4. There is an association among sclerosing cholangitis of Types II, III, or IV, sclerosing sialoadentitis, and retroperitoneal fibrosis.

For diagnosis, criterion 1 must be present together with criteria 2 and/or 3 and/or 4.

In the cases with no enlargement of the pancreas, more than 1 of the remaining three criteria (2~4) must be present.

*Some AIP cases show no enlargement of the pancreas.

(Gastrointest Endosc 2007, 65: 99-108).

Those cases of AIP diagnosed in Europe and the USA, on the other hand, showed two subsets of unique pathological findings [24, 25]. One exhibited lymphoplasmacytic sclerosing pancreatitis and the other, idiopathic duct-centric chronic pancreatitis or AIP with a granulocytic epithelial lesion. Both reports showed that the latter occured predominantly in a group of patients who are younger and more commonly suffering from ulcerative colitis and Crohn's disease.

In order to make a precise diagnosis of AIP, we made diagnostic criteria by modifying the Japanese version 2003 [6]. First, IgG4 is the most usefull marker in AIP and should be incorporated not only into the serological test but also into the pathological findings. Second, the association between characteristic sclerosing cholangitis of Types II, III, and IV and systemic extrapancreatic lesions (sclerosing sialoadenitis, retroperitoneal fibrosis, and others) is useful in a diagnosis for AIP (Table16).

Conclusion

Characteristic imaging features of AIP are diffuse narrowing of the main pancreatic duct with an irregular wall, enlargement of the pancreas. However, with the increasing number of AIP cases, various imaging findings atypical to the classical definition of AIP are being encountered. The most important diagnostic factor is clinician awareness of the concept of AIP and associated systemic extrapancreatic lesions, and the measurement of serum IgG4. Sclerosing cholangitis is the most frequently associated disease with AIP. Therefore, we propose the concept of " autoimmune sclerosing cholangiopancreatitis".

References

[1] Etemad B, Whitcomb DC. Chronic pancreatitis: diagnosis, classification, and new genetic developments. *Gastroenterology*. 2001 Feb;120(3):682-707.

[2] Sarles H, Sarles JC, Camatte R, Muratore R, Gaini M, Guien C, et al. Observations on 205 confirmed cases of acute pancreatitis, recurring pancreatitis, and chronic pancreatitis. *Gut*. 1965 Dec;6(6):545-59.

[3] Yoshida K, Toki F, Takeuchi T, Watanabe S, Shiratori K, Hayashi N. Chronic pancreatitis caused by an autoimmune abnormality. Proposal of the concept of autoimmune pancreatitis. *Digestive diseases and sciences*. 1995 Jul;40(7):1561-8.

[4] Horiuchi A, Kaneko T, Yamamura N, Nagata A, Nakamura T, Akamatsu T, et al. Autoimmune chronic pancreatitis simulating pancreatic lymphoma. *The American journal of gastroenterology*. 1996 Dec;91(12):2607-9.

[5] Uchida K, Okazaki K, Konishi Y, Ohana M, Takakuwa H, Hajiro K, et al. Clinical analysis of autoimmune-related pancreatitis. *The American journal of gastroenterology*. 2000 Oct;95(10):2788-94.

[6] Member of the Criteria Committee for Autoimmune Pancreatitis of the Japan Pancreas Society. Diagnosis criteria for autoimmune pancreatitis by the Japan Pancreas Society. *J. Jpn Panc. Soc.*2002; 17; 585–587.

[7] Nakazawa T, Ohara H, Sano H, Ando T, Imai H, Takada H, et al. Difficulty in diagnosing autoimmune pancreatitis by imaging findings. *Gastrointestinal endoscopy.* 2007 Jan;65(1):99-108.

[8] Horiuchi A, Kawa S, Hamano H, Hayama M, Ota H, Kiyosawa K. ERCP features in 27 patients with autoimmune pancreatitis. *Gastrointestinal endoscopy.* 2002 Apr;55(4):494-9.

[9] Wakabayashi T, Kawaura Y, Satomura Y, Fujii T, Motoo Y, Okai T, et al. Clinical study of chronic pancreatitis with focal irregular narrowing of the main pancreatic duct and mass formation: comparison with chronic pancreatitis showing diffuse irregular narrowing of the main pancreatic duct. *Pancreas.* 2002 Oct;25(3):283-9.

[10] Kamisawa T, Egawa N, Nakajima H, Tsuruta K, Okamoto A, Kamata N. Clinical difficulties in the differentiation of autoimmune pancreatitis and pancreatic carcinoma. *The American journal of gastroenterology.* 2003 Dec;98(12):2694-9.

[11] Hirano K, Komatsu Y, Yamamoto N, Nakai Y, Sasahira N, Toda N, et al. Pancreatic mass lesions associated with raised concentration of IgG4. *The American journal of gastroenterology.* 2004 Oct;99(10):2038-40.

[12] Sahani DV, Kalva SP, Farrell J, Maher MM, Saini S, Mueller PR, et al. Autoimmune pancreatitis: imaging features. *Radiology.* 2004 Nov;233(2):345-52.

[13] Wakabayashi T, Kawaura Y, Satomura Y, Watanabe H, Motoo Y, Okai T, et al. Clinical and imaging features of autoimmune pancreatitis with focal pancreatic swelling or mass formation: comparison with so-called tumor-forming pancreatitis and pancreatic carcinoma. *The American journal of gastroenterology.* 2003 Dec;98(12):2679-87.

[14] Takayama M, Hamano H, Ochi Y, Saegusa H, Komatsu K, Muraki T, et al. Recurrent attacks of autoimmune pancreatitis result in pancreatic stone formation. *The American journal of gastroenterology.* 2004 May;99(5):932-7.

[15] Nishimura T, Masaoka T, Suzuki H, Aiura K, Nagata H, Ishii H. Autoimmune pancreatitis with pseudocysts. Journal of gastroenterology. 2004 Oct;39(10):1005-10.

[16] Montefusco PP, Geiss AC, Bronzo RL, Randall S, Kahn E, McKinley MJ. Sclerosing cholangitis, chronic pancreatitis, and Sjogren's syndrome: a syndrome complex. *American journal of surgery.* 1984 Jun;147(6):822-6.

[17] Clark A, Zeman RK, Choyke PL, White EM, Burrell MI, Grant EG, et al. Pancreatic pseudotumors associated with multifocal idiopathic fibrosclerosis. *Gastrointestinal radiology.* 1988;13(1):30-2.

[18] Levey JM, Mathai J. Diffuse pancreatic fibrosis: an uncommon feature of multifocal idiopathic fibrosclerosis. *The American journal of gastroenterology.* 1998 Apr;93(4):640-2.

[19] Ohara H, Nakazawa T, Sano H, Ando T, Okamoto T, Takada H, et al. Systemic extrapancreatic lesions associated with autoimmune pancreatitis. *Pancreas.* 2005 Oct;31(3):232-7.

[20] Nakazawa T, Ohara H, Yamada T, Ando H, Sano H, Kajino S, et al. Atypical primary sclerosing cholangitis cases associated with unusual pancreatitis. *Hepato-gastroenterology.* 2001 May-Jun;48(39):625-30.

[21] Kitagawa S, Zen Y, Harada K, Sasaki M, Sato Y, Minato H, et al. Abundant IgG4-positive plasma cell infiltration characterizes chronic sclerosing sialadenitis (Küttner's tumor). *The American journal of surgical pathology*. 2005 Jun;29(6):783-91.

[22] Yamamoto M, Takahashi H, Ohara M, Suzuki C, Naishiro Y, Yamamoto H, et al. A new conceptualization for Mikulicz's disease as an IgG4-related plasmacytic disease. *Modern rheumatology / the Japan Rheumatism Association*. 2006;16(6):335-40.

[23] Aoki S, Nakazawa T, Ohara H, Sano H, Nakao H, Joh T, et al. Immunohistochemical study of autoimmune pancreatitis using anti-IgG4 antibody and patients' sera. *Histopathology*. 2005 Aug;47(2):147-58.

[24] Zamboni G, Luttges J, Capelli P, Frulloni L, Cavallini G, Pederzoli P, et al. Histopathological features of diagnostic and clinical relevance in autoimmune pancreatitis: a study on 53 resection specimens and 9 biopsy specimens. *Virchows Arch*. 2004 Dec;445(6):552-63.

[25] Notohara K, Burgart LJ, Yadav D, Chari S, Smyrk TC. Idiopathic chronic pancreatitis with periductal lymphoplasmacytic infiltration: clinicopathologic features of 35 cases. *The American journal of surgical pathology*. 2003 Aug;27(8):1119-27.

[26] Hamano H, Kawa S, Ochi Y, Unno H, Shiba N, Wajiki M, et al. Hydronephrosis associated with retroperitoneal fibrosis and sclerosing pancreatitis. *Lancet*. 2002 Apr 20;359(9315):1403-4.

[27] Zen Y, Sawazaki A, Miyayama S, Notsumata K, Tanaka N, Nakanuma Y. A case of retroperitoneal and mediastinal fibrosis exhibiting elevated levels of IgG4 in the absence of sclerosing pancreatitis (autoimmune pancreatitis). *Human pathology*. 2006 Feb;37(2):239-43.

[28] Nakamura A, Funatomi H, Katagiri A, Katayose K, Kitamura K, Seki T, et al. A case of autoimmune pancreatitis complicated with immune thrombocytopenia during maintenance therapy with prednisolone. *Digestive diseases and sciences*. 2003 Oct;48(10):1968-71.

[29] Taniguchi T, Ko M, Seko S, Nishida O, Inoue F, Kobayashi H, et al. Interstitial pneumonia associated with autoimmune pancreatitis. *Gut*. 2004 May;53(5):770; author reply -1.

[30] Uchiyama-Tanaka Y, Mori Y, Kimura T, Sonomura K, Umemura S, Kishimoto N, et al. Acute tubulointerstitial nephritis associated with autoimmune-related pancreatitis. *Am. J. Kidney Dis*. 2004 Mar;43(3):e18-25.

[31] Komatsu K, Hamano H, Ochi Y, Takayama M, Muraki T, Yoshizawa K, et al. High prevalence of hypothyroidism in patients with autoimmune pancreatitis. *Digestive diseases and sciences*. 2005 Jun;50(6):1052-7.

[32] Saegusa H, Momose M, Kawa S, Hamano H, Ochi Y, Takayama M, et al. Hilar and pancreatic gallium-67 accumulation is characteristic feature of autoimmune pancreatitis. *Pancreas*. 2003 Jul;27(1):20-5.

[33] Uchida K, Okazaki K, Konishi Y, Ohana M, Takakuwa H, Hajiro K, et al. Clinical analysis of autoimmune-related pancreatitis. *The American journal of gastroenterology*. 2000 Oct;95(10):2788-94.

[34] Kino-Ohsaki J, Nishimori I, Morita M, Okazaki K, Yamamoto Y, Onishi S, et al. Serum antibodies to carbonic anhydrase I and II in patients with idiopathic chronic pancreatitis and Sjogren's syndrome. *Gastroenterology.* 1996 May;110(5):1579-86.

[35] Okazaki K, Uchida K, Ohana M, Nakase H, Uose S, Inai M, et al. Autoimmune-related pancreatitis is associated with autoantibodies and a Th1/Th2-type cellular immune response. *Gastroenterology.* 2000 Mar;118(3):573-81.

[36] Hamano H, Kawa S, Horiuchi A, Unno H, Furuya N, Akamatsu T, et al. High serum IgG4 concentrations in patients with sclerosing pancreatitis. *The New England journal of medicine.* 2001 Mar 8;344(10):732-8.

[37] Kamisawa T, Funata N, Hayashi Y, Tsuruta K, Okamoto A, Amemiya K, et al. Close relationship between autoimmune pancreatitis and multifocal fibrosclerosis. *Gut.* 2003 May;52(5):683-7.

[38] Nakazawa T, Kobayashi K, Ohara H, Sano H, Ando T, Yamada T, et al. Autoimmune pancreatitis associated with biliary stricture, immune thrombocytopenic purpura and lung fibrosis. *Digestive Endoscopy* 2004;16:262-5.

[39] Nakazawa T, Ohara H, Yamada T, Ando H, Sano H, Kajino S, et al. Atypical primary sclerosing cholangitis cases associated with unusual pancreatitis. *Hepato Gastroenterol* 2001;48:621-6.

[40] Erkelens GW, Vleggaar FP, Lesterhuis W, van Buuren HR, van der Werf SD. Sclerosing pancreato-cholangitis responsive to steroid therapy. *Lancet.* 1999 Jul 3;354(9172):43-4.

[41] Angulo P, Batts KP, Jorgensen RA, LaRusso NA, Lindor KD. Oral budesonide in the treatment of primary sclerosing cholangitis. *The American journal of gastroenterology.* 2000 Sep;95(9):2333-7.

[42] van Hoogstraten HJ, Vleggaar FP, Boland GJ, van Steenbergen W, Griffioen P, Hop WC, et al. Budesonide or prednisone in combination with ursodeoxycholic acid in primary sclerosing cholangitis: a randomized double-blind pilot study. Belgian-Dutch PSC Study Group. *The American journal of gastroenterology.* 2000 Aug;95(8):2015-22.

[43] Kawaguchi K, Koike M, Tsuruta K, Okamoto A, Tabata I, Fujita N. Lymphoplasmacytic sclerosing pancreatitis with cholangitis: a variant of primary sclerosing cholangitis extensively involving pancreas. *Human pathology.* 1991 Apr;22(4):387-95.

[44] Lazaridis KN, Wiesner RH, Porayko MK, Ludwig J , Larusso NF.: Primary sclerosing cholangitis. *Schiff's Diseases of the Liver.* 8th ed.Philadelphia : Lippincott-Raven, 1999:649-78.

[45] Okazaki K, Chiba T. Autoimmune related pancreatitis. *Gut.* 2002 Jul;51(1):1-4.

[46] Loftus EV, Jr., Harewood GC, Loftus CG, Tremaine WJ, Harmsen WS, Zinsmeister AR, et al. PSC-IBD: a unique form of inflammatory bowel disease associated with primary sclerosing cholangitis. *Gut.* 2005 Jan;54(1):91-6.

[47] Sano H, Nakazawa T, Ohara H, et al. Clinicopathological features of inflammatory bowel diseases in patients with primary sclerosing cholangitis [in Japanese]. *Kan Tan Sui.* 2002;45:77–84.

[48] Uchida N, Ezaki T, Fukuma H, Tsutsui K, Kobara H, Matsuoka M, et al. Concomitant colitis associated with primary sclerosing cholangitis. *Journal of gastroenterology*. 2003;38(5):482-7.

[49] Pearson RK, Longnecker DS, Chari ST, Smyrk TC, Okazaki K, Frulloni L, et al. Controversies in clinical pancreatology: autoimmune pancreatitis: does it exist? *Pancreas*. 2003 Jul;27(1):1-13.

[50] Yoshida H, Tanaka S, Nagayama Y, et al. Autoimmune pancreatitis associated with ulcerative colitis [in Japanese]. *J. Gastroenterol Imaging*. 2002;4:66–74.

[51] Epstein O, Chapman RW, Lake-Bakaar G, Foo AY, Rosalki SB, Sherlock S. The pancreas in primary biliary cirrhosis and primary sclerosing cholangitis. *Gastroenterology*. 1982 Dec;83(6):1177-82.

[52] Palmer KR, Cotton PB, Chapman M. Pancreatogram in cholestasis. *Gut*. 1984 Apr;25(4):424-7.

[53] Borkje B, Vetvik K, Odegaard S, Schrumpf E, Larssen TB, Kolmannskog F. Chronic pancreatitis in patients with sclerosing cholangitis and ulcerative colitis. *Scandinavian journal of gastroenterology*. 1985 May;20(4):539-42.

[54] Fausa O, Kolmannskog F, Ritland S. The pancreatic ducts in primary biliary cirrhosis and sclerosing cholangitis. *Scand. J. Gastroenterol. Suppl*. 1985;107:32-5.

[55] Schimanski U, Stiehl A, Stremmel W, Theilmann L. Low prevalence of alterations in the pancreatic duct system in patients with primary sclerosing cholangitis. *Endoscopy*. 1996 May;28(4):346-9.

[56] Takikawa H, Manabe T. Primary sclerosing cholangitis in Japan--analysis of 192 cases. *Journal of gastroenterology*. 1997 Feb;32(1):134-7.

[57] Ishimaru H, Matsuda T, Igarashi R, et al. Primary sclerosing cholangitis associated with the submandibular adenitis, chronic pancreatitis and diabetes mellitus. *Jpn. Arch. Intern. Med.* 1984;31:25–34.

[58] Kyokane K, Ichihara T, Horisawa M, Suzuki N, Ichihara S, Suga S, et al. Successful treatment of primary sclerosing cholangitis with cyclosporine and corticosteroid. *Hepato-gastroenterology*. 1994 Oct;41(5):449-52.

[59] Uehara T, Hamano H, Kawa S, Sano K, Honda T, Ota H. Distinct clinicopathological entity 'autoimmune pancreatitis-associated sclerosing cholangitis'. *Pathology international*. 2005 Jul;55(7):405-11.

[60] Delbet P;Retrecissement du choledoque: Cholecystduodenostomie: *Bull. Mem. Soc. Nat.* 1924;50P:1144-1159.

[61] Wiesner RH, Porayko MK, Larusso NF, et al. Primary sclerosing cholangitis. *Schiff's Diseases of the Liver*. 7th ed.Philadelphia : Lippincott-Raven, 1993:411-426.

[62] Lindor KD, Larusso NF.: Primary sclerosing cholangitis. In; Schiff ER,et al eds. *Schiff's Diseases of the Liver*. 9th ed.Philadelphia : Lippincott WilliamsandWilikins, 2003:673-84.

[63] MacCarty RL, LaRusso NF, Wiesner RH, Ludwig J. Primary sclerosing cholangitis: findings on cholangiography and pancreatography.*Radiology* 1983;149:39-44.

[64] Majoie CB, Reeders JW, Sanders JB, Huibregtse K, Jansen PL. Primary sclerosing cholangitis: a modified classification of cholangiographic findings. *AJR*. 1991 Sep;157(3):495-7.

[65] Craig DA, MacCarty RL, Wiesner RH, Grambsch PM, LaRusso NF. Primary sclerosing cholangitis: value of cholangiography in determining the prognosis. *AJR.* 1991 Nov;157(5):959-64.

[66] Hirano K, Shiratori Y, Komatsu Y, Yamamoto N, Sasahira N, Toda N, et al. Involvement of the biliary system in autoimmune pancreatitis: a follow-up study. *Clin. Gastroenterol. Hepatol.* 2003 Nov;1(6):453-64.

[67] Nishino T, Toki F, Oyama H, Oi I, Kobayashi M, Takasaki K, et al. Biliary tract involvement in autoimmune pancreatitis. *Pancreas.* 2005 Jan;30(1):76-82.

[68] Nakazawa T, Ohara H, Sano H, Aoki S, Kobayashi S, Okamoto T, et al. Cholangiography can discriminate sclerosing cholangitis with autoimmune pancreatitis from primary sclerosing cholangitis. *Gastrointestinal endoscopy.* 2004 Dec;60(6):937-44.

[69] Nakazawa T, Ohara H, Sano H, Ando T, Okamoto T, Takada H, et al. Differential diagnosis of biliary involvement with autoimmune pancreatitis and primary sclerosing cholangitis [in Japanese]. *Kan Tan Sui.* 2005 50(4):635-644.

[70] Kazumori H, Ashizawa N, Moriyama N, Arima N, Hirakawa K, Adachi K, et al. Primary sclerosing pancreatitis and cholangitis. *Int. J. Pancreatol.* 1998 Oct;24(2):123-7.

[71] Kuroiwa T, Suda T, Takahashi T, Hirono H, Natsui M, Motoyama H, et al. Bile duct involvement in a case of autoimmune pancreatitis successfully treated with an oral steroid. *Digestive diseases and sciences.* 2002 Aug;47(8):1810-6.

[72] Hamano H, Kawa S, Uehara T, Ochi Y, Takayama M, Komatsu K, et al. Immunoglobulin G4-related lymphoplasmacytic sclerosing cholangitis that mimics infiltrating hilar cholangiocarcinoma: part of a spectrum of autoimmune pancreatitis? *Gastrointestinal endoscopy.* 2005 Jul;62(1):152-7.

[73] Zen Y, Harada K, Sasaki M, Sato Y, Tsuneyama K, Haratake J, et al. IgG4-related sclerosing cholangitis with and without hepatic inflammatory pseudotumor, and sclerosing pancreatitis-associated sclerosing cholangitis: do they belong to a spectrum of sclerosing pancreatitis? *The American journal of surgical pathology.* 2004 Sep;28(9):1193-203.

[74] Nakazawa T, Ohara H, Sano H, Ando T, Joh T. Schematic classification of sclerosing cholangitis with autoimmune pancreatitis by cholangiography. *Pancreas.* 2006 Mar;32(2):229.

[75] Zen Y, Kitagawa S, Minato H, Kurumaya H, Katayanagi K, Masuda S, et al. IgG4-positive plasma cells in inflammatory pseudotumor (plasma cell granuloma) of the lung. *Human pathology.* 2005 Jul;36(7):710-7.

[76] Zen Y, Kasahara Y, Horita K, Miyayama S, Miura S, Kitagawa S, et al. Inflammatory pseudotumor of the breast in a patient with a high serum IgG4 level: histologic similarity to sclerosing pancreatitis. *The American journal of surgical pathology.* 2005 Feb;29(2):275-8.

[77] Kamisawa T, Okamoto A. Autoimmune pancreatitis: proposal of IgG4-related sclerosing disease. *Journal of gastroenterology.* 2006 Jul;41(7):613-25.

In: Pancreatitis Research Advances
Editor: William C. Langley, pp. 233-258
ISBN: 978-1-60021-883-5

Chapter VII

Chronic Pancreatitis and the Development of Pancreatic Cancer

M. Hermanova[*1], *J. Trna*[2], *P. Dite*[2], *A. Sevcikova*[2], *J. Feit*[1] *and I. Zavrelova*[1]

[1] Department of Pathology, Masaryk University and University Hospital Brno

[2] Department of Gastroenterology, Masaryk University and University Hospital Brno

Abstract

The link between chronic inflammation and the development of cancer has been known for a number of years. Both, hereditary and sporadic forms of chronic pancreatitis represent inflammatory disorders associated with an increased risk of developing pancreatic cancer.

Pancreatic inflammation is associated with production of reactive oxygen species (ROS), cytokine release, and upregulation of pro-inflammatory transcription factors. Mediators of the inflammatory pathways (e.g., NF-κB and COX-2) have been shown to induce genetic damage, cell proliferation and inhibition of apoptosis in pancreas.

The oncogenesis of pancreatic ductal adenocarcinoma is a multistep process characterized by the progression from normal ductal epithelium through the spectrum of PanIN (pancreatic intraepithelial neoplasia) lesions to invasive ductal adenocarcinoma. PanIN lesions harbour a number of well-defined genetic alterations. The progression from normal ductal epithelium through mild to severe dysplasia is characterized by the sequence of genetic changes including activating K-*ras* point mutations, the overexpression of *HER-2/neu*, and the inactivation of *p16, p53, Smad4/DPC4,* and *BRCA2* tumor suppressor genes. PanIN lesions are more frequently present in patients with chronic pancreatitis than in the general population. It has been suggested that

* Corresponding author: Marketa Hermanova, M.D., Ph.D. Department of Pathology, University Hospital Brno, Jihlavska 20. 625 00 Brno. Czech Republic. marherman@post.cz. phone: +420532233635. fax: +420532232005

PanINs represent a possible link between chronic pancreatitis and pancreatic cancer. p16 alterations were demonstrated in a significant number of PanIN lesions in chronic pancreatitis not associated with pancreatic cancer, and were suggested to indicate high risk precursors in chronic pancreatitis that might progress to pancreatic cancer.

Pancreatic inflammation seems to represent an early step in the development of malignancy with genetic alterations occuring as a manifestation of the prolonged inflammatory process. Suppression of inflammation and oxidative damage using a large spectrum of treatment strategies (e.g. anti-cytokine vaccines, inhibitors of pro-inflammatory COX-2 and NF-κB pathways, and anti-oxidants) was suggested as potentially useful for prevention or treatment of pancreatic neoplasia.

Keywords: *chronic pancreatitis, pancreatic cancer, inflammation, carcinogenesis, chemoprevention.*

1. Introduction

The relationship between chronic inflammation and the development of cancer has been recognized for years, and observed in a number of gastrointestinal neoplasms. For example, there is a well established and extensively reported increased risk of colorectal cancer in patients with inflammatory bowel disease involving the colon, and the risk increases with the severity and duration of the disease. Associations between *Helicobacter pylori* infection of the stomach and gastric cancer, chronic viral hepatitis and hepatocellular carcinoma, esophagitis and esophageal carcinoma, liver fluke infection and cholangiocarcinoma, etc. are also well known. Chronic pancreatitis represents a progressive inflammatory disorder of the pancreas leading to irreversibile morphological changes and the permanent impairment of the exocrine and endocrine functions. In the Western world, chronic pancreatitis is usually associated with excessive and long-term alcohol consumption, but also with several other causes. There is still a large group of patients, where the exact cause of this disease is unknown. The term idiopathic pancreatitis is used for these cases. There is no apparent and known underlying cause of the disease in up to 30 % of patients with chronic pancreatitis. Patients with a positive family history suggesting a genetic basis of the disease are excluded from this group of chronic pancreatitis. Hereditary pancreatitis represents a rare disease, which accounts for less than 1 % of all cases of chronic pancreatitis. Several epidemiological studies revealed that both, hereditary and sporadic forms of chronic pancreatitis are associated with an increased risk of developing pancreatic cancer compared with the general population [1-4]. The pathogenesis of cancer is a complex and multifactorial process characterized by the sequence of acquired or inherited genetic alterations.

Recent studies repeatedly demonstrated that similar mediators of chronic inflammatory processes and downstream effectors are present in chronic pancreatitis and pancreatic cancers. Mediators of inflammatory pathways (e.g. cyclooxygenase 2 (COX-2), nuclear factor kappa B (NF-κB), 5-lipooxygenase (5-LOX), interleukin-8 (IL-8) etc.) are known to play an important role in carcinogenesis of pancreatic carcinoma and represent a key link between chronic inflammation and cancer [5-7].

The knowledge of the role of chronic inflammation in the carcinogenesis of pancreatic cancer could lead to the development of new therapeutic strategies for patients with chronic pancreatitis at risk of pancreatic cancer.

2. Risk of Pancreatic Adenocarcinoma in Chronic Pancreatitis

Recent epidemiological studies revealed an increased risk of pancreatic cancer in patients with chronic pancreatitis. Patients with sporadic chronic pancreatitis are 10 - 20 times more likely to develop pancreatic cancer compared to age matched control. The lifetime risk of developing pancreatic cancer in patients with sporadic chronic pancreatitis is estimated to be 1.8 % after 10 years, and 4 % after 20 years, respectively [1-4]. Hereditary pancreatitis represents a rare disease, which accounts for less than 1 % of all cases of chronic pancreatitis, and is caused by the mutation of cationic trypsinogen (*PRSS 1*) gene. Hereditary pancreatitis is defined as an autosomal dominant disease with a penetrance of approximately 80 %. This genetically based disorder is characterized by multiple episodes of acute pancreatitis and a high incidence of pancreatic cancer. Patients suffering from hereditary pancreatitis have an estimated 50- to 70- fold increased relative risk of pancreatic cancer [8]. Recent genetic studies revealed an association between chronic pancreatitis and the serine protease inhibitor Kazal type 1 (*SPINK1*, also called pancreatic secretory trypsin inhibitor; *PST1*) gene, and the cystic fibrosis transmembrane conductance regulator (*CFTR*) gene. Smoking increases the risk of pancreatic cancer in patients with both sporadic and hereditary chronic pancreatitis [9]. Smokers have a 2- to 3-fold risk of pancreatic cancer if compared to non-smokers and the risk remains elevated up to two decades after cessation of smoking. Cigarette smoking is an independent risk factor in alcohol associated and idiopathic pancreatitis, and was reported to accelerate the development and progression of chronic pancreatitis. Tabacco smoking induces chronic inflammation and accelerates the development and progression of chronic pancreatitis independent of etiology. Cigarette smoking is likely to contribute to pancreatic carcinogenesis via the activation of inflammatory response [10].

3. Oncogenesis of Pancreatic Cancer: Current Model of Progression

Pancreatic cancer represents the fifth leading cause of cancer-related death in Western countries, second only to colon cancer among malignancies of the digestive tract. Despite improved diagnostic and therapeutic modalities, pancreatic cancer still has a very poor prognosis. The letality of pancreatic cancer almost equals its incidence and the 5-year survival rate is less than 10 % [11-13]. Pancreatic cancer is usually advanced at the time of presentation and the detection of premalignant pancreatic lesions and earlier detection of malignancy in high-risk patients may improve the clinical outcome of the disease using current treatment modalities. Defining the molecular pathology of premalignant early neoplastic lesions could provide important information for the development of early detection and diagnostic strategies. Characterisations and understanding of the molecular alterations that lead to development of pancreatic cancer is therefore necessary, and could impact on the outcome for patients at risk of pancreatic cancer or already suffering from this disease.

Pancreatic intraepithelial neoplasias (PanINs) are thought to be the most common morphologically distinct precursor lesions of ductal adenocarcinoma of the pancreas [14, 15].

PanIN lesions were defined as neoplastic non-invasive epithelial proliferations in the smaller caliber pancreatic ducts, and were divided into three grades based on the degree of architectural and cytonuclear atypia revealed. Normal epithelium progresses into the PanIN-1A lesion previously described as flat ductal hyperplasia (characterized as a flat lesion composed of tall columnar cells with basally located nuclei and supranuclear vacuole of mucin). PanIN-1B lesion, previously described as ductal papillary hyperplasia, is characterized by a papillary, micropapillary or basally pseudostratified architecture. Cytologically, the morhology is identical to PanIN-1A. Architecture of PanIN-2 is mostly papillary, rarely flat. The lesion shows mild to moderate cytonuclear atypia (formerly termed as ductal papillary hyperplasia with atypia), and progresses to PanIN-3, previously severe ductal dysplasia, atypical hyperplasia or carcinoma in situ. PanIN-3 lesions are thought to be at the highest risk of progressing to invasive carcinoma. The current accepted model of pancreatic cancer progression from normal cuboidal and low columnar ductal epithelium to pancreatic cancer includes the series of these PanIN lesions [16,17]. Recent studies repeatedly demonstrated this process of progression from normal epithelium to cancer through the series of PanINs as a result of genetic aberrations sequence. Increasing histologic grades of PanINs are associated with the accumulation of genetic alterations in cancer-related genes [13,16]. Activation of oncogenes and inactivation of the tumor suppressor genes play a key role in carcinogenesis of pancreatic cancer. Activating point mutations in codon 12 of the K-*ras* oncogene have been reported in 70 to 100 % pancreatic carcinomas studied [18,19], and were also demonstrated in PanIN lesions associated with invasive adenocarcinoma suggesting true neoplastic origin of these lesions [20,21]. Inactivation of tumor suppressor gene *p53* was reported in 50-75 % of pancreatic adenocarcinomas. Loss of the function of the *CDKN2A* tumor suppressor gene, which encodes p16^{INK4a}, occurs in up to 95 % of pancreatic adenocarcinoma [22,23], and alterations of p16^{INK4a} were demonstrated in noninvasive precursor lesions [24]. Another tumor suppressor gene *SMAD4/DPC4* is inactivated in approximately 50 % of pancreatic cancers, compared to <10 % in other tumor types [25]. *SMAD4* inactivation represents a late event in oncogenesis of pancreatic cancer. There are no alterations of Smad4 expression revealed in low-grade PanIN lesions, and there is loss of Smad4 expression in 30-40 % of high grade PanIN-3 lesions. Alterations of *BRCA2* gene, the gene for the transforming growth factor (TGF)-β receptor, *MKK4* and the *LKB1/STK11* gene were demonstrated less frequently in pancreatic cancer [26].

4. PanIN Lesions in Chronic Pancreatitis

PanIN lesions are more frequently present in patients with chronic pancreatitis than in the general population [27,28]. The study of Volkholz with colleagues demonstrated the presence of lesions today called PanINs in 40 % of pancreata with chronic pancreatitis. Pancreatic inflammation seems to represent an early step in the development of malignancy with genetic alterations occuring as a manifestation of the prolonged inflammatory process. Some of the above described genetic alterations have been previously identified in chronic pancreatitis tissues, but at much lower frequency. Activating point mutations in codon 12 of K-*ras* oncogene were identified in 0-40 % of patients suffering from chronic pancreatitis among the studies, and these mutations were demonstrated in 4.4 % of PanINs associated with chronic pancreatitis. The mutations were identified in cigarette smoking patients with chronic pancreatitis, and the frequency of these mutations was similar to that of normal pancreas from smokers without pancreatitis [21, 29, 30]. Similarly, alterations of *p53* tumor suppressor gene expression are very rare in chronic pancreatitis associated duct lesions [21].

The $p16^{INK4a}$ tumor suppressor gene is abrogated in almost all infiltrating ductal adenocarcinoma of the pancreas. The $p16^{INK4a}$ tumor suppressor gene is inactivated in 40 % of pancreatic cancers by homozygous deletions, in 40 % by an intragenic mutation coupled with loss of the second allele, and in 15-20 % by hypermethylation of the p16 promoter [31]. Moreover, the rate of $p16^{INK4a}$ inactivations increases with increasing PanIN grade. Immunohistochemical study revealed the loss of p16 immunostaining in 30 % of PanIN-1 lesions, in 55 % of PanIN-2 lesions, and in 70 % of PanIN-3 lesions associated with invasive pancreatic adenocarcinoma. However, $\mathrm{p16}^{\mathrm{INK4a}}$ alteration was also demonstrated in significant number of PanINs in chronic pancreatitis not associated with pancreatic cancer [32,33]. Gerdes [33] revealed the loss of p16 expression in 40 % of PanIN lesions identified within chronic pancreatitis specimens. But, none of non-PanIN tissues showed the loss of p16 expression. The mutational analysis of $p16^{INK4a}$ gene was performed and no mutations were revealed. Inactivating hypermethylation of $p16^{INK4a}$ promoter was identified in two of the ten specimens with PanIN lesions. Therefore, the $p16^{INK4a}$ alterations, especially inactivating promoter hypermethylations, were for the first suggested to be possible indicators of high-risk precursors in chronic pancreatitis that might progress to invasive cancer. The second study of Rosty et al. [32] showed loss of p16 expression in 0 % of PanIN1A, 11 % of PanIN-1B, 16 % of PanIN-2, and 40 % of PanIN-3 lesions. All of the PanINs analyzed within this study showed normal *SMAD4/DPC4* expression. The expressions of p16 and Smad4 were determined by immunohistochemistry, the study supported the findings of Gerdes et al., and suggested that $p16^{INK4a}$ alterations may contribute to the predisposition of patiens with chronic pancreatitis to develop invasive pancreatic ductal adenocarcinoma. $p16^{INK4a}$ might represent an attractive genetic marker for the detection of high risk precursor lesions in the group of patients with chronic pancreatitis.

Proliferative activity in PanINs of chronic pancreatitis resection specimen was also studied, and direct correlation between the *Ki-67* labeling index and the grade of dysplasia was found [34]. These results correlate with known genetic alterations found in chronic pancreatitis, especially with the above described $p16^{INK4a}$ inactivation. Cyclin dependent kinase $\mathrm{p16}^{\mathrm{INK4a}}$ acts as a key regulator cell cycle progression at the G1/S phase transition point. Thus, inactivation of $p16^{INK4a}$ should contribute to increased proliferative acitivity [35]. Moreover, the results supported the currently accepted pancreatic progression model of carcinogenesis, and suggested these markers to be possible efficient tools for an identification of a high-risk lesion.

5. Role of Pancreatic Fibrosis: Fibrogenesis in Chronic Pancreatitis and Pancreatic Cancer Stroma

Both chronic pancreatitis and pancreatic cancer are accompanied by fibrogenesis with a formation of fibrotic stroma. Progressive replacement of pancreatic tissue with connective tissue results in an exocrine and endocrine insufficiency of the gland. In chronic pancreatitis, the dense fibrotic stroma contains inflammatory cells, proliferating myofibroblasts, and cytokines. Within the stromal elements, the macrophages and other inflammatory cells are the main effectors of chronic inflammation and initiate the process of fibrogenesis in chronic pancreatitis. These cells and mediators such as transforming growth factor-β1 (TGF-β1), fibroblast growth factor-β (FGF-β), platelet derived growth factor (PDGF), tumor necrosis factor-α (TNF-α), IL-1, and IL-6 were shown to be responsible for the transformation of pancreatic stellate cells into the proliferating myofibroblasts [36,37], which produce the proteins of extracellular matrix such as collagen type I, collagen type III, and fibronectin.

In pancreatic cancer, the desmoplastic reaction forms fibrotic tumor stroma that provides a number of inflammatory mediators and growth factors, which contribute to tumor growth, invasiveness of tumors and metastases. The fibrotic stroma in chronic pancreatitis strongly resembles pancreatic cancer stroma histologically, but differences between chronic pancreatitis and pancreatic cancer fibrotic stroma gene expression profiles were reported. Patterns of gene expression within the fibrosis in chronic pancreatitis tissue and pancreatic cancer stroma were studied and increased expressions of matrix metalloproteinase 2 (MMP-2), a proinvasive factor for tumor cells, and of epidermal growth factor (EGF) were revealed in pancreatic cancer stroma when compared with stromal cells in chronic pancreatitis [5]. Additionally, the expression of epidermal growth factor receptor (EGFR) was higher in tumor cells than in the pancreatic cancer stroma suggesting the relationship between tumor stroma and adjacent structures of carcinoma. EGF produced within the pancreatic cancer stroma may activate the signaling pathway downstream from EGFR on the surface of the tumor cells. Fibrotic stroma that results from chronic inflammation was shown as a possible source of growth factors that can facilitate the tumor progression and invasiveness. Moreover, NF-κB was demonstrated to increase the MMP-2 expression after stimulation with reactive oxygen species (ROS), [38]. Interactions between NF-κB and MMP-2 also support the important role of inflammation with fibrotic stroma formation in pancreatic cancer development.

6. Inflammatory Mechanisms Involved in Carcinogenesis of Pancreatic Cancer

6.1. Nuclear Factor Kappa B

Nuclear factor kappa B (NF-κB) represents an evolutionally conserved family of ubiquitously expressed transcription factors. Expression of NF- κB is activated by various stimuli such as reactive oxygen intermediates, hypoxia, cytokines, bacterial or viral products,

UV radiation and many others. The family comprises of five defined members NF-κB1 (p50), NF-κB2 (p52), Rel A (p65), c-Rel and RelB. Members of the family share Rel Homology Domain (RHD) in their structures. RHD is responsible for NF-κB dimerisation (most frequently heterodimerisation of p65 and p50), interactions with NF-κB inhibitory proteins comprising I-κB family, and DNA-binding. These interactions result in the sequestration of NF-κB in the cytoplasm of the cells, which is followed by a nuclear translocation of the activated NF-κB and activation of a number of genes with subsequent expression of pro-inflammatory and pro-oncogenic molecules such as inducible nitric oxide (iNOS), COX-2, cyclin D1, IL-8 and others (Figure 1). Some stimulators of NF-κB activations, such as IL-1 and TNF-α, are up-regulated by NF-κB activation, suggesting an autoregulatory loop that can potentiate the inflammatory response.

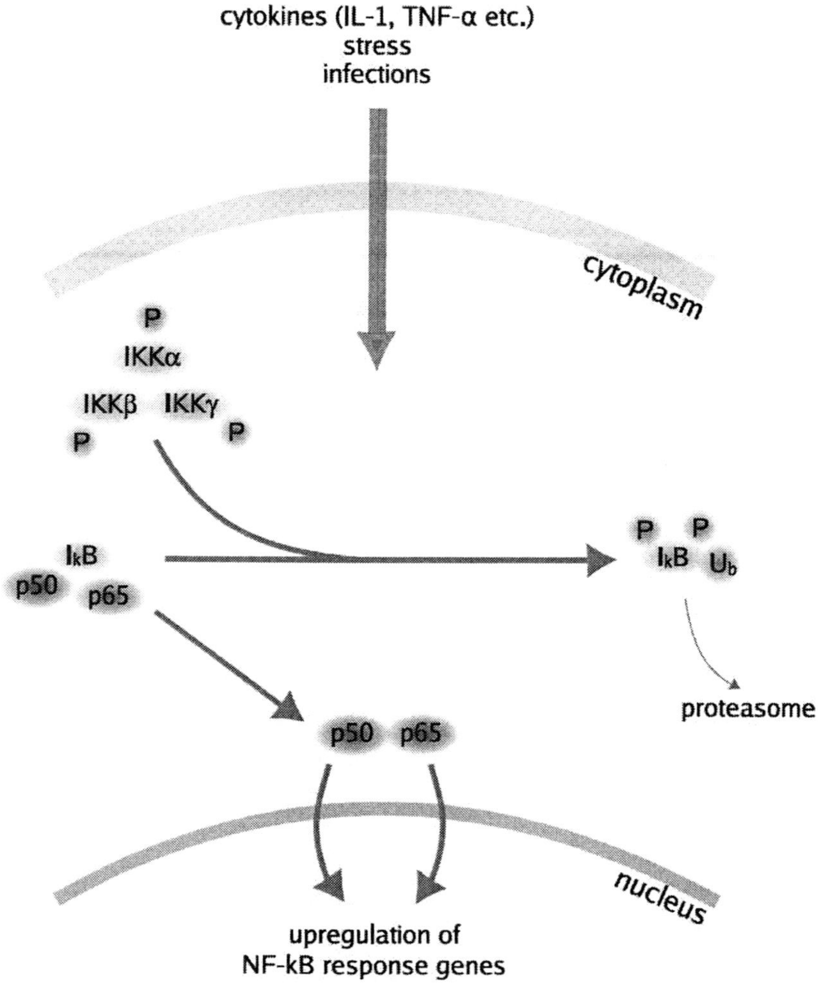

Figure 1. The NF- κB pathway. In response to various stimuli (such as cytokines, stress, infections), IKK kinases phosporylate inhibitory proteins known as IκB, which results in their ubiquitination and degradation by proteasome. The degradation of IκB results in the translocation of NF- κB dimer (the most frequent combination of p50/p65) into the nucleus where it acts as a transcription factor which activates the expression of specific genes involved in the processes of inflammation and carcinogenesis.

Upregulation and constitutive activation of NF-κB was described in several human malignancies including malignancies of gastrointestinal tract such as colorectal carcinoma and hepatocellular carcinoma [39]. Upregulation and constitutive activation of NF-κB has been revealed in a number of different human pancreatic cancer cell lines (e.g. BxPC-3, PANC-1, MiaPaCa2), [40-42]. NF-κB was repeatedly shown to promote pancreatic cell growth via inhibition of apoptosis [40]. NF-κB is activated in more than two third of human pancreatic cancers. Suppression of NF-κB activity is followed by the restoration of pancreatic cell kinetics, mainly by normalisation of the suppressed apoptosis in pancreatic cancer [43].

Moreover, the NF-κB is able to induce the expression of the mitogenic cyclin D1, a regulatory protein of cell cycle, by which NF-κB can promote pancreatic cancer growth [44]. Cyclin D1 overexpression occurs in up to 68 % of pancreatic cancer, where it is associated with poor clinical outcome [45], and was described also in premalignant ductal lesions. The study of Farrow et al. revealed the increased expression of another activator of cell cycle progression, cyclin E1 in pancreatic adenocarcinoma tumor cells but also in ductal cells of chronic pancreatitis specimens compared with normal pancreatic cells. Additionally, expression of the cyclin dependent kinase (cdk) inhibitor $p27^{kip1}$ was highest in chronic pancreatitis ductal cells and almost absent in normal pancreatic cells and tumor cells of pancreatic adenocarcinoma. Coexpression of cyclin E1 and $p27^{kip1}$ may prevent cyclin E1-induced proliferation in chronic pancreatitis ductal cells, but high expression of cyclin E1 and reduced expression of $p27^{kip1}$ present in pancreatic carcinoma favor cell proliferation [5].

Proangiogenic potential of NF-κB related to the IL-8 is discussed bellow. NF-κB and IL-8 have been shown to be implicated in increasing angiogenic potential of pancreatic cancer cells via up-regulation of the proangiogenic vascular endothelial growth factor (VEGF), [5,46,47]. Xiong et al. showed that NF-κB activity blockade significantly inhibited the *in vitro* and *in vivo* expressions of the major proangiogenic molecules VEGF and IL-8 and decreased tumor vascular formation showing that the supressed tumorigenicity by NF-κB blockade is due to impaired angiogenic potential of the tumor cells [47].

6.2. Cyclooxygenases

Prostaglandin H2 synthase – cyclooxygenase (COX) is an enzyme, which is involved in the conversion of arachidonic acid to prostaglandins (Figure 2). Two COX isoformes, COX-1 and COX-2, have been identified to date. COX-1 is constitutively expressed in many tissues, and is involved in prostaglandin synthesis under physiological conditions. The second isoform, COX-2, is not constitutively expressed under physiological conditions, but its expression is induced by various stimuli. Growth factors, cytokines (e.g. IL-1, TNF-α) and other mediators of inflammation are known inductors of COX-2 expression. Several reports demonstrated the key role of COX-2 in pathological processes, such as inflammation and carcinogenesis. Increased expression of COX-2 was observed in variety of tumors: in carcinomas of colon, lung, breast, oesophagus, bladder, and prostate [48]. Recent studies repeatedly described an increased expression of COX-2 in pancreatic carcinomas. Increased expression of COX-2 was demonstrated in 56 - 90 % of pancreatic adenocarcinomas among the studies [49]. The mechanism by which COX-2 promotes pancreatic tumor cell growth is not completely clear. Several studies suggested potential involvement of COX-2 pathwas in the regulation of tumor associated angiogenesis and cell growth in pancreatic cancer. COX-2 was demonstrated to inhibite apoptosis, promote cell proliferation and to induce the expression of VEGF [50-53].

Up-regulation and increased expression of COX-2 in duct epithelium was demonstrated in tissues of patients with chronic pancreatitis. Moreover, significant correlation between the COX-2 expression in chronic pancreatitis tissues and frequency of acute attacks of pancreatitis was revealed, supporting the hypothesis that COX-2 is involved in inflammatory response in chronic pancreatitis and in the progression of this chronic inflammatory disease [54] . The study of Koliopanos et al. revealed intense immunostaining of ductal cells in tissues of both early and advanced-stage chronic pancreatitis.

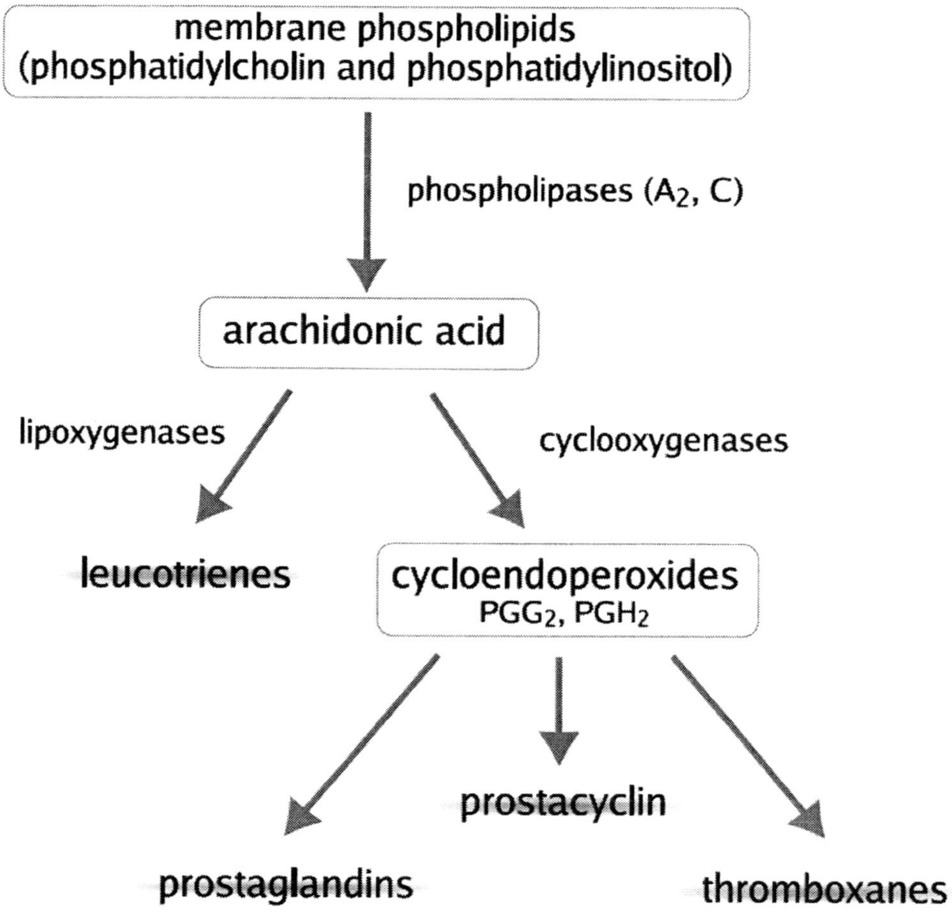

Figure 2. The lipooxygenase and cyclooxygenase pathway. Membrane phospolipids are converted to arachidonic acid through the action of phospolipases, which is further metabolised through cyclooxygenase and lipooxygenase pathways. The cyclooxygenases convert the arachidonic acid to unstable cylcloendoperoxides, which are converted to prostaglandins, prostacyclin and thromboxanes. The lipoxygenases metabolise arachidonic acid through hydroperoxyeicosatetraenoic acids (HPETEs) to leukotrienes.

Additionally, the islet cells displayed strong immunopositivity for COX-2 in early stages of chronic pancreatitis, whereas the islets in advanced-stage chronic pancreatitis displayed a variable COX-2 immunostaining, which was associated with the distribution of insulin-positive cells and with the clinical diabetes mellitus status. COX-2 immunopositivity in pancreatic islet cells was decreased or absent in diabetic patients. These findings again supported the role of COX-2 in the pathogenesis of exocrine and endocrine damage in chronic panreatitis [55]. Albazas et al. supported the previously suggested [54,55] constitutive expression of COX-2 in a population of islet cells, probably B-cells [56]. However, in duct epithelium, the increased immunostaining in chronic pancreatitis did not reach the statistical significance compared with the duct epithelium of a normal pancreas. Two studies of Maitra and Albazaz evaluated the COX-2 expression in premalignant PanIN lesions of pancreatic resection specimen. Expression of COX-2 in PanIN lesions in chronic pancreatitis was not studied separately within these studies [56,57]. They demonstrated the increased expression of COX-2 in PanINs if compared to expressions in normal ducts, and showed the significant correlation between the level of COX-2 expression and the severity of the PanIN lesion. A significant increase of COX-2 expression was shown between normal ducts and PanINs, as well as between low grade (1A and 1B) and high grade (2 and 3) PanINs. They supported the possible role of COX-2 in carcinogenesis of pancreatic ductal adenocarcinoma. It has been suggested that PanINs represent the possible link between chronic pancreatitis and pancreatic cancer and COX-2 may represent the possible therapeutic target for potential chemoprevention in patients with chronic pancreatitis and pancreatic ductal adenocarcinoma using selective COX-2 inhibitors [56, 57].

6.3. Lipooxygenases

The family of lipooxygenases (LOX) comprises of four enzymes, 5-LOX, 8-LOX, 12-LOX, and 15-LOX, nomenclature of which is dependent on their ability to insert oxygen at carbon 5, 8, 12 and 15, respectively, of the arachidonic acid molecules. Hydroperoxyeicosatetraenoic acids (HPETEs) represent the products of this conversion that are further metabolised to form leukotrienes (LT), (Figure 2). The 5-LOX pathway was suggested to play an important role in pancreatic carcinogenesis. 5-HPETE and LTB4, which represent products and biological mediators of 5-LOX, were shown to promote pancreatic cancer cell growth [58], whereas 5-LOX inhibitors and LTB4 receptors antagonists inhibit pancreatic cancer cell growth *in vivo* and *in vitro* by inducing apoptosis through the mitochondrial pathway [59]. 5-LOX overexpression was reported in a significant number of human pancreatic adenocarcinomas with intense immunostaining in cancer cells, and in ductal and islet cells in pancreatic tissues adjacent to the structures of adenocarcinomas. Strong immunostaining was also observed in a significant proportion of ductal cells of chronic pancreatitis specimens, but not in ducts of normal tissue obtained from multiorgan donors [60]. 5-LOX was found to be expressed in all grades of human pancreatic intraepithelial neoplastic lesions. The strong immunostaining was observed in more than 90 % of the ductal cells in all grades of PanIN lesions [61]. There was no correlation between the intensity of immunostaining and the grade of PanIN lesion. The 5-LOX expression was shown in PanIN lesions of both, chronic pancreatitis and pancreatic cancer specimens. These results were supported by experiments in two animal models of pancreatic adenocarcinoma, *N*-nitrosobis(2-oxopropyl)amine (BOP)-treated hamsters and EL-Kras transgenic mice. Marked expreession of 5-LOX was observed in all PanIN lesions obtained from these animal models [61].

An intense immunostaining of islet cells was identified in a significant proportion of pancreatic specimens, all from patiens with pancreatic adenocarcinoma. Islets from normal pancreas or chronic pancreatitis were not stained. Lipooxygenase metabolites also influence insulin secretion. The observation of 5-LOX upregulation in islets adjacent to the structures of pancreatic cancer may bring important information for the understanding of the relationship between pancreatic cancer and diabetes [60].

The reported findings brought the evidence that 5-LOX play an important role in development of pancreatic adenocarcinoma. 5-LOX activation seems to represent a very early event in carcinogenesis of pancreatic cancer. 5-LOX overexpression was observed markedly up-regulated in almost all low grade PanIN lesions, suggesting a 5-LOX up-regulation to be an earlier event when compared to COX-2 up-regulation. 5-LOX up-regulation was observed in PanIN lesions of chronic pancreatitis and pancreatic adenocarcinoma specimens, suggesting that both group of patients could benefit from potential chemopreventive therapy.

6.4. Nitric Oxide Synthases

Nitric oxide (NO) is a free radical and an important mediator of inflammation and carcinogenesis [62, 63]. The nitric oxide synthases (NOS) are a group of enzymes resposible for the conversion of *L*-arginin and molecular oxygen to NO and *L*-citrulline. There are three isoforms of NOS. Neuronal NOS (nNOS or NOS1) and endothelial NOS (eNOS or NOS3) are expressed constitutively, and produce low amounts of NO involved in regulation of some vascular functions and neurotransmission. Inducible nitric oxide synthase (iNOS or NOS2) uses oxidative stress of NO (a free radical) to be used by macrophages in immune defence [64]. However, iNOS is also expressed in certain types of cancer cells. Its role in carcinogenesis is not fully understood, but sustained induction of iNOS in chronic inflammation may be mutagenic, through NO-mediated DNA damage or hindering DNA repair [65]. iNOS produces NO, which was shown to be involved in the regulation of interleukin 8 (IL-8) expression, and its contribution to the progression of human pancreatic cancer was suggested [66]. NO was demonstrated to enhance COX activity (COX-1 and COX-2) and it was suggested that in conditions in which both NOS and COX systems are present, there is an NO-mediated increased production of proinflammatory prostaglandins [67]. The data suggested direct interactions between NO and COX causing an increase in the enzymatic activity of COX. Using immunohistochemistry or Western blotting, a significant proportion of pancreatic adenocarcinoma displayed expression of iNOS [68, 69]. Surprisingly, NO induced a G1-arrest followed by apoptosis was demonstrated in pancreatic carcinoma cell lines [70]. It was suggested, that the generation of high levels of NO with potential induction of endogenous reactive nitrogene intermediates might contribute to the induction of apoptosis and tumor growth inhibition [71]. Moreover, the study of Wang et al.

showed that low levels of iNOS and NO are associated with higher metastatic potential, whereas high levels are not, showing the double-edged roles of nitric oxide production in carcinogenesis of pancreatic cancer [72].

6.5. Cytokines

Endogeneous inflammatory cytokines are aberrantly produced in many malignances and serve as autocrine growth factors or as indicators of immune response to the tumors. Increased levels of IL-6, IL-8, IL-10, IL-1, and tumor necrosis factor α (TNF- α) have also been reported in pancreatic cancer and have been shown to be implicated in diverse processes that are relevant to pancreatic carcinoma, including cachexia, asthenia, and tumor growth [73,74]. IL-1 was suggested to be a growth factor for pancreatic carcinoma, but its effects seem to be balanced by the presence of a specific receptor antagonists (IL-1RA). The poor clinical outcome of some patiens might be explained by low levels of IL-1RA [73]. Recent studies repeatedly suggested that IL-6 is involved in the manifestations of pancreatic carcinoma. The correlation between high levels of IL-6 and poor performance status was observed, and IL-6 was suggested to be an independent prognostic factor for poor survival in pancreatic cancer. IL-10 may also act as an autocrine growth factor and high levels of this cytokine were also correlated with poor survival, poor performance status and advanced disease stage [73]. In addition to its inflammatory role, IL-8 represents a chemokine that may stimulate tumor growth directly through its proangiogenic effect, and overexpression of IL-8 was demonstrated in about 70 % of human pancreatic cancer cell lines [46]. Based on gene array analyses, expression of IL-8 was observed to be more than 9-fold in the cells isolated from chronic pancreatitis when compared with normal pancreatic tissue. Additionally, gene array analysis demonstrated decreased expression of IκB (an inhibitor of NF-κB) in chronic pancreatitis ductal cell compared with ducts of normal pancreatic tissue supporting the posibility of the activation of NF-κB in chronic pancreatitis [5]. NF-κB activation requires the expression of its subunits and kinases allowing the translocation of NF-κB to the nucleus followed by induction of transcription of pro-inflammatory and oncogenic factors. Increased immunostaining of both the p50 NF-κB subunit and IKKα kinase (a protein that allows activation of NF-κB) was demonstrated in chronic pancreatitis and pancreatic cancer; in contrast with minimal to no immunostaining identified in normal pancreas [5]. These results supported the concept that a common pathway for pancreatic cancer development may be through a chronic inflammatory process (Figure 3).

The study of Duell et al. suggested that polymorphisms in some cytokine/chemokine genes are associated with having a history of pancreatitis, particularly as a possible early manifestation of pancreatic cancer. These genes may be important determinants of pancreatic cancer in the presence of pancreatitis. This study represents the first study evaluating the genetic variation in cytokines and chemokines in relation to inflammation and the risk of pancreatic cancer [74].

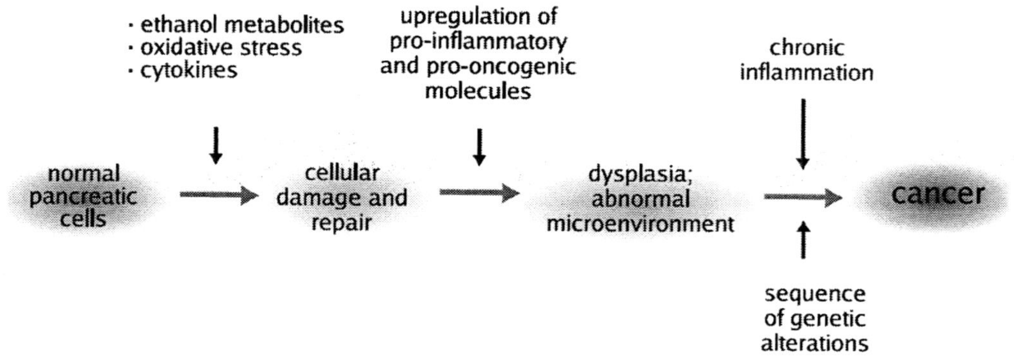

Figure 3. Chronic pancreatitis and pancreatic cancer: proposed mechanisms between inflammation and neoplasia. Continuous cellular damage and repair with increased cell turnover and increased probability of genetic damage may contribute to malignant transformation of the cells. The development of the abnormal microenvironment represented by stromal elements play also a key role in this transformation.

6.6. Reactive Oxygene Species and DNA Damage

Oxidative stress contributes to the pathogenesis of chronic pancreatitis. Chronic inflammatory processes produce an excess of reactive oxygen species (ROS), reactive nitrogen oxide species (RNOS) and DNA-reactive aldehydes from lipid peroxidation (LPO), such as *trans*-4hydroxy-2-nonenal (HNE) and malondialdehyde (MDA). Its genotoxic and mutagenic effect was extensively studied. Oxidative and LPO-derived DNA damage were suggested to play a key role in the development of human cancers, especially those types that have an inflammatory component in their etiopathogenesis. Up-regulations of oxidative stress response enzymes, such as iNOS, COX-2, and LOX, were shown to lead to the overproduction of ROS, RNOS and etheno-DNA adducts in animal models [75]. Up-regulations of these enzymes led not only to direct stimulation of cell growth, but also to an overproduction and accumulation of LPO-derived DNA damage [76]. Increased oxidative stress and LPO have been reported in chronic pancreatitis. In the pancreas of chronic pancreatitis patients, increased levels of etheno-DNA adducts were found. Promutagenic etheno-DNA adducts were shown to be generated as a consequence of chronic inflammation not only in the tissues of chronic pancreatitis patients but also in tissues of patients suffering from Crohn´s disease and ulcerative colitis. Etheno-DNA adducts were suggested to be a driving force of malignancy in cancer-prone inflammatory diseases [77]. Elevated levels of oxidative DNA adducts and MDA were observed in human pancreatic tumor tissue [78], and these findings supported the concept of the role of oxidative stress in the development of pancreatic cancer.

7. Chemoprevention of Pancreatic Cancer – Potential Treatment Strategies

Carcinogenesis of pancreatic cancer, closely related to chronic pancreatitis, is a multistep process characterized by many genetic and epigenetic changes. Multiple functional pathways are involved in this progression to cancer. Some of them may represent ideal targets for chemoprevention and/or pancreatic cancer treatment. Novel treatment strategies directed at the inflammatory mechanisms that may be involved in carcinogenesis of pancreatic cancer are discussed.

7.1. Targeting NF-κB

There are several possible approaches to inhibit the NF-κB signaling pathway. Salicylates and corticosteroids are known to inhibit the function of NF-κB non-specifically. More specific potential treatment strategies include proteasome inhibitors, inhibitors of IκB ubiquitin ligase, gene transfers of of IκB superrepressors, the blockade of NF-κB transcription using antisense oligonucleotides, delivery of IKK inhibitors etc. Anti-oxidants were also suggested since ROS are known to activate NF-κB [79].

Sodium salicylates inhibited NF-κB activation, enhanced TNF-α induced apoptosis [80], and decreased proliferation and induced G1 cell cycle arrest in human pancreatic cancer cell lines [81]. Aspirin and sodium salicylate inhibited the activity of IKKβ that is required to activate the NF-κB *in vitro* and *in vivo* [82]. Sulindac, a NSAID agent that is related both structurally and pharmacologically to indomethacin displayed growth inhibitory and anti-inflammatory properties, in part due to its ability to decrease prostaglandin synthesis by the inhibiting the activity of COXs. Moreover, sulindac mediated decrease of IKKβ activity was demonstrated [83]. Another potent inhibitor of NF-κB, sulfasalazine, which is commonly used as an anti-inflammatory agent, sensitizes pancreatic cancer cells to anti cancer drugs, in particular to etoposide *in vivo* by inhibition of NF-κB [84]. Glucocorticoids, as a part of their non-specific effect, induce synthesis of the NF-κB inhibitor IκBα and therefore limit the activation of NF-κB [85]. NF-κB essential modulator IKKγ (NEMO/ IKKγ) plays a key role in the activation of the NF-κB pathway in response to proinflammatory stimuli. Targeting oligomerization state of the NEMO proteins using NEMO-binding domain peptides represents a promising chemopreventive strategy [86]. The activation of NF-κB is controlled by proteasome-mediated degradation of its endogeneous polypeptide inhibitor IκBα. The effect of the proteasome inhibitors (e.g. PS-341 – Bortezomib/Velcade) was studied and growth inhibition of human pancreatic tumors via direct effects on tumor cells and indirect effects on the tumor vasculature was observed [87].

In many aspects, NF-κB represents a highly promising therapeutic target for the chemoprevention of pancreatic cancer but future studies are necessary for better understanding of the safety and clinical efficacy of these possible novel therapeutic strategies.

7.2. Targeting Cyclooxygenase-2

Up-regulation of COX-2 has been demonstrated in pancreatic cancer and premalignant lesions as well. Increasing expression of COX-2 demonstrated in PanIN lesions od chronic pancreatitis and tissue adjacent to pancreatic cancer is an important finding, since it suggests that COX-2 could represent a potential chemopreventive target at a non-invasive stage of pancreatic carcinogenesis, especially in chronic pancreatitis. COX-2 inhibition may also represent a feasible treatment strategy in patients with additional risk factors for pancreatic cancer such as smoking and diabetes. Recent studies demonstrated an inverse correlation between incidence of colon cancer and the use of non-steroidal anti-inflammatory drugs (NSAIDs), [88]. NSAIDs are widely used therapeutic agents effect of which is primarily achieved through COX inhibition. NSAIDs are either nonselective, affecting both COX isoforms (e.g. aspirin, ibuprofen, diclofenac) or selective, targeting only COX-2 (e.g. sulindac, celecoxib, rofecoxib). COX-2 is considered to be one of the downstream mediators of NF-κB, and COX-2 expression is regulated, in part by NF-κB. Thus, inhibition of NF-κB may also reduce COX-2 activity.

Conflicting results have been obtained from studies that have examined the relationship between NSAIDs use and the incidence of pancreatic cancer. The study of Anderson and colleagues, which included 28.256 participants, demonstrated that women who used aspirin had a 43 % lower risk of pancreatic cancer compared with those who did not use aspirin. Furthermore, the association was dose dependent, and women who took aspirin 2-5 times a week had a 53 % lower risk, and those who took aspirin 6 or more times a week had 60 % lower risk of pancreatic cancer when compared with women who never took aspirin [89]. Other studies showed no decreased risk of pancreatic cancer in association with aspirin use [90], and the study of Schernhammer and colleagues suggested an increased risk of pancreatic cancer in women with long-term regular use of aspirin [91]. Meta-analysis summarizing the data from several epidemiological studies did not support these findings and demonstrated no association between the use of aspirin or NSAIDs and the risk of pancreatic cancer [92]. Studies evaluating the risk of pancreatic cancer in chronic pancreatitis patients in a relationship to COX inhibitors use are not available. However, decreased incidence of pancreatic cancer was demonstrated in animal models after the administration of both non-selective and selective COX-inhibitors [93, 94].

Focused on molecular targeting therapy for pancreatic cancer, recent studies have shown the inhibition of of cell growth in both COX-2 positive and COX-2 negative pancreatic tumor cell lines *in vivo* and *in vitro* using both NSAIDs and COX-2 selective inhibitors [95-97]. However, the inhibition was significantly greater in COX-2 upregulated pancreatic cancer cell lines. Downregulation of vascular endothelial growth factor expression and reduction of angiogenesis and metastasis was achieved through the treatment of pancreatic cancer cells with selective COX-2 inhibitor celecoxib [98]. The presented data have indicated an antiproliferative, antiangiogenic, and proapoptotic effect of COX inhibitors and suggested that COX-2 may become a promising chemotherapeutic target for chemoprevention and the treatment of pancreatic cancer [95-98].

7.3. Targeting 5-Lipooxygenase

Marked expression of 5-LOX has been demonstrated in pancreatic adenocarcinomas and in all grades of PanIN lesions from chronic pancreatitis and pancreatic cancer tissues [60,61]. Expression of 5-LOX was already demonstrated in low-grade PanIN lesions and up-regulation of 5-LOX seems to be an earlier event when compared with expression of COX-2. Moreover, no difference in immunostaining intensity was evident between the different grades of PanIN lesions and expression of 5-LOX seems to be consistent in all patients [60]. Therefore, 5-LOX was suggested to be a potential target for chemoprevention of pancreatic cancer. Both COX-2 and 5-LOX enzymes are involved in arachidonic acid pathway and dual inhibitors of COX-2 and 5- LOX such as licofelone were suggested as a potential effective chemopreventive agent [99,100].

Intracellular tyrosine kinases, MEK/ERK and PI3 kinase/AKT pathways were reported to be involved in 5-HETE (5-LOX metabolite) stimulated pancreatic cancer cell proliferation [101,102]. It was demonstrated that blockade of the 5-LOX pathway of arachidonic acid metabolism pathway inhibits pancreatic cancer cell proliferation and also induces apoptosis [102,103]. In human pancreatic cancer xenografts, expressions of antiapoptotic proteins Bcl-2 and Mcl-1 were significantly decreased after LOX inhibitors treatment while the levels of pro-apoptotic protein bax was increased [103]. These results suggested the LOX inhibitors are also likely to be valuable also for molecular targeting therapy of pancreatic cancer.

7.4. The Role of Nitric Oxide in Chemoprevention

Nitric oxide (NO) is a free radical, which is produced by NO synthase (NOS), and required for many physiological functions. However, sustained induction of the iNOS in chronic inflammation may be mutagenic, and potentially carcinogenic [65]. The role of NO in stimulation of tumor growth and metastasis may also be triggered by activation of COX-2 as discussed above [67]. Low levels of iNOS and NO were reported to be associated with higher metastatic potential of pancreatic cancer, whereas high levels were not, suggesting the double-edged roles of NO production in pancreatic carcinogenesis [72]. Additionaly, high levels of NO were demonstrated to have a pro-apoptotic role and induce G1 arrest [71]. These observations have led to a theory that the combination of COX inhibitors and the donation of NO could be followed by the inhibition of cell proliferation and induction of apoptosis. Nitric-oxide-donating NSAIDs were suggested as potential chemopreventive agents against pancreatic cancer. In animal model of pancretic cancer (BOP-treated hamsters), nitric oxide donating aspirin (NO-ASA) reduced the incidence and multiplicity of pancreatic cancer. NO-ASA arrested the transition from PanIN2 to PanIN3 lesion and carcinoma, significantly decreased the proliferation/apoptosis ratio and suppressed the activation of NF-κB throughout PanIN lesions and carcinomas, most significantly in PanIN1B and PanIN2 lesions. The COX-2 expression was significantly decreased in PanIN3 lesions and carcinomas after the treatment with NO-ASA [104]. These results showed that NO-ASA profoundly prevented pancreatic cancer and modulated multiple molecular targets in this animal model whereas conventional NSAIDs had no such effects. NO-ASA also inhibited the growth also of colon, prostate, lung, skin, leukaemia and breast cancer cells, and was shown to be more potent than traditional ASA [105]. NO-donating NSAIDs seem to be a highly promising agent for the chemoprevention and/or treatment of cancer.

7.5. Cytokine-Targeted Therapy

Therapeutic strategies focused on antagonizing the cytokines, which are likely to play a role in carcinogenesis of pancreatic cancer are under investigaton. The use of monoclonal antibodies or other inhibitors is extensively examined. IL-8, up-regulation of which seems to play an important role in carcinogenesis of pancreatic cancer, represents a potential therapeutic target. Fully human anti-interleukin-8 antibody (ABX-IL-8) is available, and has shown anti-angiogenic activity, suppressed the tumor growth and metastatic potential of human melanoma cells [106]. These results were supported by the study of Mian and colleagues who observed the tumor growth inhibition in orthotopic bladder cancer xenografts via down-regulation of matrix metalloproteinases and NF-κB after treatment with this antibody [107]. ABX-IL-8 was suggested as a modality to treat melanoma, bladder cancer and other solid tumors either alone or in combination with conventional chemotherapy or other anti-tumor agents [106,107]. Novel cytokines, IL-21 and IL-23, expressed antitumor effect in the inoculated mice, and retroviral transduction of the IL-21 and IL-23 genes in human pancreatic carcinoma cells resulted in tumor growth retardation [108]. Other interleukins with known antitumor effect, IL-12 and IL-15 were also examined, and impaired tumorigenicity of human pancreatic cancer cells retrovirally transduced with IL-12 or IL-15 genes was reported suggesting the possible therapeutic potential of these cytokines [109].

7.6. Targeting Oxidative Stress

Persistent oxidative and nitrosative stress and excess of LPO induced by inflammatory processes cause an accumulation of massive DNA damage from endogeneous sources in affected organs. Reduction of oxidative stress and lipid peroxidation represents a promising therapeutic target in the chemoprevention of pancreatic cancer. The influence of antioxidative vitamins, such as vitamins A, C and E, on lipid peroxidation in animal models of pancreatic cancer (BOP-induced pancreatic cancer in Syrian hamsters) was examined, and the incidence of pancreatic cancer was decreased by vitamin A and vitamin C. All vitamins increased the activity of superoxidedismutase in pancreatic carcinomas with consecutive intracellular increase of hydrogen peroxide levels and this effect was selectively toxic for tumor cells [110]. Further experiments with this animal model of pancreatic cancer showed the effect of antioxidative vitamins A, C, and E on liver metastasis and intrametastatic lipid peroxidation. Vitamins A and E reduced the incidence of liver metastases of pancretic cancer, and the number and size of liver metastases were significantly reduced by vitamin A [111]. Chemopreventive effects of β-carotene, selenium and vitamin C were also reported. These micronutrients showed positive effects in azaserine-induced pancreatic carcinogenesis in rats

[112]. Thus, there are a number of antioxidants, which suggest that functional levels of these substances together may protect cells from the damage.

Conclusion

In conclusion, chronic pancreatitis represents an inflammatory disorder that predisposes the affected patients to pancreatic cancer. Patients with chronic pancreatitis have a markedly increased risk of pancreatic cancer compared with the general population. The mechanism by which this risk is mediated is not completely known. The roles of cytokines, reactive oxygen species, and mediators of inflammatory pathways have been extensively studied. The results demonstrated that the chronic pancreatic inflammation may play a key role in oncogenesis of pancreatic malignancy. Suppression of inflammation and oxidative damage using a large spectrum of treatment strategies may be useful for chemoprevention or treatment of pancreatic neoplasia.

References

[1] Malka, D; Hammel, P; Maire, F; Rufat, P; Madeira, I; Pessione, F; Levy, P; Ruszniewski, P. Risk of pancreatic adenocarcinoma in chronic pancreatitis. *Gut*, 2002, 51, 849-852.

[2] Lowenfels, AB; Maisonneuve, P; Cavallini, G; Ammann, RW; Lankisch, PG; Andersen, JR; DiMagno, EP; Andren-Sandberg, A; Dommelof, L. Pancreatitis and the risk of pancreatic cancer. *N. Engl. J. Med.*, 1993, 328, 1433-1437.

[3] Howes, N; Neoptolemos, JP. Risk of pancreatic ductal adenocarcinoma in chronic pancreatitis. *Gut,* 2002, 51, 765-766.

[4] Otsuki, M. Chronic pancreatitis in Japan: epidemiology, prognosis, diagnostic criteria, and future problems. *J. Gastroenterol.*, 2003, 38, 315-326.

[5] Farrow, B; Sugiyama, Y; Chen, A; Uffort, E; Nealon, W; Evers, BM. Inflammatory mechanisms contributing to pancreatic cancer development. *Ann. Surg.*, 2004, 239, 763-771.

[6] Garcea, G; Dennison, AR; Steward, WP; Berry, DP. Role of the inflammation in pancreatic carcinogenesis and the implications for future therapy. *Pancreatology,* 2005, 5, 514-529.

[7] Farrow, B; Evers, BM. Inflammation and the development of pancreatic cancer. *Surg. Oncol.*, 2002, 10, 153-169.

[8] Ulrich, CD 2nd; Kopras, E; Wu, Y; Ward S. Hereditary pancreatitis: epidemiology, molecules, mutations, and models. *J. Lab. Clin. Med.*, 2000, 136, 260-274.

[9] Lowenfels, AB; Maisonneuve, P; Whitcomb, DC; Lerch, MM; DiMagno, EP. Cigarette smoking as a risk factor for pancreatic cancer in patients with hereditary pancreatitis. *JAMA,* 2001, 286, 169-170.

[10] Malfertheiner, P; Schutte, K. Smoking-a trigger for chronic inflammation and cancer development in the pancreas. *Am. J. Gastroenterol.*, 2006, 101, 160-162.

[11] Bramhall, SR; Allum, WH; Jones, AG; Allwood, A; Cummins, C; Neoptolemos, JP. Treatment and survival in 13,560 patients with pancreatic cancer, and incidence of the disease in the West Midlands: an epidemiological study. *Br. J. Surg.,* 1995, 82, 111-115.

[12] Fernandez, E; La Vecchia, C; Porta, M; Negri, E; Lucchini, F; Levi, F. Trends in pancreatic cancer mortality in Europe , 1955-1989. *Int. J. Cancer,* 1994, 57, 786-792.

[13] Hruban, RH; Adsay, NV; Albores-Saavedra, J; Compton, C; Garett, ES; et al. The genetic basis of human cancer. In: Vogelstein B, Kinzler KW editors. *Pancreatic cancer.* New York: Mc Graw-Hill; 1996; 603-613.

[14] Maitra, A; Fukushima, N; Takaori, K; Hruban, RH. Precursors to invasive pancreatic cancer. *Adv. Anat. Pathol.,* 2005, 12, 81-91.

[15] Biankin, AV; Kench, JG; Dijkman, FP; Biankin, SA; Henshall, SM. Molecular pathogenesis of precursor lesions of pancreatic ductal adenocarcinoma. *Pathology* 2003, 35, 14-24.

[16] Hruban, RH; Wilentz, RE; Kern SE. Genetic progression in the pancreatic ducts. *Am. J. Pathol.,* 2000, 156, 1821-1825.

[17] Hruban, RH; Adsay, NV; Albores-Saavedra, J; Compton, C; Garrett, ES; Goodman, SN; Kern, SE; Klimstra, DS; Kloppel, G; Longnecker, DS; Luttges, J; Offerhaus, GJ. Pancreatic intraepithelial neoplasia: a new nomenclature and classification system for pancreatic duct lesions. *Am. J. Surg. Pathol.,* 2001, 25, 579-586.

[18] Hruban, RH; van Mansfeld, AD; Offerhaus, GJ; van Weering, DH; Allison, DC; Goodman, SN; Kensler, TW; Bose, KK; Cameron, JL; Bos, JL. K-ras oncogene activation in adenocarcinoma of the human pancreas: a study of 82 carcinomas using a combination of mutant-enriched polymerase chain reaction analysis and allele-specific oligonucleotide hybridization. *Am. J. Pathol.,* 1993, 143, 545-554.

[19] Tada, M; Omata, M; Ohto, M. Clinical application of ras gene mutation for diagnosis of pancreatic adenocarcinoma. *Gastroenterology,* 1991, 100, 233-238.

[20] Lemoine, NR; Jain, S; Hughes, CM; Staddon, SL; Maillet, B; Hall, PA; Kloppel, G. Ki-ras oncogene activation in preinvasive pancreatic cancer. *Gastroenterology,* 1992, 102, 230-236.

[21] Luttges, J; Diederichs, A; Menke, MA; Vogel, I; Kremer, B; Kloppel, G. Ductal lesions in patients with chronic pancreatitis show K-ras mutations in a frequency similar to that in the normal pancreas and lack nuclear immunoreactivity for p53. *Cancer,* 2000, 88, 2495-2504.

[22] Moskaluk, CA; Hruban, RH; Kern SE. p16 and K-ras gene mutations in the intraductal precursors of human pancreatic adenocarcioma. *Cancer Res.,* 1997, 57, 2140-2143.

[23] Schutte, M; Hruban, RH; Geradts, J; Maynard, R; Hilgers, W; Rabindran, SK; Moskaluk, CA; Hahn, SA; Schwarte-Waldhoff, I; Schmiegel, W; Baylin, SB; Kern, SE; Herman, JG. Abrogation of the Rb/p16 tumor suppressive pathway in virtually all pancreatic carcinomas. *Cancer Res.,* 1997, 57, 3126-3130.

[24] Hustinx, SR; Leoni, LM; Yeo, CJ; Brown, PN; Goggins, M; Kern, SE; Hruban, RH; Maitra, A. Concordant loss of MTAP and p16/CDKN2A expression in pancreatic intraepithelial neoplasia: evidence of homozygous deletions in a non-invasive precursor lesions. *Mod. Pathol.,* 2005, 18, 959-963.

[25] Schutte, M; Hruban, RH; Hedrick, L; Cho, KR; Nadasdy, GM; Weinstein, CL; Bova, GS; Isaacs, WB; Cairns, P; Nawroz, H; Sidransky, D; Casero, RA Jr; Meltzer, PS; Hahn, SA; Kern, SE. DPC4 gene in various tumor types. *Cancer Res.*, 1996, 56, 2527-2530.

[26] Kloppel, G; Luttges, J. The pathology of ductal type pancreatic carcinomas and pancreatic intraepithelial neoplasia: insight for clinicians. *Curr. Gastroenterol. Rep.*, 2004, 6, 111-118.

[27] Volkholz, H; Stolte, M; Becker, V. Epithelial dysplasias in chronic pancreatitis. *Virchows Arch. A Pathol. Anat. Histol.*, 1982, 396, 331-349.

[28] Tannapfel, A; Witzigmann, H; Wittekind, C. Pancreatic intraepithelial neoplasia in chronic pancreatitis. *Zentralbl Chir.* 2001, 126, 879-883.

[29] Rivera, JA; Rall, CJ; Graeme-Cook, F; Fernandez-del Castillo, C; Shu, P; Lakey, N; Tepper, R; Rattner, DW; Warshaw, AL; Rustgi, AK. Analysis of K-ras oncogene mutations in chronic pancreatitis with ductal hyperplasia. *Surgery,* 1997, 121, 42-49.

[30] Berger, DH; Chang, H; Wood, M; Huang, L; Heath, CW; Lehman, T; Ruggeri, BA. Mutational activation of K-ras in nonneoplastic exocrine pancreatic lesions in relation to cigarette smoking status. *Cancer,* 1999, 85, 326-332.

[31] Geradts, J; Hruban, RH; Schutte, M; Kern, SE; Maynard, R. Immunohistochemical p16INK4a analysis of archival tumors with deletion, hypermethylation, or mutation of the CDKN2/MTS1 gene. A comparison of four commercial antibodies. *Appl. Immunohistochem Mol. Morphol.*, 2000, 8, 71-79.

[32] Rosty, C; Geradts, J; Sato, N; Wilentz, RE; Roberts, H; Sohn, T; Cameron, JL; Yeo, CJ; Hruban, RG; Goggins, M. p16 inactivaton in pancreatic intraepithelial neoplasias (PanINs) arising in patiens with chronic pancreatitis. *Am. J. Surg. Pathol.*, 2003, 27, 1495-1501.

[33] Gerdes, B; Ramaswamy, A; Kersting, M; Ernst, M; Lang, S; Schuermann, M; Wild, A; Bartsch, DK. $p16^{INK4a}$ alterations in chronic pancreatitis – indicator for high risk lesions for pancreatic cancer. *Surgery,* 2001, 129, 490-497.

[34] Hermanova, M; Nenutil, R; Kren, L; Feit, J; Pavlovsky, Z; Dite, P. Proliferative activity in pancreatic intraepithelial neoplasias of chronic pancreatitis resection specimens: detection of a high risk lesion. *Neoplasma,* 2004, 51, 400-404.

[35] Liggett, WH Jr; Sidransky, D. Role of p16 tumor suppressor gene in cancer. *J. Clin. Oncol.*, 1998, 16, 1197-1206.

[36] Detlefsen, S; Sipos, B; Feyerabend, B; Kloppel, G. Fibrogenesis in alcoholic chronic pancreatitis: the role of tissue necrosis, macrophages, myofibroblasts and cytokines. *Mod. Pathol.*, 2006, 19, 1019-1026.

[37] Jaster, R. Molecular regulation of pancreatic stellate cell function. *Mol. Cancer,* 2004, 3, 26.

[38] Yoon, SO; Park, SJ; Yoon, SY; Yun, CH; Chung, AS. Sustained production of H(2)O(2) activates pro-matrix metalloproteinase-2 through receptor kinases/phosphatidylinositol 3-kinase/NF-κB pathway. *J. Biol. Chem.*, 2002, 277, 30271-30282.

[39] Rayet, B; Gelinas, C. Aberrant rel/nfkb genes and activity in human cancer. *Oncogene,* 1999, 18, 6938-6947.

[40] Liptay, C; Weber, CK; Ludwig, L; Wagner, M; Adler, G; Schmidt, RM. Mitogenic and antiapoptotic role of constitutive NF-kappaB/Rel activity in pancreatic cancer. *Int. J. Cancer,* 2003, 105, 735-746.

[41] Wang, W; Abbruzzese, JL; Evans, DB; Larry, L; Cleary, KR; Chiao, PJ. The nuclear factor –kappa B RelA transcription factor is constitutively activated in human pancreatic adenocarcinoma cells. *Clin. Cancer Res.,* 1999, 5, 119-127.

[42] Chandler, NM; Canete, JJ; Callery, MP. Increased expression of NF-kappa B subunits in human pancreatic cancer cells. *J. Surg. Res.,* 2004, 118, 9-14.

[43] Zhang, Z; Rigas B. NF-kappaB, inflammation and pancreatic carcinogenesis: NF-kappaB as a chemoprevention target. *Int. J. Oncol.,* 2006, 29, 185-192.

[44] Yamamoto, Y; Gaynor, RB. Therapeutic potential of inhibition of the NFκB pathway in the treatment of inflammation and cancer. *J. Clin. Invest.,* 2001, 107, 135-142.

[45] Gansauge, S; Gansauge, F; Ramadani, M; Stobbe, H; Rau, B; Harada, N; Beger, HG. Overexpression of cyclin D1 in human pancreatic carcinoma is associated with poor prognosis. *Cancer Res.,* 1997, 57, 1634-1637.

[46] Xie, K. Interleukin-8 and human cancer biology. *Cytokine Growth Factor Rev.,* 2001, 12, 375-391.

[47] Xiong, Q; Abbruzzese, JL; Lin, E; Wang, L; Zheng, L; Xie, K. NF-κB activity blockade impairs the angiogenic potential of human pancreatic cancer cells. *Int. J. Cancer,* 2004, 108, 181-188.

[48] Dannenberg, AJ; Altorki, NK; Boyle, JO; Dang, C; Howe, LR; Weksler, BB; Subbaramaiah, K. Cyclo-oxygenase 2: A pharmacological target for the prevention of cancer. *Lancet Oncol.,* 2001, 2, 544-551.

[49] Kokawa, A; Kondo, H; Gotoda, D; Ono, H; Saito, D; Nakadaira, S; Kosuge, T; Yoshida, S. Increased expression of cyclooxygenase-2 in human pancreatic neoplasms and potential chemoprevention by cyclooxygenase inhibitors. *Cancer,* 2001, 91, 333-338.

[50] Chu, J; Lloyd, FL; Trifan, OC; Knapp, B; Rizzo, MT. Potential involvement of cyclooxygenase-2 pathway in the regulation of tumor associated angiogenesis and growth in pancreatic cancer. *Mol. Cancer Ther.,* 2003, 2, 1-7.

[51] Kong, G; Kim, EK; Kim, WS; Lee, KT; Lee, YW; Lee, JK; Paik, SW, Rhee, JC. Role of cyclooxygenase-2 and inducible nitric oxide synthese in pancreatic cancer. *J. Gastroenterol. Hepatol.,* 2002, 17, 914-921.

[52] Ding, XZ; Tong, WG; Adrian, TE. Blockade of cyclooxygenase-2 inhibits proliferation and induces apoptosis in human pancreatic cancer cells. *Anticancer Res.,* 2000, 20, 2625-2631.

[53] Eibl, G; Bruemmer, D; Okada, Y; Duffy, JP; Law, RE; Reber, HA; Hines, OJ. PGE (2) is generated by specific COX-2 activity and increases VEGF production in COX-2 expressing human pancreatic cancer cells. *Biochem. Biophys. Res. Commun.,* 2003, 306, 887-897.

[54] Schlosser, W; Schlosser, S; Ramadani, M; Gansauge, F; Gansauge, S; Beger, HG. Cyclooxygenase-2 is overexpressed in chronic pancreatitis. *Pancreas,* 2002, 25, 26-30.

[55] Koliopanos, A; Friess, H; Kleeff, J; Roggo, A,;Zimmermann, A; Buchler, MW. Cyclooxygenase 2 expression in chronic pancreatitis: correlation with stage of the disease and diabetes mellitus. *Digestion,* 2001, 64, 240-247.

[56] Albazaz, R; Verbeke, CS; Rahman, SH; McMahon, MJ. Cyclooxygenase-2 expression associated with severity of PanIN lesions: a possible link between chronic pancreatitis and pancreatic cancer. *Pancreatology,* 2005, 5, 361-369.

[57] Maitra, A; Ashfaq, R; Gunn, CR; Rahman, A; Yeo, CJ; Sohn, TA; Cameron, JL; Hruban, RH; Wilentz, RE. Cyclooxygenase 2 expression in pancreatic adenocarcinoma and pancreatic intraepithelial neoplasia. *Am. J. Clin. Pathol.,* 2002, 118, 194-201.

[58] Ding, XZ; Hennig, R; Adrian, TE. Lipooxygenase and cyclooxygenase metabolism: new insight in treatment and chemoprevention of pancreatic cancer. *Mol. Cancer,* 2003, 2, 10.

[59] Tong, WG; Ding, XZ; Hennig, R; Witt, RC; Standop, J; Pour, PM; Adrian, TE. Leukotriene B4 receptor antagonist LY293111 inhibits proliferation and induces apoptosis in human pancreatic cancer cells. *Clin. Cancer Res.,* 2002, 8, 3232-3242.

[60] Hennig, R; Ding, XZ; Tong, WG; Schneider, MB; Standop, J; Friess, H; Buchler, MW; Pour, PM; Adrian, TE. 5-Lipooxygenase and leukotriene B (4) receptor are expressed in human pancreatic cancer but not in pancreatic ducts in normal tissue. *Am. J. Pathol.,* 2002, 161, 421-428.

[61] Hennig, R; Grippo, P; Ding, XZ; Rao, SM; Buchler, MW; Friess, H; Talamonti, MS; Bell, RH; Adrian, TE. 5-Lipooxygenase, a marker for early pancreatic intraepithelial neoplastic lesions. *Cancer Res.,* 2005, 65, 6011-6016.

[62] Jaiswal, M; LaRusso, NF; Shapiro, RA; Billiar, TR; Gores, GJ. Nitric oxide-mediated inhibition of DNA repair potentiates oxidative DNA damane in cholangiocytes. *Gastroenterology,* 2001, 120, 190-199.

[63] Jenkins, DC; Charles, IG; Thomsen, LL; Moss, DW; Holmes, LS; Baylis, SA; Rhodes, P; Westmore, K; Epson, PC; Moncada, S. Roles of nitric oxide in tumour growth. *Proc Natl Acad Sci USA,* 1995, 92, 4392-4396.

[64] Wu, K. Inducible isoforms of cyclooxygenase and nitric oxide synthase. *Adv. Pharmacol.,* 1995, 33, 179-207.

[65] Lala, PK; Chakraborty, C. Role of nitric oxide in carcinogenesis and tumour progression. *Lancet Oncol.*, 2001, 2, 149-156.

[66] Xiong, Q; Shi, Q; Le, X; Wang, B; Xie, K. Regulation of interleukin-8 expression by nitric oxide in human pancreatic adenocarcinoma. *J. Interferon Cytokine Res.,* 2001, 21, 529-537.

[67] Salvemini, D; Misko, TP; Masferrer, JL; Seifert, K; Currie, MG; Needleman, P. Nitric oxide activates cyclooxygenase enzymes. *Proc. Natl. Acad. Sci. USA*, 1993, 90, 7240-7244.

[68] Kasper, HU; Wolf, H; Drebber, U; Wolf, HK; Kern, MA. Expression of inducible nitric oxide synthase and cyclooxygenase-2 in pancreatic adenocarcinoma: correlation with microvessel density. *World J. Gastroenterol.,* 2004, 10, 1918-1922.

[69] Doria, D; Bertazzoni Minelli, E; Bassi, C; Falconi, M; Pederzoli, P; Franco, L. Primary human pancreatic adenocarcinomas and expression of inducible nitric oxide synthase and cyclooxygenase-2. *JOP J. Pancreas,* 2001, 2(5Suppl), 351-352.

[70] Gansauge, S; Nussler, AK; Beger, HG; Gansauge, F. Nitric oxide-induced apoptosis in human pancreatic carcinoma cell lines associated with a G1-arrest and an increase of the cyclin-dependent kinase inhibitor p21WAF1/CIP1. *Cell Growth Digger,* 1998, 9, 611-617.

[71] Hajri, A; Metzger, E; Vallat, F; Coffy, S; Flatter, E; Evrard, S; Marescaux, J; Aprahamian, M. Role of nitric oxide in pancreatic tumor growth: in vivo and in vitro studies. *Br. J. Cancer,* 1998, 78, 841-849.

[72] Wang, B; Wei, D; Crum, VE; Richardson, EL; Xiong, HH; Luo, Y; Juany, S; Abbruzzese, JL; Xie, K. A novel model system for studying the double-edged roles of nitric oxide production in pancreatic cancer growth and metastasis. *Oncogene,* 2003, 22, 1771-1782.

[73] Ebrahimi, B; Tucker, SL; Li, D; Abbruzzese, JL; Kurzrock,R. Cytokines in pancreatic carcinoma: correlation with phenotypic characteristics and prognosis. *Cancer,* 2004,101, 727-2736.

[74] Duell, EJ; Casella, DP; Burk, RD; Kelsey, KT; Holly, EA. Inflammation, genetic polymorphisms in proinflammatory genes TNF-A, RANTES, and CCR5, and risk of pancreatic adenocarcinoma. *Cancer Epidemiol Biomarkers Prev.,* 2006, 15, 726-731.

[75] Nair, J; Furstenberger, G; Burger, F; Marks, F; Bartsch, H. Promutagenic etheno-DNA adducts in multistage mouse skin carcinogenesis: correlation with lipid-catalyzed arachidonic acid metabolism. *Chem. Res. Toxicol.,* 2000, 13, 703-709.

[76] Bartsch, H; Nair, J. Accumulation of lipid peroxidation-derived DNA lesions: Potential lead markers for chemoprevention of inflammation derived malignancies. *Mutat. Res.,* 2005, 591, 34-44.

[77] Nair, J; Gansauge, F; Beger, H; Dolara, P; Winde, G; Bartsch, H. Increased etheno-DNA adducts in affected tissues of patiens suffering from Crohn´s disease, ulcerative colitis, and chronic pancreatitis. *Antioxid. Redox. Signal,* 2006, 8, 1003-1010.

[78] Li, D; Firozi, PF; Zhang, W; Shen, J; Di Giovanni, J; Lau, S; Evans, D; Friess, H; Hasan, M; Abbruzesse, JL. DNA adducts, genetic polymorphisms, and K-ras mutation in human pancreatic cancer. *Mutat Res.,* 2002, 513, 37-48.

[79] Schwartz, SA; Hernandez, A; Mark Evers, B. The role of NF-kappaB/IkappaB proteins in cancer: Implications for novel treatment strategie. *Surg. Oncol.*, 1999, 8, 143-153.

[80] McDade, TP; Perugini, RA; Vittimberga, FJ Jr; Carrigan, RC; Callery, MP. Salicylates inhibit NF-kappaB activation and enhance TNF-alpha-induced apoptosis in human pancreatic cancer cells. *J. Surg. Res.*, 1999, 83, 56-61.

[81] Perugini, RA; McDade, TP; Vittimberga, FJ Jr; Duffy, AJ; Callery, MP. Sodium salicylate inhibits proliferation and induces G1 cell cycle arrest in human pancreatic cancer cell lines. *J. Gastrointest. Surg.*, 2000, 4, 24-32.

[82] Yin, MJ; Yamamoto, Y; Gaynor, RB. The anti-inflammatory agents aspirin and salicylate inhibit the activity of I(kappa)B kinase-beta. *Nature*, 1998, 396, 77-80.

[83] Yamamoto, Y; Yin, MJ; Lin, KM; Gaynor, RB. Sulindac inhibits activation of the NF-kappaB pathway. *J. Biol. Chem.*, 1999, 274, 27307-27314.

[84] Muerkoster, S; Arlt, A; Witt, M; Gehrz, A; Haye, S; March, C; Grohmann, F; Wegehenkel, K; Kalthoff, H; Folsch, UR; Schafer, H. Usage of the NF-kappaB

inhibitor sulfasalazine as sensitizing agent in combined chemotherapy of pancreatic cancer. *Int. J. Cancer,* 2003, 104, 469-476.

[85] Beauparlant, P; Hiscott, J. Biological and biochemical inhibitors of the NF-kappaB/Rel proteins and cytokine synthesis. *Cytokine Growth Factor*, 1996, 7, 175-190.

[86] Agou, F; Courtois, G; Chiaravalli, J; Baleux, F; Coic, YM; Traincard, F; Israel, A; Veron, M. Inhibition of NF-kappa B activation by peptides targeting NF-kappa B essential modulator (nemo) oligomerization. *J. Biol. Chem.*, 2004, 279, 54248-54257.

[87] Nawrocki, ST; Bruns, CJ; Harbison, MT; Bold, RJ; Gotsch, BS; Abbruzzese, JL; Elliott, P; Adams, J; McConkey, DJ. Effects of the proteasome inhibitor PS-341 on apoptosis and angiogenesis in orthotopic human pancreatic tumor xenografts. *Mol. Cancer Ther.*, 2002, 1, 1243-1253.

[88] Howe, LR; Dannenberg, AJ. A role of cyclooxygenase-2 inhibitors in the prevention and treatment of cancer. *Semin Oncol.*, 2002, 29(3 Suppl II), 111-119.

[89] Anderson, KE; Johnson, TW; Lazovich, D; Folsom, AR. Association between nonsteroidal anti-inflammatory drug use and the incidence of pancreatic cancer. *J. Natl. Cancer Inst.,* 2002, 94, 1168-1171.

[90] Jacobs, EJ; Connell, CJ; Rodriguez, C; Patel, AV; Calle, EE; Thun, MJ. Aspirin use and pancreatic cancer mortality in a large United States cohort. *J. Natl. Cancer Inst.*, 2004 , 96, 524-528.

[91] Schernhammer, ES; Kang, JH; Chan, AT; Mischaud, DS; Skinner, HG; Giovannucci, E; Colditz, GA; Fuchs, CS. A prospective study of aspirin use and the risk of pancreatic cancer in women. *J. Natl. Cancer Inst.*, 2004, 96, 22-28.

[92] Larsson, SC; Giovannucci, E; Bergkvist, Wolk, A. Aspirin and nonsteroidal anti-inflammatory drug use and risk of pancreatic cancer: a meta-analysis. *Cancer Epidemiol. Biomarkers Prev.,* 2006, 15, 2561-2564.

[93] Takahashi, M; Furukawa, K; Toyoda, K; Sato, H; Hasegawa, R; Imaida, K; Hayashi, Y. Effects of various prostaglandin synthesis inhibitors on pancreatic carcinogenesis in hamsters after initiation with N-nitrosobis(2-oxopropyl)amine. *Carcinogenesis,* 1990, 11, 393-395.

[94] Wenger, FA; Kilian, M; Achucarro, P; Heinicken, D; Schimke, I; Guski, H; Jacobi, CA; Muller, JM. Effects of Celebrex and Zyflo on BOP-induced pancreatic cancer in Syrian hamsters. *Pancreatology*, 2002, 2, 54-60.

[95] Tseng, WW; Deganutti, A; Chen, MN; Saxton, RE; Liu, CD. Selective cyclo-oxygenase-2 inhibitor rofecoxib (Vioxx) induces expression of cell cycle arrest genes and slows tumor growth in human pancreatic cancer. *J. Gastrointest. Surg.*, 2002, 6, 838-843.

[96] Ding, XZ; Tong, WG; Adrian, TE. Blockade of cyclooxygenase-2 inhibits proliferation and induces apoptosis in human pancreatic cancer cells. *Anticancer Res.*, 2000, 4, 2625-2631.

[97] Molina, MA; Sitja-Arnau, M; Lemoine, MG; Frazier, ML; Sinicrope, FA. Increased cyclooxygenase-2 expression in human pancreatic carcinomas and cell lines: growth inhibition by nonsteroidal anti-inflammatory drugs. *Cancer Res.*, 1999, 59, 4356-4362.

[98] Wei, D; Wang, L; He, Y; Xiong, HQ; Abbruzzese, JL; Xie, K. Celecoxib inhibits vascular endothelial growth factor expression and reduces angiogenesis and metastasis

of human pancreatic cancer via suppresion of Sp1 transcription factor activity. *Cancer Res.*, 2004, 64, 2030-2038.

[99] Cicero, AF; Derosa, G; Gaddi, A. Combined lipooxygenase/cyclo-oxygenase inhibition in the elderly: the example of licofelone. *Drugs Aging*, 2005, 22, 393-403.

[100] Fiorucci, S; Meli, R; Bucci, M; Cirino, G. Dual inhibitors of cyclo-oxygenase and 5-lipooxygenase. New avenue in anti-inflammatory therapy. *Biochem. Pharmacol.*, 2001, 62, 1433-1438.

[101] Ding, XZ; Tong, WG; Adrian, TE. Multiple signal pathways are involved in the mitogenic effect of 5(S)-HETE in human pancreatic cancer. *Oncology*, 2003, 285-294.

[102] Tong, WG; Ding, XZ; Talamonti, MS; Bell, RH; Adrian, TE. LTB4 stimulates growth of human pancreatic cancer cells via MAPK and PI-3 kinase pathway. *Biochem. Biophys. Res. Commun.*, 2005, 335, 946-956.

[103] Tong, WG; Ding, XZ; Witt, RC; Adrian, TE. Lipoxygenase inhibitors attenuate growth of human pancretic cancer xenografts and induce apoptosis through the mitochondrial pathway. *Mol. Cancer Ther.*, 2002, 1, 929-935.

[104] Ouyang, N; Williams, JL; Tsioulias, GJ; Gao, J; Iatropoulos, MJ; Kopelovich, L; Kashfi, K; Rigas, B. Nitric oxide-donating aspirin prevents pancreatic cancer in a hamster tumor model. *Cancer Res.*, 2006, 66, 4503-4511.

[105] Kashfi, K; Rigas, B. Molecular targets of nitric-oxide-donating aspirin in cancer. *Biochem Soc Trans*, 2005, 33, 701-704.

[106] Huang, S; Mills, L; Mian, B; Tellez, C; McCarty, M; Yang, XD; Gudas, JM; Bar-Eli, M. Fully humanized neutralizing antibodies to interleukin-8 (ABX-IL8) inhibit angiogenesis, tumor growth, and metastasis of human melanoma. *Am. J. Pathol.*, 2002, 161, 125-134.

[107] Mian, BM; Dinney, CP; Bermejo, CE; Sweeney, P; Tellez, C; Yang, XD; Gudas, JM; McConkey, DJ; Bar-Eli, M. Fully human anti-interleukin 8 antibody inhibits tumor growth in orthotopic bladder cancer xenografts via down-regulation of matrix-metalloproteinases and nuclear factor-kappaB. *Clin. Cancer Res.*, 2003, 9, 3167-3175.

[108] Ugai, S; Shimozato, O; Yu, L; Wang, YQ; Kawamura, K; Yamamoto, H; Yamaguchi, T; Saisho, H; Sakiyama, S; Tagawa, M. Transduction of the IL-21 and IL-23 genes in human panreatic carcinoma cells produces natural killer cell-dependent and –independent antitumor effects. *Cancer Gene Ther.*, 2003, 10, 771-778.

[109] Yoshida, Y; Tasaki, K; Miyauchi, M; Narita, M; Takenaga, K; Yamamoto, H; Yaaguchi, T; Saisho, H; Sakiyama, S; Tagawa, M. Impaired tumorigenicity of human pancreatic cancer cells retrovirally transduced with interleukin-12 or interleukin-15 gene. *Cancer Gene Ther.*, 2000, 7, 324-331.

[110] Wenger, FA; Kilian, M; Ridders, J; Stahlknecht, P; Schimke, I; Guski, H; Jacobi, CA; Muller, JM. Influence of antioxidative vitamins A, C, and E on lipid peroxidation in BOP-induced pancreatic cancer in Syrian hamsters. *Prostaglandins Leukot Essent Fatty Acids*, 2001, 65: 165-171.

[111] Heukamp, I; Kilian, M; Gregor, JI; Neumann, A; Jacobi, CA; Guski, H; Schimke, I; Walz, MK; Wenger, FA. Effects of the antioxidative vitamins A, C and E on liver metastasis and intrametastatic lipid peroxidation in BOP-induced pancreatic cancer in Syrian hamsters. *Pancreatology*, 2005, 5, 403-409.

[112] Woutersen, RA; Appel, MJ; Van Garderen-Hoetmer, A. Modulation of pancreatic carcinogenesis by antioxidants. *Food Chem. Toxicol.*, 1999, 37, 981-984.

In: Pancreatitis Research Advances
Editor: William C. Langley, pp. 259-273

ISBN: 978-1-60021-883-5

Chapter VIII

Pathogenesis of Alcoholic Chronic Pancreatitis and Efficacy of Bromhexine Hydrochloride Therapy in Its Treatment

Tatsuhiro Tsujimoto*, Hitoshi Yoshiji, Hideto Kawaratani and Hiroshi Fukui

Third Department of Internal Medicine,
Nara Medical University, Kashihara, Nara, Japan

Abstract

Chronic pancreatitis is a condition characterized by histopathological features of chronic changes including irregular pancreatic fibrosis, infiltration by inflammatory cells, parenchymal degeneration and shedding, and granulation tissue, along with impaired exocrine and endocrine functions. The most common causes of chronic pancreatitis are alcohol, idiopathic diseases, and gallstones. Pancreatic stones can develop within the pancreatic duct in patients with chronic pancreatitis, and may act as an outlet barrier to the pancreatic juice. Stenosis or obstruction of the pancreatic duct leads to raised pressure within the pancreatic duct, painful episodes, and progressive destruction of the pancreatic parenchyma. Similarly, the combination of protein plugs within the pancreatic duct and viscous pancreatic juice is thought to cause painful episodes and progressive destruction of the pancreatic parenchyma. Amelioration of stenosis or obstruction of the pancreatic duct relieves pain and halts progression of pancreatitis.

Although abstinence is usually considered a prerequisite for the successful treatment of alcoholic chronic pancreatitis, we often encounter patients with recurrent attacks from the compensatory period to the transitional period. In alcoholic chronic pancreatitis, continued alcohol consumption causes changes in the digestive hormones and vagal

* Correspondence should be addressed to: Tatsuhiro Tsujimoto, M.D., Ph.D. Third Department of Internal Medicine, Nara Medical University, Shijo-cho 840, Kashihara, Nara 634-8522, Japan. Tel: 81-744-22-3051 (ext. 2314). Fax: 81-744-24-7122. E-mail: tat-tyan@xa2.so-net.ne.jp

nerve function that induce the pancreatic acinar cells to oversecrete protein, increasing the protein concentration and viscosity of the pancreatic juice, allowing protein sedimentation from the pancreatic juice with consequent formation of protein plugs within the pancreatic duct. Recently, the main constituent proteins in these protein plugs have been identified, and accordingly several therapies have been tried, such as administration of secretin formulations and endoscopic removal.

Bromhexine hydrochloride, a bronchial mucolytic, has an affinity for the pancreatic acinar cells, inducing them to secrete pancreatic juice of low viscosity. In this chapter, we outline new medical treatments for alcoholic chronic pancreatitis, and in particular, we discuss the efficacy of bromhexine hydrochloride in the treatment of conditions where protein plug formation and increased viscosity of the pancreatic juice cause bouts of pancreatitis.

Keywords: *Alcoholic chronic pancreatitis, bromhexine hydrochloride, acinar cell, duct cell, protein plug.*

Introduction

The pathogenic mechanisms of chronic pancreatitis are still unknown, and there is no diagnostic modality for accurately detecting early changes, delaying elucidation of the pathophysiology and development of effective therapies for this condition. In the clinical practice, most cases of chronic pancreatitis have pancreatic stones and advanced pancreatic exocrine and endocrine failure. We now understand that various factors interact producing a range of different pathologies, resulting in an end-stage state that at the first glance appears identical in all patients.

Chronic pancreatitis is a progressive condition of various etiologies, severity and speed of progression. Clinically, the main entities are alcoholic chronic pancreatitis, idiopathic chronic pancreatitis, and gallstone chronic pancreatitis. Idiopathic chronic pancreatitis is subdivided on the basis of the age at onset into early-onset pancreatitis and late-onset pancreatitis [1]. The clinical picture is different in the two conditions, perhaps reflecting genetic-based differences [2-6]. Other causes of chronic pancreatitis are autoimmune pancreatitis, where the underlying conditions include Sjögren's syndrome, primary sclerosing cholangitis (PSC), and primary biliary cirrhosis (PBC) [7], hyperparathyroidism [8], hyperlipidemia [9, 10], anomalous arrangements of the pancreaticobiliary ducts [11], congenital dilatation of the bile duct [12], pancreatic trauma [13], lesions around the papilla of Vater [14], and drugs [15].

As chronic pancreatitis progresses over a prolonged period, the clinical problems vary according to the stage of the disease. In the early stages, treatment is mainly targeted to pain and complications of recurrent acute pancreatitis, whereas in the later stages the main issues of treatment are pancreatic exocrine failure, diabetes mellitus, and malnutrition. The differences in the natural history of chronic pancreatitis, probably due to genetic and environmental factors [16-20], make it extremely difficult to evaluate the efficacy of therapies [21]. In fact, no treatment for chronic pancreatitis has been established yet. In this chapter, we discuss the pathogenesis of alcoholic chronic pancreatitis, mainly from the point of view of changes in the pancreatic acinar and duct cells, and highlight the recent advances in therapy using bromhexine hydrochloride. The treatment of other specific types of pancreatitis is described in other chapters.

Conclusions

1. Pathogenesis of Alcoholic Chronic Pancreatitis from the Point of View of Changes in the Pancreatic Acinar and Duct Cells

The pancreatic juice is an isotonic solution containing a high concentration of HCO_3^- and digestive enzymes. The digestive enzymes are secreted by acinar cells that constitute about 90% of the mass of the pancreas, whereas HCO_3^- and H_2O are secreted by epithelial cells lining the pancreatic ducts (duct cells). Although chronic pancreatitis is a progressive condition ultimately resulting in parenchymal destruction with consequent malabsorption and secondary diabetes mellitus, the mechanism of its onset and progression are unknown. The two main contending theories for the pathogenesis of chronic pancreatitis are the necrosis-fibrosis sequence theory, that emphasises damage to the acinar cells [22], and the small-duct theory, that emphasises duct cell dysfunction [23].

The necrosis-fibrosis sequence theory explains chronic pancreatitis as sequale of repeated attacks of focal acute pancreatitis, leading to necrosis, fibrosis and formation of small pancreatic pseudocysts, and stasis of the pancreatic juice due to stenosis of the small pancreatic ducts [22]. In terms of damage to the acinar cells, excluding fibrosis, acute and chronic pancreatitis can be considered to have similar pathogenesis. The initial event in pancreatitis is activation of the intracellular trypsin, probably due to prolonged elevation of the intracellular Ca^{2+} levels. Meanwhile, the nuclear factor κB (NF-κB), a transcription factor that induces the expression of inflammatory cytokines, is activated. Cerulein pancreatitis is an *in vitro* oedematous pancreatitis model, where isolated acinar cells are exposed to a high concentration of cholecystokinin (CCK), leading to increased protease activity associated with prolonged elevation of the intracellular Ca^{2+} levels [24]. Ethanol undergoes both oxidative and non-oxidative metabolism. Although the former was thought to be principally mediated by hepatic alcohol dehydrogenase (ADH) and CYP2E1, the presence of ADH has recently been confirmed in the acinar cells. Oxidative stress and intracellularly produced acetaldehyde are thought to trigger the cellular damage. Simultaneous administration of CCK and ethanol at relatively low concentrations to isolated acinar cells resulted in intracellular production of trypsinogen activation peptide (TAP) [26] and activation of NF-κB [27]. Fatty acid ethyl ester (FAEE), the product of non-oxidative metabolism of ethanol, is also cytotoxic. The pancreatic FAEE activity is many times greater than that in the liver, and a relationship was found between gene polymorphism for carboxylester lipase (CEL), an enzyme that catalyses FAEE, and the onset of alcoholic chronic pancreatitis [28)]. Addition of the FAEE palmitoleic acid ethyl ester to the acinar cells reportedly induces elevation of the intracellular Ca^{2+} levels via activation of inositol triphosphate receptors and inhibition of the Ca^{2+} pump by exhaustion of the ATP levels [29].

In contrast, the small-duct theory holds that increased protein secretion by the acinar cells and reduced production of HCO_3^- and H_2O by the duct cells lead to formation of protein plugs within the intralobular and interlobular pancreatic duct, that develop into pancreatic stones through deposition of calcium carbonate. Subsequently, stasis of the pancreatic juice causes necrosis and fibrosis of the pancreatic tissue upstream of the obstruction [23]. This theory holds that the pathophysiology of chronic pancreatitis is different from that of acute pancreatitis, and that acute episodes of alcoholic pancreatitis occur on top of pre-existing chronic pancreatitis. Reduced volumes and reduced levels of HCO_3^- are noticed in the early stages of chronic pancreatitis, suggesting that the impaired function of the pancreatic duct cell cystic fibrosis transmembrane conductance regulators (CFTR), which are responsible for HCO_3^- secretion, is involved in the etiology of this disease [30].

Ito cells, also known as hepatic stellate cells, have been identified as specific storage cells for vitamin A [31-33], an reportedly play a pivotal role in liver fibrosis [34,35]. In 1998, Apte *et al.* [36] and Bechem *et al.* [37] isolated and cultured similar cells from the rat and human pancreas. The central role of these pancreatic stellate cells in the progression of pancreatic fibrosis, an important factor in the progression of chronic pancreatitis, is under investigation (Figure 1). Immediately after isolation, the pancreatic stellate cells can be identified by their typical morphology, with multiple projections and sparse cytoplasm that comprise vitamin A-containing lipid droplets. With culture of successive generations, these cells become activated, lose their lipid droplets and projections, and change their phenotype to become activated myofibroblast-like cells with abundant cytoplasm and strongly express α-smooth muscle actin (α-SMA). Proliferation of these culture-activated pancreatic stellate cells increases in response to stimulation by platelet-derived growth factor (PDGF), and production of extracellular matrix such as collagen increases in response to transforming growth factor-β (TGF-β). The expressions of chemokines such as monocyte chemoattractant protein-1 (MCP-1), and extracellular matrix proteins such as intercellular adhesion molecule-1 (ICAM-1), are induced by cytokines such as interleukin-1β (IL-1β) and tumor necrosis factor-α (TNF-α) [38, 39].

Some *in vitro* experiments using culture-activated pancreatic stellate cells confirmed the mechanism of ethanol-related pancreatic fibrosis. The pancreatic stellate cells reportedly have ADH activity, and induction of this enzyme by ethanol induces intracellular oxidation of ethanol to acetaldehyde. The resultant oxidative stress directly stimulates the pancreatic stellate cells, possibly promoting proliferation and collagen production [40]. Stimulation of culture-activated rat pancreatic stellate cells with ethanol and acetaldehyde promoted the activity of the transcription factor, activator protein-1 (AP-1), and through intracellular signal transduction activated the extracellular signal-regulated kinase (ERK) 1/2, c-Jun N-terminal kinase/stress-activated protein kinase (JNK/SAPK), and p38 MAP kinase [41]. Furthermore, ethanol and acetaldehyde reportedly increased the procollagen gene expression by pancreatic stellate cells. Specific activation of these signal transduction pathways completely inhibited the antioxidant, N-acetyl-cysteine (NAC), and the increased procollagen expression also inhibited NAC and the p38 MAP kinase inhibitor, 4-(4-fluorophenyl)-2-(4-methylsulfinylphenyl)-5-(4-pyridyl)imidazole (SB203580). We can therefore conclude that ethanol and acetaldehyde induce the intracellular oxidative stress, activating AP-1 and p38 and promoting fiber synthesis. Although fibrosis is no more than a single component of a complex pathogenic process, studies of the pancreatic stellate cells are promising to develop new therapies for chronic pancreatitis.

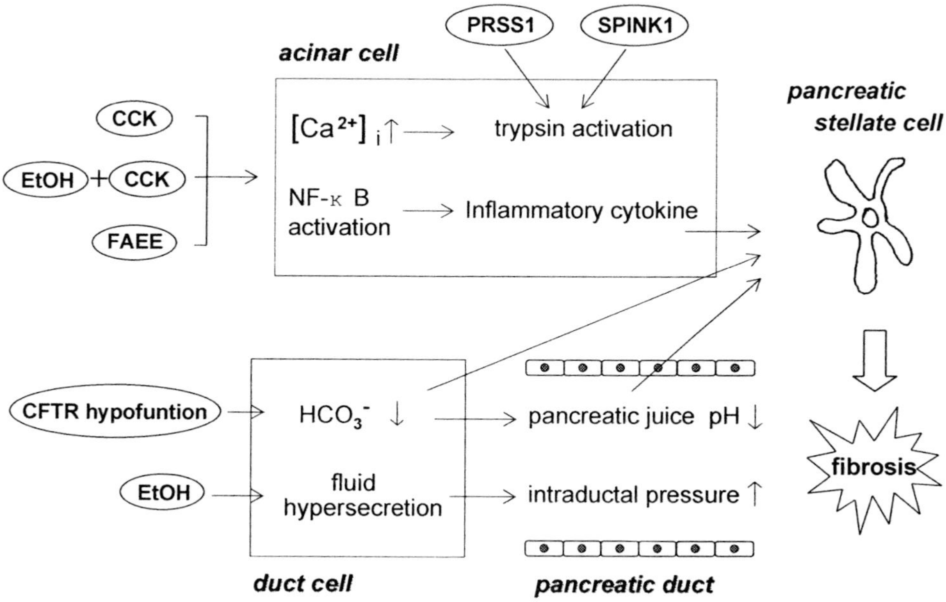

Figure 1. Pathogenesis of chronic pancreatitis.

2. Bromhexine Hydrochloride

Bromhexine hydrochloride (Figure 2) is an alkaloid derived from an Indian herbal plant adhatoda vasica. Its molecular formula is $C_{14}H_{20}Br_2N_2 \cdot HCl$, its molecular weight is 412.59, and its chemical formula is 2-amino-3, 5-dibromo-*N*-cyclohexyl-*N*-methylbenzylaminemonohydrochlorid. Its pharmacological activities comprise stimulation of serous secretions via activation of in the bronchial mucosa [42] and breaking down acid mucoproteins, the cause of sputum viscosity [43, 44]. As it facilitates sputum clearance, bromhexine hydrochloride has been widely used as an expectorant in the clinical field since its development in 1963.

3. Use of Bromhexine Hydrochloride in the Treatment Of Sjögren's Syndrome

Sjögren's syndrome is a chronic inflammatory condition characterised by reduced production of saliva and tears [45, 46]. These exocrine dysfunctions result from infiltration of the affected glands by lymphocytes and plasma cells [47]. It presents various clinical manifestations, usually including dryness of the mouth and eyes, and sometimes parotid enlargement, arthralgia and muscle weakness [47-49].

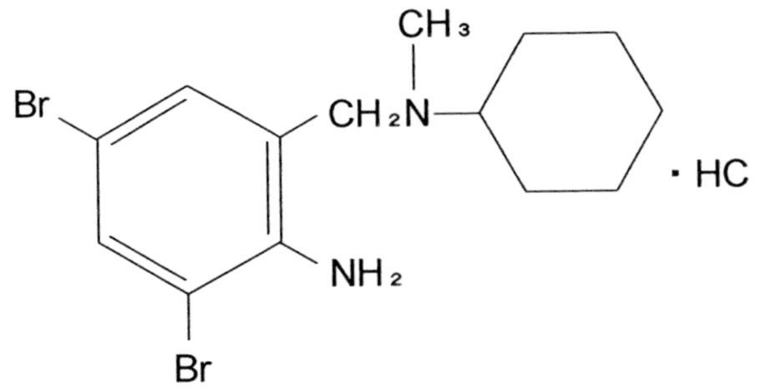

Figure 2. Structural formula of bromhexine hydrochloride.

The most common and major complaint is mucosal dryness. Isager *et al.* were the first to administer bromhexine hydrochloride, to patients with Sjögren's syndrome and chronic bronchitis, finding improvement of the oral and ocular symptoms after 2 or 3 days of treatment [50]. Subsequently, a dose-dependent lacrimal secretory effect for bromhexine hydrochloride was noticed, but it was ineffective in promoting the salivary secretion [51]. Bromhexine hydrochloride reportedly not only increased the amount of tear production, but also improved the lysozyme and albumin levels within the lacrimal secretions [52]. Subsequent animal studies [53] and clinical trials [54] have confirmed the efficacy of bromhexine hydrochloride relieving dry eye symptoms.

4. Rate of Transfer of Bromhexine Hydrochloride into the Pancreas

Initially, autoradiography was used to examine the tissue distribution of bromhexine hydrochloride following intravenous administration. Accumulation of bromhexine hydrochloride was noticed in the adipose tissue, liver, lung, kidney, the adrenal, lacrimal and pituitary glands, and the pineal body [55]. A study on the transfer of bromhexine hydrochloride into pancreatic tissue and the pancreatic juice in rats and dogs revealed a high concentration of bromhexine hydrochloride in the pancreatic tissue, and that these levels particularly in rats were maintained for a much longer period than in the blood or hepatic tissue, indicating a high affinity of bromhexine hydrochloride for the pancreas. In dogs, there was little direct transfer of bromhexine hydrochloride into the pancreatic juice [56]. These results suggested that its mucolytic action might be useful in the treatment of pancreatitis.

5. Efficacy of Bromhexine Hydrochloride Therapy in the Treatment of Alcoholic Chronic Pancreatitis

Alcoholic chronic pancreatitis is the most common type of chronic pancreatitis. Although abstinence is always considered a prerequisite for the successful treatment of alcoholic chronic pancreatitis, some patients cannot abstain from alcohol, and experience recurrent attacks. For these patients, it is important to provide detailed explanations concerning the pathophysiology and prognosis of chronic pancreatitis, advise them to reduce their alcohol consumption or have alcohol-free days, and ensure their compliance with the follow-up.

The common features of alcoholic chronic pancreatitis include the formation of stones and protein plugs within the pancreatic duct [57, 58], elevated mucoprotein levels in the pancreatic juice [59, 60], increased viscosity of the pancreatic juice [61, 62], and protein sedimentation in the pancreatic juice [63, 64]. The main constituent proteins in these protein plugs have been identified [65], and several therapies have been tried; e.g., administration of secretin formulations [66] and somatostatin analogues [67, 68], as well as endoscopic removal [69, 70] and extracorporeal shock wave lithotripsy (ESWL) [71, 72].

Few basic and clinical studies were done on the chemical breakdown of protein plugs and pancreatic stones. A thorough *in vitro* study using an experimental model investigated calcium deposition within the pancreas to stone formation within the pancreatic juice [73, 74]. Accordingly, citric acid, a calcium chelator, was selected as a pancreatic litholytic, and a 50-mg pancreatic stone was dissolved *in vitro* after 25 days in a solution of 3.9 mM/L citric acid, corresponding to a concentration of 749 μg/mL in the pancreatic juice following injection of citric acid into the canine duodenum [75]. Administration of citric acid (5.3~10.6 g/day) to 17 patients with pancreatic stones achieved reduction in size in 7, and reduction in number in 2 [76]. In the clinical practice, citric acid therapy has some problems, including its taste, large volume to drink, need for hospitalisation, and unpredictable litholytic effect.

Pancreatic litholytic therapy was attempted using orally administered trimethadione (TMO), a drug usually used to treat petit mal epilepsy [77]. TMO itself has no pancreatic litholytic activity, but its methylated metabolite, dimethadione (DMO), dissolves $CaCO_3$, the main constituent of the pancreatic stones. Problems with this therapy include difficulty in securing sufficient plasma levels of DMO to achieve sufficient litholysis (minimum: 300 μg/mL) [78] and adverse reactions including diplopia, Stevens-Johnson syndrome, and systemic lupus erythematosus (SLE).

Bromhexine hydrochloride has a high rate of transfer and high affinity for the pancreas in rats and dogs, and directly acts on the acinar cells to produce a low-viscosity pancreatic juice [56]. Clinically, in the patients with mucin-producing pancreatic tumors that experienced repeated attacks of pancreatitis, bromhexine hydrochloride improved the clinical manifestations, normalised the serum pancreatic enzymes, and reduced the viscosity of the pancreatic juice, thus indicating its efficacy in dissolving mucoprotein plugs [79]. A similar efficacy of bromhexine hydrochloride was noticed in the treatment of mucin-producing bile duct tumors [80]. In another study, protein plugs disappeared when bromhexine hydrochloride was administered to patients with idiopathic chronic pancreatitis for four and a half months [81].

Accordingly, we conducted a study on 12 patients (11 men, 1 woman; mean age: 59.1 years) with alcoholic chronic pancreatitis who, despite treatment with camostat mesilate (600 mg/day), digestive enzymes and H_2-receptor antagonists, experienced recurrent attacks of pancreatitis and could not abstain from alcohol. Anticipating a litholytic effect and a wash-out effect within the pancreatic juice, we added bromhexine hydrochloride (12 mg/day orally for 6 months), and investigated its effects on the clinical manifestations, pancreatic enzyme levels, pancreatic endocrine and exocrine functions, and lysis of protein plugs and pancreatic stones. Simultaneously, a control group of 12 patients (10 men, 2 women; mean age: 63.2 years) received a similar therapy but without bromhexine hydrochloride for six months [82, 83]. The main results were as follows. 1) The epigastric pain and back pain exacerbated in 4 subjects (33%) in the control group, did not change in 7 (58%), and improved in 1 (8%), whereas in the bromhexine group, these pains significantly improved in 8 subjects (67%), somewhat improved in 3 (25%), and did not change in 1 (8%). 2) No improvement in the pancreatic enzymes (serum amylase, lipase, trypsin, elastase 1, and urinary amylase) was seen in the control group, in contrast to the significant improvement in the bromhexine group (Figure 3). 3) There was no significant change in levels of fecal chymotrypsin, a marker of the pancreatic exocrine function, in the control group, in contrast to the significant improvement in the bromhexine group (Figure 4). 4) The changes in pancreatic diabetes mellitus were examined as an indicator of the pancreatic endocrine function. Pancreatic diabetes mellitus was diagnosed in 9 subjects (75%) in the control group and 8 (67%) in the bromhexine group, and could be controlled with diet, exercise, and sulfonylurea (SU) medication.

The mean HbA1c levels in the control group were 6.63±0.83% before treatment and 6.82±1.01% after 6 months of treatment, and 6.42±0.77% and 6.33±0.69%, respectively, in the bromhexine group, without significant differences between the two groups. 5) The protein plugs did not disappear in the control group. In the bromhexine group, they could be identified in the main pancreatic duct by endoscopic retrograde pancreatography (ERP) before treatment and disappeared after 6 months of treatment, and the tail side patency of the main pancreatic duct also improved (Figure 5). The pancreatic stones increased in number in some subjects in the control group. In the bromhexine group, the stones neither disappeared nor increased in size or number. Therefore, when treating patients with alcoholic chronic pancreatitis, we cannot expect that bromhexine hydrochloride will improve the pancreatic endocrine function or dissolve the pancreatic stones.

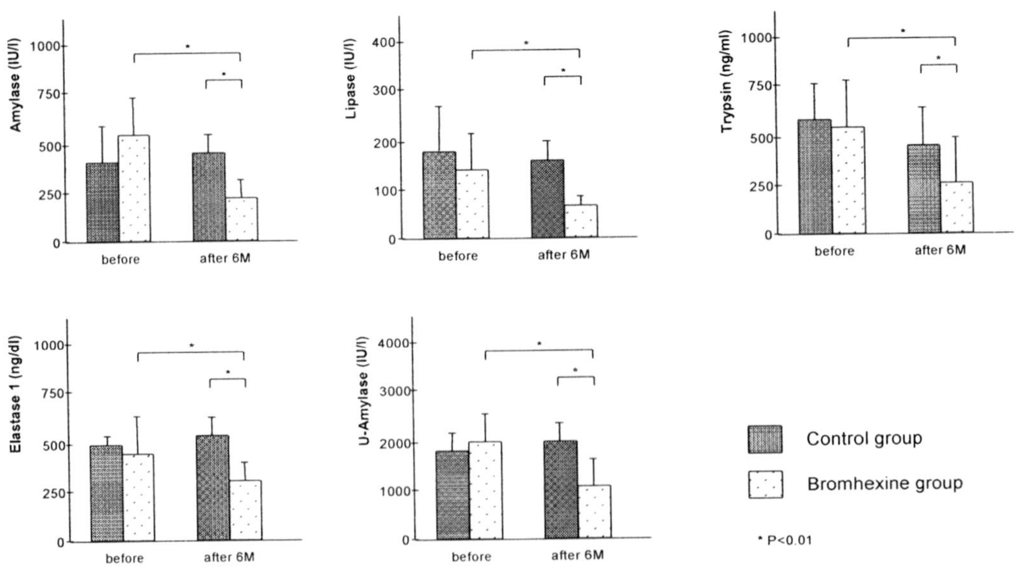

Figure 3. Pancreatic enzymes (serum amylase, lipase, trypsin, elastase 1, and urinary amylase) in the control group and bromhexine group.

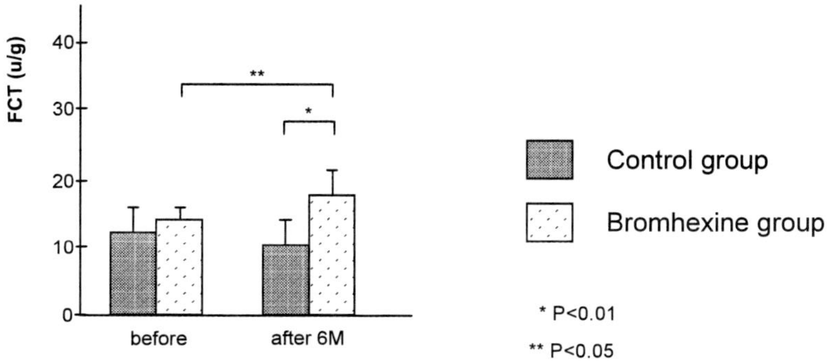

Figure 4. Fecal chymotrypsin in the control group and bromhexine group.

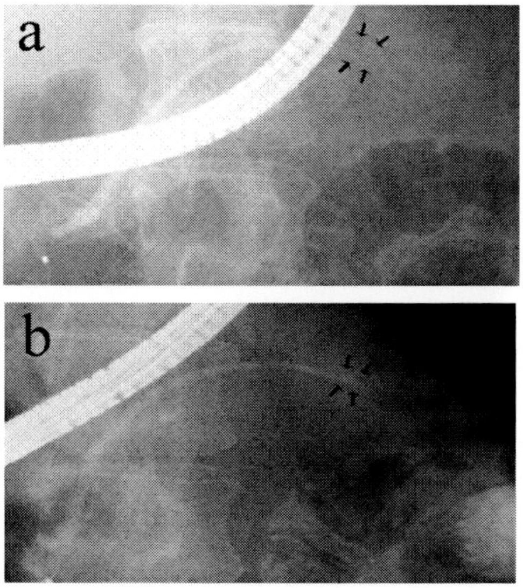

Figure 5. A: Endoscopic retrograde pancreatography (ERP) image before bromhexine hydrochloride therapy. The main pancreatic duct in the body is dilated, and there is a small transparent object, probably a protein plug, within the lumen (arrow). The main pancreatic duct lumen from the dilation toward the tail appears irregular. B: ERP image after six months of bromhexine hydrochloride therapy. The dilation of the main pancreatic duct in the body improved and the small transparent object disappeared. The irregularity of the main pancreatic duct lumen improved, too.

It will act directly on the acinar cells, which comprise the pancreatic exocrine gland, to secrete a low-viscosity pancreatic juice, relieving the stasis of the pancreatic juice, thereby improving the clinical manifestations, pancreatic enzymes, and pancreatic exocrine function, as well as dissolving and washing out the protein plugs.

Abstinence is a definitive prerequisite for the successful treatment of alcoholic chronic pancreatitis. Bromhexine hydrochloride, although not a curative therapy for alcoholic chronic pancreatitis, is effective in halting or delaying the progression of the disease, and improving the patient's quality of life. Figure 6 shows the authors' therapeutic regimen for alcoholic chronic pancreatitis, and our ranking of the various therapies. The effects of bromhexine hydrochloride are best seen in combination with a firm base of life style modification, including diet and abstinence from alcohol, as well as non-pharmacological and pharmacological therapies. Bromhexine hydrochloride is a promising new therapeutic modality for alcoholic chronic pancreatitis, where protein plug formation, increased mucoprotein levels, and increased viscosity of the pancreatic juice are implicated in the recurrent episodes of acute pancreatitis.

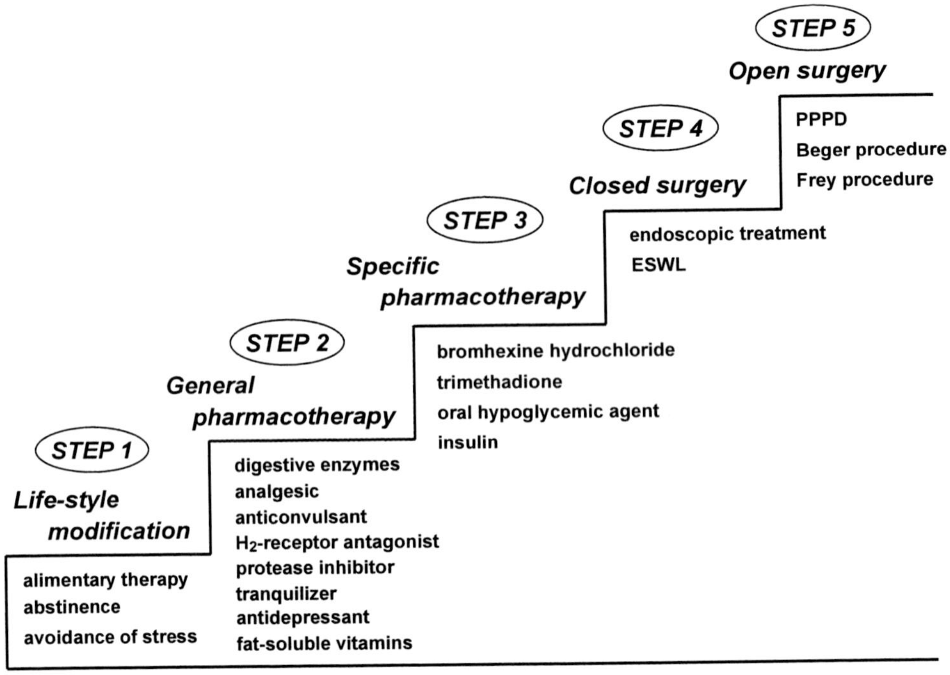

Figure 6. Treatment regimen for alcoholic chronic pancreatitis.

In conclusion, alcoholic chronic pancreatitis is a refractory chronic pathologic entity with a prolonged natural course, and alleviation of the clinical manifestations or disappearance of protein plugs in no way represents a cure. We emphasise that the treatment of this condition requires long-term general health care, while maintaining a good doctor-patient relationship.

References

[1] Layer P, Yamamoto H, Kalthoff L, Clain JE, Bakken LJ, DiMagno EP. The different courses of early- and late-onset idiopathic and alcoholic chronic pancreatitis. *Gastroenterology* 1994; 107: 1481-1487.

[2] Comfort MW, Steinberg AG. Pedigree of a family with hereditary chronic relapsing pancreatitis. Gastroenterology 1952; 21: 54-63.

[3] Ulrich CD; Consensus Committees of the European Registry of Hereditary Pancreatic Diseases, Midwest Multi-Center Pancreatic Study Group, International Association of

Pancreatology. Pancreatic cancer in hereditary pancreatitis: consensus guidelines for prevention, screening and treatment. *Pancreatology* 2001; 1: 416-422.

[4] Witcomb DC, Gorry MC, Preston RA, Furey W, Sossenheimer MJ, Ulrich CD, et al. Hereditary pancreatitis is caused by a mutation in the cationic trypsinogen gene. *Nat. Genet.* 1996; 14: 141-145.

[5] Etemad B, Whitcomb DC. Chronic pancreatitis: Diagnosis, classification, and new genetic developments. *Gastroenterology* 2001; 120: 682-707.

[6] Naruse S, Kitagawa M, Ishiguro H, Fujiki K, Hayakawa T. Cystic fibrosis and related diseases of the pancreas. *Best Pract. Res. Clin. Gastroenterol.* 2002; 16: 511-526.

[7] Okazaki K, Uchida K, Matsushita M, Takaoka M. Autoimmune pancreatitis. *Internal. Med.* 2005; 44: 1215-1223.

[8] Smith MD, Pawlak M, Pantanowitz DP, Botha RJ. Hyperparathyroidism and chronic pancreatitis. *S. Afr. J. Surg.* 1999; 37: 12-14.

[9] Fortson MR, Freedman SN, Weber PD 3rd. Clinical assessment of hyperlipidemic pancreatitis. *Am. J. Gastroenterol.* 1995; 90: 2134-2139.

[10] Yadav D, Pitchumoni CS. Issues in hyperlipidemic pancreatitis. *J. Clin. Gastroenterol.* 2003; 36: 54-62.

[11] Kamisawa T, Matsukawa M, Amemiya K, Tu Y, Egawa N, Okamoto A, et al. Pancreatitis associated with pancreaticobiliary maljunction. *Hepatogastroenterology* 2003; 50: 1665-1668.

[12] Darras T, Bernard A, Carlier L, Collette JM. A case of congenital dilatation of the common bile duct associated with chronic pancreatitis. *J. Belge. Radiol.* 1985; 68: 442-443.

[13] Bradley EL 3rd. Chronic obstructive pancreatitis as a delayed complication of pancreatic trauma. *HPB Surg.* 1991; 5: 49-59.

[14] Stolte M, Waltschew A. The papilla of Vater and chronic pancreatitis. *Hepatogastroenterology* 1986; 33: 163-169.

[15] Runzi M, Layer P. Drug-induced pancreatitis: facts and fiction. *Pancreas* 1996; 13: 100-109.

[16] Ammann RW, Akovbiantz A, Largiader F, Schueler G. Course and outcome of chronic pancreatitis. Longitudinal study of a mixed medical-surgical series of 245 patients. *Gastroenterology* 1984; 86: 820-828.

[17] Ammann RW, Muellhaupt B. The natural history of pain in alcoholic chronic pancreatitis. *Gastroenterology* 1999; 116: 1132-1140.

[18] Miyake H, Harada H, Kunichika K, Ochi K, Kimura I. Clinical course and prognosis of chronic pancreatitis. *Pancreas* 1987; 2: 378-385.

[19] Hayakawa T, Kondo T, Shibata T, Sugimoto Y, Kitagawa M. Chronic alcoholism and evolution of pain and prognosis in chronic pancreatitis. *Dig. Dis. Sci.* 1989; 34: 33-38.

[20] Lankisch PG, Lohr-Happe A, Otto J, Creutzfeldt W. Natural course in chronic pancreatitis. Pain, exocrine and endocrine pancreatic insufficiency and prognosis of the disease. *Digestion* 1993; 54: 148-155.

[21] DiMagno EP. Toward understanding (and management) of painful chronic pancreatitis. *Gastroenterology* 1999; 116: 1252-1257.

[22] Kloppel G, Maillet B. The morphological basis for the evolution of acute pancreatitis into chronic pancreatitis. *Virchows Arch. A Pathol. Anat. Histopathol.* 1992; 420: 1-4.

[23] Sahel J, Sarles H. Modifications of pure human pancreatic juice induced by chronic alcohol consumption. *Dig. Dis. Sci.* 1979; 24: 897-905.

[24] Raraty M, Ward J, Erdemli G, Vailleant C, Neoptolemos JP, Sutton R, et al. Calcium-dependent enzyme activation and vacuole formation in the apical granular region of pancreatic acinar cells. *Proc. Natl. Acad. Sci. USA* 2000; 97: 13126-13131.

[25] Haber PS, Apte MV, Applegate TL, Norton ID, Korsten MA, Pirola RC, et al. Metabolism of ethanol by rat pancreatic acinar cells. *J. Lab. Clin. Med.* 1998; 132: 294-302.

[26] Lu Z, Karne S, Kolodecik T, Gorelick FS. Alcohols enhance cerulein-induced zymogen activation in pancreatic acinar cells. *Am. J. Physiol. Gastrointest. Liver Physiol.* 2002; 282: G501-G507.

[27] Gukovskaya AS, Hosseini S, Satoh A, Cheng JH, Nam KJ, Gukovsky I, et al. Ethanol differentially regulates NF-κB activation in pancreatic acinar cells through calcium and protein kinase C pathways. *Am. J. Physiol. Gastrointest Liver Physiol.* 2004; 286: G204-G213.

[28] Miyasaka K, Ohta M, Takano S, Hayashi H, Higuchi S, Maruyama K, et al. Carboxylester lipase gene polymorphism as a risk of alcohol-induced pancreatitis. *Pancreas* 2005; 30: e87-e91.

[29] Criddle DN, Murphy J, Fistetto G, Barrow S, Tepikin AV, Neoptolemos JP, et al. Fatty acid ethyl esters cause pancreatic calcium toxicity via inositol triphosphate receptors and loss of ATP synthesis. *Gastroenterology* 2006; 130: 781-793.

[30] Steward MC, Ishiguro H, Case RM. Mechanisms of bicarbonate secretion in the pancreatic duct. *Annu. Rev. Physiol.* 2005; 67: 377-409.

[31] Ito T, Nemoto M. Über die Kupfferschen Sternzellen und die "Fettspeicherungszellen" ("fat storing cells") in der Blutkapillarenwand der menschlichen Leber. *Okajimas Folia Anat. Jpn.* 1952; 24: 243-258 (in German).

[32] Hendriks HF, Verhoofstad WA, Brouwer A, de Leeuw AM, Knook DL. Perisinusoidal fat-storing cells are the main vitamin A storage sites in rat liver. *Exp. Cell Res.* 1985; 160: 138-149.

[33] Kent G, Gay S, Inouye T, Bahu R, Minick OT, Popper H. Vitamin A-containing lipocytes and formation of type III collagen in liver injury. *Proc. Natl. Acad. Sci. USA* 1976; 73: 3719-3722.

[34] Clement B, Grimaud JA, Campion JP, Deugnier Y, Guillouzo A. Cell types involved in collagen and fibronectin production in normal and fibrotic human liver. *Hepatology* 1986; 6: 225-234.

[35] Geerts A, Vrijsen R, Rauterberg J, Burt A, Schellinck P, Wisse E. In vitro differentiation of fat-storing cells parallels marked increase of collagen synthesis and secretion. *J. Hepatol.* 1989; 9: 59-68.

[36] Apte MV, Haber PS, Applegate TL, Norton ID, McCaughan GW, Korsten MA, et al. Periacinar stellate shaped cells in rat pancreas: identification, isolation, and culture. *Gut* 1998; 43: 128-133.

[37] Bachem MG, Schneider E, Gross H, Weidenbach H, Schmid RM, Menke A, et al. Identification, culture, and characterization of pancreatic stellate cells in rats and humans. *Gastroenterology* 1998; 115: 421-432.

[38] Masamune A, Sakai Y, Kikuta K, Satoh M, Satoh A, Shimosegawa T. Activated rat pancreatic stellate cells express intercellular adhesion molecule-1 (ICAM-1) in vitro. *Pancreas* 2002; 25: 78-85.

[39] Masamune A, Kikuta K, Satoh M, Kume K, Shimosegawa T. Differential roles of signaling pathways for proliferation and migration of rat pancreatic stellate cells. *Tohoku J. Exp. Med.* 2003; 199: 69-84.

[40] Apte MV, Phillips PA, Fahmy RG, Darby SJ, Rodgers SC, McCaughan GW, et al. Does alcohol directly stimulate pancreatic fibrogenesis? Studies with rat pancreatic stellate cells. *Gastroenterology* 2000; 118: 780-794.

[41] Masamuna A, Kikuta K, Satoh M, Satoh A, Shimosegawa T. Alcohol activates activator protein-1 and mitogen-activated protein kinases in rat pancreatic stellate cells. *J. Pharm. Exp. Ther.* 2002; 302: 36-42.

[42] Engelhorn R, Püschmann S. Pharmakologische Untersuchungen über eine Substanz mit sekretolytischer Wirkung. *Arzneim Forsch.* 1963; 13: 474-480 (in German).

[43] Bruce RA, Kumar V. The effect of derivative of vasicine on bronchial mucus. *Br. J. Clin. Pract.* 1968; 22: 289-292.

[44] Takeda H, Abe Y, Misawa M, Yanaura S, Kuroiwa Y. The role of vagal reflex in mechanism of secretagogic action of bromhexine. *Jpn. J. Phamacol.* 1984; 35: 445-450.

[45] Bloch KJ, Buchanan WW, Wohl MJ, Bunim JJ. Sjögren's syndrome. A clinical, pathological, and serological study of sixty-two cases. *Medicine* 1965; 44: 187-231.

[46] Rehman H. Sjögren syndrome. *Yonsei Med. J.* 2003; 44: 947-954.

[47] Kassan SS, Moutsopoulous HM. Clinical manifestations and early diagnosis of Sjögren's syndrome. *Arch. Intern. Med.* 2004; 164: 1275-1284.

[48] Vitali C, Bombardieri S, Jonsson R, Moutsopoulos HM, Alexander EL, Carsons SE, et al. Classification criteria for Sjögren's syndrome: a revised version of the European criteria proposed by the American-European Consensus Group. *Ann. Rheum. Dis.* 2002; 61: 554-558.

[49] Mavragani CP, Moutsopoulos NM, Moutsopoulos HM. The management of Sjögren syndrome. *Nat. Clin. Pract. Rheumatol.* 2006; 2: 252-261.

[50] Isager H, Frost-Larsen K, Manthorpe R, Westergaard L. The effect of bromhexine on the functional deficiency of the lacrimal apparatus and salivary glands in Sjögren's syndrome. *Med. Monatsschr.* 1977; 31: 582-583.

[51] Frost-Larsen K, Isager H, Manthorpe R. Sjögren's syndrome treated with bromhexine: a randomized clinical study. *Br. Med. J.* 1978; 1: 1579-1581.

[52] Manthorpe R, Frost-Larsen K, Hoj L, Isager H, Prause JU. Bromhexine treatment of Sjögren's syndrome: effect on lacrimal and salivary secretion, and on proteins in tear fluid and saliva. *Scand. J. Rheumatol.* 1981; 10: 177-180.

[53] Nanni JM, Nguyen KH, Alford CE, Robinson CP, Stewart CM, Maeda N, et al. Assessment of bromhexine as a treatment regimen in Sjögren's syndrome-like disease in the NOD (non-obese diabetic) mouse. *Clin. Exp. Rheumatol.* 1997; 15: 515-521.

[54] Oxholm P, Prause JU, Schiodt M. Rational drug therapy recommendations for the treatment of patients with Sjögren's syndrome. *Drugs* 1998; 56: 345-353.

[55] Kopitar Z, Leder O. Autoradiographic studies on the distribution of 14 C-labeled Bisolvon in the rat and mouse. *Arzneimittelforschung* 1971; 21: 914-918.

[56] Chang JH, Watanabe S, Toki F, Nishino T, Moriyoshi Y, Shiratori K, et al. Studies on the transfer of bromhexine-HCl (Bisolvon^{B}) from the blood to the pancreas in the rat and the dog. *Suizo* 1993; 8: 403-407 (in Japanese).

[57] Sarles H, Sarles JC, Camatte R, Muratore R, Gaini M, Guien C, et al. Observations of 205 confirmed cases of acute pancreatitis, recurring pancreatitis, and chronic pancreatitis. *Gut* 1965; 6: 545-559.

[58] Nakamura K, Sarles H, Payan H. Three-dimensional reconstruction of the pancreatic ducts in chronic pancreatitis. *Gastroenterology* 1972; 62: 942-949.

[59] Estevenon JP, Sarles H, Figarella C. Lactoferrin in the duodenal juice of patients with chronic calcifying pancreatitis. *Scand. J. Gastroenterol.* 1975; 10: 327-330.

[60] Wakabayashi A, Takeda Y. The behavior of mucopolysaccharide in the pancreatic juice in chronic pancreatitis. *Am. J. Dig. Dis.* 1976; 21: 607-612.

[61] Harada H, Takeda M, Yabe H, Hanafusa E, Hayashi T, Kunichika K, et al. The hexosamine concentration and output in human pure pancreatic juice in chronic pancreatitis. *Gastroenterol. Jpn.* 1980; 15: 520-526.

[62] Tympner F, Rosch W. Viscosity and trypsin activity of pure pancreatic juice in chronic pancreatitis. *Acta Hepatogastroenterol.* 1978; 25: 73-76.

[63] Harada H, Ueda O, Kochi F, Kobayashi T, Komazawa M. Comparative studies on viscosity and concentration of protein and hexosamine in pure pancreatic juice. *Gastroenterol. Jpn.* 1981; 16: 623-626.

[64] Guy O, Robles-Diaz G, Adrich Z, Sahel J, Sarles H. Protein content of precipitates present in pancreatic juice of alcoholic subjects and patients with chronic calcifying pancreatitis. *Gastroenterology* 1983; 84: 102-107.

[65] Freedman SD, Sakamoto K, Venu RP. GP2, the homologue to the renal cast protein uromodulin, is a major component of intraductal plugs in chronic pancreatitis. *J. Clin. Invest.* 1993; 92: 83-90.

[66] Tympner F, Rosch W. The treatment of chronic recurrent pancreatitis with depot secretin – a preliminary report. *Hepatogastroenterology* 1986; 33: 159-162.

[67] Buchler MW, Binder M, Friess H. Role of somatostatin and its analogues in the treatment of acute and chronic pancreatitis. *Gut* 1944; 35: S15-S19.

[68] Uhl W, Anghelacopoulos SE, Friess H, Buchler MW. The role of octreotide and somatostatin in acute and chronic pancreatitis. *Digestion* 1999; 60: 23-31.

[69] Harada H, Miyake H, Miki H, Kobayashi T, Sasaki T, Kimura I. Role of endoscopic elimination of protein plugs in the treatment of chronic pancreatitis. *Gastroenterol. Jpn.* 1982; 17: 463-468.

[70] Cremer M, Deviere J, Delhaye M, Baize M, Vandermeeren A. Stenting in severe chronic pancreatitis: results of medium-term follow-up in seventy-six patients. *Endoscopy* 1991; 23: 171-176.

[71] Sauerbruch T, Holl J, Sackmann M, Werner R, Wotzka R, Paumgartner G. Disintegration of a pancreatic duct stone with extracorporeal shock waves in a patient with chronic pancreatitis. *Endoscopy* 1987; 19: 207-208.

[72] Costamagna G, Gabbrielli A, Mutignani M, Perri V, Pandolfi M, Boscaini M, et al. Extracorporeal shock wave lithotripsy of pancreatic stones in chronic pancreatitis: immediate and medium-term results. *Gastrointest. Endosc.* 1997; 46: 231-236.

[73] Moore EW, Verine HJ. Pathogenesis of pancreatic and biliary $CaCO_3$ lithiasis: The solubility product (K'sp) of calcite determined with the Ca++ electrode. *J. Lab. Clin. Med.* 1985; 106: 611-618.

[74] Moore EW, Verine HJ. Pancreatic calcification and stone formation: a thermodynamic model of calcium in pancreatic juice. *Am. J. Physiol.* 1987; 252: G707-G718.

[75] Lohse J, Vernie HJ, Sarles H. Studies on pancreatic stones. I. In vitro dissolution. *Digestion* 1981; 21: 125-132.

[76] Sarles H, Sahel J, Laugier R. Treatment of chronic calcifying pancreatitis by oral long-term administration of citrate. Preliminary results. *Gastroenterol. Clin. Biol.* 1979; 3: 615-619.

[77] Noda A, Shibata T, Hamano H, Murase T, Hayakawa T, Horiguchi Y, et al. Trimetadione (troxidone) dissolves pancreatic stones. *Lancet* 1984; 2: 351-353.

[78] Noda A, Yano M, Ibuki E, Takeuchi K, Murayama H, Kobayashi T, et al. Comparative in vitro studies of dimethadione and citric acid for lysis of pancreatic stones. *Jpn. J. Clin. Pharmacol. Ther.* 1996; 27: 575-581.

[79] Chang JH, Takeuchi T. Effect of bromhexine in the treatment of pancreatitis accompanied by a mucin-producing pancreatic tumor. *Tan to Sui* 1991; 12: 281-285 (in Japanese).

[80] Shinohara Y, Fukuda S, Takeda K, Ikeda H, Kawaguchi M, Saitoh T, et al. A case of mucin-producing bile duct tumor which responded to bromhexine hydrochloride treatment and radiotherapy. *Tando* 1993; 7: 527-534 (in Japanese).

[81] Noda A, Ibuki E, Murayama H, Hase S. Bromhexine hydrochloride eliminates protein plugs and relieves attacks of pancreatitis. *Pancreas* 1997; 15: 209-211.

[82] Tsujimoto T, Takano M, Tsuruzono T, Hoppo K, Matsumura Y, Yamao J, et al. Mediastinal pancreatic pseudocyst caused by obstruction of the pancreatic duct was eliminated by bromhexine hydrochloride. *Internal. Med.* 2004; 43: 1034-1038.

[83] Tsujimoto T, Tsuruzono T, Hoppo K, Matsumura Y, Yamao J, Fukui H. Effect of bromhexine hydrochloride therapy for alcoholic chronic pancreatitis. *Alcohol. Clin. Exp. Res* 2005; 29: 272S-276S.

In: Pancreatitis Research Advances
Editor: William C. Langley, pp. 275-287
ISBN: 978-1-60021-883-5

Chapter IX

Expression Profiling of Chronic Pancreatitis

Deepak Hariharan and Tatjana Crnogorac-Jurcevic*
Centre for Molecular Oncology, Institute of Cancer,
Barts and the London School of Medicine and Dentistry,
Queen Mary University of London,
Charterhouse Square, London EC1M 6BQ, UK

Abstract

Chronic pancreatitis is associated with intense desmoplastic reaction, replacing normal acinar and islet cells with fibrous tissue, thus leading to exocrine and endocrine pancreatic insufficiency. The risk of developing pancreatic cancer in patients with chronic pancreatitis is well established. Clinical differentiation between the two remains difficult and establishing the diagnosis of chronic pancreatitis, in the absence of calcifications, diabetes, malabsorbtion, with equivocal imaging tests remains a challenge.

Several large-scale expression profiling technologies have recently been employed in chronic pancreatitis research, both at RNA and protein level.

Microarray technologies using high-density oligonucleotide arrays fabricated by Affymetrix Inc. (Santa Clara, CA) have implicated various genes in the pathobiology of chronic pancreatitis, including genes encoding for extracellular matrix formation, cell structural components, immune and inflammatory factors, signal transduction and regulatory molecules.

Proteomic techniques, such as immunoblotting analysis (PowerBlot, BD Biosciences, NJ), revealed 30 proteins to be deregulated in comparison between chronic pancreatitis and normal pancreas, whereas a substantial proportion of proteins were similarly dysregulated in both chronic pancreatitis and pancreatic ductal adenocarcinoma. Two dimensional gel electrophoresis (2D gels) and isotope coded affinity tagged labeling (ICAT) with mass spectrometry (MS) have also been employed, revealing additional set

* Phone: +44 (0)20 7014 0427. Fax: +44 (0)20 7014 0431. e-mail: T.C.Jurcevic@qmul.ac.uk

of proteins deregulated in chronic pancreatitis, namely several antioxidants, calcium binding proteins, proteases and catalytic enzymes.

The data obtained from such large-scale profiling approaches will lay the foundation and provide further understanding of the underlying pathophysiological processes, thus providing novel targets for diagnosis and treatment of chronic pancreatitis.

Introduction

The recent advances in large scale genomic technologies and bioinformatics, along with the completion of human genome sequencing project has enabled analysis of global gene and protein expression in cells, tissues and body fluids. Differential expression profiling has led to the discovery of a number of dysregulated genes and their products and for the first time helped uncover various molecular mechanisms underlying pathogenesis and stratification of diverse disease condition, including distinguishing between disease subtypes and development of candidate biomarkers [1-4].

Chronic pancreatitis (CP) is characterised by a progressive inflammatory process with irregular and irreversible fibrosis of the gland parenchyma, with varying degrees of dilatation of the ductal system, thus leading to exocrine and endocrine pancreatic insufficiency in the advanced stages of the disease [5]. The disease affects more males than females. Its clinical manifestations tend to appear in middle age, though it can present early or even remain asymptomatic throughout life [6]. The classic symptoms associated with CP are deep persistent abdominal pain, malabsorbtion and diabetes, and these may vary with the degree of desmoplastic change occurring in the gland. The deep anatomical location of the gland requires the use of sophisticated and expensive imaging techniques to investigate diseases relating to the pancreas. The symptoms need to be corroborated with findings on Computerised Tomography scans (CT), Endoscopic ultrasound (EUS) and Endoscopic Retrograde Choloangio Pancreatography (ERCP) which would detect the presence of calcifications, cysts, duct irregularities and parenchymal heterogeneity, thus confirming diagnosis. Pancreatic exocrine function tests in association with upper gastrointestinal endoscopy may also be used. All of the above-mentioned methods are neither sensitive nor specific and histology still remains the gold standard for diagnosing chronic pancreatitis [7]. However, the difficulty in obtaining tissue specimens along with the ethical issues of performing an invasive procedure on patients with suspected CP, combined with occasional non-representational tissue sampling represent major hurdles in achieving an accurate diagnosis.

Alcoholism has been identified as the primary cause in 66 - 80% of patients diagnosed with CP, while only 5 – 10% of alcoholics develop chronic pancreatitis. In alcoholics a prolonged, sustained, asymptomatic latent phase can last as long as 10 – 20 years and histological changes in the gland do not ensue until the alterations are fairly advanced [8-10]. In the absence of symptoms, presence of equivocal imaging and no histology, reaching a diagnosis can be extremely difficult and thus the initiation of treatment is often delayed.

In 25% of cases the cause of CP is unknown and these are further classified depending on the time of presentation either as early or late onset subtypes.

The other rarer causes of CP include hereditary pancreatitis, hyperparathyroidism, hyperlipidaemia, malnutrition, autoimmune pancreatitis, tropical pancreatitis, chronic obstructive lesions and congenital malformations of the pancreas. Of these, hereditary pancreatitis, an autosomal dominant condition, has been well studied and accounts for about 1% of CP cases [11-14]. The criteria to diagnose hereditary chronic pancreatitis undergoes constant change and currently differs in various clinical centres [11]. Therefore, a great need exists to evolve an international consensus to promote better understanding of different etiologies and various pathogenetic mechanisms involved in the development of CP.

Several studies have been undertaken to explore the genetic basis for the development of chronic pancreatitis and three major groups of gene mutations have been recognised [15-19]. Serine protease 1 (PRSS1) or cationic trypsinogen gene is mutated in 52 – 81% of patients with hereditary pancreatitis [20]. In about 50% of patients who were classified as early onset idiopathic CP, mutations of serine protease inhibitor Kazal type 1 (SPINK1) and cystic fibrosis trans-membrane conductance regulator (CFTR) gene mutations were found [21, 22]. In 20 – 55% of patients with tropical pancreatitis, SPINK1 mutations have been documented [23], while heterozygous CFTR and SPINK1 mutations play a limited role in the development of sporadic CP [24, 25].

Mutations in PRSS1 and SPINK1 cause acinar cell death by different mechanisms that include both apoptotic and non-apoptotic pathways, while CFTR mutation causes increased cytokine production leading to necrotic acinar cell death [26].

Surprisingly low number of people that are heavy alcohol consumers go on to develop CP (less than 10%), thus genetic and environmental factors were investigated [27]. As a result, a genetic polymorphism involving the detoxifying enzyme uridine 5'-diphosphate glucuronyl transferase (UGT1A7*3) was shown to increase the risk of developing alcohol-induced CP [28].

However, neither of the described gene abnormalities have until now been translated to improved identification and treatment of chronic pancreatitis due to low sensitivity and specificity associated with screening asymptomatic populations.

Several studies have shown that chronic pancreatitis is an independent risk factor for the development of pancreatic ductal adenocarcinoma (PDAC), the 4th common cause of cancer related death in the western world [29-31]. Sporadic chronic pancreatitis carries a lifetime risk of about 4% after 20 years, whereas hereditary pancreatitis carries a 53 fold increased relative risk of causing pancreatic cancer [30, 32]. The intense desmoplastic response commonly seen in both PDAC and CP makes differentiating between the two extremely difficult [33, 34].

As large scale genomic and proteomic profiling have proved beneficial in the identification of differentially regulated genes and gene products in a number of diseases, the profiling of CP and PDAC in a similar fashion could provide insight into the evolution of both diseases. This would enable better understanding of the underlying pathogenetic and pathophysiological mechanisms and thus help establish better stratifications of the two diseases. Such studies performed until date have been summarised in Table 1.

Table 1. Studies looking at expression profiling of chronic pancreatitis

Gene expression profiling			
Year	Author	Platform	Samples used for comparison
2001	Friess, H et al	Oligonucleotide array (Affymetrix)	Tissue - 8 CP, 8 PDAC and 8 N
2003	Logsdon et al	Oligonucleotide array (Affymetrix)	Tissue – 10 PDAC, 5 CP, 5 N and 7 Pancreatic cell lines
2004	Binkley et al	Oligonucleotide array (Affymetrix)	Tissue – 10 PDAC, 5 CP, 5 N and 7 Pancreatic cell lines
Protein expression profiling			
Year	Author	Platform	Samples used for comparison
2001	Valerio, A et al	MALDI-TOF/ MS	Serum –13 PDAC, 9 CP and 10 N
2004	Shen, J et al	2DE/MS	Tissue – 6 PDAC, 7 CP and 8 N
2005	Crnogorac-Jurcevic, T et al	BD PowerBlot	Tissue – 5 PDAC, 5 CP and 5 N
2007	Chen et al	ICAT/MS	Pancreatic Juice – 1CP and 10 benign cystic tumours

Gene Expression Profiling in CP

Although the prevalence of CP is much higher than that of PDAC (10-40/100,000 vs 8-12/100,000) [35, 36], due to the severity of the latter and substantial overlap between the two, the number of studies looking to examine the expression profile of CP alone is far fewer than those incorporating comparisons between CPs and PDAC.

Freiss et al [37] used HuGeneFL DNA array (Affymetrix, Santa Clara,CA) which contained 7,000 oligonucleotide sequences representing 5,600 full length human genes, to compare 8 CP, 8 PDAC and 8 normal (N) pancreatic tissue samples. RNA was extracted from whole tissue specimens and comparison revealed 157 genes to be over-expressed in CP as compared to normal tissue, of which 152 were simultaneously over-expressed in PDAC. The expression of 34 genes was decreased in PDAC and CP, taking the total number of dysregulated genes in CP to 191. A set of 5 genes which include mucin 6 (MUC6), germline oligomeric matrix protein (COMP), tryptase (TPSB1), rearranged immunoglobulin lambda light chain (IgGλ) and cysteine rich secretory protein-3 (CRISP-3) were identified as significantly up-regulated in CP, when compared to PDAC and normal tissue. This study also suggested that the molecular alterations occurring in CP might be precancerous as the vast set of deregulated genes (186) was also present in PDAC.

Andrianifahanana et al undertook reverse transcriptase polymerase chain reaction (RT-PCR) analysis to look at MUC6 expression in chronic pancreatitis, pancreatic tumour and pancreatic cancer cell lines [38]. MUC6 was highly expressed in all chronic pancreatitis patients, and to a lesser extent in patients with cancer. It was also seen in well and moderately differentiated cancer cell lines (CAPAN1 and BxPC3), thus MUC6 alone was unable to clearly differentiate CP from pancreatic cancer. The expression of COMP and CRISP-3 proteins were also studied and found to be moderate to highly expressed in CP as compared to tumour samples and normal tissue [39, 40]. As the expression of these proteins was again not exclusive to CP, their use in diagnosis of chronic pancreatitis would be limited.

In a slightly larger study Logsdon et al used HuGeneFL oligonucleotide arrays (Affymeterix, Santa Clara, CA) with 7,129 probe sets interrogating 6,800 genes [41]. A common cluster of 322 probe sets was identified, which were highly expressed both in PDAC and CP (after the comparisons between expression profiles of tissue from N, CP, and PDAC), 461 probe sets were noted to be highly expressed when CP was compared to normal samples and 735 probe sets were over-expressed when pancreatic cancer was compared to normal. The common set identified seemed to account for the intense desmoplasia common to PDAC and CP. Deducting the commonly expressed probe sets from highly expressed genes between CP and normal samples gives a set of 139 probes purely up-regulated in CP [41]. This set is, however, not available for further examination.

In the follow up study by the same group, Binkley et al [34] investigated the molecular elements of fibrosis by analysing the previously obtained data [41]. They used a deductive comparison strategy where genes expressed in normal tissue and in pancreatic cancer cell lines were selectively eliminated from those expressed in PDAC and CP. A set of 107 genes was identified in this manner, most of which were found to encode for extracellular matrix proteins, signalling molecules, immune and inflammation modulation. Cadherin 11 type 2 (CDH11), thrombospondin 2 (THBS2), fibronectin 1 (FN1) and apolipoprotein C1 (APOC1) showed high level of expression in pancreatic cancer and CP, and were selected for further study using RT-PCR and immunohistochemistry (IHC). RT-PCR confirmed the enhanced expression of these genes in PDAC and CP, while IHC demonstrated that they were localized to the stromal compartment. The study also identified α smooth muscle actin (α SMA), platelet derieved growth factor receptors α and β (PDGFR α and β), matrix metalloproteinase 2 (MMP2) and collagens type I and III (COL1A1 and COL3A1). All these genes were previously shown to be associated with activated pancreatic stellate cells and localized to the stromal compartment [42-45]. The isolation and characterisation of pancreatic stellate cells (PSCs) has much improved our understanding of cellular basis of desmoplasia [46]. Fibrosis results from an imbalance of collagen synthesis and degradation [47], with tumour growth factor β (TGFβ) playing an important role in development of desmoplastic reaction [48] and matrix metalloproteinases (MMPs) being a key to extracellular matix degradation [47]. Ethanol and oxidative metabolite acetaldehyde activates PSCs leading to release of cytokines, TGFβ, tissue inhibitors of metalloproteinases 1, 2 (TIMP 1, 2) and type1 collagen secretion [49] along with the activation of mitogen activated protein kinase (MAPK) and activated protein 1 (AP-1) pathways. These in turn cause proliferation, migration and continued secretion from PSCs, thus sustaining fibrosis [50].

Protein Expression Profile in CP

Proteomics is defined as the study of proteins encoded by the genome [51]. As proteins form the biochemical basis for most diseases, proteomic technologies are being increasingly applied to identify new diagnostic and prognostic disease markers as well as new therapeutic targets [52].

The studies to evaluate protein levels in CPs were designed in much the same way as the transcriptomic studies described above; investigators have used several platforms to explore protein expression profile of PDAC using CP and normal samples for comparison. Valerio et al compared the mass spectral peaks obtained by analysing sera from patients suffering from CP, pancreatic cancer and healthy individuals using a matrix associated laser desorbtion ionisation reflex time of flight instrument (MALDI-TOF) [53]. The authors found several peaks in low molecular weight fractions (mass/charge -1310, 2135, 2411, 2585, 3591, 3973, 4299) rich in ionic species that were seen purely in diseased sera (both CP and PDAC) and not in healthy controls. The study was unable to show peaks that differed between CP and PDAC, although the relative abundance of few fragments was higher in cancer as compared to chronic pancreatitis [53].

Shen et al used 2 dimensional polyacrylamide gel electrophoresis (2D-PAGE) followed by mass spectrometry (MS) to identify 40 differentially expressed proteins while comparing either individual samples or pools of whole tissues derived from healthy pancreata, chronic pancreatitis and pancreatic ductal adenocarcinoma [54]. Superoxide dismutase 1 (SOD1), an antioxidant protein was found over-expressed in chronic pancreatitis when compared to normal and cancerous tissue, while heat shock cognate protein 54, trypsinogen I, trypsinogen II and pancreatic amylase α2A were up-regulated in chronic pancreatitis and normal tissue when compared to pancreatic cancer specimens. The two-fold up-regulation of SOD1 in CP samples seen on 2D-PAGE/MS was confirmed by Western blot analysis in the same set of samples [54].

A PowerBlot immunoblotting analysis with approximately 900 antibodies was performed with lysates of pooled tissue obtained from patients suffering from CP, PDAC and N pancreatic tissue [55]. This study revealed 30 differentially expressed proteins between CP and N (15 up-regulated and 15 down-regulated) and 112 deregulated proteins (54 up-regulated and 48 down-regulated) when PDAC, CP and N were compared. 76 of 112 (74%) proteins were found to be commonly deregulated between CP and PDAC. Three proteins, namely ubiquitin-like, containing PHD and RING finger domains (UHRF1) and Menkes disease-associated protein (ATP7A) that were over-expressed in PDAC and absent in CP, along with aldehyde oxidase1 (AOX1), seen in CP and N and absent in PDAC were selected for further evaluation using RT-PCR and IHC.

Chen et al used a quantitative proteomic approach, isotope-coded affinity tag labelling (ICAT) followed by tandem mass spectrometry to study the profile of pancreatic juice in benign diseases of the pancreas [56]. The samples were obtained from a patient with CP and 10 patients with benign cystic neoplasms (these were treated as normal since procurement of pancreatic juice from healthy individuals through an invasive procedure such as ERCP is not ethical). Out of 72 identified proteins, 27 were differentially expressed by at least two fold (19 were up-regulated and 8 were down-regulated). The authors further compared these results with their previous study [57], where 105 proteins were identified from pancreatic cancer juice. The analysis revealed nine up-regulated proteins that were common to PDAC and CP with a further set of 18 proteins that were differentially expressed only in pancreatitis. However, none of these proteins underwent further validation.

Discussion

In the race to develop biomarkers specific for various diseases, it is vital that the results obtained from gene expression profiling studies are correlated with the differential expression seen in proteomic studies, followed with extensive validation on large sets of individual samples.

The yield of differentially expressed genes/proteins exclusive for CP is limited and there are several potential reasons for this. Dysregulated genes and proteins identified in CP are a result of very few studies undertaken to look for markers specific to chronic pancreatitis; the majority of studies performed until now (Table 1) were designed to differentiate PDAC's, with the inclusion of CP samples to either exclude or examine the set of genes/proteins that were involved in the common desmoplastic reaction. Only 2 of 7 studies evaluated looked for differential expression purely in CP [37, 56].

Furthermore, the availability of microarray platforms at the time when reviewed studies were performed led to the limited examination of the human genome. Friess et al used cDNA array examining 5,600 genes, whereas Logsdon et al and Binkley et al used slightly larger oligonucleotide arrays with 6,800 genes, thus still leaving a vast number of genes unexamined. In addition, the poor correlation between genomic and proteomic approaches that has been documented previously [58], is also exemplified here, as none of the statistically significant deregulated genes in CP were seen in any of the proteomic studies.

The technical limitations of proteomic approaches also lead to unavoidable source of bias. Valerio et al visualized peaks in serum samples of PDAC and CP using MALDI-TOF but the major drawback of the study was the lack of identification of obtained differential peaks. The use of 2-DE/MS approach by Shen et al was limited by the identification of high abundance proteins which is a known drawback of 2D gel-based proteomic approaches [54]. The PowerBlot approach, though more comprehensive, was based on 900 antibodies and was determined by the availability of well-optimised antibodies at the time of analysis [55]. The ICAT/MS analysis performed by Chen et al allowed for better quantitation over traditional gel based methods and identification of lower abundance proteins; however this technique is biased towards labelling peptides with cysteine residues and remains technically challenging [56]. None of the 18 proteins reported to be significantly up-regulated in CP in this study have been validated and furthermore, the results obtained from examination of secreted proteome in pancreatic juice of individuals with benign disease of pancreas are not directly comparable to the other proteomic studies performed on tissue specimens.

Several studies used pooled sampling in their analysis [54-56]. The strategy to pool samples in the proteomic experiments was utilised to reduce the large inter-individual differences arising as a result of biological variation when small number of samples are analysed. The difficulty in obtaining large number of samples in relatively rare conditions such as CP and PDAC, along with the need to obtain statistically valid data makes pooling mandatory, but results from all such studies require rigorous validation on large number of individual samples.

The inclusion criteria of CP samples where tissue was analysed was based on histology, while in the study by Valerio et al and Chen et al, serum and pancreatic juice samples, respectively, were obtained from CP patients where diagnosis was based on imaging and/or endoscopy. Specimen pooling along with inconsistent inclusion criteria form additional sources of bias.

Very few genes were found differentially expressed between CP and PDAC. The genes found to be expressed predominantly in CP, namey MUC6, COMP and CRISP-3 in the study by Friess et al [37], were subsequently found to be non-specific in the confirmatory studies [37-40]. In the 2D gel study by Shen et al, several of the proteins that were found to be over-expressed in CP (Super oxide dismutase 1, heat shock cognate protein 54, trypsinogen I, trypsinogen II and pancreatic amylase α2A), SOD1 was the only protein to be further validated by Western blot and its increased expression in CP as compared to PDAC and N was confirmed [54]. However, the difference found was only quantitative, thus this would hamper the usage of SOD1 as a marker of CP. UHRF1 and ATP7A that were validated in the immunoblotting study were chosen predominantly due to their specificity for PDAC rather than CP [55]. AOX1, which was over-expressed in CP and N and showed no expression in PDAC, when validated using IHC was found to have higher expression in normal pancreas than in CP, with a complete loss of expression in malignant pancreatic cells. Its use as a potential marker for CP therefore remains limited.

The molecular basis of fibrosis, comprising large number of common genes and proteins deregulated in CP and PDAC, was substantiated in several studies included in this review. Binkley et al [34] confirmed 4 genes (CDH 11, THBS2, FN1, APOC1) to be involved in desmoplastic reaction and in addition confirmed a host of other genes identified in the study by Friess and Logsdon et al [37, 41].

At the proteome level the overlap between CP and PDAC was also found to be considerable, with most studies reporting close to 70% of commonly deregulated proteins. In addition to desmoplastic gene products, other proteins involved in catalytic activity, transport, signal transduction and immune modulation were also found to be commonly dysregulated in CP and PDAC. Hypoxia inducible factor 1, alpha subunit (HIF1α) was the only molecule found to be commonly over-expressed at both proteomic and transcriptomic level [34, 55]. While its up-regulation in PDAC is well illustrated [59, 60] its role in the development of desmoplasia needs further evaluation.

Experimental fibrinolytic strategies using immunosuppressive agents, cyclooxygenase –2 (COX-2) inhibitors, selective 5-hydroxytryptamine (5-HT) antagonists and antioxidants have shown promising treatment responses, at least in animal models [61-64]. Anti monocyte chemoattractant protein (MCP) 1 gene therapy and nuclear hormone receptor peroxisome proliferators activated receptor γ (PPARγ) agonists (troglitazones) have shown to reduce PSCs activation, pancreatic inflammation and fibrosis in experimental animals [65, 66].

Future Perspectives

In the recent years the need to find new diagnostic and prognostic markers as well as novel therapeutic targets has led to increased use of large scale genomic and proteomics approaches thus generating vast amounts of information. The need to develop tests that will aid in early diagnosis of CP and distinguish it from PDAC is vital, hence enabling timely institution of therapy.

It is unfortunate that the possible CP markers generated in published work that was reviewed here have largely remained unverified. Further studies examining biomarkers specific to CP in tissue and particularly body fluids are urgently needed, and the capacity to verify and validate these markers on a large number of samples needs improvement. As the technology for biomarker discovery continues to develop, there exists a need to evolve an International consensus on establishing and developing standardized sample procurement and analysis protocols. Large collaborative efforts from laboratories with similar interests worldwide would need to be initiated in order to verify and validate results on large sample numbers. Consensus on establishing a panel of markers rather than single molecules specific to CP is required along with the use of techniques that would be able to assay large numbers of clinical specimens (blood, urine, pancreatic juice) at different stages of the disease. This will not only enable in depth understanding of the disease process, but would also lead to new improved diagnostic methods and identification of effective therapeutics targets, which would if not cure, delay the onset and stop the progression of the disease.

References

[1] Alizadeh, A.A., et al., Distinct types of diffuse large B-cell lymphoma identified by gene expression profiling. *Nature,* 2000. 403(6769): p. 503-11.

[2] Bittner, M., et al., Molecular classification of cutaneous malignant melanoma by gene expression profiling. *Nature*, 2000. 406(6795): p. 536-40.

[3] Golub, T.R., et al., Molecular classification of cancer: class discovery and class prediction by gene expression monitoring. *Science*, 1999. 286(5439): p. 531-7.

[4] Ramaswamy, S., et al., A molecular signature of metastasis in primary solid tumors. *Nat. Genet.*, 2003. 33(1): p. 49-54.

[5] Naruse, S., M. Kitagawa, and H. Ishiguro, Molecular understanding of chronic pancreatitis: a perspective on the future. *Mol. Med. Today*, 1999. 5(11): p. 493-9.

[6] Lowenfels, A.B., et al., Prognosis of chronic pancreatitis: an international multicenter study. International Pancreatitis Study Group. *Am. J. Gastroenterol.,* 1994. 89(9): p. 1467-71.

[7] DiMagno, M.J. and E.P. DiMagno, Chronic pancreatitis. *Curr. Opin. Gastroenterol.*, 2004. 20(5): p. 444-51.

[8] Etemad, B. and D.C. Whitcomb, Chronic pancreatitis: diagnosis, classification, and new genetic developments. *Gastroenterology*, 2001. 120(3): p. 682-707.

[9] Banciu, T., et al., Prevalence of chronic (latent) pancreatitis in hospitalized chronic consumers of alcohol. *Rom. J. Intern. Med.,* 1991. 29(1-2): p. 49-53.

[10] Andersen, B.N., et al., Incidence of alcoholic chronic pancreatitis in Copenhagen. *Scand. J. Gastroenterol.*, 1982. 17(2): p. 247-52.

[11] Rosendahl, J., et al., Hereditary chronic pancreatitis. *Orphanet J. Rare Dis.,* 2007. 2: p. 1.

[12] Pfutzer, R., et al., Novel cationic trypsinogen (PRSS1) N29T and R122C mutations cause autosomal dominant hereditary pancreatitis. *Gut*, 2002. 50(2): p. 271-2.

[13] Ferec, C., et al., Mutations in the cationic trypsinogen gene and evidence for genetic heterogeneity in hereditary pancreatitis. *J. Med. Genet.*, 1999. 36(3): p. 228-32.

[14] Gorry, M.C., et al., Mutations in the cationic trypsinogen gene are associated with recurrent acute and chronic pancreatitis. *Gastroenterology*, 1997. 113(4): p. 1063-8.

[15] Gaiser, S., et al., Expression of mutated cationic trypsinogen reduces cellular viability in AR4-2J cells. *Biochem. Biophys. Res. Commun.*, 2005. 334(2): p. 721-8.

[16] Ohmuraya, M., et al., Autophagic cell death of pancreatic acinar cells in serine protease inhibitor Kazal type 3-deficient mice. *Gastroenterology*, 2005. 129(2): p. 696-705.

[17] Lempinen, M., et al., Mutations N34S and P55S of the SPINK1 gene in patients with chronic pancreatitis or pancreatic cancer and in healthy subjects: a report from Finland. *Scand. J. Gastroenterol.*, 2005. 40(2): p. 225-30.

[18] Kume, K., et al., Mutations in the serine protease inhibitor Kazal Type 1 (SPINK1) gene in Japanese patients with pancreatitis. *Pancreatology*, 2005. 5(4-5): p. 354-60.

[19] Weiss, F.U., et al., Complete cystic fibrosis transmembrane conductance regulator gene sequencing in patients with idiopathic chronic pancreatitis and controls. *Gut*, 2005. 54(10): p. 1456-60.

[20] Whitcomb, D.C., et al., Hereditary pancreatitis is caused by a mutation in the cationic trypsinogen gene. *Nat. Genet.*, 1996. 14(2): p. 141-5.

[21] Noone, P.G., et al., Cystic fibrosis gene mutations and pancreatitis risk: relation to epithelial ion transport and trypsin inhibitor gene mutations. *Gastroenterology*, 2001. 121(6): p. 1310-9.

[22] Witt, H., et al., Mutations in the gene encoding the serine protease inhibitor, Kazal type 1 are associated with chronic pancreatitis. *Nat. Genet.*, 2000. 25(2): p. 213-6.

[23] Rossi, L., et al., SPINK1/PSTI mutations are associated with tropical pancreatitis in Bangladesh. A preliminary report. *Pancreatology*, 2001. 1(3): p. 242-5.

[24] Schneider, A., et al., Limited contribution of the SPINK1 N34S mutation to the risk and severity of alcoholic chronic pancreatitis: a report from the United States. *Dig. Dis. Sci.*, 2003. 48(6): p. 1110-5.

[25] Pezzilli, R., et al., Mutations of the CFTR gene in pancreatic disease. *Pancreas*, 2003. 27(4): p. 332-6.

[26] Dimagno, M.J., et al., A proinflammatory, antiapoptotic phenotype underlies the susceptibility to acute pancreatitis in cystic fibrosis transmembrane regulator (-/-) mice. *Gastroenterology*, 2005. 129(2): p. 665-81.

[27] Dufour, M.C. and M.D. Adamson, The epidemiology of alcohol-induced pancreatitis. *Pancreas*, 2003. 27(4): p. 286-90.

[28] Ockenga, J., et al., UDP glucuronosyltransferase (UGT1A7) gene polymorphisms increase the risk of chronic pancreatitis and pancreatic cancer. *Gastroenterology*, 2003. 124(7): p. 1802-8.

[29] Malka, D., et al., Risk of pancreatic adenocarcinoma in chronic pancreatitis. *Gut*, 2002. 51(6): p. 849-52.

[30] Howes, N. and J.P. Neoptolemos, Risk of pancreatic ductal adenocarcinoma in chronic pancreatitis. *Gut*, 2002. 51(6): p. 765-6.

[31] Talamini, G., et al., Incidence of cancer in the course of chronic pancreatitis. *Am. J. Gastroenterol.*, 1999. 94(5): p. 1253-60.

[32] Rosty, C., et al., p16 Inactivation in pancreatic intraepithelial neoplasias (PanINs) arising in patients with chronic pancreatitis. *Am. J. Surg. Pathol.*, 2003. 27(12): p. 1495-501.

[33] Ruszniewski, P., et al., The diagnostic dilemmas in discrimination between pancreatic carcinoma and chronic pancreatitis. *Gut,* 2004. 53(5): p. 771.

[34] Binkley, C.E., et al., The molecular basis of pancreatic fibrosis: common stromal gene expression in chronic pancreatitis and pancreatic adenocarcinoma. *Pancreas,* 2004. 29(4): p. 254-63.

[35] Lin, Y., et al., Nationwide epidemiological survey of chronic pancreatitis in Japan. *J. Gastroenterol.*, 2000. 35(2): p. 136-41.

[36] Wong, T., et al., Molecular diagnosis of early pancreatic ductal adenocarcinoma in high-risk patients. *Pancreatology,* 2001. 1(5): p. 486-509.

[37] Friess, H., et al., Identification of disease-specific genes in chronic pancreatitis using DNA array technology. *Ann. Surg.,* 2001. 234(6): p. 769-78; discussion 778-9.

[38] Andrianifahanana, M., et al., Mucin (MUC) gene expression in human pancreatic adenocarcinoma and chronic pancreatitis: a potential role of MUC4 as a tumor marker of diagnostic significance. *Clin. Cancer Res.,* 2001. 7(12): p. 4033-40.

[39] Liao, Q., et al., COMP is selectively up-regulated in degenerating acinar cells in chronic pancreatitis and in chronic-pancreatitis-like lesions in pancreatic cancer. *Scand. J. Gastroenterol.*, 2003. 38(2): p. 207-15.

[40] Liao, Q., et al., Preferential expression of cystein-rich secretory protein-3 (CRISP-3) in chronic pancreatitis. *Histol. Histopathol.,* 2003. 18(2): p. 425-33.

[41] Logsdon, C.D., et al., Molecular profiling of pancreatic adenocarcinoma and chronic pancreatitis identifies multiple genes differentially regulated in pancreatic cancer. *Cancer Res.*, 2003. 63(10): p. 2649-57.

[42] Bachem, M.G., et al., Identification, culture, and characterization of pancreatic stellate cells in rats and humans. *Gastroenterology*, 1998. 115(2): p. 421-32.

[43] Linder, S., et al., Immunohistochemical expression of extracellular matrix proteins and adhesion molecules in pancreatic carcinoma. *Hepatogastroenterology*, 2001. 48(41): p. 1321-7.

[44] Schneider, E., et al., Identification of mediators stimulating proliferation and matrix synthesis of rat pancreatic stellate cells. *Am. J. Physiol. Cell Physiol.,* 2001. 281(2): p. C532-43.

[45] Iacobuzio-Donahue, C.A., et al., Exploring the host desmoplastic response to pancreatic carcinoma: gene expression of stromal and neoplastic cells at the site of primary invasion. *Am. J. Pathol.,* 2002. 160(1): p. 91-9.

[46] Apte, M.V., et al., Pancreatic stellate cells are activated by proinflammatory cytokines: implications for pancreatic fibrogenesis. *Gut,* 1999. 44(4): p. 534-41.

[47] Arthur, M.J., Collagenases and liver fibrosis. *J. Hepatol.,* 1995. 22(2 Suppl): p. 43-8.

[48] Desmouliere, A., et al., Transforming growth factor-beta 1 induces alpha-smooth muscle actin expression in granulation tissue myofibroblasts and in quiescent and growing cultured fibroblasts. J. *Cell Biol.,* 1993. 122(1): p. 103-11.

[49] Shek, F.W., et al., Expression of transforming growth factor-beta 1 by pancreatic stellate cells and its implications for matrix secretion and turnover in chronic pancreatitis. *Am. J. Pathol.*, 2002. 160(5): p. 1787-98.

[50] Kikuta, K., et al., 4-hydroxy-2, 3-nonenal activates activator protein-1 and mitogen-activated protein kinases in rat pancreatic stellate cells. *World J. Gastroenterol.*, 2004. 10(16): p. 2344-51.

[51] Wilkins, M.R., et al., From proteins to proteomes: large scale protein identification by two-dimensional electrophoresis and amino acid analysis. *Biotechnology* (N Y), 1996. 14(1): p. 61-5.

[52] Verrills, N.M., Clinical proteomics: present and future prospects. *Clin. Biochem. Rev.*, 2006. 27(2): p. 99-116.

[53] Valerio, A., et al., Serum protein profiles of patients with pancreatic cancer and chronic pancreatitis: searching for a diagnostic protein pattern. *Rapid. Commun Mass. Spectrom.*, 2001. 15(24): p. 2420-5.

[54] Shen, J., et al., Protein expression profiles in pancreatic adenocarcinoma compared with normal pancreatic tissue and tissue affected by pancreatitis as detected by two-dimensional gel electrophoresis and mass spectrometry. *Cancer Res.*, 2004. 64(24): p. 9018-26.

[55] Crnogorac-Jurcevic, T., et al., Proteomic analysis of chronic pancreatitis and pancreatic adenocarcinoma. *Gastroenterology*, 2005. 129(5): p. 1454-63.

[56] Chen, R., et al., Comparison of pancreas juice proteins from cancer versus pancreatitis using quantitative proteomic analysis. *Pancreas*, 2007. 34(1): p. 70-9.

[57] Chen, R., et al., Quantitative proteomic profiling of pancreatic cancer juice. *Proteomics,* 2006. 6(13): p. 3871-9.

[58] Tian, Q., et al., Integrated genomic and proteomic analyses of gene expression in Mammalian cells. *Mol. Cell Proteomics*, 2004. 3(10): p. 960-9.

[59] Kitada, T., et al., Clinicopathological significance of hypoxia-inducible factor-1alpha expression in human pancreatic carcinoma. *Histopathology*, 2003. 43(6): p. 550-5.

[60] Shibaji, T., et al., Prognostic significance of HIF-1 alpha overexpression in human pancreatic cancer. *Anticancer Res.*, 2003. 23(6C): p. 4721-7.

[61] Okamoto, T., et al., FTY720, an immunosuppressant, attenuates chronic pancreatitis in rats by suppressing T-cell infiltration. *Pancreas*, 2005. 30(3): p. e64-70.

[62] Reding, T., et al., A selective COX-2 inhibitor suppresses chronic pancreatitis in an animal model (WBN/Kob rats): significant reduction of macrophage infiltration and fibrosis. *Gut,* 2006. 55(8): p. 1165-73.

[63] Ogawa, T., et al., Effects of R-102444 and its active metabolite R-96544, selective 5-HT2A receptor antagonists, on experimental acute and chronic pancreatitis: Additional evidence for possible involvement of 5-HT2A receptors in the development of experimental pancreatitis. *Eur. J. Pharmacol.*, 2005. 521(1-3): p. 156-63.

[64] Yoo, B.M., et al., Novel antioxidant ameliorates the fibrosis and inflammation of cerulein-induced chronic pancreatitis in a mouse model. *Pancreatology,* 2005. 5(2-3): p. 165-76.

[65] Zhao, H.F., et al., Anti-monocyte chemoattractant protein 1 gene therapy attenuates experimental chronic pancreatitis induced by dibutyltin dichloride in rats. *Gut,* 2005. 54(12): p. 1759-67.

[66] Shimizu, K., et al., Troglitazone inhibits the progression of chronic pancreatitis and the profibrogenic activity of pancreatic stellate cells via a PPARgamma-independent mechanism. *Pancreas*, 2004. 29(1): p. 67-74.

In: Pancreatitis Research Advances
Editor: William C. Langley, pp. 289-315
ISBN: 978-1-60021-883-5

Chapter X

An Inside into the Physiopathogenesis of Acute and Chronic Pancreatitis

Marcelo Gustavo Binker and Laura Iris Cosen-Binker*
RHC-LICB Biomedical Research Institute,
Buenos Aires, Argentina
Programa de Estudios Pancreáticos", Hospital de Clínicas,
Universidad de Buenos Aires, Argentina
Cátedra de Gastroenterología y Enzimología Clínica –
Departamento de Bioquímica Clínica,
Facultad de Farmacia y Bioquímica,
Universidad de Buenos Aires, Argentina

Abstract

The morphologic pattern of cell death, whether through an apoptotic or necrotic process, plays an important role in the degree of severity of an acute pancreatitis episode. In cases of biliary acute pancreatitis, which clinically is the most frequent (70%), a complex interrelationship of factors determine its main characteristics and probable outcome. Marked by the patient's genetic background and the *immuno-neuro-endocrine* peculiarities, closely similar types of injury may induce either a mild (edematous) or a very serious (necrotizing) episode of *pancreatic inflammation*.

This review was prompted by our conviction that in biliary acute pancreatitis duodeno-pancreatic autonomic-arc-reflexes induce, through several mechanisms (ischemia-reperfusion, free-oxygen-radicals) the expression and release of different types of cytokines, that either favour or abrogate the inflammatory response. This modulation is dependant of *adrenal glucocorticoids*, the last link of the *hypothalamic-pituitary-adrenal (HPA) axis*. This *immune-neuro-endocrine interaction* is set in motion by the cytokines themselves that prompt the fore-mentioned feedback loop between the *pancreatic immune system and the neuro-endocrine-system.*

* Correspondence: Laura Iris Cosen-Binker, Biochemical Dr, PhD. laura.cosen.binker@utoronto.ca. labcosen@hotmail.com

Undoubtedly, genetically determined features of both the immunocytes, primarily the neutrophils granulocytes, and the neuro-endocrine apparatus, must play a pivotal influence in delineating the degree of reactivity of the pancreatic inflammatory response. It is probable that a blunted *HPA axis* response contributes to an episode of acute necrotizing pancreatitis. The same might occur in cases with genetically determined over-reactive immunocytes. In both clinical settings, the administration of glucocorticoids might have a sound justification.

Keywords: *acute pancreatitis – chronic pancreatitis – glucocorticoids – neuro-endocrine interactions.*

Summary

An overview of apoptosis disclosed that this is a highly evolutionary process for deleting senescent, damaged, redundant and deleterious cells from the organism. Its dysregulation can lead to hyperplasia or atrophy. The morphologic patterns of cell death, necrosis and apoptosis are described. In coagulative necrosis the basic outline of the cell is preserved. Liquefactive necrosis is characteristic of focal bacterial infections. In caseous necrosis, fragmented coagulated cells appear as amorphous granular. In fat necrosis, grossly chalky white areas are observed. In apoptosis, the cell is smaller in size and chromatin aggregates peripherally into dense masses. The cell shows surface blebbing and then undergoes fragmentation into membrane-bound apoptotic bodies, which are phagocytosed by adjacent healthy cells, either parenchymal cells or macrophages. The biochemical feature of apoptosis implies changes in the plasma membrane phospholipid orientation, i.e., phosphatidilserine is translocated to the outer leaflet of the plasma membrane, presumably for phagocytic recognition. Members of the caspase protease family lead to the structural changes of apoptosis. Its induction is related to Fas receptor/Fas ligand interactions. Fas receptor is a member of the nerve growth factor. Several growth factor signaling cascades regulate apoptosis. Transcription factors function as "third messengers" in the signaling cascades. Based on their DNA-binding domain, two families are distinguished: homeo-box and zinc-finger. In the pancreatic gland, the exocrine cells express receptors that display preferred mechanism for signaling. The EGF and CCK receptors mediate proliferative cascades.those of the TGF arrest the cell cycle and induce apoptosis. In acute pancreatitis, as well as in chronic pancreatitis, tubular complexes appear by a dedifferentiation process. In the former, they are reversible structures; instead, they are persistent in the latter. In severe acute pancreatitis, as observed following obstruction of the opossum common bile-pancreatic duct, marked necrosis but very little apoptosis is found. In mild acute pancreatitis, as evoked by obstructing the rat common bile-pancreatic duct, very little necrosis and high degree of apoptosis. The severity of acute pancreatitis is inversely related to the degree of apoptosis. The induction of this process could be of clinical value. The apoptotic process can be changed to necrosis by infiltrating neutrophils. This may be modified by endogenous glucocorticoids through the suppression of chemical mediators and/or cytokines that work as chemo attractants to leukocytes. In acute pancreatitis, activation of the hypothalamic-pituitary-adrenal-axis may be self-guarding against necrosis.

In chronic pancreatitis, overexpression of the TGFβ-Regulated zinc-finger encoding gene induces fibrous scarring in part mediated by the apoptotic clearance or pancreatic acinar cells.

A sound approach to treatment of acute pancreatitis in the future seems to be centered on trying to reduce the leukocyte infiltration of the pancreatic gland and promote through pharmaceutical means the apoptotic procession the neutrophils, a pivotal agent of the acute pancreatic inflammation. The idea that acute necrotizing pancreatitis might be limited to a genetically determined excessive reaction of the leukocytes is discussed. Also, the mechanisms by which glucocorticoids might exert a beneficial effect are also analyzed. But how, following pancreatic injuries, neuro-endocrine-immune interactions, in which the hypothalamic-pituitary-adrenal axis plays a pivotal role, determine the type and degree of severity of pancreatic inflammation.

I. Introduction

This review was prompted by new knowledge, primarly in the field of acute pancreatic inflammation, in what concerns the influence exerted by the patterns of cell death, apoptosis and necrosis, in the severity of the exocrine pancreatic lesion. Besides, how the relative proportional involvement of each of these processes varies in the different models of acute pancreatitis. In addition, a new approach of our former postulation that the speed at which the phenomenon of "supramaximal ecbolic stimulation" develops influences the triggering of apoptosis or necrosis. Indeed, if the "supramaximal" stimulation of the acinar cells evolves slowly, the apoptotic pattern of the cell death predominates and this probably sets the stage to developing either chronic pancreatitis or chronic pancreatopathy. If, on the contrary, the supranormal ecbolic stimulation of the acinar cells develops at a fast pace, then the histopathologic picture of the pancreatic lesions is dominated by necrosis and this determines an episode of acute pancreatitis. This can occur on a normal pancreatic gland, or else, superimposed on a background of chronic pancreatitis.

Also, an analysis is made of the immunologic-neuro-endocrine loop that, essentially, is the one that depicts the interrelationships between the immunocytes' secretory agents, the cytokines with the hypothalamic-pituitary-adrenal (HPA) axis. The counter-regulation exerted by the adrenal glucocorticoids upon the cytokines is examined. The different pro and anti-inflammatory cytokines are described. Another factor that is discussed is that of the influence exerted by certain genetic traits. It is known today that these factors influence decisively upon the reactivity of the fore-mentioned immune-neuro-endocrine loop.

Finally it is analysed the value of glucocorticoids both as preventive as well as therapeutic agents of an episode of biliary acute pancreatitis.

II. Morphologic Pattern of Cell Death

The term apoptosis was introduced in 1972.Cell death by apoptosis is a highly conserved evolutionary process for deleting senescent, damaged, redundant and deleterious cells from the organism [1]. Rates of apoptosis are paired with rates of mitosis so that epithelial cell numbers remain constant and tissue homeostasis is maintained (Figure 1).

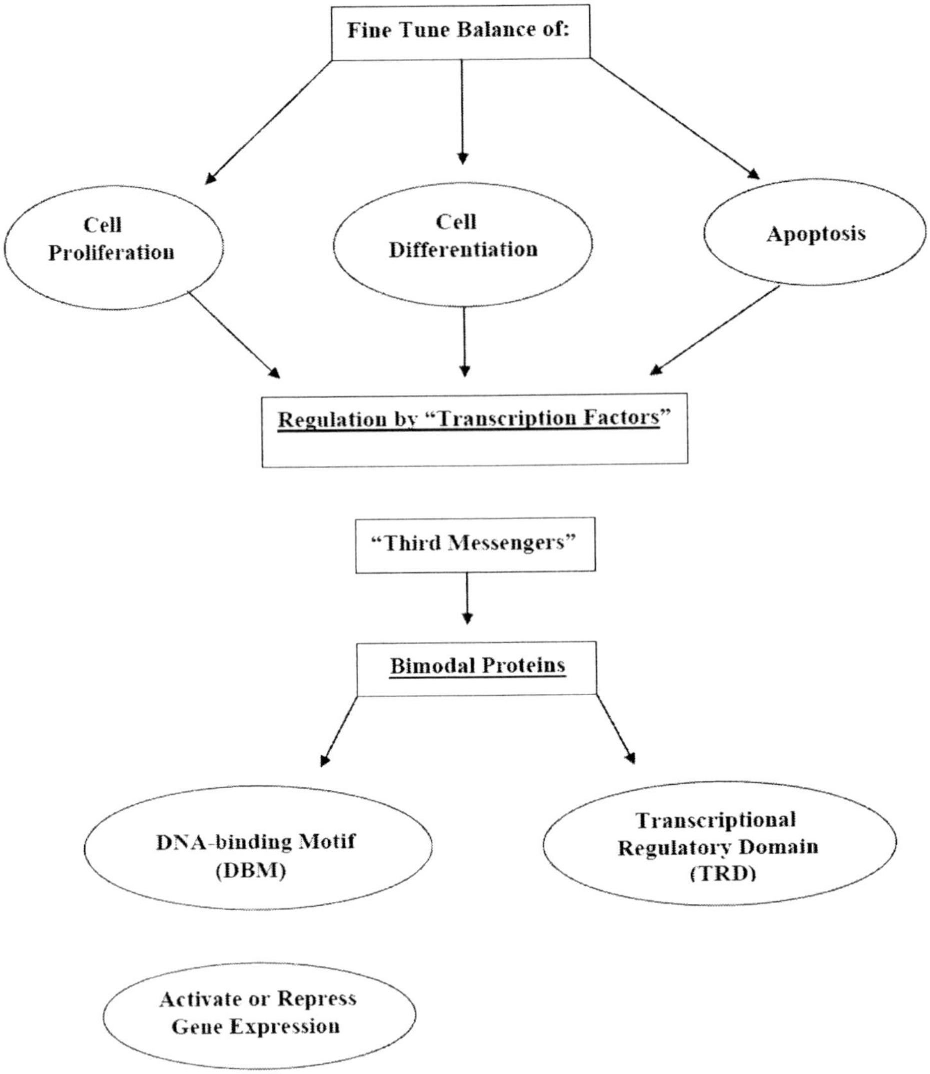

Figure 1.

Given the widespread and critical role of apoptosis in physiology, it is not surprising that dysregulation of apoptosis occurs frequently during pathophysiological disturbances. Indeed, several key concepts have recently emerged with respect to the dysregulation of apoptosis in pathophysiological processes, making a review focused on the pancreatic gland timely and topical.

First, tissue hyperplasia and atrophy can result from inhibition or potentiation of apoptosis, respectively.

Second, pathophysiological processes can trigger the cellular apoptotic machinery leading to rapid and extensive cell death and tissue dysfunction.

Failure of apoptosis to delete genetically altered cells appears to contribute to malignant transformation.

The therapeutic corollaries of these concepts are that: 1) inhibition of apoptosis may prevent tissue injury and/or promote tissue regeneration and restitution; 2) induction of apoptosis in dysplastic processes may be approach to prevent malignant transformation, and 3) conversion of necrotic inflammatory injury to an apoptotic non-inflammatory process may ameliorate disease processes.

Today it is accepted that apoptosis is responsible for numerous physiologic and pathologic events, including the following: a) The programmed destruction of cells during embryogenesis and metamorphosis; b) hormone-dependent involution in the adult, such as endometrial cell breakdown during menstrual cycle, ovarian follicular atresia in the menopause and the regression of the lactating breast after weaning; c) cell death in tumors, most frequently during regression but also in tumors with active cell growth; d) death of immune cells, both B and T lymphocytes after cytokine depletion,as well as the deletion of auto-reactive T cells in the developing thymus; e) pathologic atrophy in parenchymal organs after duct obstruction,such as occurs in the pancreas, parotid gland and kidney; f) cell death induced by cytotoxic T cells, such as in cellular immune rejection and graft versus host disease;g) cell injury in certain viral diseases,as fro example in viral hepatitis in which apoptotic cell fragments in the capable of producing necrosis,but when given in low doses,including mild thermal injury,radiation,cytotoxic anticancer drugs,and possibly hypoxia,induce apoptosis. There are two morphologic patterns of cell death: necrosis and apoptosis (Figure 2).

Necrosis, or coagulation necrosis, is the more common type of cell death after exogenous stimuli, occurring after such stresses as ischemia and chemical injury. It is manifested by severe cell swelling or cell rupture, denaturation and coagulation of cytoplasmatic proteins and breakdown of cell organelles.

Apoptosis is a more regulated event. It is designed for the normal elimination of unwanted cell populations during embryogenesis and in various physiologic processes. It also occurs, however, under pathologic conditions, in which it is sometimes accompanied by necrosis. Its chief morphologic features are chromatin condensation and fragmentation.

Although the mechanisms of necrosis and apoptosis differ, there is overlap between these two processes.

A) Necrosis

This is one of the two morphologic expressions of cell death. Its characteristics changes result from the progressive degradative action of enzymes on the lethally injured cell. Two concurrent processes are involved: 1) enzymatic digestion of the cell, 2) denaturation of proteins.

The catalytic enzymes are derived either from the lysosomes of the death cells,in which case the enzymatic digestion is referred to as autolysis,or from the lysosomes of immigrant leukocytes,termed heterolysis.Depending on whether denaturation of proteins or enzymatic digestion is ascendant,one of two patterns of cell necrosis develops.In the former instance,coagulative arises.In the latter,progressive catalysis of cell structures leads to the so-called liquefactive necrosis.Both of these two processes require hours to develop.

The necrotic cells show increased eosinophilia, attributable in part to loss of the normal basophilia imparted by the RNA in the cytoplasm and, in part, due to the increased binding of eosin to denatured intracytoplasmatic proteins. The cells may have a more glossy homogenous appearance than that of normal cells, mainly as a result of the loss of glycogen particles. When enzymes have digested the cytoplasmatic organelles, the cytoplasm becomes vacuolated and appears moth eaten. Finally, calcification of the death cells may occur. By electron microscopy, necrotic cells are characterized by overt discontinuities in plasma and organelle membranes, marked dilatation of mitochondria with the appearance of large amorphous densities, intracytoplasmic myelin figures, amorphous eosinophilic debris and aggregates of fluffy material, probably representing denatured protein.

Nuclear changes appear in the form of one of three patterns. The basophilia of the chromatin may fade (karyolisis), a change that presumably reflects DNAse activity. A second pattern is piknosis, characterized by nuclear shrinkage and increased basophilia. Here the DNA apparently condenses into a solid, shrunken basophilic mass. In the third pattern, known as kariorrhexis, the piknotic, or partially piknotic nucleus undergoes fragmentation. With the passage of time the nucleus in the necrotic cell totally disappears.

Once the necrotic cells have undergone the early alterations described above, the mass of necrotic cells may have several morphologic patterns: coagulative necrosis, liquefactive necrosis, or, in special circumstances, caseous necrosis and fat necrosis (Figure 2).

a) *Coagulative Necrosis:* implies preservation of the basic outline of the coagulated cell for a span of at least some days. Presumably, the injury, or the subsequent increasing intracellular acidosis, denatures not only structural proteins but also enzymes and so blocks the proteolysis of the cell. This process is characteristic of the hypoxic death of cells in all tissues, save the brain.
b) *Liquefactive Necrosis:* It results from autolysis or heterolysis. It is characteristic of focal bacterial infections because bacteria constitute powerful stimuli to the accumulations of white cells.
c) *Caseous Necrosis:* This term is derived from the gross appearance (white and cheese) of the area of necrosis. Histologically, the necrotic focus appears as amorphous granular debris seemingly composed of fragmented coagulated cells enclosed within a destructive inflammatory border known as granuloma.
d) *Enzymatic Fat Necrosis:* This is characterized by focal areas of destruction of fat resulting from abnormal release of activated pancreatic lipases into the substance of the pancreas and the peritoneal cavity. In this condition enzymes liquefy fat cell membranes and the activated lipases split the trygliceride esters contained within the fat cells. The released fatty acids combine with calcium to produce grossly visible chalky white areas. Histologically, the necrosis takes the form of foci of shadowy outlines of necrotic fat cells with basophilic calcium deposits surrounded by an inflammatory reaction.

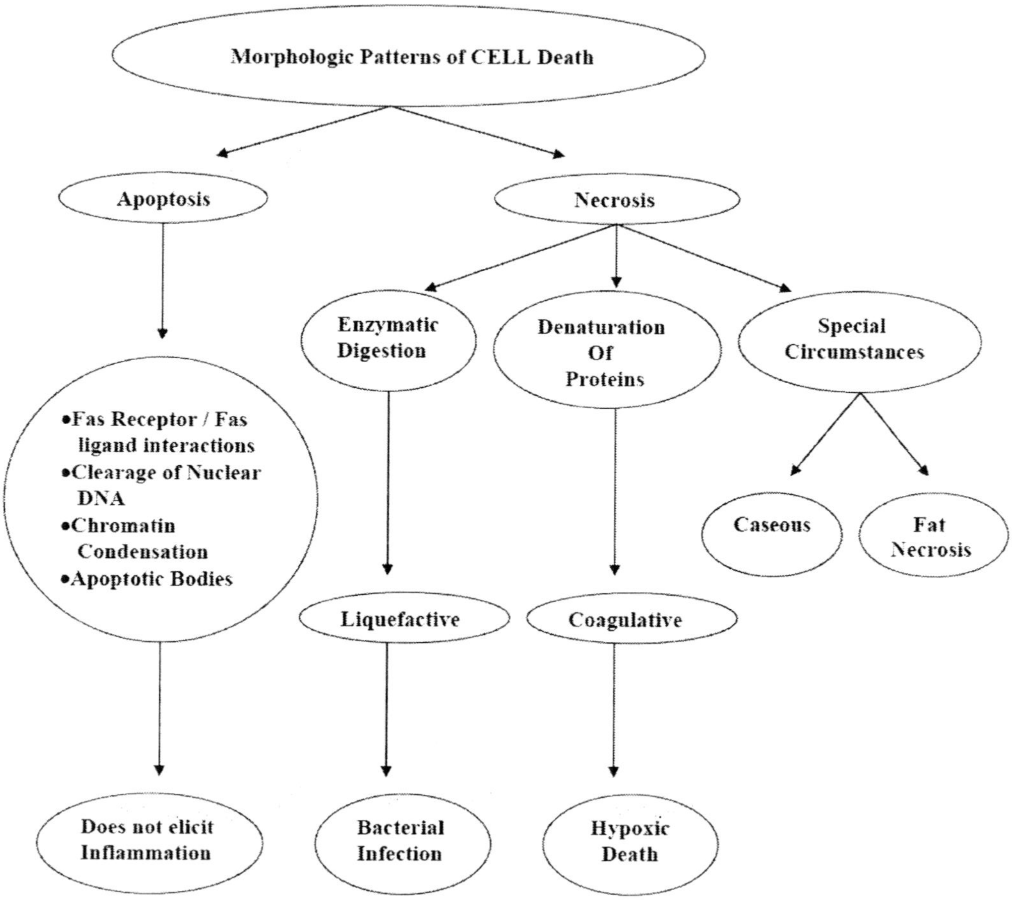

Figure 2.

B) Apoptosis

This morphologic pattern of cell death should be differentiated from the common coagulative necrosis (Figure 2).

The following morphologic features characterize cells undergoing apoptosis:

a) *Cell Shrinkage*: The cell is smaller in size. The cytoplasm is dense. The organelles are more tightly packed.
b) *Chromatin Condensation:* This is the most characteristic feature of apoptosis. The chromatin aggregates peripherally under the nuclear membrane, into well-delimited dense masses of various shapes and sizes. The nucleous itself may break-up, producing two or more fragments.
c) *Formation of Cytoplasmic Blebs and Apoptotic Bodies*: The apoptotic cell first shows surface blebbing, then undergoes fragmentation into a number of membrane-

bound apoptotic bodies composed of cytoplasma and tightly packed organelles with or without a nuclear fragment.

d) *Phagocytosis of Apoptotic Cells or Bodies*: This is carried-out by adjacent healthy cells, either parenchymal cells or macrophages. The apoptotic bodies are rapidly degraded within lysosomes, the adjacent cells migrate or proliferate to replace the space occupied by the now deleted apoptotic cell.

Histologically, in tissues stained with hematoxylin and eosin, apoptosis involves single cells or small clusters of cells. The apoptotic cell appears as round or oval mass of intensely eosinophilic cytoplasm with dense nuclear chromatin fragments. Because the cell shrinkage and formation of apoptotic bodies are rapid and the fragments are quickly phagocytosed, degraded or extruded into the lumen, considerable apoptosis may occur in tissues before it becomes apparent in histologic sections. In addition, apoptosis, in contrast to necrosis, does not elicit inflammation, making it more difficult to detect histologically.

III. Mechanism of Apoptosis

A number of mechanisms appear to be established. The characteristic chromatin condensation is associated with cleavage of nuclear DNA, occurring at the linker regions between nucleosomes to produce a series of fragments. This fragmentation is mediated by a calcium-sensitive endonuclease.

The alteration in cell volume and shape has been ascribed, in part, to the induction of transglutamase activity. This enzyme causes extensive cross-linking of cytoplasmatic proteins, forming a shell under the plasma membrane similar to that of keratinised squamous cells.

The phagocytosis of apoptotic bodies by macrophages and other cell types is mediated by receptors on these cells, which bind and engulf the apoptotic cell.

The speedy phenomenon of phagocytosis is thought to limit the release of intracellular constituents into the extra-cellular space. Because this is limited, the inflammatory response to the dead cell is postulated to be inexistent. However, apoptosis may not be as "silent" as presumed. For example, hepatocyte apoptosis is associated with the appearance of hepatocyte intracellular enzymes in circulation.

The biochemical features of apoptosis identified to date include changes in the plasma membrane phospholipid orientation, alterations of intracellular ion homeostasis, activation of proteases and endonucleases with cleavage of proteins and DNA, respectively, intracellular generation of ceramide via sphingomyelinase, and activation of transglutaminase. Phosphatidylserine is located predominantly on the inner or cytoplasmic face of the plasma membrane in healthy cells, however, early in apoptosis; phosphatidylserine is translocated to the outer leaflet of the membrane, presumably for phagocytic recognition [1]. The externalization of phosphatidylserine can be readily detected using fluorecently labeled annexin V, which has strong affinity for phosphatidylserine.

Increases in cytosolic free calcium and magnesium and decreases in cytosolic pH and potassium have been implicated as mechanisms contributing to apoptosis.

A variety of proteases have been implicated in apoptosis, including members of the caspase family. Caspase protease cascade, analogous to the coagulation protease cascade, has been suggested as a mechanism leading to the structural changes of apoptosis.

The intracellular signaling pathways for apoptosis have not yet been completely delineated. However; the Fas receptor/Fas ligand pathway of apoptosis has been elucidated more fully and remains the best characterized model of apoptosis.

Fas receptor/Fas ligand interactions are important inducers of apoptosis, as for example in hepatocytes. The Fas receptor is a member of the nerve growth factor receptor family. Binding of the receptor by Fas ligand results in apoptosis of the cells expressing the Fas receptor. The latter is expressed in high numbers of cytotoxic T lymphocytes. In a variety of liver diseases, Fas receptor is up-regulated, as for example in viral hepatitis and alcohol-induced liver disease [2]. In hepatitis-C positive patients, Hepatocyte apoptosis occurs via T-cell mediated Fas pathway [1].

IV. Regulation of Apoptosis in the Pancreatic Gland

During the development of the pancreas, both acini and ducts are formed from the proliferation and differentiation of a poorly characterized ductular-like precursor cell. In addition, programmed cell death also appears to be an important process for maintaining an appropriate number of the different pancreatic cell populations throughout development. Thus, normal pancreatic morphogenesis requires a fine-tuned balance of cell proliferation, differentiation and apoptosis (Figure 1).

Studies performed during the last decade have revealed that several growth factor signaling cascades regulate apoptosis, cell proliferation and differentiation in a variety of different cell types. In addition, other factors influence proteins that function downstream of these signaling pathways, known as transcription factors, influence the growth, differentiation and apoptosis phenomena (Figure 1).

Transcription factors function as "third messengers" in the signaling cascades. They are bimodular proteins composed of a DNA-binding motif (DBM) and a transcriptional-regulatory domain (TRD). Once in the nucleus of the cell, transcriptional factors can bin to DNA regulatory sequences through the DBM.Thus, they can either activate or repress gene expression [3] (Figure 1).

The transcription factor proteins have been classified into families based on the structure of their DNA-binding domain, such as the homeobox and the zinc-finger proteins. It has been shown that these transcription factors play regulatory role in organogenesis from insects to vertebrates [3]. That mutations in these genes, and/or their aberrant expressions, can give rise to neoplasic transformation. Besides, several members of these two families are indeed expressed in the pancreas.

Exocrine pancreatic cell populations express a large number of receptor on the cell surface for binding growth factors and gastrointestinal hormones. These receptors can be grouped into different structural families that display a preferred mechanism for signaling:

tyrosine-kinase receptors (eg.,EGF receptor),G-protein-coupled receptors (eg.,CCK Receptor) and serine/threonine-kinase receptor (eg.,TGF).

The EGF receptor and CCK receptors mediate proliferative cascades or regulate functions that are characteristics of differentiated pancreatic cells, such as secretion. In contrast,those of the TGF can arrest the cell cycle and induce apoptosis [4] (Figure1).

V. Apoptosis in Pancreatic Duct Obstruction

TDT-mediated d-UTP-biotin nick end labeling (TUNEL) is a method that allows visualizing apoptosis by specific labeling of DNA strand breaks. This method is based on the specific binding of terminal deoxynucleotidyl-transferase (TDT) to 3'-OH ends of fragmented DNA [5].

With the above method TUNEL it has been shown that following duct obstruction acinar cells progressively disappear and islet tissue is preserved in mammals. On the basis of the microscopic findings, it is considered that the acinar cell death is due to apoptosis. What is interesting is that the TUNEL method detects directly apoptotic cells before their fragmentation.

It is noteworthy that solely pancreatic acinar cells are involved in apoptosis after duct ligation. Ductal and islet do not participate in this cell death process.

VI. Apoptosis, Tubular Complexes, Acute and Chronic Pancreatitis and Exocrine Pancreas Regeneration

In an acute pancreatitis episode three major findings deserve emphasis: first, pancreatic cells reorganize their genetic program; second, stem cells forming tubular complexes appear during the regenerative period; third, many pancreatic cells activate is their apoptotic program [6] (Figure 3-4).

The first step in the formation of tubular complexes is the dilatation of the acinar lumen and a decrease in cell height. Thereafter, a progressive disappearance of secretory granules is observed and, concomitantly, the endoplasmic reticulum becomes less abundant, giving a duct-like appaerence to the acinar cells. When the degranulation is completed, the tubular complexes appear as cylindrical tubes, sometimes connected with a wide empty lumen.

It is now clear that cells forming tubular complexes that appear during acute pancreatitis, as well as in chronic pancreatitis, are derived from the acinar cells by a dedifferentiation process as demonstrated by light microscopy and ultramicroscopy.

The acinar origin of the tubular complexes is supported by the fact that cells express an acinar cell specific antigen [6] (Figure 4).

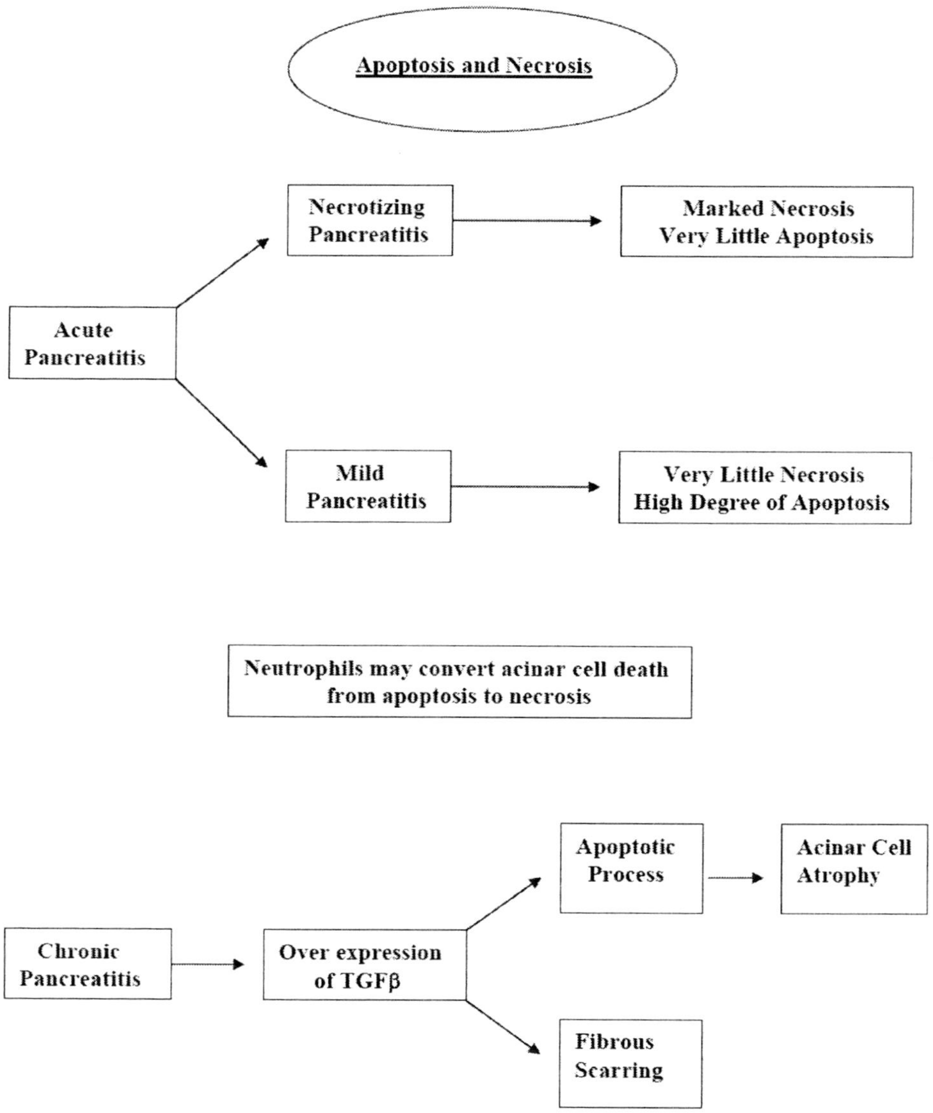

Figure 3.

Arias and Bendayan [7] have shown, in-vitro, that acinar cells retain a morphogenetic plasticity, and, on particulate stimulation, can change their commitment pattern toward that of the duct cells phenotype.

That cells forming the tubular complexes have returned to a protodifferentiated stage is supported by the fact that villin, which is a marker of the embryonic pancreas, is localized to these structures which are similar to the ones observed in the embryonic pancreas. This is confirmed by reports stating that acinar, ductular, alfa and beta islet cells can derive from cells of the tubular complexes [8] (Figure 4).

It is noteworthy that in acute pancreatitis there are reversible structures. Instead, they are persistent in chronic pancreatitis and in some experimental models of acute pancreatitis ("pseudo-chronic tubular complexes").

As the "pseudo-chronic tubular complexes" are localized close to obstructed ducts draining pathological areas, the suggestion has been formulated that persistence of "pseudo-chronic" lesions following bile salts or trypsin injection into the bile-pancreatic canal are owing to ductal structures.

According to Iovanna [6], the persistent "tubular complexes" of "chronic pancreatitis" or cystic fibrosis have a similar physiopathology to "pseudo-chronic" lesions observed in that model of acute pancreatitis. They could be consequence of complete or partial obstruction of the pancreatic ducts by stones or protein plugs. It is possible that these lesions persist because the ducts remain obstructed. Another possibility is that after acute pancreatitis, but not in chronic pancreatitis, there are activation of growth factor(s) or cytokines within the pancreas acting in an autocrine, paracrine or yuxtacrine manner to induce exocrine cell proliferation and differentiation.

When there are obstacles to the normal flow of pancreatic juice into the gut, the regenerative capacity of the pancreas is arrested [8]. This is re-established when the obstruction is overcome. This was shown by our experiments in dogs [9]. Indeed, in canines in which the pancreatic ducts had been ligated and transacted for periods varying from 1 to 7 weeks, after wich, duct continuity had been restored by direct end-to-end microsurgical ductal anastomoses, sequential biopsies and repeated testings of the maximal secretory capacity of the pancreas with secretin and pancreozymin indicated that secretory functional return paralleled histological recovery.

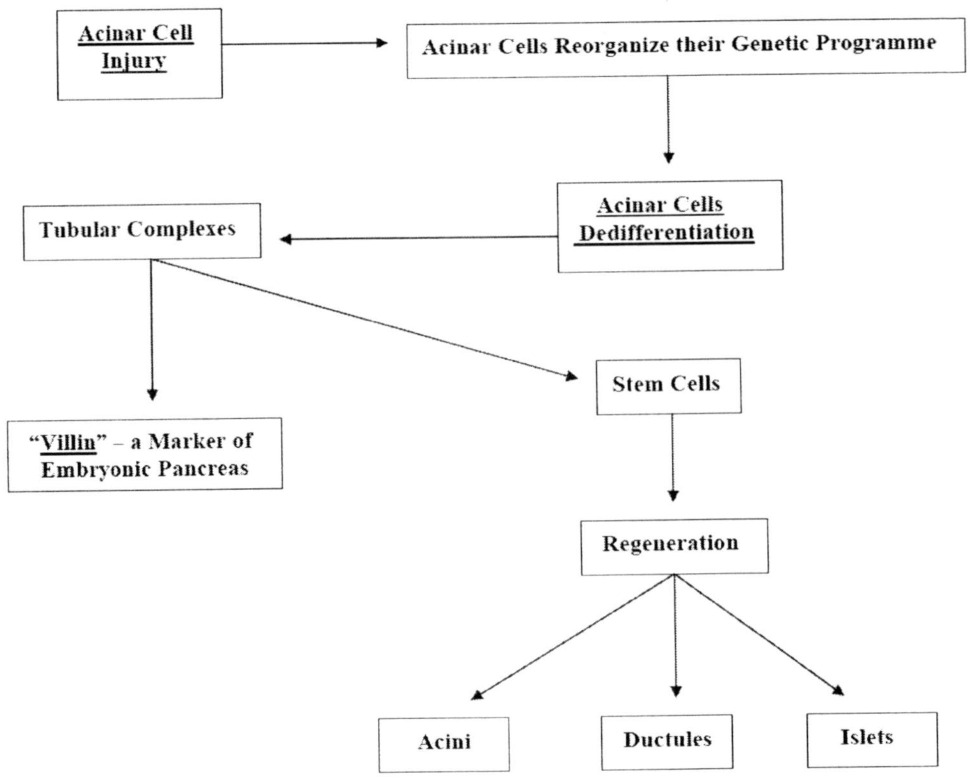

Figure 4.

In these experiments it was quite evident that complete recovery of secretion was seen only in animals in which pancreatic ductal continuity, as indicated by pancreatography, had been completely successful.

Other suggestive findings, confirmatory of the above described, are those reported Shaw and Latimer [10]. These authors implanted isolated pancreatic ductal segments,1 to 2 cm in length,under the serosa of the duodenum in partially or completely pancreatectomized dogs.After a delay of 8 weeks these ductal autographs became vascularized and underwent varying degrees of cellular differentiation with regeneration of parenchymal tissue,i.e.,ductals,pancreatic acini and islets.The transplanted regenerating duct system often re-established continuity with the gut lumen.When continuity was not achieved,regeneration appeared to be arrested and secretory detritus accumulated and distended the transplanted tissue.

VII. Relationship between Severity, Necrosis and Apoptosis in Different Models of Experimental Acute Pancreatitis

The group of Steer [11] has tried to elucidate those factors that determine the severity of an attack of acute pancreatitis. Severe pancreatitis was induced by: 1) obstructing the opossum common bile-pancreatic duct, 2) by administering to mice 12 hourly injections of a supramaximally stimulating dose of cerulein, 3) by feeding young female mice a choline-deficient ethionine-supplemented diet.

In each of these models of severe pancreatitis, marked necrosis but very little apoptosis was found.

In contrast, when mild pancreatitis was induced (obstructing the rat common bile-pancreatic duct, or by infusing rats with a supramaximally stimulating dose of cerulein) very little necrosis and a high degree of apoptosis was found (Figure 3).

The fact that the severity of acute pancreatitis is inversely related to the degree of apoptosis suggests that this type of cell death may be a teleologically beneficial response to acinar cell injury in general and especially in acute pancreatitis.

According to the above authors, apoptosis in the pancreas, unlike in other organs, such as the involuting breast or prostate, can be associated with mild evidence of inflammation, such as: edema and/or infiltration by inflammatory cells. This mild inflammation may indicate that apoptotic acinar cells, in contrast to other types of cells, release digestive enzymes and/or chemotactic factors, which can induce mild inflammation. Clearly, however, the degree of inflammation and, therefore, the severity of pancreatitis are significantly less in situations associated with acinar cell apoptosis than under conditions associated with acinar cell necrosis.

The group of Steer [11] emphasizes then notion that medications or other interventions that favour the development of apoptosis may minimize the severity of pancreatitis, and they could, therefore be of substantial clinical value.

Jones and Gores [1] point-out that neutrophils may convert the process of acinar cell death from apoptosis to necrosis. They, like the group of Steer [11],emphasize the concept that pharmacological induction of pancreatic apoptosis during the early stages of acute pancreatitis provides a new therapeutic strategy for the treatment of this disease (Figure 3).

Another potential pharmacological approach would include prevention of neutrophil infiltration of the pancreas.

In contrast to acute pancreatitis, chronic pancreatitis is characterized by acinar cell atrophy and replacement of the gland architecture with fibrotic tissue. Acinar cell atrophy likely occurs through an apoptotic process. In that sense it is known that TGFβ is capable of inducing fibrogenesis in pancreatic tissue and conceivably replacement of acinar tissue by fibrous scarring is in part mediated by the apoptotic clearence of pancreatic acinar cells [1] (Figure 3).

The role of TGFβ in inducing acinar cell apoptosis as well as fibrous scarring in-vivo remains unknown. However, over-expression of the TGFβ regulated zinc-finger encoding gene, TIEG, induces apoptosis in pancreatic epithelial cells [1]. Thus, it is highly likely that TGFβ can induce pancreatic cell apoptosis. Contrariwise, it is interesting that inhibition of TGFβ-induced apoptosis may be important in pancreatic carcinogenesis.

It is our view that in alcoholic pancreatitis the speed at which the phenomenon of supraoptimal ecbolic stimulation develops influences whether necrosis or apoptosis plays a predominant role in evoking pancreatic lesions. The former would prevail when the above process in intense and abrupt. This might be the case in those episodes of acute pancreatitis that quite often are observed superimposed on a background of chronic alcoholism following a heavy meal, generally associated with a high alcoholic intake. We have characterized this type of pancreatitis as due to a hyperfunction of the "trigger zone" (antro-duodenum) of the pancreatic "revolver" [12].

Apoptosis prevails when the "supranormal ecbolic stimulation" of the acinar pancreocytes develops slowly and progressively.

It is our hypothesis that the ethanol-evoked loss or impairment of the negative component of pancreatic innervation (failure of PP secretion) has a crucial role in the triggering of the characteristic lesions of alcoholic pancreatitis. This would lead to the pancreon's supranormal ecbolic stimulation via an elevated intrapancreatic cholinergic tone and enhanced ecbolic response to CCK [13, 14] (Figure 5).

The cholinergic tone (Ach) and CCK stimulation after activating specific receptors on the plasma membranes of the acinar cells induce enzyme exocitosis through an increase in cytosolic Ca^{2+}. Supranormal concentration of this cation elicits damage to the cell. At the ultrastructural level, the formation of large vacuoles has been shown in the Golgi region. Further, a crinophagic phenomenon, that is, the fusion of the contents of both the zymogen granules and lysosomes is observed. These cytoplasmic vacuoles, in a subsequent step, are extruded through the basolateral membranes into the pancreatic interstitium.

Excessive elevation of cytosolic Ca^{2+} induces disappearance of microvilli, the appearance of "cytoplasmic lakes" of zymogen material surround by a membrane, and the disaggregation and disruption of the filamentous system.

It is of interest, that cAMP, the major intracellular second messenger of secretin and VIP prevents these morphologic changes.

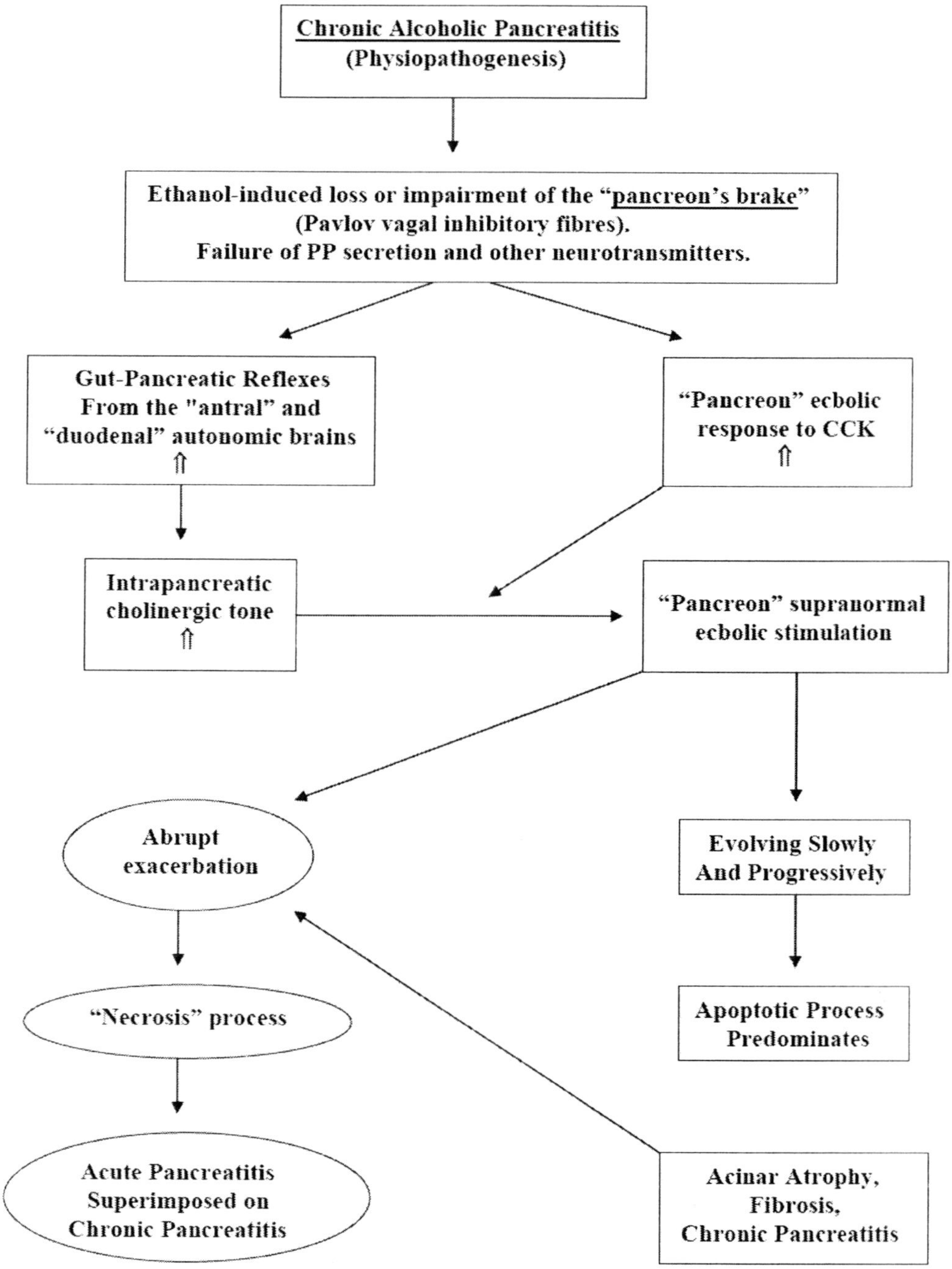

Figure 5.

When the above described modifications evolve slowly, leading to acinar fat deposition and then to cellular damage, acinar cell dedifferentiation ("pseudotubules"), or acinar atrophy with fibrotic replacement, the apoptotic process might have a predominant involvement.

In contrast, when the chronic alcoholic suddenly drinks to excess or indulges in a copious meal rich in protein and fat, an excessive supranormal ecbolic stimulation of abrupt onset, high intensity, and relatively short duration follows and may trigger disruption of the cellular organelles involved in protein synthesis with a resultant extrusion of enzymes through the basolateral membranes of the acinar cells into the pancreas interstitium. This sequence of events, plus the participation of neutrophils characteristic of necrosis, leads to an episode of acute pancreatitis (Figure5).

VIII. Biliary Acute Pancreatitis: Influence of Necrosis or Apoptosis in Its Prognosis

The acute pancreatitis episodes that are triggered by biliary tract stones or blood clots (hemobilia) that migrate into the duodenum or get impacted in the Vaterian region and also by endoscopic maneuvers at Oddi's sphincter (sphincterotomy, sphinctero-manometry, cholangio-pancreatography) can be encompassed as biliary acute pancreatitis. We have postulated that in its physiopathogenesis autonomic-arc-reflexes play a significant role [15]. Their interruption by local anesthetic instillation into the duodenum might be able to attenuate the severity of the pancreatic inflammation by preserving pancreatic microcirculation thus reducing the chances of release of free oxygen radicals, cytokines and agents of the neurogenic inflammation cascade. In fact, what local anesthetic instillation into the duodenum would do is prevent or at least reduce the acinar cell necrosis process with all the consequences that this implies [15] (Figures 5-6).

In different animal species, attempts have been tried to mimic the main features of human biliary acute pancreatitis. The most common approach has been to obstruct the bile-pancreatic ducts. In most species, primarily dogs and rats, duct obstruction leads only to atrophy of the exocrine pancreas. An exception is the opposum. This animal has been chosen because its bilio-pancreatic ductal anatomy is remarkably similar to that of humans as it has a single terminal pancreatic duct before entry into the duodenum.

Studies by Senninger et al [16] have indicated that ligation of the opposum bile-pancreatic duct at its point of insertion into the duodenum leads to hemorrhagic pancreatitis with a mortality of 100% by the end of 2 weeks. In these experiments, evidence of pancreatic injury was noted within 3 days of duct ligation. Progression to severe pancreatitis was observed 7 days after duct ligation.

Lerch et al [17] have repeated these studies. According to them, macroscopic and microscopic evidence of acute pancreatitis can be detected after 24 hours of ligating the opposum bilio-pancreatic duct. At the light microscopic level, changes observed included loss of acinar cell polarity, necrosis of acinar cells and perilobular fat necrosis. In fact, marked changes of acinar cells are observed within 3 hours of duct obstruction.

Dilatation of RER, loss of acinar cell polarity, and alterations of the apical plasmalemma are the leading morphologic features. Over the next 3 hours, these changes become apparent and progressively increasing numbers of acinar cell with evidence of acinar cell necrosis, including disruption of the apical plasmalemma, can be detected. The basolateral membranes, including junctional complexes, remain intact. Fat necrosis, primarily localized to areas at the periphery of lobules, it first observed 12 hours after duct obstruction, evidence of periductal inflammation can first be detected.

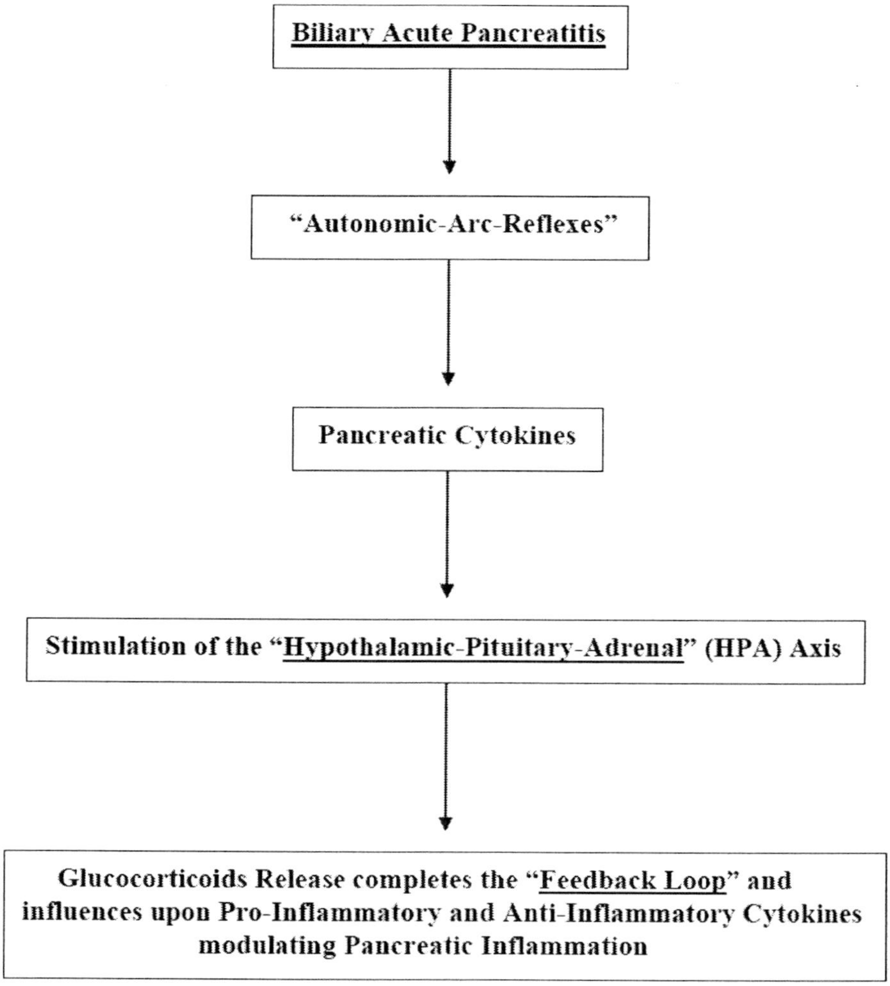

Figure 6.

The above group of authors has postulated that the first identifiable changes of acute pancreatitis involve the acinar cells. The periductal inflammation and fat necrosis is only detected several hours after the acinar cell necrosis is evident.

From their whole series of test in the opossum, Lerch et al [17] have concluded that pancreatic duct obstruction is the critical event that triggers acute pancreatitis and that neither bile duct obstruction nor reflux of bile into the pancreatic duct are important determining factors. In another set of tests performed by Runzi et al [18], it was observed that decompression of the obstructed opossum bilio-pancreatic ductal system can favourably affect the course of biliary acute pancreatitis by preventing the increase in severity of reversible as well as irreversible changes that occur during continued ductal obstruction.

The above findings would seem to support the practice of early interventions, endoscopic or surgical, directed at removing persistently obstructing stones in patients with gallstone pancreatitis.

Doi et al [5] have analysed, employing molecular biological methods whether acinar cell deletion following pancreatic duct obstruction in rats is due to apoptosis. Through the visualization of DNA fragmentation of acinar cell nuclei by the TUNEL method, they confirmed that acinar cells are exclusively involved in apoptosis after pancreatic duct ligation. TUNEL-positive nuclei in acinar cells appeared 12 hours after pancreatic duct ligation. The number of TUNEL-positive nuclei reached the maximum at day 2, and then decreased by day 5. The histology and tissue amylase evaluation showed that no functioning acinar cells remained after day 3.

From the above results, it can be easily inferred that apoptosis is dominantly involved in the acinar cell deletion after pancreatic duct ligation.

The intriguing dilemma remaining to be solved in humans is whether necrosis or apoptosis is the mechanism of acinar cell death predominated. The speculation is warranted that this could be linked to the peculiar neuro-endocrine status of the patient at the time when the acute pancreatitis episode is triggered.

An experimental finding that provides support to the above postulation is that reported by Kimura et al [19]. Indeed, these authors have put in evidence, in the rat, the influence of a variable intrapancreatic "steroid tonus" on the percentage indexes of acinar cell apoptosis in different circumstances.

According to Kimura et al [19], adrenalectomy might cause a defect in the suppression of cytokine production, leading to marked infiltration of inflammatory cells. The apoptotic process can be changed to necrosis by infiltrating neutrophils. Therefore, endogenous glucocorticoids may modify the pathological features of pancreatitis by suppressing the production of chemical mediators and/or cytokines that work as chemoattractans of leukocytes. Thus, the increased secretion of endogenous glucocorticoids during pancreatitis through the activation of the hypothalamic-pituitary-adrenal axis may form a self-guard against acinar cell destruction during acute pancreatitis (Figure 6).

IX. Neural Immune-Hormone-Interactions

Sternberg [20] has stressed the new advances in the Neuro-Immune-Hormone-Interactions.Peripheral cytokines, released by autonomic arc-reflexes in the pancreatic gland, stimulate a variety of central nervous system (CNS) functions, including neuro-endocrine responses, behavioural patterns, sleep and fever. They do so through several routes, including by directly crossing the blood barrier, by stimulating second messengers, and via the vagus nerve.

Peripheral cytokines stimulate ACTH release from the anterior pituitary. Hypothalamic-arginine-vasopressing can act as co-stimulator with corticotropin-releasing hormone to ACTH.Pituitary ACTH stimulates the adrenal glands to release glucocorticoids, which suppress inflammation, completing this counter-regulatory feedback loop.

A feature to take into account is that corticosteroids are anti-inflammatory agents that suppress both cellular and humeral responses. They affect a number of factors involved in the process of tissue inflammation (Figure 7). They significantly elevate C1 esterase inhibitor levels. The later inhibitor has been shown to suppress trypsin activation, which may subsequently lessen the severity of pancreatitis [21]. A number of enzymes are also produced as pancreatitis develops, including phospholipase A_2. This enzyme is inhibited by the protein lipomodulin whose synthesis is induced by corticosteroids. The consequence is a diminished synthesis of prostaglandins and leukotrienes. These substances seem to play an important role in acute pancreatitis [22] (Figure 7).

Another detail to be stressed is that although the therapeutic actions of glucocorticoids are largely attributed to their anti-inflammatory and immunosuppressive effects, they have been implicated in enhancing tissue and cellular protection. This protective action is mediated by induction of heat-shock-proteins (hsp), that protects epithelial cells against oxidant-induced stress [23-24] (Figure 7).

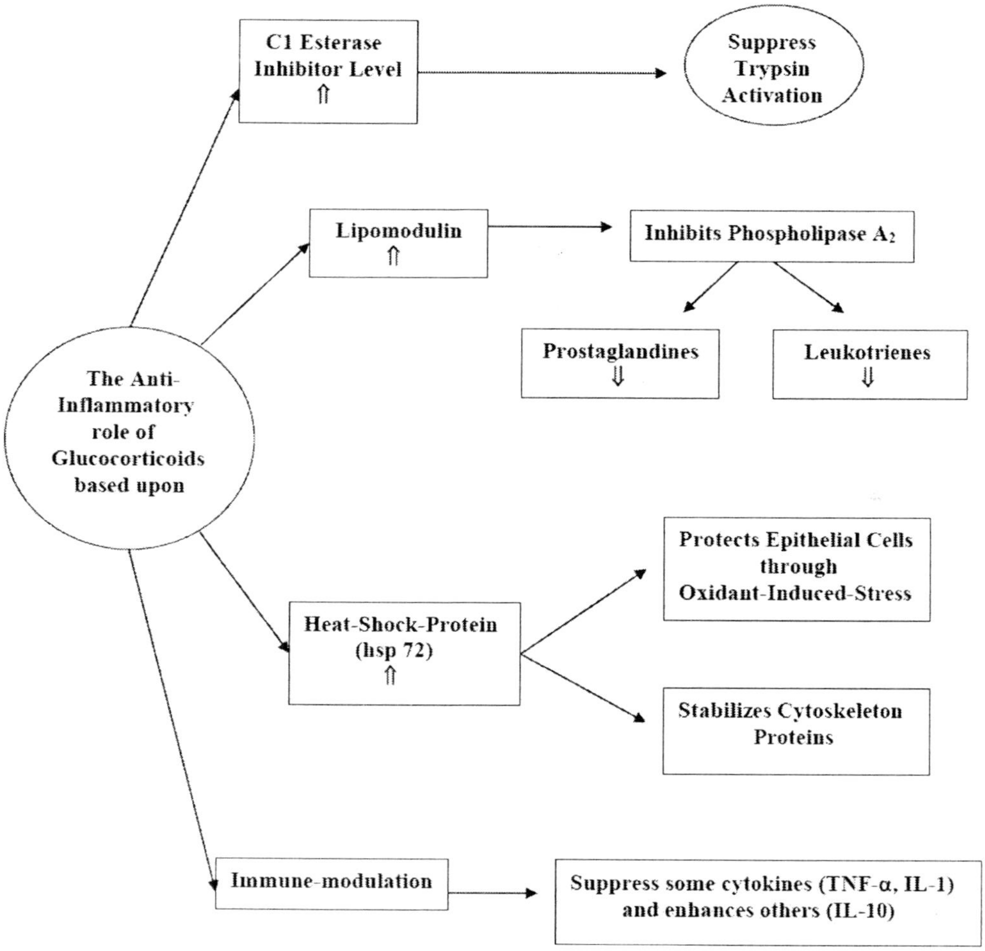

Figure 7.

The mechanism of glucocorticoids' cellular protection may involve stabilization of key intracellular proteins by hsp 72. Indeed, hsp 72 associates with and stabilizes cytoskeleton proteins under conditions of thermal and oxidant-induced stress [25].

It should be pointed out that initially it was thought that glucocorticoids were largely immunosuppressive [20]. However, more recent studies indicate that they are more accurately classed as immunomodulatory, although their overall effect is still immunosuppressive. Thus, glucocorticoids do not uniformly suppress production of all cytokines. They selectively suppress some, while stimulating others. In human blood cytokine stimulation and glucocorticoids suppression assay, some cytokines show differential sensitivity to glucocorticoid suppression, being TNFα, IL-1, IL-12 the most sensitive and IL-6 relatively resistant to glucocorticoid suppression [26-28] (Figure 3).

The mechanism by which glucocorticoids exert these differential effects on cytokine production and suppression has not been ascertained. However, it is known that glucocorticoids generally exert their effects through binding to a soluble cytoplasmatic receptor, displacing hsp and moving to the nucleus [29]. Once there, the ligand-receptor complex binds directly to DNA binding sites, or GRIs, and induces protein synthesis. By interfering with availability of transcription factors directly, such as by competition with NFκB binding sites, or indirectly, by induction of the NFκB binding protein, IκB, glucocorticoids can downregulate protein synthesis. It is likely that similar mechanism exists for cytokine production and suppression [26,30-31].

In addition to the neuro-hormonal routes by which the CNS can modulate immune function, there is also a rich network of innervation of immune organs that plays an important role in local immune regulation, either at sites of inflammation or in immune organs as cell traffic through them. Virtually all immuno organs, including the spleen, thymus, bone marrow and lymph nodes are densely innervated by various components of the autonomic and peripheral nervous system. In these anatomical connections, nerve endings and immune cells are in close apposition. In general, neuropeptides, neuro-hormones and neurotransmitters, such as vasoactive-intestinal-polypeptide (VIP), substance P, released at sites of inflammation have a pro-inflammatory, immunostimulatory effect.

It should be stressed that physiological and pathophysiological effects of the signaling of the CNS by the immune system, and the countermodulation of the immune system by the CNS are profound and are just beginning to be understood.

A fact to be pointed out is that inflammatory autoimmune diseases in humans are associated to a blunted HPA axis response.

The fore-mentioned interactions that now are being better ascertained and understood provide a rationale understanding why, at least in some acute pancreatitis episodes, the administration of glucocorticoids may be a life saving therapeutical measure. These cases are probably those in which due to a favourable genetic background the patient's leukocytes overreact and the HPA axis counter-regulatory responses are not efficient enough to temperate the acute inflammation.

All the above considerations seem to validate the idea that in order that an acute necrotizing pancreatitis could develop it would be necessary that the injurious agent/s impinges on a host with a genetically predisposing background [26] (Figure 8).

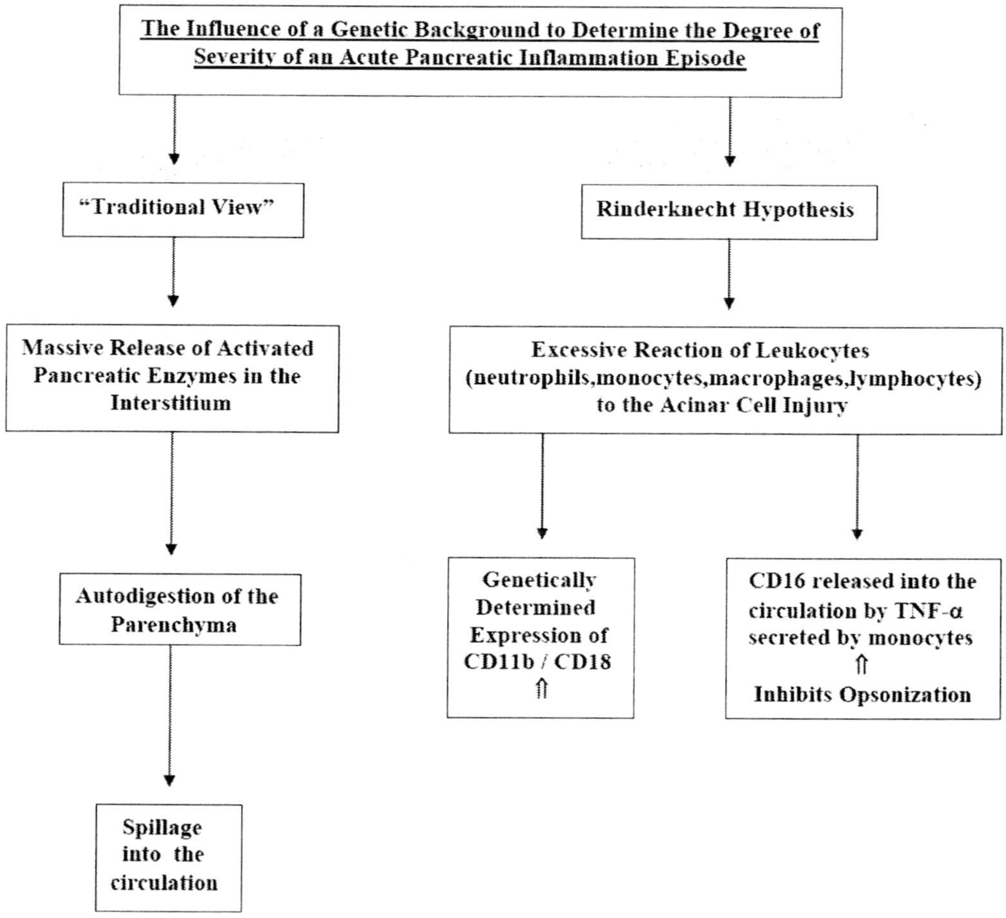

Figure 8.

This review allows the inference that the approach to future research efforts should be directed to elucidate the neurons-immune interactions, the finding of new genetic markers that might put in evidence an overactive immune system, and the evaluation of those therapeutic strategies capable of putting a break to an exaggerate inflammatory response.

As to cytokines, their expression in most normal healthy tissues is very low. However, cytokine production increases during "tissue stress" as a result of cellular challenges, including rapid cellular growth, tissue remodeling, infection or trauma. The particular cytokines produced in response to a threat to tissue homeostasis depends on the nature of the threat, the cellular or tissue type being threatened and the hormone milieu [32].

Cytokines interact between them. Pro-inflammatory cytokines, TNFα and IL-1 stimulate other cytokines, as well as each other, IL-6, IL-8, IL-9, macrophage-inflammatory-protein. Anti-inflammatory cytokines, such as, IL-4, IL-10 and IL-13 abrogate the production of many pro-inflammatory cytokines. Although many cytokines have been shown to influence the HPA axis secretory activity, most have focused on Il-1, Il-6 and TNFα. There is substantial evidence for the critical role of medullary cathecolaminergic innervation of the hypothalamus in the activation of the HPA axis in response to systemic IL-1 [27-28,33].

Recent evidence shows that an intact vagus is critical for the elaboration of CNS responses to abdominal/peritoneal inflammation. Thus, subdiaphragmatic truncal vagotomy several days before intraperitoneal lipopolysacharides administration reduces sickness behavior and hyperalgesia. The vagus is a neural afferent route by which inflammation within the peritoneal cavity can influence the brain [20]. The vagus also appears to play a role in the activation of the HPA axis in response to peripheral lipopolysacharides or cytokines. In rats truncal vagotomy attenuates the rise in plasma ACTH and corticosterone concentrations produced by intraperitoneal IL-1bβ. Vagotomy interferes with the activating signal to the neuroendocrine hypothalamus. Similarly, truncal vagotomy blocks the rise in plasma corticosterone caused by intraperitoneal TNFα.

X. Glucocorticoids and Pancreas, Steroids Revisited

A "bi-directional communication" may occur between the immune and neuro-immune systems, thus, the increased secretion of endogenous glucocorticoids during acute pancreatitis may play an important role in mitigating the pathological course of the disease. This is shown by the study that analyses the effects of adrenalectomy or cerulein-induced pancreatitis and Pfeffer-induced pancreatitis [19]. These experiments have clarified the following:

a) Secretion of endogenous corticosterone increased during the course of both models of experimental acute pancreatitis.
b) Adrenalectomy aggravated the pathological features of the experimental-evoked pancreatitis. In the Pffefer-induced studies, it result in higher mortality.
c) The aggravation of pancreatitis in adrenalectomized rats was accompanied by high levels of serum IL-8.
d) Not only the severity of pancreatitis and the mortality but also the elevated IL-8 in adrenalectomized rats with pancreatitis were suppressed by exogenous hydrocortisone.

All the previous findings suggest that adrenocortical function may be activated during acute pancreatitis and that the increased secretion of endogenous glucocorticoids may play an important role in mitigating the pathological course of this disease.

According to previous studies [34-35] adrenocortical steroids have critical effects on both the acinar and the centro-acinar-ductal segments of the "pancreon" units, but the worsening of both cerulein and Pffefer-induced acute pancreatitis elicited by adrenolectomy is not caused by metabolic changes in acinar cells due to a depletion of glucocorticoids but caused by the absence of steroidal inhibitory effects on the inflammation. Therefore, the secretion of endogenous glucocorticoids during acute pancreatitis seems to be an important intrinsic mechanism of suppressing the deterioration of the inflammatory lesions, regardless of the cause.

Toyota et al [19] show that the aggravation of pancreatitis by adrenalectomy was accompanied by a marked elevation of IL-8 in serum. It has been inferred that Il-8, which is produced locally in pancreatic tissues, may be primarily responsible for the marked infiltration of neutrophils into the pancreas and the development of edema, acinar cell injury, and interstitial hemorrhage observed in adrenalectomized rats. The latter changes are suppressed by the administration of glucocorticoids. Because glucocorticoids inhibit the production of numerous cytokines, the alleviation of pancreatitis in adrenalectomized rats by steroid replacement may be caused by infiltration of the activation of the cytokine network.

We have previously reported that the treatment with glucocorticoids depends on two parameters (DOSE and TIME) to achieve an effective and beneficial therapeutic action. The administration of hydrocortisone in the short-term closed-duodenal-loop model in Wistar rats, leads to four different circumstances [36]:

1. *Effective and beneficial* results when using a *dose of 4 mg/kg in previous form,* 30 minutes before inducing acute pancreatitis;as the pathology evolved towards mild or moderate.From this situation it is deduced that hydrocortisone stimulated the synthesis of anti-inflammatory factors (IL-10, IL-12, IκBα, lipocortin-1, etc.)[37-38] required to counteract the inflammatory cascade and cytoprotective ones like hsp while blocking the synthesis of pro-inflammatory factors [39].
2. *Inefficient results* when using *doses inferior to 4 mg/kg in previous form.*It is deduced that this dosage was insufficient to achieve a good induction in the expression of anti-inflammatory factors.
3. *Harmful results:* a) When using *higher doses than 4 mg/kg in previous form,* since hydrocortisone possibly made prevail its adverse immune-suppressor effects over cytoprotective immune-modulation. b) When using hydrocortisone in a *posterior form.* This administration time was ineffective as the inflammatory cascade was already unchained unable to induce immune-modulation when having to act on an altered *HPA axis;* under these conditions the averse effects were accentuated such as coagulation disorders favouring hemorrhage.

The preceding facts support the concept of an optimum "DOSE and TIME". The use of glucocorticoids (low dose-previous time) can be considered as a preventive factor.

When glucocorticoids interact with the glucocorticoid-receptor (GR) they can induce genomic effects and non-genomic effects. In genomic effects the union of GR to DNA by a trans-activation mechanism stimulates the synthesis of anti-inflammatory proteins but this is also the pathway followed in the generation of adverse effects associated to glucocorticoids. In non-genomic effects the GR inhibits by trans-repression the action of pro-inflammatory transcription factors (Nf-κB, AP-1, CREB) decreasing in this way the synthesis of pro-inflammatory proteins [29,31,40-42]. That is why trans-repression must be favoured stimulating the anti-inflammatory action while trying to achieve the right balance in trans-activation expression to avoid adverse effects.

Weiner et al [22] have also shown an overall decrease in the incidence of post-ERCP in patients receiving pre-ERCP corticosteroids in the form of two doses of methylprednisolone administered 12 hours and 2 hours prior to the procedure.

Our physiopathogenetic hypothesis of acute pancreatitis, primarily of the biliary acute variety, is that autonomic-arc-reflexes triggered at the peri-Vaterian duodenum, elicit through the mechanism of ischemia-reperfusion and release of free oxygen radicals, the unchaining of the cytokine cascade [15]. The latter is responsible of trying to keep intact or of restoring tissue homeostasis. This is achieved primarily by activating the HPA axis, which through the release of adrenal glucocorticoids modulates the pancreatic inflammatory response. Thus, it is logical to infer that when the HPA axis is somewhat blunted the acute pancreatic inflammation has enhanced chances of being necrotizing.

Similarly, in those patients that due to a genetically appropriate background, present immunocytes that overreact to tissue injury making the normal counter-regulatory role of the HPA axis inefficient to attenuate the pancreatic inflammatory response.

XI. The Genetic Determinants

According to several reports [26], the high mortality of acute necrotizing pancreatitis may be related to an aggressive immunological defensive system of the host rather than to autodigestion of the gland. As it is well known, the classical hypothesis is centered on the idea that the acute necrotizing pancreatitis episode results from the massive release of activated pancreatic enzymes into the interstitium followed by autodigestion of the parenchyma and systemic complications owing to spillage of the pancreatic enzymes into circulation. According to Rinderknecht [26] the fatal outcome of necrotizing pancreatitis is primarily due to excessive reaction of leukocytes (neutrophils, monocytes/macrophages, plateles, lymphocytes) to the initial injury. In this type of reaction, genetic factors may play an important role. Several findings have been observed, one of them is an enhanced expression of the adhesion/complement receptor CD11b? CD18. Another is the high expression of CD16, the neutrophil low affinity receptor for IgG. Release of CD16 molecules into circulation, where it inhibits opsonization and promotes sepsis, is mediated by TNFα secreted by monocytes. It is interesting that the level of TNFα and IL-1 secretion by these cells is linked to the expression of genetically encoded polymorphism of the mayor histocompatibility antigen, MHC-II (HLA-DR). Remarkably, heterozygotes are higher secretors of these cytokines than homozygotes and, therefore, at greater risk of developing pancreatic necrosis and sepsis.

In addition to the above, the behaviour of both monocytes and lymphocytes determine the perspectives of an acute inflammatory episode. An upward or downward trend of HLA-DR expression by monocytes is highly correlated with the course of the illness. Patients that show an uncomplicated recovery from an initial acinar cell injury are those whose T-lymphocytes reveal an increased MHC-II expression and the monocytes disclose a recovery of an initial depressed MHC-II expression.

Rinderknecht [26] suggests that future research in acute pancreatitis should focus on elucidating genetically linked aberrant host responsiveness and its correction. Discovery of more accessible genetically encoded markers would be invaluable in the design of prophylactic measures and therapies (Figure 8).

References

[1] Jones, B.; Gores, G. Physiology and pathophysiology of apoptosis in epithelial cell of the liver, pancreas and intestine. *Am. J. Physiol.*, 273:G1174-G1188, 1997.

[2] Mi, L.; Mak, K.; Lieber, C. Alcohol-induced apoptosis of hepatocytes and its modulation by polyenylphosphatidilcholine (PPC) in a rat model. *Mt. Sinai J. Med.*, 66(5):366(A),1999.

[3] Ponta, H.; Cato, B.; Herrlick, P. Interference of specific transcription factors. *Biochim. Biophys. Acta*, 1129:255-261, 1992.

[4] Urrutia, R. Exploring the role of homeobox and zinc finger proteins in pancreatic cell proliferation, differentiation and apoptosis. *Int. J. Pancreatol.*, 22(1):1-14,1997.

[5] Doi, R.; Wada, M.; Hosotani, R.; Lee-Jeon, O.; Koshiba,T.; Fujimoto, K.; Mori, C.; Nakamura, N.; Shiota, K.; Imamura, M. Role of apoptosis in duct-obstruction induced pancreatic involution in rats. *Pancreas,* 14(1):39-46,1997.

[6] Iovanna, J. Dedifferentiation and apoptosis of pancreatic cells during acute pancreatitis. *Int. J. Pancreatol.,*20(2):77-81,1996.

[7] Arias,A.;Bendayan,M.Differentiation of pancreatic acinar cells into duct- like cells. *Lab. Invest.,*69:518-530,1993.

[8] Tiscornia, O.; Dreiling,D.Does the pancreatic gland regenerate? *Gastroenterol.,*51(2):267-271,1966.

[9] Tiscornia, O.; Dreiling, D. Recovery of pancreatic exocrine secretory capacity following prolonged ductal obstruction. *Annals of Surgery,*169(2):267-276,1966.

[10] Shaw, J.; Latimer, E. Regeneration of pancreatic tissue from the transplanted pancreatic duct in the dog. *Am. J. Physiol.,*76:49-53,1926.

[11] Kaiser, A.; Saluja, A.; Sengupta, A.; Saluja, M.; Steer, M. Ralationship between severity,necrosis and apoptosis in five models of experimental acute pancreatitis. *Am. J. Physiol.*, 269:C1295-C1304,1995.

[12] Tiscornia, O.; Dreiling, D. Physiopathogenic hypothesis of alcoholic pancreatitis: Supranormal ecbolic stimulation of the "pancreon" units secondary to the loss of the negative component of pancreas innervation. *Pancreas,*2(5):604-612,1987.

[13] Tiscornia,O.;Celener,D.;Perec,C.;Lehmann,E.;CrestamC.; Dreiling,D.Physiopathogenic basis of alcoholic pancreatitis:The effects of elevated cholinergic tone and increased "pancreon" ecbolic response to CCK. *Mt. Sinai J. Med.,*50:369-387,1983.

[14] Tiscornia,O.;Perec,C.;Celener,D.;Cresta,M.;Tumilasci,O.;Lehmann,E.;Dreiling,D.The relationship of hyperactivity of the duodenal autonomic nervous brain and enhanced "pancreon" secretory response to CCK in Chronic alcoholism. *Mt. Sinai J. Med.,*51:650-663,1984.

[15] Cosen-Binker, L.; Binker, M.; Negri,A.; Tiscornia, O. Acute Pancreatitis:Possible initial triggering mechanism and prophylaxis. *Pancreatol.,*3(6):445-456,2003.

[16] Senninger,N.;Moody,F.;Coelho,J.;Van Buren,D.The role of biliary obstruction in the pathogenesis of acute pancreatitis in the opossum. *Surgery,*99:688-693,1986.

[17] Lerch, M.; Saluja, A.; Dawra, R.; Ramarao, P.; Saluja, M.; Steer, M. Acute necrotizing pancreatitis in the opossum:earliest morphologic changes involve acinar cells. *Gastroenterol.,*103:205-213,1992.

[18] Runzi, M.; Saluja, A.; Lerch, M.; Dawra, R.; Nishino, H.; Steer, M. Early ductal decompression prevents the progression of biliary pancreatitis: An experimental study in the opossum. *Gastroenterol.*,105:157-164,1993.

[19] Kimura,K.;Shimosegawa,T.;Sasano,H.;Abe,R.;Satoh,A.;Masamone,A.;Korizumi,M.;Nagura,H.; Toyota,T.Endogenous glucocorticoids decrease the acinar cell sensitivity to apoptosis during cerulein pancreatitis in rats.Gastroenterol.,114:372-381,1998.

[20] Sternberg, E. Neural-immune interaction in health and disease. *J. Clin. Invest.,*100:2641-2647,1997.

[21] Yamaguchi, H.; Weidenbach, H.; Adler, G. Combined treatment with C1 esterase inhibitor and antithrombin improves survival in severe acute experimental pancreatitis. *Gut*, 40:531-535,1997.

[22] Weiner, G.; Geenen, J.; Hogan, W.; Catalano, M. Use of corticosteroids in the preventive of post-ERCP pancreatitis. *Gastrointest. Endoscopy*, 42:579-583,1995.

[23] Shäfer, C.; Williams, J. Stress kinases and heat shock proteins in the pancreas:possible roles in normal function and disease. *J. Gastroenterol.*, 35:1-9,2000.

[24] Santoro, M. Regulation of the stress response by heat shock factors. *Biochem. Pharmacol.*,59:1-63,2000.

[25] Urayama, S.; Musch, M.; Rataky, V.; Madonna, M.; Straus, D.; Chang, E. Dexamethasone protection of rat epithelial cells against oxidant injury is mediated by induction of heat shock protein. *J. Clin. Invest.*,102:1860-1865,1998.

[26] Rinderknecht, H. Genetic determinants of mortality in acute necrotizing pancreatitis. *Int. J. Pancreatol.*,16(1):11-15,1994.

[27] Blinman, T.; Gokovsky, I.; Gukovskaya, S. Pancreatic acinar cells express a variety of cytokines that are regulated in experimental pancreatitis. *Gastroenterol.*, 112:A429,1997.

[28] Kusske, A.; Rongione, A.; Reber,H.Cytokines and acute pancreatitis. *Gastroenterol.*, 110:639-642,1996.

[29] Kornberg, R. Eukaryotic transcriptional control. *Millenium Issue TCB*, 9:1679-1687,1999.

[30] Caldenhoven, E.; Liden, S.; Wissinik, A. Negative cross-talk between Rel A and the glucocorticoid receptor:a possible mechanism for the anti-inflammatory action of glucocorticoids. *Mol. Endocrinol.*, 9:401-412,1995.

[31] Auphan, N.; Di Donato, J.; Rosetti, C. Immunosuppression by Glucocorticoids: Inhibition of Nf-κB activity through Induction of I kappa B synthesis. *Science*, 270:286-290, 1995.

[32] Turnbull, A.; Rivier, C. Regulation of the hypothalamic-pituitary adrenal axis by cytokines actions and mechanisms of action. *Physiological Reviews*, 79(1):1-50,1999.

[33] Norman, J.; Franz, M.; Messina, J.IL-1 receptor antagonist decreases severity of experimental acute pancreatitis. *Surgery,* 117:648-655,1995.

[34] Tiscornia, O.; Hansky, J.; Dreiling, D.; Janowitz, H. The adrenal cortex and external pancreatic secretion in the dog. *J. Mt. Sinai Hosp.*, 32(5):551-561,1964.

[35] Tiscornia, O.; Dreiling, D. The effect of hypophysiotomy on canine pancreatic function. *Surgery,* 60(4):883-890,1966.

[36] Cosen-Binker, L.; Binker, M.; Negri,A.;Tiscornia,O.Experimental Model in Wistar Rat-Glucocorticoid Treatment profile. *Dig. Dis. Sci.,* 48(8):1453-1464,2003.

[37] Abe, R.;S himosigawa, T; Toyota,T. The role of endogenous glucocorticoids in rat experimental models of acute pancreatitis. *Gastroenterol.*,109:933-943,1995.

[38] Rangione, A.; Kusske, A.; Kwan, K. IL-10 reduces the severity of acute pancreatitis in rats. *Gastroenterol.*, 112:960-967,1997.

[39] Van Laethem, J.; Marchant, A.; Delvaux, A.IL-10 prevents necrosis in murine experimental acute pancreatitis. *Gastroenterol.*, 108:1917-1922,1995.

[40] Sheinman, R.; Cogswell, P.; Lofquist, A.; Baldwin, A. Role of transcriptional activation of IκB in mediation of immunosuppression by glucocorticoids. *Science,* 270:283-286,1995.

[41] Scheinman, K.; Gualberto, C.; Jewll, J. Characterization of the mechanism involved in the transrepression of Nf-κB by activated glucocorticoid receptors. *Moll. Cell Biol.*, 15:943-953,1996.

[42] Herrlich, P. Cross-talk between glucocorticoid receptor and AP-1. *Oncogene*, 20:2465-2475,2001.

In: Pancreatitis Research Advances
Editor: William C. Langley, pp. 317-335
ISBN: 978-1-60021-883-5

Chapter XI

Acute Pancreatitis: Topics of Interest

Yong-Song Guan**, Qing He, Ying Hu, Ming-Quan Wang, Lin Yang and Zi La
West China Hospital of Sichuan University,
Chengdu, China, 610041
State Key Laboratory of Biotherapy, West China Hospital,
West China Medical School, Sichuan University,
Gaopeng Street, Keyuan Road 4, Chengdu, 610041, China

Abstract

Acute pancreatitis (AP) has been drawing attention of many medical practitioners and researchers for more than a century. Much attention has been paid to its exact pathophysiological mechanism, which is still not completely understood. Nevertheless, our understanding of the mechanistic processes that mediate the pathobiologic responses of pancreatitis is rapidly evolving in recent years. In addition, we now have initial evidence for potential treatment strategies for this disorder. Testing treatment strategies will lead to improved therapies and outcomes for patients with AP. Novel imaging techniques have been developed and appliced in diagnosis and severity grading of AP. Proinflammatory and anti-inflammatory cytokines have certain values in predicting the outcome of AP, and have shown promising in combination immunotherapy to decrease sepsis mortality in animal studies. For a given case, a multidisciplinary decision as treatment strategy is necessary to be made to benefit the sufferer by an early standard management.

* Correspondence: Dr. Yong-Song Guan, State Key Laboratory of Biotherapy, West China Hospital, West China Medical School, Sichuan University, Gaopeng Street, Keyuan Road 4,Chengdu, 610041, China. Phone: 86-28-85421008. Fax: 86-28-85538359. E-mail: yongsongguan@yahoo.com.

Abbreviations (Alphabetic)

ANP, acute necrotic pancreatitis;
AP, acute pancreatitis;
APACHE, Acute Physiologic and Chronic Health Evaluation;
[Ca2+]i, intracellular free calcium ions;
COX, cyclooxygenase;
ERCP, endoscopic retrograde cholangiopancreatography;
ERK, extracellular signal-regulated kinases;
HIV, human immunodeficiency virus;
ICK, inflammatory cytokine;
IL, interleukin;
JNK, C-Jun N-terminal kinases;
MIF, macrophage migration inhibitory factor;
MODS, multiple organ dysfunction syndrome;
MOF, multiple organ failure;
MRCP, magnetic resonance cholangiopancreatography;
MRI, magnetic resonance imaging;
MSOF, multisystem organ failure;
NF-κB, nuclear factor kappa B;
PAR-2, protease activated receptor-2;
PCT, procalcitonin;
PSTI, pancreatic secretory trypsin inhibitor;
SAPS, simplified acute physiology score;
SGE, spoiled gradient-echo;
SIRS, systemic inflammatory response syndrome;
SP, severe pancreatitis;
TNF-α, tumor necrosis factor-alpha;
vATPase, vacuolar adenosine triphosphatase;

1. Introduction

Acute pancreatitis (AP) has an incidence of approximately 40 cases per year per 100,000 adults [1]. It is usually self-limited; however, 10% to 20% of patients suffering from it will progress to severe pancreatitis (SP). The mortality rate among patients with SP may approach 30% when they progress to multisystem organ failure (MSOF). As an emergency, AP is frequently encountered in the clinical departments such as Surgery and Internal Medicine. In the United States, emergency department visits for AP are rising [2]. For management of AP, especially SP, one factor is becoming more and more important, that is to choose the right time of intervention [3]. In many centers, the management of AP is still based on speculative and unproven paradigms [4], so evidence-based analysis provides new insight into many aspects of interest. Studies suggest that the indications for antibiotic prophylaxis and surgery as well as other interventions need further clinical trials [4,5]. Clinically, AP has been classified as mild or severe types (Atlanta classification) [6,7]. Incidence and etiology of AP as well as percentage of the severe type show large regional differences [1,8-10]. At the present time, available diagnostic and therapeutic methods apply even highly advanced technology or devices; however, this disease still results in numerous complications and quite frequently in lethal outcome, leaving several topics of interest in the field of research.

1.1. Brief History

In ancient times, the pancreas was neglected in general, both as an organ and as a place of disease [11]. It is said [12] that the pancreas was firstly described by Herophilus of Chalcedon in about 300 BC, and the organ was named by Rufus of Ephesus in about 100 AD. However, it is proved that Aristotle (384-322 BC) had used the word pancreas before Herophilus. In Aristotle's *Historia Animalium*, there is a line saying "another to the so-called pancreas." It is considered that the words "so-called pancreas" imply that the word pancreas had been popular at the time of Aristotle, but it had not been authorized yet as an anatomical term. However, the word pancreas presumably has been accepted as an anatomical term since Herophilus.

The anatomical basis was first created in the 17th century [11,13]. In 1642, Johann Georg Wirsung (1589-1643), the prosector of Padua, Italy, discovered the human pancreatic duct [13] during the dissection of an executed murderer. And this duct is named after him as the main duct of Wirsung. In 1689, Johann Conrad Brunner (1653-1727) induced temporary diabetes mellitus in an experiment in pancreatectomized dogs [14]. In 1889, Reginald Fitz firmly established pancreatitis as a disease entity [11]. In 1963, the first Marseilles Symposium promoted a clinic pathologic classification of pancreatitis [15]. In 1984, the second Marseilles Symposium revised that classification [15]. At last, in 1992, the Atlanta Symposium [7] set up a clinically based classification system for acute pancreatitis. In recent years, as the imaging modalities [16] are becoming increasingly sophisticated, the classification of pancreatitis is expected in further refinements.

1.2. Status Quo

Between 1993 and 2003, emergency department visit rate for AP per 10,000 U.S. population increased from 4.9 visits to 10.9[2].

The diagnosis of AP is based on clinical examination as described by Fitz in 1889 and on laboratory tests. Amylase [17] and lipase [18] levels in the blood (hyperamylasemia and hyperlipasemia) are the most useful of the latter. The severity of AP is classically graded by the Ranson [19] and Imrie [20] scores, both systems are specific for AP but request 48 hours for a prognosis to be defined. Non-specific prognostic scores such as Acute Physiologic and Chronic Health Evaluation (APACHE) II [19, 20] and simplified acute physiology score (SAPS)[21] avoid such a delay. At the present, CT [22] is the reference diagnostic method whenever pathologic proof of the disease is lacking, magnetic resonance imaging (MRI) also plays a role in the evaluation of benign pancreatic disease [23], and such imaging information substantiates the prognostic value of the bioclinical scores.

The mild form [6, 7] is also known as edematous pancreatitis, because there is edematous swelling of the pancreas combined with tiny foci of interstitial (fat) necrosis. Severe or necrotizing pancreatitis [6, 7] shows large areas of often hemorrhagic necrosis of the pancreatic and particularly the peripancreatic tissue. Approximately half of the deaths in AP occur because of multiple organ failure (MOF) [24,25] or septic complications.

1.3. Perspectives

Recent studies suggest that single biologic markers such as C-reactive protein [21] and trypsinogen activation peptides [26] may soon allow a simple and early assessment of the prognosis. New imaging modalities and novel applications of existing techniques will play an important role in the management of pancreatic diseases, including acute and chronic pancreatitis [22].

When systemic inflammatory response syndrome (SIRS)[27] goes to MODS and MOF, the mortality becomes high, ranging from 30-80% depending on the number of failed organs [25]. Multiple therapeutic agents are to be tried to prevent MODS and SIRS. And therapies antagonizing inflammatory cytokines (ICKs) [28] are drawing attention, as they play an important role in the progression of AP into SP.

2. Mechanisims of Pathogenesis

The two major etiological factors [9] responsible for AP are alcohol and cholelithiasis (biliary stones). Other risk factors include endoscopic retrograde cholangiopancreatography（ERCP）, surgery, therapeutic drugs, human immunodeficiency virus (HIV) infection, hyperlipidemia, and biliary tract anomalies. Idiopathic AP[29] is defined as AP in which the etiological factor cannot be specified.

2.1. Difficulties in Uncovering the Mechanisms of Pancreatitis

The pathogenesis of AP involves the interplay of local and systemic immune responses that are often difficult to characterize, particularly when results from animal models are used as a foundation for human trials [1]. None of these models resemble closely [29] the clinical situation where quite different degrees of severity usually occur, ranging from mild edematous pancreatitis to severe necrotizing pancreatitis. On the other hand, in spite of significant progress in the understanding of molecular events in experimental pancreatitis, knowledge of these mechanisms has not yet been translated into therapeutic strategies useful in humans.

2.2. Interplay of Local and Systemic Immune Responses

AP is an inflammatory disorder that develops a complex series of immunological events [30]. The critical players of this interaction include some proinflammatory cytokines [1]. Cytokines are regulatory proteins, such as the interleukins and lymphokines that are released by cells of the immune system and act as intercellular mediators in the generation of an immune response. The causes of immune responses to AP are various; some authors [31] even reported a case of necrotizing pancreatitis that developed following combined hepatitis A and B vaccination.

2.3. Calcium Ions

A large, sustained increase in intracellular free calcium ions ([Ca2+]i) in acinar cells may play a key role in the pathogenesis of AP[32,33]. A calcium signal is an impetuous increase in concentration of calcium ions (Ca2+) in the cytosol, the aqueous part of the cytoplasm within which various particles and organelles are suspended. Such signals are critical to the control of many important functions of the body, and in gland cells they are responsible for regulation of secretion. As a particular type of cell, the pancreatic acinar cell is responsible for the secretion of the enzymes crucial for the digestion of food. Ca2+ signals control diverse activities [34], not only the normal enzyme secretion, but also growth (cell division) and programmed cell death (apoptosis). The cell is able to localize Ca2+ signals [34] to certain regions in enabling Ca2+ to perform these multiple functions, by creating high local concentrations of Ca2+ (microdomains), which differ from the cytoplasmic average. Patterns of Ca2+ signals can be created different in space and time, which allow specific cellular responses to be evoked [32]. For [Ca2+]i increases, the origin and duration rather than their extent or vacillating nature, determine whether the cell will secrete or die [33]. An abnormal [Ca2+]i increase can trigger trypsin activation, acinar cell damage and AP. Animal experiments demonstrated that serum pancreatic enzyme elevation as well as trypsinogen activation was significantly reduced by pretreatment of animals with calcium chelator [35] and that calcium chelators inhibit radical-induced trypsin activation as well as cell necrosis and apoptosis[33]. Therefore, an inhibition of pathological [Ca2+]i release may have a therapeutic potential of AP.

2.4. Activation of Trypsinogen

Although the pathogenesis of AP has not yet been explained clearly, a common feature is the premature activation of trypsinogen [29] within pancreatic tissues, which triggers autodigestion of the gland. For further understanding of pancreatic intracellular digestive enzyme activation [36-39], the pathophysiologic concept of AP is concentrated on early events inside acinar cells including activation of trypsin. Under normal conditions, trypsin activity is properly suppressed in the pancreatic acinar cells [38], when a small amount of trypsinogen changes into active trypsin and the latter is inactivated by pancreatic secretory trypsin inhibitor (PSTI). This process is as a first line of defense to prevent damage to pancreatic acinar cells. However, when there is excessive stimulation to pancreatic acinar cells, activated trypsin can overwhelm PSTI; a series of events will follow and result in the activation of various proteolytic enzymes that cause damage to cells. Trypsin is secreted from the pancreatic acinar cells and activates protease activated receptor-2 (PAR-2), which is present at high densities on the luminal surfaces of pancreatic acinar cells and duct cells. Activation of PAR-2 leads to the production of cytokines. The actions of trypsin, PSTI and PAR-2 are strongly connected with each other in the pancreas. During AP, trypsin and its specific receptor, PAR-2, play an important role in cytokine production and the consequent development of distant organ injury [39].

2.5. Research into the Cellular Subunits

Vacuolar adenosine triphosphatase (vATPase) [40] is a multiprotein complex that carries protons across cellular membranes. Proenzyme or zymogen denotes any of a group of compounds that are inactive precursors of enzymes and require some change (such as the hydrolysis of a fragment that masks an active enzyme) to become active. Activation of zymogens within the pancreatic acinar cell is an early feature of AP [41, 42]. Supramaximal concentrations, agonist-induced zymogen activation requires vATPase activity [42]. Activation of the vATPase requires assembly of the soluble subunits on the membrane subunits, and conditions that cause protease activation in the acinar cell also cause the same assembly [41]. Supraphysiologic concentrations of cholecystokinin [42] cause intrapancreatic zymogen activation and pancreatitis. Translocation of a soluble subunit to membrane-bound organelles, a marker of vATPase activation, was observed in an *in vitro* model of AP. In addition, inhibitors [40] of vATPase block this protease activation. Ethanol and butanol sensitize the acinar cell to cholecystokinin-induced zymogen activation, and vATPase inhibitors also blocked this activation. Activation of the vATPase may be central to the pathologic activation of proteases in the acinar cell and may also modulate the sensitizing effects of alcohols. It is proposed [41] that vATPase-mediated acidification of zymogen-containing organelles stimulates pathologic zymogen activation in the pancreatic acinar cell.

2.6. Molecular Aspects

Recent advances [29] in basic research suggest that etiologic factors including cyclooxygenase-2 [43], substance P, and angiotensin II may have novel roles in this disease. There are at least 2 isoforms of cyclooxygenases (COX). COX-2 is stimulated by proinflammatory cytokines and inhibited by anti-inflammatory mediators. One study [43] concluded that the treatment with a COX-2 inhibitor might lower serum levels of at least two cytokines, but the potential benefits of this effect are still unclear. Substance P [29] is a neuropeptide located in the nerve endings throughout the body and is released into the gap where it acts via the neurokinin receptor 1 to mediate pain. When pancreatitis develops, there is an increase in substance P levels as well as neurokinin receptor 1 on pancreatic acinar cells. In vivo study [44] demonstrated that substance P mediated pancreatic microcirculatory dysfunction during the development of AP, and that blockage of substance P receptor attenuated substance P-induced pancreatic microcirculatory dysfunction. The pancreas contains a local renin-angiotensin system, it has been demonstrated [45] that exogenous addition of angiotensin II can stimulate a dose-dependent release of digestive enzymes from the acinar cells, and administration of selective angiotension receptor antagonist significantly inhibited the acinar digestion enzyme secretion in both normal and pancreatitis-induced acini.

3. Early Diagnosis of the Severe Type

AP is an inflammatory condition of the pancreas manifested by abdominal pain and elevated pancreatic enzymes in the blood [43]. AP is characterized [29] by edema, acinar cell necrosis, hemorrhage, and severe inflammation of the pancreas. SP may lead to SIRS and MODS, which account for the high mortality rate of AP. The Atlanta classification should no longer be used to describe computed tomography findings in AP [3].

3.1. The Lethal Toxicity of Pancreatic Ascites Fluid

Ascites fluid is known to be important in the clinical progression of AP [46]. The inflammatory necrotizing process takes place in the retroperitoneal area during the early phase of AP [47], and several pro-inflammatory mediators including cytokines are released locally by overactivated neutrophils and monocytes/macrophages among other cells. Cytokines are a family of low-molecular weight proteins (16-25 KiloDalton) that are secreted by a multitude of cells, including macrophages and monocytes [27]. The drained liquid around the pancreas may containe cytokines, protease, vasoactive substances and bacterial contamination, with lethal toxicity. Ascitic fluid reflects cell death responses such as necrosis and apoptosis [36] in AP, early peritoneal aspiration of the fluid and measurement of trypsinogen activation peptides may be used as a means of severity assessment and identification of pancreatic necrosis. Careful comparative analysis of peritoneal exudate, plasma and lymph with regards to the mediators may provide essential pathophysiological clues helpful for consideration of antimediator therapy in the early attack of AP [47]. CT is helpful [48] for aspiration of localized fluid and endoscopic ultrasound-guided fine-needle aspiration of ascites frequently identifies ascites missed by other imaging studies.

3.2. Leptin and Adiponectin Levels

Cytokines [28] that are secreted by adipose tissue are termed as adipokines or adipocytokines, including leptin, adiponectin and TNF-α. Leptin is a hormone that influences endocrine and exocrine functions of the pancreas and regulates feeding behaviors and energy metabolism. Adiponectin is also a protein hormone that modulates a number of metabolic processes, including glucose regulation and fatty acid catabolism. These two adipokines also regulate the course of systemic inflammation [49, 50]. Because SP is characterized by lipase-induced peripancreatic fat cell necrosis, leptin and adiponectin have been studied as to see that whether they could serve as potential markers predicting peripancreatic necrosis and severity in SP. However, studies yielded controversial results [49, 50] in the correlation between plasma levels of adiponectin and leptin on admission and disease severity.

3.3. Imaging Modalities

In AP, a modification of the standard computed tomography severity index, which places greater emphasis on extrapancreatic complications, has shown superior correlation with various patient outcome measures [16]. Contrast-enhanced ultrasound has shown promise in evaluating the severity of AP [22]. Optical coherence tomography [22] permits high-resolution imaging of tissue microstructures using a probe that can be inserted into the duct of Wirsung through a standard ERCP catheter. This intraductal optical coherence tomography is now feasible for investigating main pancreatic duct strictures [51]. Multidetector-row computed tomography has some advantages [52] in diagnosing the inflammatory lesions and grading severity of pancreatitis. Contrast enhanced ultrasonography [52] may prove to be a useful way to judge the degree of inflammation and fibrosis in autoimmune pancreatitis and to monitor response to steroid therapy. Improvements in positron emission tomography/computed tomography scans [52] may be helpful for differentiating malignant from benign in localized lesions.

MRI is comparable with CT in staging AP, with advantage in analysis of pancreatograms and textural changes of the parenchyma helpful in diagnosing chronic pancreatitis over AP [52]. Precontrast breath-hold spoiled gradient-echo (SGE) imaging is sensitive [53] for the detection of AP. MRI is effective as a problem-solving modality so that it can be used as a valuable tool in the assessment of the full spectrum of pancreatic diseases. Although MRI [23] and magnetic resonance cholangiopancreatography (MRCP) are most often used to evaluate the liver and bile duct, technical advances such as the use of secretin stimulation also allow for high-quality imaging of the pancreas and pancreatic ductal system. Secretin-stimulated MRCP (S-MRCP) can aid the diagnosis of acute and chronic pancreatitis, and delineate ductal pathology such as benign strictures and duct leaks.

3.4. Other Laboratory Tests

Patients with AP exhibit with elevated levels of pancreatic digestive enzymes [29] in blood and urine, including amylase and lipase. Infection of pancreatic necrosis has a high incidence and mortality rate, so early diagnosis and prediction of infection in necrotizing pancreatitis are extremely important [54-56]. Soluble receptor proteins [54] derived from the macrophage-monocyte lineage promote the ICK response early in AP. The concentration of 24-hour plasma macrophage migration inhibitory factor (MIF) has prognostic utility in predicting ANP [54]. Procalcitonin (PCT) and IL-6 serum levels were elevated very early in patients who eventually developed necrosis infection [55, 56]. However, a review of the clinical studies suggests that we still do not have an optimal model, a single morphologic or laboratory marker reliably predicting the individual course of AP still awaits discovery [37].

3.5. Fine Needle Aspiration Biopsy

There are no specific signs or symptoms to differentiate sterile necrosis from infected. This can only be confirmed by CT- or ultrasound-guided aspiration of necrotic material or peripancreatic fluid collections [56, 57].

4. Treatment of the Severe Type

The standard treatment for AP is still based on supportive care [43]. Currently, there is inadequacy [10] in management of severe cases, there was poor use of objective severity stratification (19%), low admission rates to a high dependency unit or intensive care unit (67%), and only 33% of patients had computed tomography. Early enteral nutrition in SP is not only capable of cutting down infectious complications but may also reduce mortality [3].

MOF [24], MODS, and the SIRS are problems of medical progress and intensive care units and require prevention of organ failure through excellent patient care. Whether blockade of mediators or treatment of the manifestations of diseases or injuries will have substantial impact remains to be learned. A single magic bullet for complex and diverse illnesses is not likely to appear or to be successful [24]. The difference between SIRS and sepsis is the absence or presence of a focus of infection [27]. AP is one of the non-infective causes of SIRS. What is interesting is that more and more evidence [3] indicates that antibiotic-prophylaxis is not capable of preventing infectious complications in SP. New approaches have to be found to counteract these severe complications, on the basis of understanding of the control of microcirculatory disturbances in AP [36].

Probiotic-prophylaxis is being considered as an alternative with promising experimental results [3]. Systematic use of broad spectrum antibiotics has been recommended in patients with infection of necrosis but may induce serious side effects [55]. A combination of PCT and IL-6 thresholds could be helpful in identifying a subgroup of patients in whom antibiotic prophylaxis is likely to be ineffective.

Surgical intervention for infected (peri-) pancreatic necrosis is increasingly being postponed [3]. Minimally invasive strategies are being considered as a full alternative for necrosectomy by laparotomy in infected (peri-) pancreatic necrosis [3]. Percutaneous interventional radiology [46] can be indicated for the abscess drainage in cases with acquired peripancreatic infection. On the basis of encouraging animal experiments early percutaneous or surgical peritoneal lavage with or without the addition of antiproteases can be carried out in human AP [47], to wash out potential toxic mediators from the peritoneal cavity before they gain access to the systemic circulation. The procedure of percutaneous peripancreatic drainage can be guided by CT [48], and in certain cases the percutaneous drainage is sufficient for the total recovery of ANP, in other cases can be used to postpone surgery. Interventional treatment using large-bore percutaneous catheters to perform percutaneous necrosectomy, fragmentation of necrotic pancreatic tissue with a snare catheter and dormia basket, and aspiration has been reported [57].

There are several benefits of enteral feeding on outcome of AP [36]. Understanding of the role of the pancreatic neural system in regulating the microcirculation as well as the pain associated with the disorder is helpful for the strategy of medication [36].

5. Management of Pancreatitis with Biliary Origin

Gallstones are the commonest cause of AP in developed countries [58-60]. The diagnosis of biliary pancreatitis is often readily established, as the cause of the disease is the presence of stones in the common bile duct. A prompt diagnosis requires a high degree of suspicion and clinical shrewdness shown by keen insight [55]. Common bile duct lithiasis can result in not only AP, but also acute purulent cholangitis, raising the difficulty at bedside in detecting the primary lesion that leads the systemic inflammatory response.

The patients can be managed supportively and undergo laparoscopic cholecystectomy with intraoperative cholangiography during their initial hospitalization to prevent recurrence [58]. If necessary, laparoscopic common bile duct exploration can be performed. There is a hypothesis that early endoscopic intervention, performed on patients with acute gallstone pancreatitis and biliopancreatic obstruction, reduces systemic and local inflammation. However, the role of early endoscopic intervention, in the treatment of acute biliary pancreatitis, remains controversial [3, 5].

One study [3] suggested that, in biliary pancreatitis, early endoscopic retrograde cholangiography with sphincterotomy (within 48 h) is beneficial in case of ampullary obstruction, although it may be withheld in the event of negative endoscopic ultrasound.

Another study [5] concluded that that early endoscopic intervention reduces systemic and local inflammation in patients with acute gallstone pancreatitis and biliopancreatic obstruction lacks evidence, and if acute cholangitis can be safely excluded, early endoscopic intervention is not mandatory and should not be considered a standard indication, because most patients by early conservative management had persisting bile duct stones at elective biliary surgery and no significant differences were observed between conservative management and endoscopic intervention as for mean organ failure score, complications, overall morbidity and mortality.

There seems to be a role for S-MRCP in the assessment of pancreatic function and (possibly) sphincter of Oddi dysfunction. When endoscopic or surgical therapy is planned, S-MRCP can help to establish a diagnosis as well as offer a "road map" to guide therapy [23]. S-MRCP is noninvasive and almost entirely without risk to the patient, which gives it a distinct advantage over traditional endoscopic methods of diagnosis for conditions such as pancreas divisum and other ductal pathology. The information provided by S-MRCP, obtained before endoscopic or surgical therapy is attempted, can assist the patient and physician in making a fully informed decision with regard to the risks and probable benefits of any planned intervention.

Experiments suggest that pancreatic duct obstruction rapidly changes the physiological response of the exocrine pancreas to a (Ca2+)-signaling pattern that has been associated with premature digestive enzyme activation and the onset of pancreatitis, both of which can be prevented by administration of an intracellular calcium chelator [35].

Rectal diclofenac [36, 61] given immediately after ERCP can reduce the incidence of AP induced by the procedure of ERCP.

6. Cellular Factors and Inhibitors

In AP, serum and intracellular levels of some inflammatory cytokines (ICKs), such as interleukin (IL) -1, IL-6, IL-8 and tumor necrosis factor-alpha (TNF-α), are markedly increased [1, 28, 38] with positive correlation to the severity of disease. Cytokines are important components of the immune system, act as messages between cells [27], and are involved in many pathological aspects of the cascade leading to SIRS and ultimately MODS. Cytokine secretion is a very closely regulated process and expression of most cytokines is modulated by transcription factors such as nuclear factor kappa B (NF-κB)[30]. And the blockage of inflammatory mediators reduces the severity and enhances therapeutic effects of SP. In 1994, Viedma et al first reported [62] that serum levels of various ICKs were remarkably elevated only in SP and ANP, while in edematous AP, localized inflammation was the essential manifestation without large quantity of ICKs entering the blood stream. Subsequently, other authors [50, 54] observed results as the same. Obvious elevation of ICKs has also been positively correlated to ANP and MODS development. When serum ICKs were correlated to Ransen and APACHE scores, they were also confirmed as specific for predicting the severity, MOF, total mortality and the hospitalization duration of AP.

The sites of ICKs' production [63] seem critical to the explanation of local or systemic damages by AP. However, such production sites have not been identified until 1994. Animal experiments of AP resulted that IL-1, TNF and IL-6 are manufactured in parenchymal pancreas. In addition, other animal experiments revealed that, in AP, IL-1 and TNF are produced not only locally in the pancreas, but also systemically [64], including in tissues of the spleen, the lungs and the liver. What is importantly different is that, ICKs are always produced several hours or days earlier in the pancreas than in other sites, and this is of course dependent on the speed of pancreatitis development. Such observations are helpful for the elucidation of the roles of IL-1 and TNF in resulting in MOF. For example, it is believed currently that the development of acute respiratory distress syndrome is directly associated with the production of IL-1 and TNF in pulmonary parenchyma [64].

6.1. Role of ERK, p38, and JNK

Extracellular signal-regulated kinases (ERKs)[65,66] are widely expressed and are involved in the regulation of meiosis, mitosis, and postmitotic functions in differentiated cells. Many different stimuli, including growth factors, cytokines, virus infection, ligands for heterotrimeric guanine nucleotide-binding protein (G protein)-coupled receptors, transforming agents, and carcinogens, activate the ERK pathway. P38 mitogen-activated protein kinases [65] are a class of mitogen-activated protein kinases, which are responsive to stress stimuli, such as cytokines, ultraviolet irradiation, heat shock, and osmotic shock, and are involved in cell differentiation and apoptosis. C-Jun N-terminal kinases (JNKs)[66] are mitogen-activated protein kinases, which are responsive to stress stimuli, such as cytokines, ultraviolet irradiation, heat shock, and osmotic shock, and are involved in cell differentiation and apoptosis. JNK1 and JNK2 are ubiquitinous distributed and JNK3 is found in neuronal tissue. The JNK1 is involved in inflammatory conditions and cytokine production. ERK, p38, and JNK as stress kinases, play an important role in acinar cell cytokine production. [citation needed]

6.2. The Proinflammatory Cytokines

Proinflammatory cytokines IL-1beta, TNF-α, IL-6, IL-8, and platelet activating factor (PAF) have certain values in predicting the outcome of AP [67]. Severe sepsis is characterized by an overwhelming production of proinflammatory cytokines. While cytokines trigger a beneficial inflammatory response that promotes local coagulation to confine tissue damage, the excessive production of these proinflammatory cytokines can be even more dangerous [27] than the original stimulus, overcoming the normal regulation of immune response and producing pathological inflammatory disorders as notably seen in sepsis. During acute severe pancreatitis, the pro- and anti-inflammatory cytokine response occurred early and persisted in the systemic circulation for several days [68,69].

6.3. The Anti-Inflammatory Cytokines

The anti-inflammatory cytokines [1] IL-10, as well as TNF-soluble receptors and IL-1 receptor antagonist, have also been shown to be intimately involved in the inflammatory response to AP. IL-10, also known as human cytokine synthesis inhibitory factor (CSIF), is an anti-inflammatory cytokine, capable of inhibiting synthesis of pro-inflammatory cytokines like Interferon-gamma, IL-2, IL-3 and TNF-α by cells such as macrophages and the Type 2 T helper cells. However, it is also stimulatory towards certain T cells, mast cells and B cells. Inhibition of TNF or IL-1 alone has not improved sepsis survival in human clinical trials; therefore, it has been suggested that blockade of both may be successful. Animal study [70] revealed that combination immunotherapy with soluble tumor necrosis factor receptors plus IL-1 receptor antagonist decreased sepsis mortality.

6.4. Other Compounds

Other compounds [1] implicated in disease pathogenesis in experimental models include complement, bradykinin, nitric oxide, reactive oxygen intermediates, substance P, and higher polyamines. Complement activation regulators may participate in the pathogenesis of pancreatic inflammation. Downregulation of complement activation regulators expression may be one of the causes of pancreatic necrosis. IL-4 treatment may control SP aggravation by enhancing expression of complement activation regulators in pancreas and decreasing pancreatic necrosis [69]. Polyamines [71] are required for optimal growth and function of cells. Regulation of their cellular homeostasis is therefore tightly controlled. Acute induction of regulatory enzyme for polyamine catabolism leads to pancreatic inflammation, suggesting that sufficient pools of higher polyamine levels are essential to maintain pancreatic integrity.

7. Rare Complications

7.1. Splenic Lesions

Splenic lesions complicated from AP are with a very low incidence and thus often neglected. However, such lesions strongly imply the severity of the condition. The pseudocyst of the pancreas is a frequent complication of AP, but the splenic involvement [72] from the pancreatic pseudocyst is uncommon. Splenectomy and distal pancreatectomy should be performed to remove the cysts. CT is useful for detection and follow-up of these complications [73]. The presence of infarction of spleen, fluid in capsule, hemorrhage in spleen tissue or under capsule, and pseudoaneurysm of the splenic artery should be correlated with the symptoms. Most splenic parenchymal complications of pancreatitis regress spontaneously and may be managed conservatively. Surgical indication is based mainly on clinical findings.

7.2. Abdominal Hemorrhage

Bleeding from the pancreas itself and surrounding arteries [74] is the common cause of massive abdominal hemorrhage in AP patients. Small arteries of the pancreas are invaded and damaged in the processes of pancreatic parenchymal necrosis, destruction of ducts, and exudation of pancreatic juice in autodigestion. Breakdown of small arteries or burst of pseudoaneurysms results in abdominal hemorrhage. In CT images, when scanning is enhanced with contrast, aneurysms in the celiac trunk or the splenic artery can be revealed as enlarged vessel cross section, circular with high intensity and synchronously enhanced with the abdominal aorta. The rupture site can be accurately revealed by digital substraction angiography [72, 74]. Another major cause of massive abdominal hemorrhage in AP patients is portal hypertension with varices [75] resulted from venous thrombosis in portal, splenic and superior mesenteric veins and their tributaries. Hemorrhage has been observed most frequently occurring from splenic vein and at the bifurcation of the portal vein near the pancreas. The reason is that as the splenic vein is very close to the body and tail of the pancreas, with pancreatic tissue necrosis and formation of pseudocysts in the region, together with release of pancreatic enzymes, infection and other factors, the splenic vein may become embolized or compressed, leading back flow of splenic venous blood, firstly to the short gastric vein, then to the left and right gastric vein, and finally to the portal vein. When a pseudoaneurysm or a pseudocyst hemorrhages acutely, transcatheter arterial blockade [74] can control the hemorrhage and improve the hemodynamic status of the patient before surgery.

8. Conclusion

AP is one of the emergencies frequently confronted in clinical practice. Its pathogenesis has not been elucidated completely yet, and this elucidation is subject to the continuous efforts of the researchers in clinical and basic sciences. The clinical outcome of AP is dependent on the presence of necrosis and systemic complications. The significant advances in our understanding of the molecular aspects of AP will provide theoretical and experimental bases for the development of novel strategies of management. For the clinical practitioners, it is of great importance to distinguish as early as possible the severe form from the mild. For SP cases, a multidisciplinary decision as treatment strategy is necessary to be made with participation of internists, surgeons, critical care specialists, nutritionists and other specialized experts, taking advantages of available high technology approaches and sophisticated modalities, to benefit the sufferers by an early standard management, and to reduce the mortality of this disease.

References

[1] Granger J, Remick D. Acute pancreatitis: models, markers and mediators. *Shock,* 2005 Dec;24 Suppl 1:45-51.

[2] Fagenholz PJ, Castillo CF, Harris NS , Pelletier AJ, Camargo CA Jr. National study of United States emergency department visits for acute pancreatitis, 1993-2003. *BMC Emerg. Med.,*2007Jan 22;7:1.

[3] Besselink MG, van Santvoort HC, Witteman BJ, Gooszen HG; for the Dutch Acute Pancreatitis Study Group. Management of severe acute pancreatitis: it's all about timing. *Curr. Opin. Crit. Care,* 2007 Apr;13(2):200-6.

[4] Heinrich S, Schafer M, Rousson V, Clavien PA. Evidence-based treatment of acute pancreatitis: a look at established paradigms. *Ann. Surg.,* 2006 Feb;243(2):154-68.

[5] Oria A, Cimmino D, Ocampo C, Silva W, Kohan G, Zandalazini H, Szelagowski C, Chiappetta L. Early endoscopic intervention versus early conservative management in patients with acute gallstone pancreatitis and biliopancreatic obstruction: a randomized clinical trial. *Ann. Surg.,* 2007 Jan;245(1):10-7.

[6] Kloppel G. Acute pancreatitis. *Semin. Diagn. Pathol.,* 2004 Nov;21(4):221-6.

[7] Bradley EL 3rd. A clinically based classification system for acute pancreatitis. Summary of the International Symposium on Acute Pancreatitis, Atlanta, Ga, September 11 through 13, 1992. *Arch. Surg.,* 1993 May;128(5):586-90.

[8] Gislason H, Horn A, Hoem D, Andren-Sandberg A, Imsland AK, Soreide O, Viste A. Acute pancreatitis in Bergen, Norway. A study on incidence, etiology and severity. *Scand. J. Surg.,* 2004;93(1):29-33.

[9] Sekimoto M, Takada T, Kawarada Y, Hirata K, Mayumi T, Yoshida M, Hirota M, Kimura Y, Takeda K, Isaji S, Koizumi M, Otsuki M, Matsuno S; JPN. JPN Guidelines for the management of acute pancreatitis: epidemiology, etiology, natural history, and outcome predictors in acute pancreatitis. *J. Hepatobiliary Pancreat. Surg.*, 2006;13(1):10-24.

[10] Toh SK, Phillips S, Johnson CD. A prospective audit against national standards of the presentation and management of acute pancreatitis in the South of England. *Gut,* 2000 Feb;46(2):239-43.

[11] Busnardo AC, DiDio LJ, Tidrick RT, Thomford NR. History of the pancreas. *Am. J. Surg.,* 1983 Nov;146(5):539-50.

[12] Tsuchiya R, Fujisawa N. On the etymology of "pancreas". *Int. J. Pancreatol.,* 1997 Jun; 21 (3): 269-72.

[13] Howard JM, Hess W, Traverso W. Johann Georg Wirsung (1589-1643) and the pancreatic duct: the prosector of Padua, Italy. *J. Am. Coll Surg.,* 1998 Aug;187(2):201-11.

[14] Keck FS, Pfeiffer EF. The first experimental diabetes mellitus. *Acta Diabetol. Lat.,* 1989 Jan-Mar;26(1):79-81.

[15] Chavez Rossell M. History of the pancreas and the evolution of concepts and classification of pancreatitis. *Rev. Gastroenterol Peru,* 2002 Jul-Sep;22(3):243-7.

[16] Nichols MT, Russ PD, Chen YK. Pancreatic imaging: current and emerging technologies. *Pancreas,* 2006 Oct;33(3):211-20.

[17] Honda K, Itaba S, Mizutani T, Sumida Y, Kanayama K, Higuchi N, Yoshinaga S, Akiho H, Kawabe K, Arita Y, Ito T, Nakamura K, Takayanagi R. An increase in the serum amylase level in patients after peroral double balloon enteroscopy: an association with the development of pancreatitis. *Endoscopy,* 2006 Oct;38(10):1040-3.

[18] Tomonari A, Takahashi S, Takasugi K, Ooi J, Tsukada N, Konuma T, Iseki T, Tojo A, Asano S. Pancreatic hyperamylasemia and hyperlipasemia in association with cytomegalovirus infection following unrelated cord blood transplantation for acute myelogenous leukemia. *Int. J. Hematol.,* 2006 Dec;84(5):438-40.

[19] Yeung YP, Lam BY, Yip AW. APACHE system is better than Ranson system in the prediction of severity of acute pancreatitis. *Hepatobiliary Pancreat. Dis. Int.,* 2006 May;5(2):294-9.

[20] Liu TH, Kwong KL, Tamm EP, Gill BS, Brown SD, Mercer DW. Acute pancreatitis in intensive care unit patients: value of clinical and radiologic prognosticators at predicting clinical course and outcome. *Crit. Care Med.,* 2003 Apr;31(4):1026-30.

[21] Dajak M, Ignjatovic S, Majkic-Singh N, Lausevic Z, Bukumirovic V. Prognostic value of phospholipase A2 group II, C-reactive protein and Simplified Acute Physiological Score II in intensive care patients. *Clin. Lab.,* 2006;52(78):387-92.

[22] Kwon RS, Scheiman JM. New advances in pancreatic imaging. *Curr. Opin. Gastroenterol.,* 2006 Sep;22(5):512-9.

[23] Kinney TP, Punjabi G, Freeman M. Technology insight: applications of MRI for the evaluation of benign disease of the pancreas. *Nat. Clin. Pract. Gastroenterol. Hepatol.,* 2007 Mar;4(3):148-59.

[24] Baue AE. Multiple organ failure, multiple organ dysfunction syndrome, and the systemic inflammatory response syndrome -where do we stand? *Shock,* 1994 Dec;2(6):385-97.

[25] Baue AE, Durham R, Faist E. Systemic inflammatory response syndrome (SIRS), multiple organ dysfunction syndrome (MODS), multiple organ failure (MOF): are we winning the battle? *Shock,* 1998 Aug;10(2):79-89.

[26] Allen HS, Steiner J, Broussard J, Mansfield C, Williams DA, Jones B. Serum and urine concentrations of trypsinogen activation peptide as markers for acute pancreatitis in cats. *Can. J. Vet. Res.*, 2006 Oct;70(4):313-6.

[27] Matsuda N, Hattori Y. Systemic inflammatory response syndrome (SIRS): molecular pathophysiology and gene therapy. *J. Pharmacol. Sci.,* 2006 Jul;101(3):189-98.

[28] Closa D, Motoo Y, Iovanna JL. Pancreatitis-associated protein: from a lectin to an anti-inflammatory cytokine. *World J. Gastroenterol.,* 2007 Jan 14;13(2):170-4.

[29] Chan YC, Leung PS. Acute pancreatitis: animal models and recent advances in basic research. *Pancreas,* 2007 Jan;34(1):1-14.

[30] Shi C, Zhao X, Lagergren A, Sigvardsson M, Wang X, Andersson R. Immune status and inflammatory response differ locally and systemically in severe acute pancreatitis. *Scand. J. Gastroenterol,* 2006 Apr;41(4):472-80.

[31] Shlomovitz E, Davies W, Cairns E, Brintnell WC, Goldszmidt M, Dresser GK. Severe necrotizing pancreatitis following combined hepatitis A and B vaccination. *CMAJ,* 2007 Jan 30;176(3):339-42.

[32] Petersen OH, Burdakova N. The specificity of Ca2+ signalling. *Acta Physiol. Hung.,* 2002;89(4):439-50.

[33] Niederau C, Luthen R, Klonowski-Stumpe H, Schreiber R, Soika I, Sata N, Bing H, Haussinger D. The role of calcium in pancreatitis. *Hepatogastroenterology,* 1999 Sep-Oct;46(29):2723-30.

[34] McCarron JG, Chalmers S, Bradley KN, MacMillan D, Muir TC. Ca2+ microdomains in smooth muscle. *Cell Calcium.*, 2006 Nov-Dec;40(5-6):461-93.

[35] Mooren FCh, Hlouschek V, Finkes T, Turi S, Weber IA, Singh J, Domschke W, Schnekenburger J, Kruger B, Lerch MM. Early changes in pancreatic acinar cell calcium signaling after pancreatic duct obstruction. *J. Biol. Chem.*, 2003 Mar 14;278(11):9361-9.

[36] Pandol SJ. Acute pancreatitis. *Curr. Opin. Gastroenterol.*, 2006 Sep;22(5):481-6.

[37] Weber CK, Adler G. Acute pancreatitis. *Curr. Opin. Gastroenterol.*, 2001 Sep;17(5):426-9.

[38] Hirota M, Ohmuraya M, Baba H. The role of trypsin, trypsin inhibitor, and trypsin receptor in the onset and aggravation of pancreatitis. *J. Gastroenterol.*, 2006 Sep;41(9):832-6.

[39] Maeda K, Hirota M, Kimura Y, Ichihara A, Ohmuraya M, Sugita H, Ogawa M. Proinflammatory role of trypsin and protease activated receptor 2 in a rat model of acute pancreatitis. *Pancreas*, 2005 Jul;31(1):54-62.

[40] Gorelick FS, Shugrue CA, Kolodecik TR, Thrower EC. Vacuolar adenosine triphosphatase and pancreatic acinar cell function. *J. Gastroenterol. Hepatol.,* 2006 Oct;21 Suppl 3:S18-21.

[41] Waterford SD, Kolodecik TR, Thrower EC, Gorelick FS.Vacuolar ATPase regulates zymogen activation in pancreatic acini. *J. Biol. Chem.*, 2005 Feb 18;280(7):5430-4.

[42] Gorelick FS. Alcohol and zymogen activation in the pancreatic acinar cell. *Pancreas*, 2003 Nov;27(4):305-10.

[43] de Almeida JL, Jukemura J, Coelho AM, Patzina RA, Machado MC, da Cunha JE. Inhibition of cyclooxygenase 2 in experimental severe acute pancreatitis. *Clinics*, 2006 Aug;61(4):301-6.

[44] Ito Y, Lugea A, Pandol SJ, McCuskey RS. Substance P mediates cerulean induced pancreatic microcirculatory dysfunction in mice. *Pancreas,* 2007 Jan;34(1):138-43.

[45] Tsang SW, Cheng CH, Leung PS. The role of the pancreatic rennin-angiotensin system in acinar digestive enzyme secretion and in acute pancreatitis. *Regul. Pept.,* 2004 Jul 15;119(3):213-9.

[46] Sugimoto M, Takada T, Yasuda H, Nagashima I, Amano H, Yoshida M, Miura F, Uchida T, Isaka T, Toyota N, Wada K, Takagi K, Kato K. The lethal toxicity of pancreatic ascites fluid in severe acute necrotizing pancreatitis. *Hepatogastroenterology*, 2006 May-Jun;53(69):442-6.

[47] Dugernier T, Laterre PF, Reynaert MS. Ascites fluid in severe acute pancreatitis: from pathophysiology to therapy. *Acta Gastroenterol. Belg.,* 2000 Jul-Sep;63(3):264-8.

[48] Szentkereszty Z, Kerekes L, Hallay J, Czako D, Sapy P.CT guided percutaneous peripancreatic drainage: a possible therapy in acute necrotizing pancreatitis. *Hepatogastroenterology,* 2002 Nov-Dec;49(48):1696-8.

[49] Tukiainen E, Kylanpaa ML, Ebeling P, Kemppainen E, Puolakkainen P, Repo H. Leptin and adiponectin levels in acute pancreatitis. *Pancreas*, 2006 Mar;32(2):211-4.

[50] Schaffler A, Landfried K, Volk M, Furst A, Buchler C, Scholmerich J, Herfarth H. Potential of adipocytokines in predicting peripancreatic necrosis and severity in acute pancreatitis: Pilot study. *J. Gastroenterol. Hepatol.*, 2007 Mar;22(3):326-34.

[51] Testoni PA, Mariani A, Mangiavillano B, Arcidiacono PG, Di Pietro S, Masci E. Intraductal optical coherence tomography for investigating main pancreatic duct strictures. *Am. J. Gastroenterol.*, 2007 Feb;102(2):269-74.

[52] Kwon RS, Brugge WR. New advances in pancreatic imaging. *Curr. Opin. Gastroenterol,* 2005 Sep;21(5):561-7.

[53] Pamuklar E, Semelka RC. MR imaging of the pancreas. *Magn. Reson. Imaging Clin. N. Am.,* 2005 May;13(2):313-30.

[54] Rahman SH, Menon KV, Holmfield JH, McMahon MJ, Guillou JP. Serum macrophage migration inhibitory factor is an early marker of pancreatic necrosis in acute pancreatitis. *Ann. Surg.,* 2007 Feb;245(2):282-9.

[55] Riche FC, Cholley BP, Laisne MJ, Vicaut E, Panis YH, Lajeunie EJ, Boudiaf M, Valleur PD. Inflammatory cytokines, C-reactive protein, and procalcitonin as early predictors of necrosis infection in acute necrotizing pancreatitis. *Surgery,* 2003 Mar;133(3):257-62.

[56] Dambrauskas Z, Pundzius J, Barauskas G. Predicting development of infected necrosis in acute necrotizing pancreatitis. *Medicina (Kaunas),* 2006;42(6):441-9.

[57] Zorger N, Hamer OW, Feuerbach S, Borisch I. Percutaneous treatment of a patient with infected necrotizing pancreatitis. *Nat. Clin. Pract. Gastroenterol. Hepatol.*, 2005 Jan;2(1):54-7.

[58] Larson SD, Nealon WH, Evers BM. Management of gallstone pancreatitis. *Adv. Surg.*, 2006;40:265-84.

[59] Alexakis N, Neoptolemos JP. Algorithm for the diagnosis and treatment of acute biliary pancreatitis. *Scand. J. Surg.*, 2005;94(2):124-9.

[60] Nealon WH, Bawduniak J, Walser EM. Appropriate timing of cholecystectomy in patients who present with moderate to severe gallstone associated acute pancreatitis with peripancreatic fluid collections. *Ann. Surg.*, 2004 Jun;239(6):741-9; discussion 749-51.

[61] Murray B, Carter R, Imrie C, Evans S, O'Suilleabhain C. Diclofenac reduces the incidence of acute pancreatitis after endoscopic retrograde cholangiopancreatography. *Gastroenterology,* 2003 Jun;124(7):1786-91.

[62] Viedma JA, Perez-Mateo M, Agullo J, Dominguez JE, Carballo F. Inflammatory response in the early prediction of severity in human acute pancreatitis. *Gut,* 1994 Jun;35(6):822-7.

[63] Hughes CB, Henry J, Kotb M, Lobaschevsky A, Sabek O, Gaber AO. Up regulation of TNF alpha mRNA in the rat spleen following induction of acute pancreatitis. *J. Surg. Res,* 1995 Dec;59(6):687-93.

[64] Dugernier TL, Laterre PF, Wittebole X, Roeseler J, Latinne D, Reynaert MS, Pugin J. Compartmentalization of the inflammatory response during acute pancreatitis: correlation with local and systemiccomplications. *Am. J. Respir. Crit. Care Med.*, 2003 Jul 15;168(2):148-57.

[65] Samuel I, Zaheer A, Fisher RA. In vitro evidence for role of ERK, p38, and JNK in exocrine pancreatic cytokine production. *J. Gastrointest. Surg.*, 2006 Dec;10(10):1376-83.

[66] Dabrowski A. Exocrine pancreas; molecular basis for intracellular signaling, damage and protection- Polish experience. *J. Physiol. Pharmacol.*, 2003 Dec;54 Suppl 3:167-81.

[67] Chen CC, Wang SS, Lee FY, Chang FY, Lee SD. Proinflammatory cytokines in early assessment of the prognosis of acute pancreatitis. *Am. J. Gastroenterol.*, 1999 Jan;94(1):213-8.

[68] Brivet FG, Emilie D, Galanaud P. Pro- and anti-inflammatory cytokines during acute severe pancreatitis: an early and sustained response, although unpredictable of death. Parisian Study Group on Acute Pancreatitis. *Crit. Care Med.*, 1999 Apr;27(4):749-55.

[69] Zhang C, Ge CL, Guo RX, He SG. Effect of IL-4 on altered expression of complement activation regulators in rat pancreatic cells during severe acute pancreatitis. *World J Gastroenterol,* 2005 Nov 21;11(43):6770-4.

[70] Remick DG, Call DR, Ebong SJ, Newcomb DE, Nybom P, Nemzek JA, Bolgos GE. Combination immunotherapy with soluble tumor necrosis factor receptors plus interleukin 1 receptor antagonist decreases sepsis mortality. *Crit. Care Med.*, 2001 Mar;29(3):473-81.

[71] Alhonen L, Parkkinen JJ, Keinanen T, Sinervirta R, Herzig KH, Janne J. Activation of polyamine catabolism in transgenic rats induces acute pancreatitis. *Proc. Natl. Acad. Sci. USA,* 2000 Jul 18;97(15):8290-5.

[72] Wong SR, Lee KT, Kuo KK, Chen JS, Ker CG, Sheen PC. Pancreatic pseudocyst involving the spleen. *Kaohsiung J. Med. Sci,* 1998 Aug;14(8):524-7.

[73] Rypens F, Deviere J, Zalcman M, Braude P, Van de Stadt J, Struyven J, Van Gansbeke D. Splenic parenchymal complications of pancreatitis: CT findings and natural history. *J. Comput. Assist. Tomogr.,* 1997 Jan-Feb;21(1):89-93.

[74] Savastano S, Feltrin GP, Antonio T, Miotto D, Chiesura-Corona M, Castellan L. Arterial complications of pancreatitis: diagnostic and therapeutic role of radiology. *Pancreas,* 1993 Nov;8(6):687-92.

[75] Singhal D, Kakodkar R, Soin AS, Gupta S, Nundy S. Sinistral portal hypertension. A case report. *JOP,* 2006 Nov 10;7(6):670-3.

In: Pancreatitis Research Advances
Editor: William C. Langley, pp. 337-348
ISBN: 978-1-60021-883-5

Chapter XII

Acute Severe Hyperlipidemic Pancreatitis: Management, Follow Up and Prevention

A. V. Kyriakidis[*1], *M. Pyrgioti*[2] *and B. Raitsiou*[2]
[1]Surgery Department, General Hospital of Amfissa,
Fokida Greece and ICU General Hospital Athens Sismanogleion,
Athens Greece,
[2]ICU General Hospital Athens Sismanogleion,
Athens Greece

Abstract

Acute severe hyperlipidemic pancreatitis although a rare condition (accounts for a small percentage 1.3-3.8% of the cases of acute pancreatitis) is a severe condition with considerable morbidity. It seems that this condition becomes more and more often. Severe acute hyperlipidemic pancreatitis has a clinical course, which is characterized by an early toxic phase with organ dysfunction, acute pain due to triglycerides in circulation and may usually need the hospitalization in Intensive Care Unit. Plasmapheresis is an important procedure that should be done in these patients, resulting in acute regression of pain and improvement of their clinical course. Plasmapheresis is better to be applied the first 24 hours to provide maximal benefits and to be repeated as needed till triglyceride levels fall to normal levels. Afterwards these patients should be classified according to their lipidemic profile and treated with appropriate free fat diet and subsequent statin therapy. It seems important to these patients when triglyceride levels remain high during follow up although treatment, that plasmapheresis should be done prior to the attack of acute pancreatitis in order to prevent it. Acute pancreatitis involves a complex cascade of events. It is discussed that plasmapheresis should be done in order to decrease the effect of this cascade through the elimination of activated proteases, cytokines that are released by neutrophils and other inflammatory mediators.

* Author of correspondence: Alexandros V.Kyriakidis, Frouriou 95 ,GR-33100 Amfissa Fokida Greece, Tel +302265072265 ,e-mail: alkidi@hotmail.com

Hyperlipidemic Pancreatitis- Pathogenesis

Hyperlipidemia and especially severe primary and secondary triglyceridemia is a cause of acute pancreatitis. Hyperlipidemic pancreatitis accounts for 1.3-3.8% of the cases of acute pancreatitis.[1,2] It is a rare condition in contrast with the other major etiological causes, gallstones and alcohol corresponding to 80% of all cases.[2] It has considerable morbidity and is important to find the etiologic factors involved as it is treatable and recurrences can be avoided and prevented.[3] The disease presents a similar clinical pattern as the other causes of acute pancreatitis. Medical history, clinical presentation, slightly elevated amylase, elevated triglycerides and evidence of pancreatitis on ultrasound and dynamic CT establish the diagnosis of hyperlipidemic pancreatitis.

Acute pancreatitis usually develops in patients with triglyceride levels >11.3 mmol/l and associated lipidemia [4]. Hyperlipidemic pancreatitis accounts approximately up to 21% in patients suffering from familial hyperlipoproteinemia types I, IV, and V according to the classification of Frederickson and the presence of these types of hyperlipidemia indicates an increased risk.[5] High TGLs seem to play an important aggravating or promoting role for pancratitis in patients with types IV and V. A primary causal role has so far been exclusively demonstrated for the type I form. This type of hyperlipidemia includes the onset of attacks of recurrent pancreatitis in childhood and may also include hepatosplenomegaly, hyperchylomicronemia, lipemia retinalis and eruptive xanthomas. Due to its chylomicron content, type I hyperlipidemia has an adverse effect on the rheologic properties of blood and this results in acute pancreatitis possibly through ischemia and shock. Patients with type V hyperlipoproteinemia usually have no lipoprotein lipase activity with normal apoprotein C-II levels or the opposite depending on their genotype. Clearance of triglycerides carrying lipoproteins is reduced, lipoprotein lipase activity may be normal and hepatic very low-density lipoprotein may be higher. For the optimal lipoprotein lipase activity apoprotein C-II should be functional. Patients who are diabetic, obese and hyperuricemic often suffer from type V hyperlipidemia that is more common than the other types. Attacks of pancreatitis in these patients occur in adulthood and their TGLs are lower than in patients with type I. Alcohol consumption is usually combined with types IV and V hyperlipidemia. Patients with alcohol –induced pancreatitis are more frequently hyperlipidemic than patients with biliary pancreatitis. [6] There have been reported a few cases of type IIb hyperlipidemic pancreatitis. This type usually doesn't have increased chylomicrons. It is a dominant inherited genetic disorder and doesn't manifest the subjective symptom before combining vascular complication such a coronary artery disease [7].

There are patients with normal TGLs who had an attack of acute pancreatitis at least 6 months earlier. These patients had impaired clearance of serum TGLs after an oral fat tolerance test.[8] Their impaired clearance was not related to the presence of diabetes, alcohol consumption or biliary lithiasis. A TGL tolerance test has been suggested to detect patients who could suffer from an attack of acute pancreatitis after a hyperlipidemic diet and alcohol consumption. In another study the same authors state this abnormal oral fat test may be due to an impaired clearance of chylomicron remnants after an episode of acute pancreatitis. This strongly suggests that a relatively common and preexisting defect in lipid metabolism may be important for the pathogenesis of the disease [8].

Hyperlipidemic Pancreatitis and Drugs

Hypertriglyceridemia can be caused by several drugs and this can induce hyperlipidemic pancreatitis. Usually these are synthetic oestrogens (like oestrogen-progesterone contraceptives, some hypotensive drugs (non cardioselective b-blockers and thiazidic diuretics), corticosteroids, retinoids, tamoxifen, cyclosporine, enzyme inductors and iodine products.[9] Especially as far as it concerns tamoxifen it seems that the activity of lipoprotein lipase and hepatic triglyceride lipase which are enzymes of triglyceride metabolism decreased when this medicine is used for treatment. Hypertriglyceridemia is also induced when isotretinoin is used for example in cases of acne. This phenomenon is reversed with cessation of therapy [10-12].

Hyperlipidemic Pancreatitis and Pregnancy

Pancraetitis due to severe hypertriglyceridemia is a rare but serious complication of pregnancy .It occurs usually in the second and third semester and carries a high risk of death for the mother and the fetus. Except the existence of gallstones, which is considered to be the first reason for pancreatitis in pregnancy, hypertriglyceridemia should also be taken under consideration since it can be treated. During the second trimester of pregnancy plasma cholesterol rises. In addition the levels of triglycerides increase during prenancy especially in the third trimester. This is due to enhanced adipose tissue lipolysis, high flux of VLDLs into circulation and reduction of removal of TGLs due to reduction of lipoprotein lipase activity. Plasma excange seems to rapidly and safely reduce triglycerides from the circulation with drammatic and unexpectedly rapid resolution of severe pancreatitis in women with severe gestational hyperlipidemic pancreatitis. Usually in these women exists an underlying Fredrickson's type V or III hyperlipoproteinemia exacerbated by pregnancy [13-15].

Laboratory Results in Hyperlipidemic Pancreatitis

Hyperlipidemia may produce multiple spurious laboratory results, which complicate the diagnosis and management of pancreatitis. The patients who suffer from acute severe hyperlipidemic pancreatitis usually have spuriously normal amylase levels as a result of the suppression of enzymatic activity by the patient's serum due to hypertriglyceridemia. Patients with hypertriglyceridemia may have a more insidious course of disease progression than other patients with acute pancreatitis, resulting in normalization of amylase levels when they seek for medical help. Serum lipase is not masked by hypertriglyceridemia so it is used in hyperlipidemic pancreatitis and in those cases of suspected pancreatitis when amylase values are normal. Warshaw et al [16] suggested the presence of a circulating inhibitor of amylase distinct from the serum lipids, in the serum and urine of patients with acute hyperlipidemic pancreatitis. In addition hyperlipidemia can mask anemia, by high hemoglobin levels and can be presented wit hyponatremia. When TGLs are above 1000mg/dl both VLDL and chylomicrons are present. Brunzell et al demonstrated that the appearance of chylomicrons was a marker for severely impaired triglyceride metabolism showing massive accumulation of triglyceride –rich lipoprotein in serum. The presence of chylomicrons must be confirmed. One simple test is the observation of a layer of chylomicrons at the top of the plasma stored overnight at 4° in a refrigerator, the so-called refrigerator test. When patient shows hypertriglyceridemia it is practical to measure serum amylase levels using diluted serum or plasma samples [17-22].

Mechanisms of Induction of Hyperlipidemic Pancreatitis

The mechanisms by which hyperlipidemia induces acute severe pancreatitis have not yet been elucidated. One concept is the damage of acinar cells caused by free fatty acids. The hydrolysis by pancreatic lipase of triglycerides results in a high concentration of free fatty acids, which cause an inflammatory reaction in the pancreas. The presence of pancreatic phospholipase, lipoprotein phospholipids and cytotoxic lysolecithins enhances this procedure. The pancreatic enzymes are activated, released and their passage into the interstitial region of the pancreatic tissue results in autodigestion and consequent morphological damage. Another mechanism suspected is that trypsinogen could be activated by acidosis due to the presence of fatty acids, or the fatty acids may disturb the microcirculation of the pancreas via detrimental effects on the vessel endothelium [23, 24].

Clinical Course

The clinical course of hyperlipidemic pancreatitis is not different from pancreatitis of other causes. [6] The clinical course consists of an early toxic phase with distant organ dysfunction of various degrees, lasting approximately 2 weeks and a second phase with local and regional complications. Signs of sepsis could appear on day 3 to day 21-17. [25,26] When necrotic tissue is infected early, the two phases are often superimposed. [27] Around 80% of deaths from acute pancreatitis are caused by septic complications and it is often difficult to seperate systematic inflammatory response syndrome and sepsis in patients with severe acute pancreatitis [25].

Clinical Profile

The clinical profile of a patient with hyperlipidemic pancreatitis includes impaired lipid levels combined with other risk factors such as diabetes, alcohol or drugs.[5] Acute pancreatitis secondary to hyperlipidemia is characterized by three manifestations. The first is poorly controlled diabetes with a history of hypertriglyceridemia. The second is alcohol-associated pancreatitis with hypertriglyceridemia or lactescent serum on admission. The third type of pancreatitis occurs in the non- diabetic, non-obese patient with drug- or diet-induced hypertriglyceridemia (15-20%) [28].

Treatment

Treatment in patients with severe hyperlipidemic pancreatitis in the acute phase does not differ from acute pancreatitis of other causes. This includes intravenous aggressive fluid replacement that is essential due to third space loses. Pain management is essential. Since the administration of opiates has been associated with spasm of the sphincter of Oddi and their use is questioned, meperidine was used for the analgesia of the patients. Although theoretically epidural anesthesia may be effective cerebral dysfunction and /or coagulation abnormalities are obstacles for the insertion of the epidural catheter. Oxygen supplementation and restoration of fluid and electrolyte balance could also be essential. Depending on initial assessment observation of the patient could be in the intensive care unit or in the medical unit. Noninvasive or invasive ventilation is applied when needed and long-term mechanical ventilation may require tracheostomy. If the shock persists despite the volume replacement then vasoconstrictors are used. All the patients should be under continous respiratory and cardiovascular monitoring [28, 29].

Insulin and Heparin

The main characteristic for hyperlipidemic pancreatitis treatment is the reduction of plasma triglycerides during the acute phase as well as after the episode to reduce recurrences. In many cases the administration of heparin and /or insulin is used as an efficient alternative to reduce triglyceride levels. Insulin promotes tissue uptake of lipids, it enhances lipoprotein lipase activity in the muscle and the adipose tissue. It is observed that insulin in insulin dependent diabetic patients corrects hypertriglyceridemia. Short acting insulin lowers triglyceride levels and so reduces the risk of acute pancreatitis. There has been disaggreement about the role of insulin in the regulation of VLDL triglyceride secretion. Some authors state that it may accumulate secretion and others that it may be inhibitory or without effect. Insulin seems to inhibit VLDL triglyceride secretion and favors the accumulation of TGL within the cells. There is also an inhibitory effect of insulin on VLDL triglyceride secretion by liver cells. The reduction in serum TGL when insulin is administered to patients with either type I or type II diabetes and primary hypertriglyceridemia is consisted with an inhibitory effect of insulin on TGL secretion. A major contribution to this effect is the reduction in serum fatty acid levels or effects on lipoprotein lipase levels. Heparin is an effective lipase-releasing agent. It releases lipoprotein lipase from tissues and this accelerates the removal of TGLs from the blood and promotes the clearing of lipemia.

Heparin and insulin stimulate lipoprotein lipase activity and accelerate chylomicron degradation [30-33]. It could also contribute to the decrease of serum triglyceride level. Besides this effect on blood triglyceride, it could also improve microcirculation and prevent activation of neutrophils activity [34]. Polymorphonuclear cells (PMN) could play an important role in the deterioration of severe acute pancreatitis, especially release of elastase (PMNE), which would lead to persistent pancreatic necrosis and acute lung injury [35].

Antihyperlipidemic Drugs and Diet

Antihyperlipidemic medications are used to maintain relatively low TGLs like fluvastatin or lipanthyl. The dietary fat constriction is extremely important in patients with hyperlipidemic pancreatitis. In acute phase of hyperlipidemic pancreatitis as in pancreatitis of other causes, withdrawal of enteral nutrition per os is the standard measure because it prevents the stimulation of pancreatic secretions. The nutritional support is important because failure to achieve a positive nitrogen balance is associated with an increased mortality in patients with SAP. Total parental nutrition is essential but in cases of hyperlipidemic pancreatitis it is advisable to omit high concentrations of glucose and lipid emulsions. [36-38] The rapid progression to enteral feeding using a nasojejunal tube has proven both possible and effective, because enteral feeding helps to maintain the gut mucosal barrier and even decrease the infective complications of the pancreatitis. Although enteral feeding according to studies seems to be important, it is avoided because enteral nutrition contains lipids in different amounts. The use of parenteral feeding in cases of severe hyperlipidemic pancreatitis is extremely essential and importat at least until triglycerides normalize. [39] Parenteral nutrition offers a safe and flexible treatment option by providing pancreatic rest and controlling serum triglycerides concentrations while maintaining nutrirional support.

Antibiotic Therapy

Infection is considered to be the single and most important risk factor for mortality in patients with severe acute hyperlipidemic pancreatitis as in acute pancreatitis generally. The role of pre-emptive antibiotic treatment has attracted considerable interest. Questions include the use of antibiotics in the management of these patients, the selection of patients most likely to benefit, the optimal choice and timing, fungal infection and prophylaxis [40] Usually prophylactic antibiotic therapy is given due to the severity of such a condition and the risk of infection. The recommended treatment is quinolone with metronidazole or monotherapy imipranem/cilastatin for at least 2 weeks. There are also used cephalosporins of 2nd and 3rd generation [41-43].

Plasmapheresis

Experience with plasmapheresis, lipid apheresis and extracorporeal lipid elimination is limited in patients with hyperlipidemic pancreatitis. [5] Plasmapheresis is an established treatment for familial hypercholesterolemia. In non-selective plasmapheresis, the patient's plasma is replaced by salt-free human albumin or fresh –frozen plasma. TGLs are drammatically reduced and the risk of pancreatitis is decreased [44]. Plasmapheresis also seems to change cytokine –anticytokine patterns since cytokines and their endogenous antagonists are released from inflammatory cells during acute pancreatitis. [45] The benefit of plasmapheresis might also relate to the direct elimination of excessive plasma proteases associated with acute pancreatitis. This procedure is a symptomatic therapy since it does not eliminate the source of pathogenic factors. [4] It reduces TGL within a few hours but also decreases the accompanying plasma hyperviscosity. However prompt relief of abdominal pain is obtained. In a study by Piolot et al [46], the regular use of plasmapheresis in patients with severe hypertriglyceridemia and reccurence acute pancreatitis prevented further episodes of pancreatitis. Another study stated that plasma exchange should be performed for the treatment of hypertriglyceridemic necrotizing pancreatitis immediately after its onset. Yen et al showed in 13 of 17 hypertriglyceremic patients with hyperlipidemic acute pancreatitis that plasmapheresis is aneffective method to clear lipids and enzymes from plasma in a single session. Lenertz et al found that rapidly initiated plasmapheresis effectively reduced TG and cholesterol levels in five patients with hyperlipidemic pancreatitis [47-51].

As a formalized therapeutic guideline for hyperlipidemic severe acute pancreatitis by Mao et al there is a reference in Penta association therapy which seems to be effective and consists of blood purification, antihyperlipidemic agents, low molecular weight heparin, insulin and topical application of Pixiao (a traditional Chinese medicine) over the whole abdomen [52].

In 2000, the Pancreatic Disease Therapy Center considered a therapeutic strategy aiming at hyperlipidemic severe acute pancreatitis that was based on the concepts that hyper-triglyceride, fatty acid and inflammatory mediators were the pathological mechanism of deterioration of hyperlipidemic severe acute pancreatitis. Principles of the strategy included rapid lowering serum triglyceride, blocking of induction pancreatic damage by pro-inflammatory mediators, preventing recurrence by the use of antihyperlipidemic agents, promoting self- absorption of pancreatic pseudocyst. These measures are widely used but still there are a 15% of patients that cannot be cured [52,53].

Follow Up

During their stay the patients should be classified according to their lipidemic profil Plasmapheresis is applied the first 24 hours to provide maximal benefits and when triglycerides remain at high levels patients undergo plasmapheresis and the subsequent days so as to lower triglyceride levels. So the next days during hospitalization patients continue with symptomatic treatment, plasmapheresis and free fat parenteral nutrition. When acute phase is over, patients continue with free fat enteral nutrition and antihyperlipidemic medication like fluvastatinor lipanthyl or gemfibrozil and maintain the target TGL level less than 1000mg/dl. Insulin and heparin are stopped because intermittent insulin therapy fails in maintaining TGLlevel below 1000mg/dl. It is possible that insulin –induced enhancement of LPL activity is a transient phenomenon that wears off after several weeks of treatment. The need for injection, potential hypoglycemic effect and variation of the TGL level during the long-term use of insulin are factors against long-term insulin therapy. Other concerns for long-term use of insulin include the adverse effect of hyperinsulinemia on VLDL, LDL, and HDL levels [54, 39].

Prevention

For the prevention of other episodes of hyperlipidemic pancreatitis patients need to institute therapeutic life changes, like cessation of alcohol, weight loss, exercise and diet including elimination of sugar-sweetened beverages. Total fat intake should be restricted. Restricting simple carbohydrates and increasing dietary fiber are important adjuncts that can lower TGLs substantially. Omega 3 fatty acids in large amounts (10 or more g/day) lower TGL 40% or more. Exercise can have a drammatic impact on TGL levels and may increase HDL-c slightly. Secondary causes of hypertriglyceridemia should be treated and corrected like poorly controlled diabetes mellitus, nephrotic syndrome, alcoholism, hypothyroidism and medications such as protease inhibitors, corticosteroids, estrogens, b-blockers and thiazide diuretics. TGL levels respond well to dietary control and increased exercise. This should be the first line nonparmacological therapy. Some suggested that drugs to lower TGL should be used conservatively and are only indicated when TGL> 4.5mmol/l (>400mg/dl) after dietary methods have failed or if other risk factors are present. Nicotinic acid lower TGL directly by inhibiting adipose tissue lipases, thus reducing substrate for availability for VLDL-C synthesis. Reductions of 20-40% have been seen. Fibrates have a higher potency reucing TGL levels by 20-25%. Statins reuce TGLlevels indirectly by enhancing the expression of LDL-C receptors in the liver and by inhibiting VLDL-C and LDL-C synthesis via the reduction of apo B. Omega 3 and fish oil supplements could also be used [55, 56]. Plasmapheresis could also be used as a procedure for prevention of pancreatitis by elimination of TGLs when other measures have failed but still remais unclear because experience is limited.

It should be reffered that are studies that use plasmapheresis in acute severe necrotic pancreatitis of other origin too. Acute pancreatitis involves a complex cascade of events. Plasmapheresis seems to decrease the effect of this cascade through elimination of activated proteases, cytokines that are released by neutrophils and other inflammatory mediators. Some authors refer that after the performance of plasmapheresis in patients with acute severe necrotic pancreatitis there was reduction of endotoxenemia and facilitates the effectiveness of treatment. Blood purification methods have been used for treatment of organ failure in patients with severe pancreatitis [57, 58, 59, 60].

In conclusion hyperlipidemic pancreatitis secondary to hypertriglyceridemia has been apparently increased in recent years and it has high mortality in its severe form. Thus it is essential its treatment and prevention. Efforts have been made by the pancreatic disease specialists for a formalized therapeutic guideline, which includes supportive treatment, free fat nutrition, antiyperlipidemic drugs insulin and heparin. Substantial role seems to have palsmapheresis for the treatment but also the prevention of recurrences.

References

[1] Toskes P. Hyperlipidemic Pancreatitis. *Gastr. Clin. N. Am.* 1990;19:783-791.

[2] Karne S, Golerick F: Etiopathogenesis of acute pancreatitis. *Surg. Clin. North Am.* 1999;79;699-709.

[3] M.W. Büchler, W. Uhl, P. Malfertheiner, M.G. Sarr. *Diseases of the Pancreas*. Edition 2004 S.Karger AG. pp. 1-58.

[4] Yeh JH, Chen JH, ChiuHC; Plasmapheresis for hyperlipidemic pancreatitis. *J. Clin. Apheresis.* 2003;18:181-185.

[5] Yadav D, Pitchumoni CS: Issues in hyperlipidemic pancreatitis. *J. Clin. Gastroenterol.* 2003; 26:54-62.

[6] Delakidis S, Elezoglou A: Hypercalcemia, hyperlipidemia andd rheumatic diseases: Uncommon causes inducing acute pancreatitis. *Ann. Gastroenterol.* 2000; 13:102-112.

[7] Kim BK, Kim MJ, Chang WC, Yoo KH, Shin YG, Chung CH. Recurrent acute pancreatitis in a patient withtype Iib hyperlipoproteinemia: a case report and review of the literature inKorea. *Yonsei Msd. J.* 2006 Feb28;47(1):144-7.

[8] Rollan A, Guzman S, Pimentel F et al.: Catabolism of chylomicron remnants in patients with previous acute pancreatitis.Gastroenterology 1990;98(6) :1650-1653.

[9] Stone N: Secondary causes of hyperlipidemia. *Med. Clin. North Am.* 1994;78(1):117-141.

[10] Mc Arthur KE: Drug-iduced pancreatitis. *Aliment Pharmacol. Ther.* 1996; 10:23-28.

[11] Wilmink T, Frick T: Drug –induced pancreatitis. *Drug safety* 1996 6/14 406-423.

[12] Frick TW, Speiser DE, Bimmler D.et al.: Druginduced pancreatitis: Further criticism. *Dig. Dis.* 1993;11:113-132.

[13] Roberts J: Hyperlipidemic gestational pancreatitis. *Gastroenterology* 1993; 104:1560-1662.

[14] Majlis S, Anguita T, Weishaupt R, Socias M.Plasmapheresis in acute pancreatitis secondary to familial hyperlipidemia in a pregnant woman. Rev. Med. Chil. 1989 Nov; 117(11):1275-8.

[15] SaravananP, Blumenthal S, Anderson C, Stein R, Berkelhammer C.Plasma exchange for drammatic gestational hyperlipidemic pancreatitis. *J. Clin. Gastroenterol.* 1996 Jun;22 (4):295-8.

[16] Warshaw AL, Bellini CA, Lesser PB: Inhibition of serum and urine amylase activity in pancreatitis with hyperlipemia. *Ann. Surg.* 1975; 182:72-75.

[17] Okenberg K., Lee M: Spuriously normal amylase levels in a patient with acute pancreatitis secondary to hypertriglyceridemia. *J. Am. Board Fam. Pract.* 1999;12:68-70.

[18] Wong EC, Butch AW, Rosenblum JL: The clinical, chemistry, laboratory and acute pancreatitis. *Clin. Chem.* 1993;39:234-243.

[19] Brunzell JD, Schrott HG.the interaction of familial and secondary causes of hypertriglyceridemia; role in pancreatitis. *Trans. Assoc. Am. Physicians.* 1973;86:245-254.

[20] Brunzell JD, Bierman EL.Chylomicronemia syndrome.Interaction of genetic and aquired hypertriglyceridemia. *Med. Clin. North Am.* 1982;66:455-468.

[21] Lesser PB, Warshaw AL Diagnosis of pancreatitis masked by hyperlipemia. *Ann. Int. Med.* 1975;82:795-798.

[22] Chait A, Brunzell JD Chylomicronemia syndrome. *Adv. Intern. Med.* 1992;37:249-273.

[23] Hofbauer B, Daluja A, Learch M:Early trypsinogen activation in acute pancreatitis. *Am. J. Physiol.* 1998;275:352-362.

[24] Mayer J, Rai B, Shoenberg M: Mechanism and role of trypsinogen activation in acute pancreatitis. *Hepatogastroenterology* 1999;46:2757-2763.

[25] Beger HG, Rau B, Mayer J, Pralle U: Natural course of acute pancreatitis. *World journal. surg.* 1997;21:130-135.

[26] Mc Kay CJ, Butter A; Natural history of organ failure in acute pancreatitis. *Pancreatology* 2003;3:111-114.

[27] Dugernier T, Reynaert M, Laterre PF: Early multi system organ failure associated with acute pancreatitis :A plea for a conservative therapeutic strategy. *Acta gastroenterol. Belg.* 2003;66:177-183

[28] Nathens AB, Curtis JR, Beale RJ et al.Management of the critically ill patient with severe acute pancreatitis. *Crit. Care Mer.* 2004;32:2524-2536.

[29] Bernhardt A, Kortgen A, Niesel H, Goertz A: using epidural anesthesia in patients with acute pancreatitis- prospective study of 121 patients. *Anaethesiol rearum*. 2002;27:16.

[30] Berger Z, Quera R, Poniachik J, Oksenberg D, Guerrero J. Heparin and insulin treatment of acute pancreatitis caused by hypertriglyceridemia. Experience of 5 cases. *Rev. Med. Chil.* 2001; 129: 1373-1378.

[31] Alazoglu H, Cindonik M, Karakan T, Sellatin U Heparin and Insulin in the treatment of hypertriglyceridemia –induced severe acute pancreatiis. *Digestive Diseases and Sciences* Vol 51, No 5 May 206 :931-933.

[32] Reaven G.M., R.L.Lemer, M.P. Stem, JW Farguliar role of insulin inendogeous hypertriglyceridemia. 1967 J Clin Invest 46:1756-1767.

[33] Steiner G Insulin regulation of triglyceride metabolism. *Atheroscler. Rev.* 1991;22:27-32.

[34] Capecchi PL, Ceccatelli L, Laghi Pasini F, Di Perri T. Inhibition of neutrophil function in vitro by heparan sulfate. *Int. J. Tissue React.* 1993; 15: 71-76.

[35] Mao EQ, Han TQ, Tang YQ, Zhang SD, Zhang SD. Polymorphonuclear elastase is the major causative factor in acute lung injury complicating severe acute pancreatitis in rats. *Zhonghua Xiaohua Zazhi* 1998; 18: 207-209.

[36] O'Keefe SJ , Lee RB, Anderson FP, Gennings C, Abou –AssiS, Clore J, Heuman D, Chey W. Physiological effects of entera and parenteral feeding on pancreatobiliary secretion in humans. *Am. Physiol.* 2003;284:627-636.

[37] Imre CW, Carter CR, McKay CJ. E.Enteral and Parenteral nutrition in acute pancreatitis. *Best Pract. Res. Clin. Gastroenterol.* 2002;16:391-397.

[38] Kalfarentzos F, Kehagias J, Mead N, Kokkinis K, Gogos CA. Enteral nutrition is superior to parental nutrition in severe acute pancreatitis ;results of a randomized prospective trial. *Br. J. Surg.* 1997;84:1665-1669.

[39] Kyriakidis A.V, Karydakis P. Neofytou N, Pyrgioti M, Vasilakakis D, Digenis P, Antsaklis G: Plasmapheresis in the management of acute severe hyperlipidemic pancreatitis: report of five cases. *Pancreatology* 2005;5:201-204.

[40] Garg PK, Khannas S, Bohidar NP, Kapil a, Tandon RK. Incidence, spectrum and antibiotic sensitivity pattern of bacterial infections among patients with acute pancreatitis. *J. Gastroenterol. Hepatol.* 2001;16:1055-1059.

[41] Gloor B,Muller CA, WorniM, Stahel PF, Redaellic , Uhl W, Buchler MW; pancreatic infection in severe pancreatitis. The role of fungus and multiresistant organisms. *Arch. Surg.* 2001;136:592-596.

[42] Golub R, Siddigi F, Pohl D: Role of antibiotics in acute pancreatitis. A metaanalysis. J *Gastrointest. Surg.* 1998;2:496-503.

[43] Sharma VK, Howden CW; Prophylactic antibiotic administration reduces sepsis and mortality in acute necrotizing pancreatitis; a meta –analysis. *Pancreas* 2001;22:28-31.

[44] Keller C: LDL –apheresis: Results of longterm treatment and vascular outcome. *Atherosclerosis* 1991;86:1-8.

[45] Schomerlich J: Interleukins in acute pancreatitis. *Scand. J. Gastroenterol. Suppl.* 1996;219:37-42.

[46] Piolot A, Nadler F, Cavallero E, Coquard JL, Jacotot B: Prevention of recurrent acute pancreatitis in patients with severe hypertriglyceridemia: Value of regular plasmapheresis. *Pancreas* 1996;13:96-99.

[47] Furuya T, Komatsu M, Takahashi K,et al.:Plasma exchange for hypertriglyceridemic acute necrotizing pancreatitis: Report of two cases. *Ther. Apheresis* 2002;6:454.

[48] Kyriakidis A.V. , Raitsiou B, Sakagianni A, Harisopoulou V, Pyrgioti M, Panagopoulou A, Vasilakis N, Lambropoulos S Management of acute severe hyperlipidemic pancreatitis. *Digestion* 2006 ;73(4) 205-268.

[49] Yeh JH, Chen JH, Chiu HC Plasmapheresis for hyperlipidemic pancreatitis. *J. clin. Apher.* 2003;18(4):181-5.

[50] Lennertz A, Parhofer K, Samtleben W, Bosch T. Therapeutic plasma exchange in patients with chylomicronemia syndrome complicated by acute pancreatitis. *Ther. Apher.* 1999;3:227-233.

[51] GC Nikou, CH Toubanakis, G Poulakou, EJ Giamarellou –Bourboulis, D Stamatakis , N.Katsilambros. Lipapheresis in the management of hyperlipidemic pancreatitis:Our experience in a series of 7 patients. *Annals of Gastroenterology* 2005;18(3):336-340.

[52] En-Qiang Mao, Yao-Qing Tang, Sheng-Dao Zhang :Formalized therapeutic guideline for hyperlipidemic severe acute pancreatitis. *World J. Gastroenterol.* 2003 November ;9(11):2622-2626.

[53] Gronroos JM, Nylamo EI. Mortality in acute pancreatitis in Turku University Central Hospital 1971-1995. *Hepatogastroenterology* 1999; 46: 2572-2574.

[54] Athyros VG, Giouleme OI, Nikolaidis NL et al Long term follow up of patients with acute hyperlipidemia induced pancreatitis. *J. Clin. Gastroenterol.* 2002;34:472-475.

[55] Pearson TA, Laurora I, Chiu H, Katonek S.The lipid treatment assessment projsct (L-TAP) *Arch. Intern. Med.* 2000;160:459-67.

[56] Haffner SM: Management of dyslipidemia in adults with diabetes. *Diabetes care* 1998;21:160-7886.

[57] Romanichishen AF, Chalenko VV, Dubchenko SG, Pastukhova NK , Zoikov AG Extracorporeal hemocorrection in acute pancreatitis. *Vest. Khir. Im. I. Igrek.* 2000;159(4)70-3.

[58] Pupelis G, Austrums E, Snippe K Blood purification methods for the treatment of organ failure in patients with severe pancreatitis. *Zentralbl. Chir*. 2001 Oct;126(10):780-4.

[59] Papagoras D, Giamarellos-Bourboulis EJ, Kanara M, Douridas G,Paraskevopoulos I, Antzaklis G, Karayannacos P, Giamarellou H. Pancreatic concentrations of cefepime in experimental necrotizing pancreatitis. *J. Chemother*. 2003 Feb;15(1):43-6.

[60] Terekhov NT, Stankov AV Plasmapheresis i the complex tratment of acute pancreatitis. *Klin. Khir*. 1989;(11):38-40.

In: Pancreatitis Research Advances
Editor: William C. Langley, pp. 349-360

ISBN: 978-1-60021-883-5

Chapter XIII

Critical Role of Inflammatory Mediators in Acute Pancreatitis

Madhav Bhatia*
Department of Pharmacology, National University of Singapore, Singapore.

Abstract

Acute pancreatitis is a common clinical condition. The exact mechanisms by which diverse etiological factors induce an attack are still unclear but once the disease process is initiated common inflammatory and repair pathways are invoked. Acute pancreatitis is an inflammatory disorder, and inflammation not only affects the pathogenesis but also the course of the disease. Acinar cell injury early in acute pancreatitis leads to a local inflammatory reaction; if marked this leads to a systemic inflammatory response syndrome (SIRS). An excessive SIRS in acute pancreatitis leads to distant organ damage and multiple organ dysfunction syndrome (MODS), which is the primary cause of morbidity and mortality in this condition. Recent studies by us and other investigators have established the critical role played by inflammatory mediators such as TNF-α, IL-1β, IL-6, IL-8, CINC/GRO-α, MCP-1, PAF, IL-10, CD40L, C5a, ICAM-1, MIP1-α, RANTES, substance P, and hydrogen sulfide in acute pancreatitis and the resultant MODS. This chapter intends to present an overview of the role of inflammatory mediators in the pathogenesis of acute pancreatitis and associated MODS.

Introduction

Acute pancreatitis (AP) is a common clinical condition with potentially devastating consequences. It is one of the most frequent causes of acute inflammatory states in the

* Address for correspondence: Madhav Bhatia, Ph.D. Department of Pharmacology, National University of Singapore, Yong Loo Lin School of Medicine, Centre for life Sciences, 28 Medical Drive, Singapore 117456; Tel. (65)-6516-8256; Fax. (65)- 6775-7674; email. mbhatia@nus.edu.sg

abdomen. About 40 cases of AP per 100,000 adults are reported every year [1]. At present, there is no treatment against severe acute pancreatitis, other than supportive critical care [2]. The main etiological factors of AP are biliary disease leading to ductal obstruction and excessive alcohol consumption. Other minor factors include hyperlipidemia, viral infection, drugs, and hypercalcemia [3]. The incidence of the disease differs geographically; however, the death rate of the disease has remained high at 8-13 % over the past 20 years. The severity of AP can vary from mild to severe in different cases. Majority of the patients (80 %) suffer mild pancreatitis, which is self-limiting and recover in few days. The other 20 % may require intensive care treatment for haemorrhagic and necrotic lesions of the pancreas with a mortality rate of 40 %. High incidence of death is due to the systemic inflammatory response syndrome (SIRS) leading to multiple organ failure [1-3].

An important characteristic feature of acute pancreatitis is the pancreatic inflammation with excessive recruitment of leukocytes. Inflammatory mediators appear to play a critical role in the pathogenesis of pancreatitis and more so of the subsequent inflammatory response [1-4]. Inflammatory mediators believed to participate in the pathophysiology of this condition include: Tumor necrosis factor-α (TNF-α), Interleukin-1β (IL-1β), Interleukin-6 (IL-6), platelet activating factor (PAF), intercellular adhesion molecule-1 (ICAM-1), interleukin-8 (IL-8), growth related oncogene-α/cytokine-induced neutrophil chemoattractant (GRO-α/CINC), monocyte chemoattractant protein-1 (MCP-1), interleukin 10 (IL-10), complement component C5a, substance P, hydrogen sulfide (H_2S), and neutral endopeptidase (NEP) [1-5].

TNF-α and IL-1β

Tumor necrosis factor-α (TNF-α) and interleukin-1β (IL-1β) are derived predominantly from activated macrophages and act via specific cell membrane bound receptors. Levels of both these pro-inflammatory mediators are elevated upon the onset and during the progress of acute pancreatitis [6, 7]. Naturally occurring soluble TNF receptors (sTNFR) and interleukin-1 receptor antagonist (IL-1ra), by neutralizing the activity of TNF-α and IL-1β respectively, act as anti-inflammatory mediators [6]. Intrapancreatic TNF-α and IL-1β are detectable one hour following induction of acute pancreatitis and levels increase rapidly over the following six hours [6, 7]. Both TNF-α and IL-1β are thought to play an important role in acute pancreatitis.

Combined infusions of TNF-α and IL-1β have synergistic pro-inflammatory effects. Using knockout mice deficient in IL-1 type 1 receptors, TNF type 1 receptors, or both, it has been shown that IL-1β and TNF-α make an equivalent contribution to the severity of an attack. Preventing the activity of both cytokines concurrently has no additional effect on the degree of pancreatitis but does attenuate the systemic stress response and is associated with an additional but modest decrease in mortality [7]. Numerous investigators have employed specific antagonists to TNF-α or IL-1β in experimental models of acute pancreatitis. Examples of this approach include the use of an anti-TNF-α antibody, soluble type 1 TNF receptor and IL-1ra [7, 8]. Blockade of the IL-1 receptor before or soon after induction of pancreatitis is associated with decreased severity of pancreatitis and reduced intrinsic pancreatic damage. Also, neutralization of TNF-α with a polyclonal antibody significantly reduces the severity of acute pancreatitis in the rats [8].

IL-6

Interleukin 6 (IL-6) is produced by a wide range of cells including monocytes/macrophages, endothelial cells, fibroblasts and smooth muscle cells in response to stimulation by endotoxin, IL-1β and TNF-α [1-3]. IL-6 levels are raised in patients with acute pancreatitis and correlate with disease severity [9]. Transgenic mice overexpressing IL-6 are more susceptible to acute pancreatitis, and in these mice a monoclonal anti-IL-6 antibody has a protective effect [10].

IL-10

Interleukin-10 (IL-10) is an anti-inflammatory cytokine. Its plasma levels are elevated in animal models of endotoxemia and inhibit the release of pro-inflammatory cytokines (i.e. IL-1β, IL-6 and TNF-α) from monocytes/macrophages thus preventing subsequent tissue damage. IL-10 also stimulates production of the naturally occurring IL-1 receptor antagonist (IL-1ra) and release of the soluble p75 TNF receptor [11].

IL-10 it believed to have a protective role in acute pancreatitis. In normal subjects IL-10 is not measurable in serum, but in acute pancreatitis levels are markedly raised within the first 24 hours of an attack followed by a steady decline over the following few days Administration of IL-10 in experimental acute pancreatitis reduces the local inflammatory response and subsequent mortality [12]. In a study, prophylactic administration of IL-10 to patients undergoing therapeutic endoscopic retrograde cholangiopancreatography (ERCP) reduced the incidence of pancreatitis (pain and hyperamylasemia) from 24.4 % to 6.8 %. Only two patients had severe acute pancreatitis, i.e. developed organ failure or had an in patient stay greater than ten days. Therefore it is at present uncertain if IL-10 will reduce the severity of acute pancreatitis in patients with severe disease form other causes [13].

PAF

Platelet activating factor (PAF) is a low molecular weight phospholipid, which acts via specific cell surface receptors that have been identified on numerous cells and tissues including platelets, leukocytes and endothelial cells [1-3]. Isolated pancreatic acini have been reported to synthesize PAF and pancreatic tissue concentrations rise during the course of an attack. In animal models intra-peritoneal or intravascular injection can bring about or increase the severity of acute pancreatitis [14]. Blood and pulmonary tissue levels also rise co-ordinately indicating that PAF is a key mediator of the systemic inflammatory response [14].

Specific PAF antagonists have been evaluated in experimental models with varying success. Prophylactic treatment with these antagonists causes a reduction in local inflammation and acinar cell necrosis, in several experimental models of acute pancreatitis [15, 16]. In a recent study using a model of severe acute pancreatitis induced by infusion of bile salts into the pancreatic duct in combination with caerulein administered intravascularly, treatment with lexipafant, a PAF antagonist had no effect on survival or local inflammation [16].

PAF is inactivated by the enzyme platelet activating factor acetylhydrolase (PAF-AH). In severe acute pancreatitis induced by the ligation of combined biliopancreatic duct in the opossum, there was significant protection against acute pancreatitis and associated lung injury by treatment with PAF-AH [17].

Despite promising results from a phase II clinical study, in a large multicenter phase III study lexipafant failed to reduce organ failure or mortality in severe acute pancreatitis [18]. Further development of lexipafant as a therapy for acute pancreatitis has since been abandoned [19]. It is noteworthy that some experimental studies had also shown lack of effect of lexipafant. Nevertheless, large multicenter studies such as these demonstrate that it is possible to investigate the potential of anti-inflammatory mediator therapy in the clinic.

CD40L

CD40, a member of the tumor necrosis factor (TNF) receptor family, is expressed on the membrane of a variety of cells, including B-lymphocytes, monocytes, dendritic cells, and biliary epithelial cells. CD40 binds to its ligand CD40L (also referred to as CD154) to mediate major immunoregulatory signals. Although CD40L expression was previously thought to be restricted to activated T lymphocytes, this cell surface protein has been detected in various cell types, including macrophages, smooth muscle and endothelial cells. In pancreatic tissue from control mice and caerulein-treated mice, the expression of both CD40 and CD40L was detected on the acinar cell surface. Interestingly, pancreatitis and pancreatitis-associated lung injury were markedly decreased in mice deficient in CD40L compared with wild-type mice, suggesting an important pro-inflammatory role of CD40L in the pathogenesis of acute pancreatitis and associated lung injury [20].

ICAM-1

Intercellular adhesion molecule-1 (ICAM-1; CD54) is an inducible protein expressed on the surface of endothelial cells. Under physiological conditions, ICAM-1 is not constitutively expressed or is expressed at low levels in most tissues; during inflammation its levels are upregulated [1-3]. It has recently been reported that ICAM-1 is present on rat pancreatic acinar cells, is upregulated by caerulein and mediates direct binding of neutrophils to acinar cells [21]. ICAM-1 was also upregulated in pancreas of rats with experimental pancreatitis induced by supramaximal doses of caerulein [21]. ICAM-1 knockout mice are protected against acute pancreatitis and associated lung injury, pointing to an important role for ICAM-1 in the development of pancreatitis and subsequent organ damage [22]. The protective effect of ICAM-1 gene deletion does not differ from that seen following neutrophil depletion in the choline-deficient, ethionine supplemented (CDE) diet model of acute pancreatitis [23]. Indeed neutrophil depletion in ICAM-1 knockout mice affords no additional protection [22]. Blocking ICAM 1 has been shown to have a protective effect against local and systemic organ damage in different experimental models of acute pancreatitis [24]. These results suggest that ICAM-1 deficiency interferes with neutrophil recruitment and supports the concept of a therapeutic strategy directed against neutrophil migration and activation.

C5a

C5a is a potent anaphylatoxin and chemoattractant that is generated from C5 as part of both the classic and alternate pathways of complement activation. C5a, acting via C5aR on target cells, is generally believed to serve as a "complete" proinflammatory mediator. We evaluated the role of C5a in a model of pancreatitis and systemic injury after pancreatitis using two independent but complementary approaches. In the first, mice that do not express C5aR were used, whereas in the second set of experiments, mice that do not express C5 were employed. The results of both studies were similar, i.e., interruption of C5a action either by deletion of its receptor or by deletion of its parent protein resulted in a worsening of pancreatitis. The severity of pancreatitis-associated lung injury was also increased when C5a action was rendered inoperative [25].

Chemokines

Leukocyte chemotaxis in acute pancreatitis is a well-orchestrated process that involves a number of proteins, including pro-inflammatory cytokines, adhesion molecules, matrix metalloproteinases and the large cytokine subfamily of chemotactic cytokines - the chemokines [1-3]. Numerous chemokines have now been identified as inflammatory mediators with potent leukocyte activating properties and many of them have been shown to be involved in the patho-physiological process of experimental acute pancreatitis.

Chemokines have been divided into four major sub-groups: C, CC, CXC and CX_3C, on the basis of the position and spacing of N-terminal cysteine residues [1-3]. Historically, CC chemokines (such as MCP-1, MIP-1α, RANTES) have been believed to act principally upon monocytes, and CXC chemokines which contain a three amino acid ELR motif at the amino terminal end (such as IL-8, GRO-α, ENA-78) are believed to act upon neutrophils. Recent work by us, as well as other investigators, has, however, shown that these narrow definitions are no longer valid [26-28].

Mob1, a CXC rat chemokine, was shown to be elevated within one hour of induction of acute pancreatitis in the rat by caerulein hyperstimulation [29]. We have recently shown that pancreatic acinar cells produce the CC chemokine MCP-1 and that treatment with supramaximally stimulating doses of caerulein causes an upregulation of MCP-1 production. Caerulein-induced stimulation of chemokine production is regulated via NF-κB and Ca^{2+} [4].

Levels of IL-8, GRO-α, and ENA-78 (epithelial-derived neutrophil-activating peptide 78) are raised in clinical acute pancreatitis and are predictors of disease severity [30,31]. The chemokines are an ideal target for anti-inflammatory therapy.

The best characterized of the rat CXC chemokines is CINC (cytokine-induced neutrophil chemoattractant), the homologue of the human chemokine GRO-α (growth related oncogene-α). Circulating levels of CINC are raised in experimental acute pancreatitis [32] and treatment with neutralizing antibody against CINC protects rats against acute pancreatitis-associated lung injury [33]. Furthermore, treatment with antileukinate, a hexapeptide antagonist of the CXCR2 chemokine receptor, protects mice against acute pancreatitis and associated lung injury [34]. We have also shown that in knockout mice, the deletion of the MIP-1α/ RANTES receptor CCR1 decreased the pulmonary damage seen in severe acute pancreatitis. There was little protection against pancreatic damage [26]. Similarly, treatment with Met-RANTES, a CCR1 antagonist, protected mice against acute pancreatitis-associated lung injury, with little protection against pancreatic damage [28]. In a recent study, we have shown that treatment a small molecule CCR1 antagonist BX 471 protects mice against acute pancreatitis and associated lung injury [35]. These studies show the critical role of chemokines in the pathogenesis of acute pancreatitis and associated lung injury.

There are over 50 different chemokines and over 20 different receptors, with overlapping functions. Despite the complexity and apparent redundancy of this system, it is reasonable to believe that specific chemokine receptor antagonists that interfere with leukocyte migration and activation could be useful in acute pancreatitis.

Substance P and Neutral Endopeptidase

Substance P is an 11 amino acid neuropeptide that is released from nerve endings in many tissues. Subsequent to its release, substance P binds to neurokinin-1 (NK1) receptors on the surface of effector cells and in addition to being a mediator of pain it has been shown to play an important role in inflammation. In a recent study, we have shown the presence of substance P in the pancreas and of NK1 receptors on pancreatic acinar cells in mice [36]. On induction of pancreatitis, there is a several fold upregulation of pancreatic substance P levels and of NK1 receptors on pancreatic acinar cells [36]. Moreover, knockout mice deficient in NK1 receptors are protected against pancreatitis. Interestingly, these mice are almost completely protected against pancreatitis-associated lung injury [36]. In a subsequent paper, we have shown for the role of preprotachykinin-A (PPT-A) gene products (e.g. substance P and neurokinin-A) in the pathogenesis of acute pancreatitis and associated lung injury [37]. NK1 receptors bind other peptides in addition to substance P, not all of which are derived from the PPT-A gene. In this study, we found that knockout mice deficient in the PPT-A gene were protected against acute pancreatitis and associated lung injury [37]. Furthermore, both prophylactic, and therapeutic, treatment with CP-96345, an antagonist of the NK1 receptor, protected mice against acute pancreatitis and associated lung injury [38]. These three papers clearly show that PPT-A gene products, acting via NK1 receptors, are critical pro-inflammatory mediators in acute pancreatitis and the associated lung injury. In a more recent study, we have shown a differential regulation of tachykinins and tachykinin receptors in the pancreas and lungs in acute pancreatitis [39]. These early results point to a differential regulation of inflammation in the pancreas and lungs, an interesting concept that merits further study.

The results showing a pro-inflammatory role of substance P in acute pancreatitis are further substantiated by the observation that knockout mice deficient in neutral endopeptidase (NEP), the enzyme that hydrolyses substance P thereby terminating its action, are more susceptible to experimental acute pancreatitis and associated lung injury [40,41].

These results demonstrate the critical role played by substance P in the pathogenesis of acute pancreatitis and point to a potential therapeutic approach against this clinical condition.

Substance P and Chemokines

Some studies have also shown that substance P can induce the synthesis of chemokines. In the first study on the interaction of substance P and chemokines in acute pancreatitis, we have recently shown an interaction of SP with chemokines in pancreatic acinar cells [42]. SP was found to stimulate chemokine synthesis in pancreatic acinar cells [42]. When pancreatic acini were stimulated with SP, we found a dose dependent increase in the synthesis of MCP-1, MIP-1α as well as MIP-2. Furthermore, we found that SP-induced chemokine synthesis was mediated by NFκB activation. Pretreatment of acinar cells with an NFκB inhibitory peptide was found to abolish SP- induced chemokine synthesis, thereby showing that the stimulatory effect of SP was specific to chemokine synthesis through the NFκB pathway. This is the first direct evidence of the role of substance P, acting via NK-1R present on mouse pancreatic acini, in inflammation and points to the mechanism by which SP contributes to inflammation in acute pancreatitis [42].

We have shown that there are temporally and spatially selective chemokine responses in CCK secretagogue caerulein-induced acute necrotizing pancreatitis in mice. CC chemokines MCP-1 and MIP-1α and CXC chemokine MIP-2 are elevated after AP induction. Time-dependent, tissue-specific analysis of their mRNA and protein expression suggested that they are early mediators in the AP and they mediate local as well as systemic inflammatory responses. In contrast, another CC chemokine RANTES is only involved in local pancreatic inflammation at a later stage of the disease. Either prophylactic or therapeutic treatment with a potent selective NK-1R antagonist CP-96,345 significantly suppressed caerulein-induced increase in MCP-1, MIP-1α and MIP-2 expression but had no apparent effect on RANTES expression [43]. The suppression effect of CP-96,345 on MCP-1, MIP-1α and MIP-2 expression was further confirmed by immunohistochemistry. This suggests that chemokine immunoreactivity is localized to acinar cells, infiltrating leukocytes in the pancreas, alveolar macrophages, and epithelial and endothelial cells in the lungs [43]. Our data suggests SP, probably by acting via NK-1R upon various chemokine-secreting cells in the pancreas and lungs, stimulates the release of chemokines that aggravate local AP and the development of its systemic sequelae.

H_2S

The toxic effect of H_2S on living organisms has been recognized for nearly three hundred years. However, growing evidence has accumulated in recent years which suggests that H_2S is formed naturally in mammalian tissues and exhibits a range of biological and physiological functions. Cystathionine-γ-lyase (CSE), which utilizes L-cysteine as substrate, is the enzyme responsible for the production of H_2S in mammalian vascular tissues. In a recent paper, we have shown the presence of H_2S synthesizing enzyme activity and CSE (as determined by mRNA signal) in the pancreas. Also, prophylactic, as well as therapeutic, treatment with the CSE inhibitor, DL-propargylglycine (PAG), significantly reduced the severity of caerulein-induced pancreatitis and associated lung injury [44]. This study has shown H_2S as a novel inflammatory mediator that plays a key role in acute pancreatitis and associated lung injury.

H_2S and Substance P

In a recent study, we have investigated the involvement of substance P and neurogenic inflammation in H_2S-induced lung inflammation. Intraperitoneal administration of NaHS, an H_2S donor, to mice caused a significant increase in circulating levels of substance P in a dose-dependant manner. H_2S alone could also cause lung inflammation, as evidenced by a significant increase in lung myeloperoxidase activity and histological evidence of lung injury. Maximum effect of H_2S on substance P levels and on lung inflammation was observed 1 h after NaHS administration. At this time, a significant increase in lung levels of TNF-α and IL-1β was also observed. In substance P deficient mice, the preprotachykinin-A (PPT-A) knockout mice, H_2S did not cause any lung inflammation. Furthermore, pretreatment of mice with the NK1 receptor antagonist CP-96,345 protected mice against lung inflammation caused by H_2S. Depleting neuropeptide from sensory neurons by capsaicin significantly reduced the lung inflammation caused by H_2S. In addition, pretreatment of mice with capsazepine, an antagonist of the transient receptor potential vanilloid (TRPV)-1, protected mice against H_2S-induced lung inflammation. These results demonstrate a key role of substance P and neurogenic inflammation in H_2S-induced lung injury in mice. A possible interaction between H_2S and substance P in acute pancreatitis will be the subject of future studies.

Conclusion

Significant progress has been made in recent years in our awareness on the role of inflammatory mediators in the pathogenesis of acute pancreatitis. In most of the studies, experimental animal models were used, while early clinical studies show clinical relevance of these findings. An understanding of the elucidation of the key mediators of inflammation in acute pancreatitis and associated MODS coupled with the discovery of specific inhibitors is likely to make it possible to develop clinically effective anti-inflammatory therapy for this, as yet incurable, clinical condition.

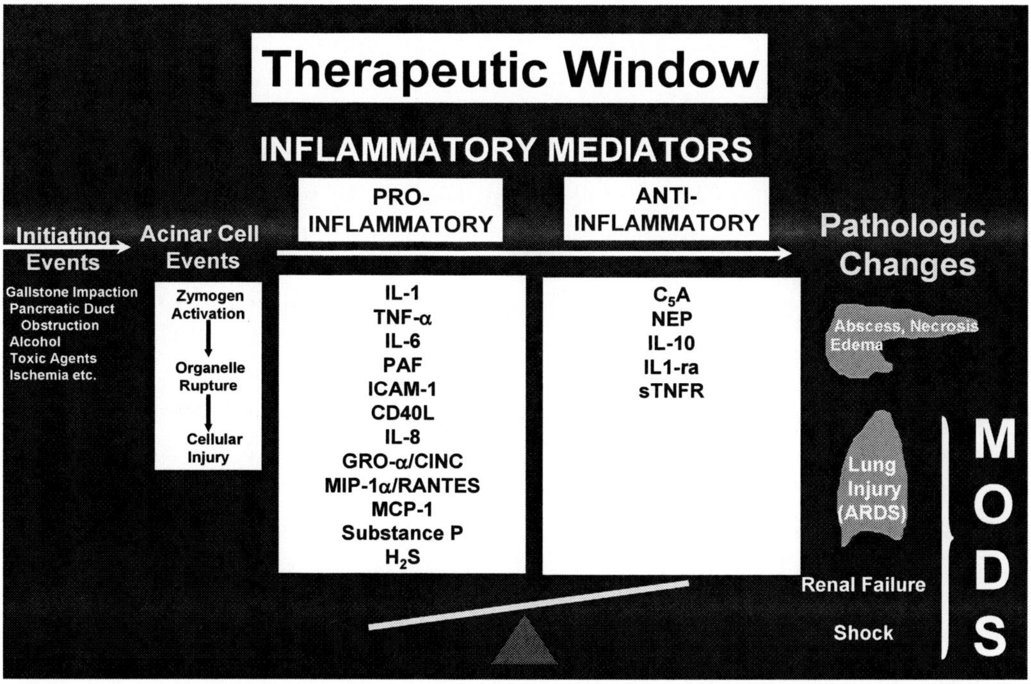

Figure 1. Schematic diagram of inflammatory mediators in the pathogenesis of acute pancreatitis. Activation of various digestive enzymes in acinar cells leads to autodigestion of the pancreas and release of inflammatory mediators. When the inflammatory reaction is severe, it leads to pathological damages in various organs such as pancreas, lung and kidney and eventually death. The final severity of acute pancreatitis is determined by an interplay of these pro- and anti-inflammatory mediators. The time between symptom onset in acute pancreatitis and the development of distant organ dysfunction provides an ideal therapeutic window in this condition.

Acknowledgement

The author would like to acknowledge grant support from National Medical Research Council, Biomedical Research Council, and Academic Research Fund.

References

[1] Bhatia, M., et al. Inflammatory mediators in acute pancreatitis. *J. Pathol.* 2000;190:117-125.

[2] Bhatia, M., and Moochhala, S. Role of Inflammatory Mediators in the Pathophysiology of Acute Respiratory Distress Syndrome. *J. Path.* 2004; 202: 145-156.

[3] Bhatia, M., et al. Pathophysiology of acute pancreatitis. *Pancreatology*. 2005. 5: 132-144.

[4] Bhatia, M., et al. MCP-1 but not CINC synthesis is increased in rat pancreatic acini in response to cerulein hyperstimulation. *Am. J. Physiol. Gastrointest. Liver Physiol.* 2002;282:G77-G85.

[5] Bhatia, M. Inflammatory response on the pancreatic acinar cell injury. *Scand. J. Surg.* 2005; 94: 97-10.

[6] Fink, G.W., and Norman, J.G. Specific changes in the pancreatic expression of the interleukin 1 family of genes during experimental acute pancreatitis. *Cytokine* 1997;9:1023-1027.

[7] Denham, W., et al. Gene targeting demonstrates additive detrimental effects of interleukin-1 and tumor necrosis factor during pancreatitis. *Gastroenterology* 1997; 113:1741-1746.

[8] Hughes, C.B. et al. Anti-TNFalpha therapy improves survival and ameliorates the pathophysiologic sequelae in acute pancreatitis in the rat. *Am. J. Surg.* 1996; 171: 274-280.

[9] Leser, H.G., et al. Elevation of serum interleukin-6 concentration precedes acute-phase response and reflects severity in acute pancreatitis. *Gastroenterology* 1991;101:782-785.

[10] Suzuki, S., et al. Induction of acute pancreatitis by cerulein in human IL-6 gene transgenic mice. *Pancreas*. 2000;21:86-92.

[11] Rongione, A.J., et al. Interleukin-10 reduces circulating levels of serum cytokines in experimental pancreatitis. *J. Gastrointest. Surg.* 1997;1:159-166.

[12] Rongione, A.J., et al. Interleukin 10 reduces the severity of acute pancreatitis in rats. *Gastroenterology* 1997;112:960-967.

[13] Deviere, J., et al. Interleukin-10 reduces the incidence of pancreatitis after therapeutic endoscopic retrograde cholangiopancreatography. *Gastroenterology* 2001;120:498-505.

[14] Konturek, S.J., et al. Role of platelet activating factor in pathogenesis of acute pancreatitis in rats. *Gut* 1992; 33: 1268-1274.

[15] Galloway, S.W., and Kingsnorth, A.N. Lung injury in the microembolic model of acute pancreatitis and amelioration by lexipafant (BB-882), a platelet-activating factor antagonist. *Pancreas* 1996; 13: 140-146.

[16] Rivera, J.A., et al. Lexipafant fails to improve survival in severe necrotizing pancreatitis in rats. *Int. J. pancreatol.* 1998; 23: 101-106.

[17] Hofbauer, B., et al. Effect of recombinant platelet-activating factor acetylhydrolase on two models of experimental acute pancreatitis. *Gastroenterology.* 1998;115: 1238-1247.

[18] Johnson, C.D., et al. Double blind, randomised, placebo controlled study of a platelet activating factor antagonist, lexipafant, in the treatment and prevention of organ failure in predicted severe acute pancreatitis. *Gut.* 2001;48:62-69.

[19] McKay, C.J. Recent developments in the management of acute pancreatitis. *Dig. Surg.* 2002;19:129-134.

[20] Frossard, J.L., et al. CD40 ligand-deficient mice are protected against cerulein-induced acute pancreatitis and pancreatitis-associated lung injury.*Gastroenterology*, 2001; 121, 184-194.

[21] Zaninovic, V., et al. Cerulein upregulates ICAM-1 in pancreatic acinar cells, which mediates neutrophil adhesion to these cells. *Am. J. Physiol. Gastrointest. Liver Physiol.* 2000;279:G666-G676.

[22] Frossard, J.L., et al. The role of intercellular adhesion molecule 1 and neutrophils in acute pancreatitis and pancreatitis-associated lung injury. *Gastroenterology.* 1999;116:694-701.

[23] Bhatia, M., et al. The effects of neutrophil depletion on a completely noninvasive model of acute pancreatitis-associated lung injury. *Int. J. Pancreatol.* 1998;24:77-83.

[24] Lundberg, A.H., et al. Blocking pulmonary ICAM-1 expression ameliorates lung injury in established diet-induced pancreatitis. *Ann. Surg.* 2001;233:213-20.

[25] Bhatia, M., et al. Complement factor C5a exerts an anti-inflammatory effect in acute pancreatitis and associated lung injury. *Am. J. Physiol. Gastrointest. Liver Physiol.* 2001;280:G974-G978.

[26] Gerard, C., et al. Targeted disruption of the beta-chemokine receptor CCR1 protects against pancreatitis-associated lung injury. *J. Clin. Invest.* 1997; 100: 2022-2027.

[27] Bonecchi, R., et al. Up-regulation of CCR1 and CCR3 and induction of chemotaxis to CC chemokines by IFN-gamma in human neutrophils. *J. Immunol.* 1999;162:474-479.

[28] Bhatia, M., et al. Treatment With Met-RANTES Reduces Lung Injury in Caerulein Induced Pancreatitis In Mice. *Br. J. Surg.* 2003; 90:698-704.

[29] Grady, T., et al. Chemokine gene expression in rat pancreas acinar cells is an early event associated with acute pancreatitis. *Gastroenterology* 1997; 113: 1966-1975.

[30] Rau, B., et al. The potential role of procalcitonin and interleukin 8 in the prediction of infected necrosis in acute pancreatitis. *Gut* 1997; 41: 832-840.

[31] Shokuhi, S., et al. Levels of the chemokines growth-related oncogene alpha and epithelial neutrophil-activating protein 78 are raised in patients with severe acute pancreatitis. *Br. J. Surg.* 2002; 89: 566-572.

[32] Brady, M., et al. Expression of the chemokines MCP-1/JE and cytokine-induced neutrophil chemoattractant in early acute pancreatitis. *Pancreas* 2002; 25: 260-269.

[33] Bhatia, M., et al. Treatment with neutralising antibody against cytokine induced neutrophil chemoattractant (CINC) protects rats against acute pancreatitis associated lung injury. *Gut* 2000; 47: 838-844.

[34] Bhatia, M., and Hegde, A. Treatment with Antileukinate, a CXCR2 chemokine receptor antagonist, protects mice against acute pancreatitis and associated lung injury. *Regul. Pept.* 2007; 138: 40-48.

[35] He, M., et al. Treatment with BX471, a non-peptide CCR1 antagonist, protects mice against acute pancreatitis-associated lung injury by modulating neutrophil recruitment. *Pancreas*. 2007 (in press).

[36] Bhatia, M., et al. Role of substance P and the neurokinin 1 receptor in acute pancreatitis and pancreatitis-associated lung injury. *Proc. Natl. Acad. Sci. USA*. 1998; 95:4760-4765.

[37] Bhatia, M., et al. Preprotachykinin-A gene deletion protects mice against acute pancreatitis and associated lung injury. *Am. J. Physiol. Gastrointest. Liver Physiol.* 2003;284: G830-G836.

[38] Lau, H.Y., et al. A key role of neurokinin 1 receptors in acute pancreatitis and associated lung injury. *Biochem. Biophys. Res. Commun.* 2005;327:509-515.

[39] Lau, H.Y., and Bhatia, M. Effect of CP96,345 on the expression of tachykinins and neurokinin receptors in acute pancreatitis. *J. Pathol.* 2006; 208: 364-371.

[40] Bhatia, M., et al. Neutral endopeptidase (NEP) plays an anti-inflammatory role in acute pancreatitis and pancreatitis-associated lung injury. *Pancreas* 1997; 15: 428.

[41] Maa, J., et al. Substance P is a determinant of lethality in diet-induced hemorrhagic pancreatitis in mice. *Surgery*. 2000;128: 232-239.

[42] Ramnath, R.D., and Bhatia, M. Substance P treatment stimulates chemokine synthesis in pancreatic acinar cells via the activation of NF-κB. *Am. J. Physiol. Gastrointest. Liver Physiol.* 2006; 291:G1113-1119.

[43] Sun, J., and Bhatia M. Blockade of neurokinin 1 receptor attenuates CC and CXC chemokine production in experimental acute pancreatitis and associated lung injury. *Am. J. Physiol. Gastrointest. Liver Physiol.* 2007 (in press).

[44] Bhatia, M., et al. Role of hydrogen sulfide in acute pancreatitis and associated lung injury. *FASEB J.* 2005;19:623-625.

[45] Bhatia, M., et al. Role of substance P in hydrogen sulfide-induced pulmonary inflammation in mice. *Am. J. Physiol. Lung Cell Mol. Physiol.* 2006; 291: L896-L904.

Index

A

B

C

D

E

F

G

H

I

J

N

Q

R

S

T

U

V

W

X

Y

Z